CORE CONCEPTS IN PHARMACOLOGY

LELAND NORMAN HOLLAND, PHD, JR

Science Chair, Division for Health, Mathematics, and Science
Pasco-Hernando Community College

MICHAEL PATRICK ADAMS, RT(R), PHD

Associate Dean for Health, Mathematics, and Science
Pasco-Hernando Community College

Prentice Hall

Upper Saddle River, New Jersey 07458

Library of Congress Cataloging-in-Publication Data

Holland, Norman, (date)
  Core concepts in pharmacology/Norman Holland, Michael Adams.
    p.; cm.
  Includes index.
  ISBN 0-13-089329-3
  1. Pharmacology—Outlines, syllabi, etc. I. Adams, Michael, (date). II. Title.
  [DNLM: 1. Pharmaceutical Preparations—Handbooks. 2. Drug Therapy—Handbooks.
QV 39 H736c 2003]
RM301.14.H655 2003
615′.1—dc21   2002017091

Publisher: Julie Levin Alexander
Assistant to Publisher: Regina Bruno
Executive Editor: Maura Connor
Senior Managing Editor: Marilyn Meserve
Development Editor: Elena Mauceri
Assistant Editor: Yesenia Kopperman
Editorial Assistant: Sladjana Repic
Director of Production and Manufacturing: Bruce Johnson
Managing Production Editor: Patrick Walsh
Production Liaison: Danielle Newhouse
Production Editor: Amy Hackett, Carlisle Publishers Services
Manufacturing Manager: Ilene Sanford
Design Director: Cheryl Asherman
Design Coordinator: Maria Guglielmo
Interior & Cover Design: Wanda España
Electronic Art Creation: Precision Graphics
Photographer: Al Dodge, AD Productions
Manager of Media Production: Amy Peltier
New Media Project Manager: Stephen Hartner
New Media Production: Jack Yensen, Synergy
Marketing Manager: Nicole Benson
Marketing Coordinator: Janet Ryerson
Production Information Manager: Rachele Strober
Composition: Carlisle Communications, Ltd.
Cover Printer: Phoenix Color
Printer/Binder: The Banta Company

Pearson Education LTD.
Pearson Education Australia PTY, Limited
Pearson Education Singapore, Pte. Ltd
Pearson Education North Asia Ltd
Pearson Education Canada, Ltd.
Pearson Educación de Mexico, S. A. de C. V.
Pearson Education—Japan
Pearson Education Malaysia, Pte. Ltd

Notice: The authors and the publisher of this volume have taken care to make certain that the doses of drugs and schedules of treatment are correct and compatible with the standards generally accepted at the time of publication. Nevertheless, as new information becomes available, changes in treatment and in the use of drugs become necessary. The reader is advised to carefully consult the instruction and information material included in the package insert of each drug or therapeutic agent before administration. This advice is especially important when using, administering, or recommending new and infrequently used drugs. The authors and publisher disclaim all responsibility for any liability, loss, injury, or damage incurred as a consequence, directly or indirectly, of the use and application of any of the contents of this volume.

DEDICATION

I would like to acknowledge the willful encouragement of Farrell and Norma Jean Stalcup. I dedicate this book to my beloved wife Karen, and my two wonderful children, Alexandria Noelle, my double-deuce daughter, and Caleb Jaymes, my number-one son.

LNH

I dedicate this book to my wife Kim and my daughter Kimberly Michelle Valiance, who supported me through the endless hours of creativity and preparation that culminated in this work.

MPA

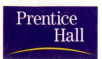
Prentice Hall

10 9 8 7 6 5 4 3 2 1
ISBN 0-13-089329-3

PROFILE DRUGS (continued)

Name of Drug	Classification	Page
interferon alfa 2 (Roferon-A, Intron-A)	Antineoplastic; biologic response modifier	370
isoniazid (INH)	Antitubercular	332
isosorbide dinitrate (Isordil)	Organic nitrate; vasodilator	223
isotretinoin 13–C is–Retinoic Acid (Accutane)	Antiacne agent; retinoid	516
levodopa (Larodopa)	Dopaminergic agonist	138
levothyroxine (Synthroid)	Hormone; thyroid	455
lidocaine (Xylocaine)	Local anesthetic	169
lindane (Kwell)	Scabicide	513
lisinopril (Prinivil) Zestoric	ACE inhibitor	222
lithium carbonate (Eskalith)	Bipolar disorder agent	126
medroxyprogesterone (Provera)	Hormone; progestin	471
methotrexate (Mexate)	Antineoplastic; antimetabolite	364
methylphenidate (Ritalin)	CNS stimulant	115
metoprolol (Lopressor)	Beta-adrenergic blocker	258
metronidazole (Flagyl)	Antiparasitic; antimalarial	349
milrinone (Primacor)	Phosphodiesterase inhibitor	226
morphine sulfate (Astramorph PF, Duramorph, and Others)	Opioid	156
naloxone (Narcan)	Opioid-blocker	157
naproxen (Naprosyn) and naproxen sodium (Aleve, Anaprox)	NSAID	304
nifedipine (Procardia)	Antihypertensive; calcium channel blocker	206
nitrous oxide	General anesthetic; gas	172
norepinephrine (Levarterenol Levophed)	Sympathomimetic; vasoconstrictor	268
nystatin (Fungizone)	Superficial antifungal	341
omeprazole (Prilosec)	Proton pump inhibitor	399
Ortho-Novum 1135 (Ethinyl Estradiol)	Hormone; oral contraceptive	468
oxymetazoline (Afrin and Others)	Sympathomimetic; decongestant	303
oxytocin (Pitocin, Syntocinon)	Hormone; oxytocic	473
penicillin G potassium (Pentids)	Antibiotic; penicillin	324
phenelzine (Nardil)	Antidepressant; MOA	120
phenobarbital (Luminal)	Anticonvulsant; barbiturate	102
phenytoin (Dilantin)	Anticonvulsant; hydantoin	104
pilocarpine (Adsorbocarpine, Ocusert, and Others)	Antiglaucoma agent; parasympathomimetic	526
potassium chloride	Electrolyte	437
prednisone (Meticorten and others)	Systemic glucocorticoid; anti-inflammatory agent	307
prochlorperazine (Compazine)	Antiemetic; phenothiazine	406
propranolol (Inderal)	Beta-adrenergic blocker	240
propylthiouracil (Propacil)	Antithyroid agent	456
quinidine (Quinidex)	Sodium channel blocker	238
nitroglyucerin (Notrostat, Nitrobid, Nitro-Dur, and Others)	Organic nitrate	252
psyllium mucilloid (Metamucil and Others)	Laxative; bulk-forming	402
raloxifene (Evista)	Hormone; estrogen antagonist	496
ranitidine (Zantac)	H2-receptor blocker	398
reteplase (Retavase)	Thrombolytic	258
salmeterol (Serevent)	Sympathomimetic; bronchodilator	383
secobarbital (Seconal)	Barbiturate	92
sibutramine (Meridia)	Anorexiant	407
sildenafil (Viagra)	Erectile dysfunction agent	476
sodium bicarbonate	Acid-base agent	435
spironolactone (Aldactone)	Diuretic; potassium-sparing	433
streptokinase (Streptase)	Thrombolytic	190
sumatriptan (Imetrex)	Antimigraine agent; triptan	160
tacrine (Cognex)	Cholineric agonist	143
tamoxifen (Nolvadex)	Antineoplastic; estrogen antagonist	368
testosterone base (Andro and Others)	Hormone; androgen	475
tetracycline HCl (Achromycin and Others)	Antibiotic; tetracycline	327
thiopental (Pentathal)	IV anesthetic	174
valproic acid (Depakene)	Anticonvulsant	104
vancomycin (Vancocin)	Antibiotic; miscellaneous	330
verapamil (Calan)	Calcium channel blocker	242
vincristine (Oncovin)	Antineoplastic; plant extract/alkaloid; mitotic inhibitor	367
warfarin (Coumadin)	Anticoagulant	188
zidovudine (Retrovir, AZT)	Antiviral; nucleoside reverse transcriptase inhibitor	346

PROFILE DRUGS

Name of Drug	Classification	Page
abciximab (ReoPro)	Antiplatelet agent; glycoprotein IIb/IIIa inhibitor	189
acetaminophen (Tylenol and others)	Analgesic; non-narcotic	159
acetazolamide (Diamox)	Antiglaucoma agent; diuretic	529
acyclovir (Zovirax)	Antiviral	347
aminocaproic acid (Amicar)	Antifibrinolytic; hemostatic	192
amiodarone (Cardarone)	Potassium channel blocker	241
amphotericin B (Fungizone)	Systemic antifungal	339
aspirin (Acetylsalicylic acid, ASA)	NSAID; salicylate	153
atenolol (Tenormin)	Beta-adrenergic blocker	253
atorvastatin (Lipitor)	Antihyperlipidemic; HMG CoA reductase inhibitor	282
atropine	Anticholinergic	75
beclomethasone (Beclovent, Beconase, Vancenase, Vanceril)	Glucocorticoid	385
benzocaine (Solarcaine and Others)	Anesthetic; topical	514
benztropine (Cogentin)	Anticholinergic	138
bethanechol (Urecholine)	Parasympathomimetic	74
calcitriol (Calcijex, Rocaltrol), Active Vitamin D	Vitamin D	494
calcium gluconate (Kalcinate)	Electrolyte; calcium supplement	493
carvedilol (Coreg)	Beta-adrenergic blocker	227
cefotaxime (Claforan)	Antibiotic; cephalosporin	326
chlorothiazide (Diuril)	Diuretic; thiazide	432
chlorpromazine (Thorazine)	Antipsychotic; phenothiazine	128
cholestyramine (Questran)	Antihyperlipidemic; bile acid resin	284
clozapine (Clozaril)	Antipsychotic; atypical	130
colchicine	Antigout agent	502
conjugated estrogens (Premarin) and conjugated estrogens with medroxyprogesterone (Prempro)	Hormone; estrogen	469
cyanocobalamin (Cyanabin and Others)	Vitamin	414
cyclobenzaprine (Cycloflex, Flexeril)	Skeletal muscle relaxant; central-acting	485
cyclophosphamide (Cytoxan)	Antineoplastic; alkylating agent	362
cyclosporine (Neoral, Sandimmune)	Immunosuppressant	309
dantrolene sodium (Dantrium)	Skeletal muscle relaxant; peripheral-acting	488
diazepam (Valium)	Benzodiazepine	88
digoxin (Lanoxin)	Cardiac glycoside	221
diltiazem (Cardizem)	Calcium channel blocker	254
diphenhydramine (Benadryl and Others)	Antihistamine	300
diphenoxylate with Atropine (Lomotil)	Antidiarrheal; opioid	404
dopamine (Dopastat, Inotropin)	Sympathomimetic; cardiotonic/inotropic agent	270
doxazosin (Cardura)	Antihypertensive; alpha1-adrenergic blocker	210
doxorubicin (Adriamycin)	Antineoplastic; antitumor antibiotic	366
enalapril (Vasotec)	Antihypertensive; ACE inhibitor	208
epinephrine (Adrenalin)	Sympathomimetic	272
erythromycin (E-mycin, Erythrocin)	Antibiotic; macrolide	328
ethosuximide (Zarontin)	Anticonvulsant; succinimide	106
etidronate (Didronel)	Biphosphonate	497
ferrous sulfate (Ferralyn and Others)	Mineral	416
fexofenadine (Allegra)	Antihistamine	300
fluoxetine (Prozac)	Antidepressant; selective serotonin reuptake inhibitor	124
fluticasone (Flonase)	Intranasal glucocorticoid	302
furosemide (Lasix)	Loop diuretic	225
gemfibrozil (Lopid)	Antihyperlipidemic; fibric acid agent	285
gentamicin (Garamycin)	Antibiotic; aminoglycoside	329
glipizide (Glucotrol)	Antidiabetic; oral hypoglycemic	452
halothane (Fluothane)	General anesthetic; volatile agent	173
heparin	Anticoagulant	187
hydralazine (Apresoline)	Antihypertensive; direct vasodilator	210
hydrochlorothiazide (HydroDiuril)	Antihypertensive; thiazide diuretic	204
hydrocortisone (Cortef, Hydrocortone)	Glucocorticoid	458
hydroxychloroquine sulfate (Plaquenil)	Antiinflammatory; antimalarial	500
imipramine (Tofranil)	Antidepressant; tricyclic antidepressant	122
insulin regular, (Humulin R, Novolin R, and Others)	Antidiabetic; insulin	449

continued on next page

CONTENTS

UNIT VI
The Endocrine and Reproductive Systems 441

UNIT VII
The Musculoskeletal System, Integumentary System, and Eyes and Ears 481

Pharmacology is one of the most challenging subjects for those embarking on careers in the health sciences. By its very nature, pharmacology is an interdisciplinary subject, borrowing concepts from a wide variety of the natural and applied sciences. Prediction of drug action, the ultimate goal in the study of pharmacology, requires a thorough knowledge of anatomy, physiology, chemistry, and pathology, as well as the social sciences of psychology and sociology. It is the interdisciplinary nature of pharmacology that makes the subject difficult to learn but also makes it fascinating to study.

This text presents pharmacology from an interdisciplinary perspective. The text draws upon core concepts of anatomy, physiology, and pathology in order to make drug therapy more understandable. This text does not assume that the student comes to the course with a strong background in the natural or applied sciences. Although it is true that many students have prerequisite courses prior to attempting introductory pharmacology, such courses may have been taken many years prior. In this text, the prerequisite science-knowledge necessary for understanding drug therapy is reviewed prior to presenting the core concepts in pharmacology.

APPROACH AND RATIONALE

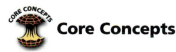 ## Core Concepts

The authors have created a concise means of communicating the most important pharmacologic information to the student. Through the use of numbered **Core Concepts,** the student can quickly identify key ideas. These core concepts are stated at the beginning of each chapter so the student gets an overview of what is to be learned. **Concept Reviews** are questions placed strategically throughout the chapter to stimulate student comprehension and retention. Also, **Concept Summaries** are repeated at the end of the chapter, which include brief summary of the important concepts.

Disease and Body System Approach

Core Concepts in Pharmacology is organized according to body systems and diseases. This clearly places the drugs in context with how they are used therapeutically. The student can easily locate all relevant anatomy, physiology, pathology, and pharmacology in the same chapter in which the drugs are discussed.

Prototype Approach to Drug Therapy

The vast number of drugs taught in a pharmacology course is staggering. To facilitate learning, a prototype approach is used in which the one or two most representa-

tive drugs in each classification are introduced in detail. **Drug Profile** boxes are used to clearly indicate these important medications.

Pharmacology as a Visual Discipline

For many students, learning can be a highly visual process. *Core Concepts in Pharmacology* is the first pharmacology text to incorporate **Mechanisms in Action,** which use computer animations to clearly demonstrate drug action. A colorful graphic of the animation is included in many of the Drug Profile boxes along with a description of the drug action. The complete animation, including audio narrations that describe each step of the mechanism, are provided on the included student CD-ROM. This text also incorporates generous use of figures and diagrams to illustrate and summarize key concepts.

Health Professions Focus

Core Concepts in Pharmacology uses an interdisciplinary approach to pharmacology that is applicable for all basic nursing and allied health professions. Practical nurses, respiratory therapists, radiographers, EMTs, paramedics, physical therapist assistants, patient care assistants, home health care workers, and those beginning the allied health occupations can benefit from the unique structure and clarity of the text. **On the Job** boxes, included in most chapters, show the student the application of pharmacology by various health professionals.

The Health Professional as Teacher

It is not sufficient for a health professional to only learn pharmacology. It is equally important to learn to communicate pharmacological knowledge to clients and other members of the public. To help the student achieve the ability to communicate pharmacology, each drug chapter contains concise **Client Teaching** boxes which apply fundamental patient care principles to pharmacology.

Holistic Pharmacology

Core Concepts in Pharmacology approaches pharmacology from a holistic perspective. Throughout the text, the relationship between lifestyle habits, such as proper body weight, exercise, and nutrition, to pharmacology are discussed. Most chapters contain a **Natural Alternative** feature which presents a popular herbal or dietary supplement that may be considered along with conventional drugs. The **FastFacts** feature puts the disease in a social and economic perspective.

Medical Terminology

Pharmacology and other medical sciences use a unique language that can be overwhelming for beginning students. In each chapter of *Core Concepts in Pharmacology* key terms are defined at the beginning of each chapter, and each term includes the page number on which the first reference to the word can be found. **Key terms** are placed in blue boldface type throughout the text. Since pronunciation of medical terms is often difficult, a phonetic pronunciation is provided for difficult key terms. Phonetic pronunciations are also provided in the index for the generic name of each drug. **Word roots** are included in the margins to help the student identify prefixes and suffixes essential to medical word-building. An **audio glossary** can be found at the Companion Website and the free Student CD-ROM.

PharMedia and PharmLinks

PharMedia is included at the beginning of each chapter. This feature guides the student to resources, interactive exercises, and animations for that chapter on the Student CD-ROM and Companion Website. PharMedia serves as a gateway to additional learning. **PharmLinks** invite the student to perform specific web activities or to consult the accompanying CD-ROM.

COMPLETE TEACHING & LEARNING PACKAGE

To enhance the teaching and learning process, an attractive media-focused supplements package for both students and faculty has been developed in close correlation with *Core Concepts in Pharmacology*. The full complement of supplemental teaching materials is available to all qualified instructors from your Prentice Hall Health Sales Representative.

Student CD-ROM. The Student CD-ROM is packaged free with each copy of the textbook. It provides thirty animations showing how drug action occurs at the cellular and system levels. These animations build upon the feature in the textbook entitled, *Mechanism in Action,* and help students visualize these difficult concepts. The CD-ROM also includes NCLEX-PN Review questions that emphasize application of care and client education related to drug administration. Students can test their knowledge and gain immediate feedback through rationales for right and wrong answers. In addition, Concept Review questions provide students an additional opportunity for applying their knowledge. Students will also find the audio glossary and objectives useful for review. Finally, the CD-ROM allows access to the Companion Website described below (internet connection required).

Student Workbook. A Student Workbook for *Core Concepts in Pharmacology* has been developed to closely parallel the text. The Workbook contains a variety of question types and a large number of practice questions and learning activities. Other study aids may be found at the Companion Website.

Instructor's Resource Manual. This manual contains a wealth of material to help faculty plan and manage the pharmacology course. It includes chapter overviews, lecture suggestions and outlines, learning objectives, a complete test bank, teaching tips, and more. The IRM guides faculty on how to assign and use the text-specific Companion Website, www.prenhall.com/holland, and the CD-ROM which accompany the textbook.

Instructor's Resource CD-ROM. This CD-ROM provides many resources in an electronic format. First, the CD-ROM includes the complete test bank in Test-Gen format. Second, it includes a comprehensive collection of images from the textbook in PowerPoint format so that faculty can easily import these photographs and illustrations into their own classroom lecture presentations. Finally, the CD-ROM provides instructors with access to the same animations which appear on the student CD-ROM, allowing faculty to incorporate these visual accents into their lectures.

Companion Website and Syllabus Manager®. Students and faculty will both benefit from the free Companion Website at www.prenhall.com/holland. This website serves as a text-specific, interactive online workbook to *Core Concepts in Pharmacology*. The Companion Website includes modules for Objectives, Audio Glossary, Chapter Summary for lecture notes, Dosage Calculations, PharmLinks, Case Studies, Care Plan activities, Drug Reviews, and more. Instructors adopting this textbook for their courses have free access to an online Syllabus Manager. The syllabus Manager hosts a wide variety of features that facilitate the students' use of the Companion Website and allows faculty to post their syllabi online for their students. For more information or a demonstration of Syllabus Manager, please contact your Prentice Hall Health Sales Representative or go online to www.prenhall.com/demo.

ACKNOWLEDGMENTS

We are grateful to all the educators who reviewed the manuscript of this text. Their insights, suggestions, and eye for detail helped us prepare a more relevant and useful book, one that focuses on the core components of learning in the field of pharmacology.

Jerri Adler, BA, AA, CMA, CMT
Lane Community College
Eugene, Ohio

Amy Bieda, MSN, RN, CPNP
Frances Payne Bolton School of Nursing, Case Western Reserve
  University
Cleveland, Ohio

Sue Biederman, BS, MS
Southwest Texas State University
San Marcos, Texas

Joseph R. Bittengle, MEd, RT(R) (ARRT)
University of Arkansas for Medical Sciences
Little Rock, Arkansas

Becky Cameron, CNC, CLNC
Midland Community College
Midland, Texas

Rose Corder, RN, BSN
San Jacinto College North
Houston, Texas

Bonnie Deister, MA, MS, BSN, RN, CMA
Broome Community College
Binghamton, New York

Connie S. Dempsey, RN, BSN, MSN
Stark State College of Technology
New Canton, Ohio

Rebecca Ensminger, RN, MSN
Valencia Community College
Orlando, Florida

Nancy Fairchild, MS, CAES, RN
Boston College School of Nursing
Chestnut Hill, Massachusetts

Rosalinda H. Giffard, MSN, RNC, CS, FNP
University of Texas at Brownsville/Texas Southmost College
Brownsville, Texas

Wanda Gifford, RN, MSN, FNP
St. Elizabeth School of Nursing

Barbara Kinsman, RN, MSN
Corning Community College
Corning, New York

Mary Beth Kiefner, MS, RN
Illinois Central College
Peoria, Illinois

Carol Ann Lammon, RN, PhD
Capstone College of Nursing, The University of Alabama
Tuscaloosa, Alabama

Renee Lewis, MS, RN, CCRN
Rose State College
Midwest City, Oklahoma

Sandra Liming, RN, MN, PhD
North Seattle Community College
Seattle, WA

Joni D. Marsh, MN, ARNP
Intercollegiate College of Nursing
Spokane, Washington

Catherine McJannet, RN, MN, CEN
Southwestern College School of Technology
Chula Vista, CA

Jennifer Ponto, RN, BSN
South Plains College
Levelland, Texas

Linda Roan, RN, MN
University of Phoenix–Colorado Campus
Colorado Springs, CO

Linda Agustin Simunek, RN, PhD, JD
Purdue University
Lafayette, Indiana

Claudia R. Stoffel, MSN, RN
Paducah Community College
Paducah, Kentucky

Patricia R. Teasley, MSN, RN, CS
Central Texas College
Killeen, Texas

Jean Ure
Rolla Technical Institute
Rolla, MO

Dr. Victoria Wetle, RN, EdD
Chemetka Community College
Salem, Oregon

When authoring a text such as this, a huge number of dedicated and talented professionals are needed to bring the initial vision to reality. At the top of the list is our Executive Editor, Maura Connor, who supplied the expert guidance and expertise to overcome innumerable hurdles to see this project to its completion. Guiding the formation of every minute detail of the text from its inception to completion and supplying great patience and innovation was Elena Mauceri, Developmental Editor. Cheryl Asherman, Design Director, and Maria Guglielmo, Design Coordinator, created a very special and incredible text design. Pat Walsh, Managing Production Editor, provided expertise on art and photography issues. Overseeing a very difficult production process with finesse and patience was Danielle Newhouse, Production Editor at Prentice Hall, and Amy Hackett at Carlisle Publisher Services. Providing the necessary expertise for our comprehensive supplement package was Yesenia Kopperman, Assistant Editor. Sladjana Repic, Editorial Assistant, did an outstanding job of managing the myriad of office details throughout the many stages of text creation.

A special thanks to the many registered nurses who provided their knowledge and wisdom to this project. Of particular note is Rita Plyer who shared some of the initial vision for this text. We also acknowledge the important contributions of Connie Dempsey, Daryle Wane and Reesa Stroker who wrote test items and helped to create an exceptional Instructor's Resource Manual.

Our thanks also to Claudia Stoffel, MSN, RN, who skillfully checked our drug tables for accuracy and developed the content for the Student CD-ROM and Companion Website.

Michael Patrick Adams, RT(R), PhD is the Associate Dean for Health, Mathematics, and Science at Pasco-Hernando Community College. He is an accomplished educator, author, and national speaker. The National Institute for Staff and Organizational Development in Austin, Texas named Dr. Adams a Master Teacher. He has been registered by the American Registry of Radiologic Technologists for over 30 years. Dr. Adams obtained his master's degree in pharmacology from Michigan State University and his doctorate in education from the University of South Florida.

Leland Norman Holland, PhD, JR is the Science Chair in the Division for Health, Mathematics, and Science at Pasco-Hernando Community College. He is actively involved in teaching and preparing students for various health professions including nursing, dentistry, and pharmacy. He comes to the teaching profession after several years involvement in basic science research at the VA Hospital in Augusta, Georgia and the Medical College of Georgia, where he received his Ph.D. in pharmacology. He has taught pharmacology for 10 years at both the undergraduate and graduate levels. One of his paramount goals as an educator is to help students achieve success, and he has assisted many in their pursuit of healthcare degrees.

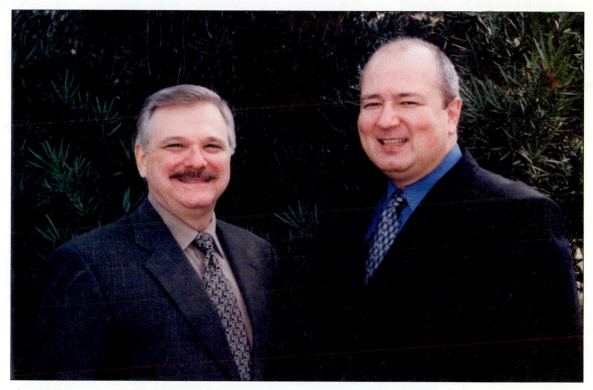

Photograph courtesy of O. Elizabeth Register.

GUIDE TO
CORE CONCEPTS IN PHARMACOLOGY

Core Concepts

Through the use of numbered **Core Concepts**, the student is able to quickly identify key ideas. These core concepts are stated at the beginning of each chapter, so that the student can get an overview of what is to be learned.

Disease and Body System Approach

The organization by **body systems and diseases** clearly places the drugs in context with how they are used therapeutically. The student is able to easily locate all relevant anatomy, physiology, pathology, and pharmacology in the same chapter in which the drugs are discussed.

Objectives

Objectives provide the student with a listing of knowledge they can expect to have upon completion of the chapter.

PharMedia

PharMedia is included at the beginning of each chapter. This feature guides the student to resources, interactive exercises, and animations for that chapter on the Student CD-ROM and Companion Website. PharMedia serves as a gateway to additional learning.

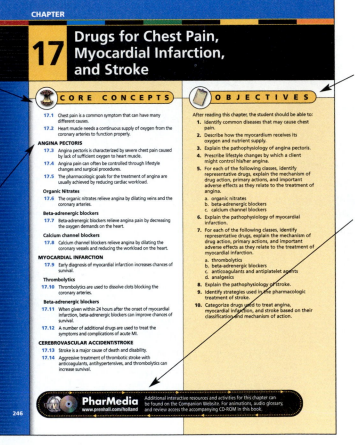

CHAPTER 17 Drugs for Chest Pain, Myocardial Infarction, and Stroke

CORE CONCEPTS

17.1 Chest pain is a common symptom that can have many different causes.

17.2 Heart muscle needs a continuous supply of oxygen from the coronary arteries to function properly.

ANGINA PECTORIS

17.3 Angina pectoris is characterized by severe chest pain caused by lack of sufficient oxygen to heart muscle.

17.4 Angina pain can often be controlled through lifestyle changes and surgical procedures.

17.5 The pharmacologic goals for the treatment of angina are usually achieved by reducing cardiac workload.

Organic Nitrates

17.6 The organic nitrates relieve angina by dilating veins and the coronary arteries.

Beta-adrenergic blockers

17.7 Beta-adrenergic blockers relieve angina pain by decreasing the oxygen demands on the heart.

Calcium channel blockers

17.8 Calcium channel blockers relieve angina by dilating the coronary vessels and reducing the workload on the heart.

MYOCARDIAL INFARCTION

17.9 Early diagnosis of myocardial infarction increases chances of survival.

Thrombolytics

17.10 Thrombolytics are used to dissolve clots blocking the coronary arteries.

Beta-adrenergic blockers

17.11 When given within 24 hours after the onset of myocardial infarction, beta-adrenergic blockers can improve chances of survival.

17.12 A number of additional drugs are used to treat the symptoms and complications of acute MI.

CEREBROVASCULAR ACCIDENT/STROKE

17.13 Stroke is a major cause of death and disability.

17.14 Aggressive treatment of thrombotic stroke with anticoagulants, antihypertensives, and thrombolytics can increase survival.

OBJECTIVES

After reading this chapter, the student should be able to:

1. Identify common diseases that may cause chest pain.
2. Describe how the myocardium receives its oxygen and nutrient supply.
3. Explain the pathophysiology of angina pectoris.
4. Prescribe lifestyle changes by which a client might control his/her angina.
5. For each of the following classes, identify representative drugs, explain the mechanism of drug action, primary actions, and important adverse effects as they relate to the treatment of angina.
   a. organic nitrates
   b. beta-adrenergic blockers
   c. calcium channel blockers
6. Explain the pathophysiology of myocardial infarction.
7. For each of the following classes, identify representative drugs, explain the mechanism of drug action, primary actions, and important adverse effects as they relate to the treatment of myocardial infarction.
   a. thrombolytics
   b. beta-adrenergic blockers
   c. anticoagulants and antiplatelet agents
   d. analgesics
8. Explain the pathophysiology of stroke.
9. Identify strategies used in the pharmacologic treatment of stroke.
10. Categorize drugs used to treat angina, myocardial infarction, and stroke based on their classification and mechanism of action.

PharMedia www.prenhall.com/holland — Additional interactive resources and activities for this chapter can be found on the Companion Website. For animations, audio glossary, and review access the accompanying CD-ROM in this book.

246

Key Terms

Key terms are defined at the beginning of each chapter, with the page number on which the first reference to the word can be found. **Key terms** are also placed in blue boldface type throughout the text.

KEY TERMS

afterload: pressure that must be overcome in order for the ventricles to eject blood from the heart / *page 216*

chronotropic effect (KRO-no-TRO-pik): change in the heart rate / *page 218*

contractility (kon-trak-TILL-eh-tee): the strength by which the myocardial fibers contract / *page 216*

dromotropic effect (dro-mo-TRO-pik): change in the conduction speed across the myocardium / *page 218*

dysrhythmia (diss-RITH-mee-uh): abnormal cardiac rhythm / *page 221*

Frank-Starling Law: the greater the degree of stretch on the myocardial fibers, the greater will be the force by which they contract / *page 216*

heart failure (HF): disease in which the heart muscle cannot contract with sufficient force to meet the body's metabolic needs / *page 215*

inotropic effect (in-oh-TRO-pik): change in the strength or contractility of the heart / *page 218*

peripheral edema (purr-IF-ur-ul eh-DEE-mah): swelling in the limbs, particularly the feet and ankles due to an accumulation of interstitial fluid / *page 216*

phosphodiesterase (fos-fo-die-ES-tur-ase): enzyme in muscle cells that cleaves phosphodiester bonds; its inhibition increases myocardial contractility / *page 224*

preload: degree of stretch of the cardiac muscle fibers just before they contract / *page 216*

refractory period (ree-FRAK-tore-ee): time during which the myocardial cells rest and are not able to contract / *page 218*

Drug Profiles

To facilitate learning, a prototype approach is used in which the one or two most representative drugs in each classification are introduced in detail. **Drug Profile** boxes are used to clearly indicate these important medications.

DRUG PROFILE:
Fluoxetine (Prozac)

Actions:

Actions of fluoxetine are attributed to its ability to selectively inhibit the reuptake of serotonin into pre-synaptic nerve terminals. It is mainly used for clinical depression, although it may also be used for obsessive-compulsive disorder and eating disorders. Actions include improved affect, mood enhancement, and reduced appetite, with maximum therapeutic effects taking several days to several weeks.

Back

Adverse Effects:

Fluoxetine may cause headaches, nervousness, insomnia, nausea, and diarrhea. Foods high in the amino acid, tryptophan should be avoided because tryptophan is the chemical precursor for serotonin synthesis. Coadministration with selegiline (Carbex, Eldepryl) may increase the risk of a hypertensive crisis. Tricyclic antidepressants administered simultaneously may produce serotonin syndrome. Serotonin syndrome is characterized by fever, confusion, shivering, sweating, and muscle spasms.

Mechanism in Action:

Fluoxetine (Prozac) is a selective serotonin reuptake inhibitor (SSRI). It acts by blocking the recycling of the brain neurotransmitter serotonin into pre-synaptic nerve terminals. At the synaptic cleft, serotonin continually binds with post-synaptic receptors and activates excitatory post-synaptic potentials (EPSPs). This is thought to restore the mental state of a depressed client to a normal level.

Mechanism in Action

Mechanism in Action features use computer animations to clearly demonstrate drug action on the student CD-ROM. A colorful graphic of the animation is included in many of the Drug Profile boxes, as well as a description of the drug action.

Drug Tables

Drug tables provide the most important information for each drug in a user-friendly format. Drugs that are profiled within that chapter are also identified with a **Profile icon**.

TABLE 9.9	Conventional Anti-psychotic Drugs	
DRUG	**ROUTE AND ADULT DOSE**	**REMARKS**
Phenothiazines		
chlorpromazine hydrochloride (Thorazine)	PO; 25–100 mg tid or qid (clients may require up to 1000 mg/day). IM/IV; 25–50 mg (max 600 mg q 4–6 hours).	Strong sedative properties; controls nausea and vomiting, dementia and hiccups not treated by any other means; for agitated patients.
fluphenazine hydrochloride (Prolixin, Permitil)	PO; 0.5–10 mg/day up to a usual max of 20 mg/day.	Also for dementia; available in IM or SC forms.
mesoridazine besylate (Serentil)	PO; 10–50 mg bid or tid; may increase up to 400 mg/day.	Strong sedative properties; also for dementia, hyperactivity, alcohol dependence, and anxiety.
perphenazine (Phenazine, Trilafon)	PO; 4–16 mg bid to qid (max 64 mg/day).	Also for dementia and nausea; available in IM and IV forms.
prochlorperazine (Compazine)	PO; 5–10 mg tid or qid.	Also for severe nausea and vomiting; available as suppositories, IM or IV forms.
promazine hydrochloride (Prozine, Sparine)	PO/IM; 10–200 mg every 4–6 hours (max 1,000mg/day).	For agitated and paranoid clients; useful in clients withdrawing from alcohol; available in IM form.
thioridazine hydrochloride (Mellaril)	PO; 50–100 mg tid; (max 800 mg/day).	Strong sedative properties; for moderate to severe depression and dementia.
trifluoperazine hydrochloride (Stelazine)	PO; 1–2 mg bid; may increase up to 20 mg/day.	Used also for dementia; use cautiously in clients with seizure disorders; available in IM form.
Phenothiazine-like Drugs		
chlorprothixene (Taractan)	PO; 75–150 mg/day (max 600 mg/day).	Prominent sedative effects; less hypotensive than phenothiazines; available in IV form.
haloperidol (Haldol)	PO; 0.2–5 mg bid or tid.	For severe psychosis, dementia, and Tourette's disorder; available in IM form.
loxapine succinate (Loxitane)	PO; Start with 20 mg/day and rapidly increase to 60–100 mg/day in divided doses (max 250 mg/day).	Also for dementia.
molindone hydrochloride (Moban)	PO; 50–75 mg/day in 3–4 divided doses; may increase to 100 mg/day in 3–4 days (max 225 mg/day).	May produce insomnia and drowsiness.
pimozide (Orap)	PO; 1–2 mg/day in divided doses; gradually increase every other day to 7–16 mg/day (max 10mg/day).	For Tourette's disorder; use cautiously in clients with seizure disorders.
thiothixene hydrochloride (Navane)	PO; 2 mg tid; may increase up to 15 mg/day (max 60 mg/day).	Also for dementia; unlabeled use as an antidepressant.

Cross-Referencing

Cross-reference icons refer the student to content in other chapters. This helps to facilitate understanding that one drug may be prescribed for several different conditions.

All of the narcotic analgesics cause physical and psychological dependence to some degree, as discussed in Chapter 5. Many practitioners have been hesitant to administer the proper amount of opioid medication for fear of causing client addiction or of producing serious adverse effects such as sedation or respiratory depression. However, attitudes have changed mainly due to organized awareness groups, which feel that the medical community has not taken seriously clients who are in excruciating pain and have not medicated properly. It should now be understood that, when used according to accepted medical practice, clients can receive the pain relief they need without fear of addiction.

Some opioids are used primarily for conditions other than pain. For example, alfentanil (Alfenta), fentanyl (Sublimaze and others), remifentanil (Ultiva), and sufentanil (Sufenta) are used for general anesthesia; these are discussed in Chapter 12.

Codeine is often prescribed as a cough suppressant and is covered in Chapter 24. Opiates of value in treating diarrhea are covered in Chapter 25.

ON THE JOB

Teamwork in an Adult Psychiatric Facility

Working in an adult psychiatric facility is often an intimidating job because of a wide range of psychiatric disorders found within one confined area. Clients will have all kinds of disorders from depression to schizophrenia, and at any time, clients may become aggressive, agitated or suicidal. One has to be alert and familiar with the ways clients might behave while being confined in such a facility. Being familiar with behavioral symptoms and the types of medications clients are taking may be critical to the well-being and safety of everyone, including the staff. The healthcare practitioner might be tasked with a one-on-one observation of a client on suicide precautions for the entire duration of his or her shift. This kind of job is a situation where everyone—from the mental health worker to the charge nurse—must work together. ■

On the Job

On the Job boxes, included in most chapters, show the student the application of pharmacology by practical nurses and various health professionals.

CLIENT TEACHING

Clients taking antidepressants need to know the following:

1. Tricyclics may increase appetite, cause dizziness with rapid change of position, and be sedating. Report dry mouth, constipation, urinary retention, or blurred vision if they occur.
2. MAO inhibitors may cause problems with sleep, agitation, dizziness when rapidly changing position, and dangerous interactions with other medications. Eating foods high in tyramine can cause a hypertensive crisis. Obtain a list of foods high in tyramine from your healthcare practitioner.
3. SSRIs may cause GI upset, dizziness, skin rash, and headache. Report these signs and symptoms to your healthcare practitioner.
4. Do not combine MAO inhibitors and SSRI antidepressants. Do not take St. John's Wort with any antidepressant. These combinations can cause serious side effects termed serotonin syndrome: confusion, mania, headache, respiratory problems, kidney failure, and possibly death.
5. Antidepressants may take one to four weeks to become fully effective.
6. Some antidepressants may decrease sexual interest or performance. If this occurs, discuss a change in medication with your healthcare practitioner.
7. If insomnia is a problem, take your medication in the morning.
8. If nausea is a problem, take your medication with food, unless ortherwise instructed.
9. Monitor your weight; an increase or a decrease may occur.
10. Avoid driving or operating machinery until you know your response to the medication. Its sedating effects can increase your risk for accidental injury.
11. Do not stop your medication without consulting your healthcare practitioner.

Clients taking anti-psychotics need to know the following:

1. It is imperative to report the development of tremors, involuntary repetitive movements, decreased muscle tone, or increased restlessness to your healthcare practitioner. These symptoms may indicate serious side effects that can be reversed if medication is changed soon after their onset.
2. If dry mouth, rapid heart rate, constipation, or urinary retention occur, consult your healthcare practitioner. An additional medication may be prescribed to relieve these signs and symptoms.
3. Avoid taking antacids with anti-psychotics: they delay or decrease anti-psychotic absorption.
4. Alcohol increases the depressant effects, so it should be avoided while taking anti-psychotics.
5. Extra protection from the sun is necessary: wear hats and sunscreen.
6. Avoid driving or operating machinery until you know your response to the medication. Its sedating effects can increase your risk for accidental injury.
7. If symptoms of your illness increase or are not relieved by the medication, contact your healthcare practitioner for guidance. Do not stop the medication unless directed to do so. ■

Client Teaching

It is not sufficient for a health professional to learn pharmacology. Just as important, is the ability to communicate this knowledge to clients and other members of the public. To help the student achieve the ability to communicate pharmacology, each drug chapter contains concise **Client Teaching** boxes that apply fundamental patient care principles to pharmacology.

Natural Alternatives

Natural Alternatives features present a popular herbal or dietary supplement that may be considered along with conventional drugs.

NATURAL ALTERNATIVES

Glutathione and Milk Thistle for the Treatment of Parkinson's Disease

The word is getting out about a natural alternative used for the treatment of Parkinson's disease: glutathione therapy. Glutathione is inexpensive and readily available; however, it is not available in oral form. IV therapy given by a qualified practitioner may dramatically reverse symptoms for up to four months. The primary role of glutathione is not to reverse neural damage after it has already begun, but to slow down the progression of damage by limiting the action of circulating free radicals. Free radicals are highly reactive molecules that are thought to produce molecular damage throughout the body, especially in vulnerable places including the brain. Glutathioine is an antioxidant, which means it is a molecular scavenger for molecules in the bloodstream that might cause serious cellular damage. Milk thistle (*Silybum marianum*) has been used to retain glutathione in the bloodstream during therapy. ■

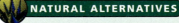

Fast Facts ADD/ADHD

- ADHD is the major reason why children are referred for mental health treatment.
- About one-half are also diagnosed with oppositional defiant or conduct disorder.
- About one-fourth are also diagnosed with anxiety disorder.
- About one-third are also diagnosed with depression.
- And about one-fifth also have a learning disability.

Source: National Mental Health Association

hyper = increased
kinetic = activity

The causes of ADD/ADHD are not clear; however, several theories have been proposed. For many years, scientists described these disorders as *minimal brain dysfunction (MBD)* and *hyperkinetic syndrome*, focusing on abnormal brain function and overactivity. More recent evidence suggests that hyperactivity may be related to dysfunction of a special group of neurotransmitters in the brain, including dopamine, norepinephrine, and serotonin. The specific location of neurotransmitter dysfunction is probably associated with the reticular activating system in the brain.

Within the past decade, experts have suggested that one-third to one-half of children diagnosed with ADD/ADHD will continue to experience symptoms of attention dysfunction in their adult years. Symptoms of ADD/ADHD in adults are similar to those of mood disorders and include anxiety, mania, restlessness, and depression. Some clients are perceived as lacking motivation and direction and have difficulty keeping a job or maintaining normal relationships with others. Frustration and problems with impulse control place the ADD/ADHD client at increased risk for alcohol and substance abuse.

PharmLink

ADULTS WITH ADD

FastFacts

The **FastFacts** feature puts the disease in a social and economic perspective.

PharmLinks

PharmLinks invite the student to perform specific web activities.

Word Roots

Word roots are included in the margins to help the student identify prefixes and suffixes essential to medical word-building. Since pronunciation of medical terms is often difficult, a phonetic pronunciation is provided for difficult terms. Phonetic pronunciations for generic drugs are provided for each generic entry in the index.

Concept Reviews

Concept Reviews are questions placed strategically throughout the chapter to stimulate student comprehension and retention.

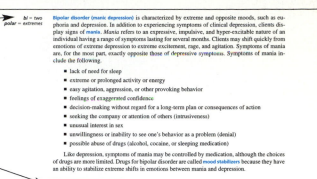

bi = two
polar = extremes

Bipolar disorder (manic depression) is characterized by extreme and opposite moods, such as euphoria and depression. In addition to experiencing symptoms of clinical depression, clients display signs of **mania**. *Mania* refers to an expressive, impulsive, and hyper-excitable nature of an individual having a range of symptoms lasting for several months. Clients may shift quickly from emotions of extreme depression to extreme excitement, rage, and agitation. Symptoms of mania are, for the most part, exactly opposite those of depressive symptoms. Symptoms of mania include the following:

- lack of need for sleep
- extreme or prolonged activity or energy
- easy agitation, aggression, or other provoking behavior
- feelings of exaggerated confidence
- decision-making without regard for a long-term plan or consequences of action
- seeking the company or attention of others (intrusiveness)
- unusual interest in sex
- unwillingness or inability to see one's behavior as a problem (denial)
- possible abuse of drugs (alcohol, cocaine, or sleeping medication)

Like depression, symptoms of mania may be controlled by medication, although the choices of drugs are more limited. Drugs for bipolar disorder are called **mood stabilizers** because they have an ability to stabilize extreme shifts in emotions between mania and depression.

Concept review 9.3

- Identify the symptoms of mania. How do manic symptoms generally compare with depressive symptoms? Give the general name used to describe drugs used to treat bipolar disorder.

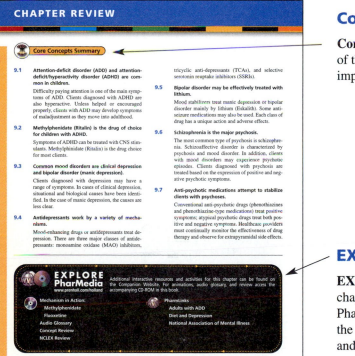

Concept Summary

Concept Summaries are repeated at the end of the chapter, with a brief summary of the important concepts.

EXPLORE PharMedia

EXPLORE PharMedia at the end of each chapter identifies specific animations, PharmLinks, and other resources available to the student on the accompanying CD-ROM and Companion Website.

ADDITIONAL ONLINE RESOURCES

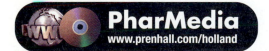

Animations

The free Student CD-ROM contains thirty animations showing how drug action occurs at the cellular and system levels. These animations build upon the feature in the textbook entitled, *Mechanism in Action*, and help students visualize these difficult concepts.

NCLEX-PN Review and Concept Review

Both the Student CD-ROM and the Companion Website offer students numerous opportunities for practicing NCLEX questions. The CD-ROM includes NCLEX-PN review questions that emphasize application of care and client education related to drug administration. For each chapter, questions are graded automatically and provide complete rationales. Students can test their knowledge and gain immediate feedback through rationales for right and wrong answers. In addition, Concept Review questions provide students an additional opportunity for checking their knowledge. Students will also find the audio glossary and objectives useful for review. The NCLEX review module on the Companion Website provides additional practice questions and allows students to email their results directly to instructors.

1   BASIC CONCEPTS IN PHARMACOLOGY

1 Introduction to Pharmacology: Drug Regulation and Approval

CORE CONCEPTS

1.1 Pharmacology is an integrated subject.

1.2 For healthcare professionals, the fields of pharmacology and therapeutics are connected.

1.3 Agents may be classified as traditional drugs, biologics, and natural alternatives.

1.4 Drugs are available by prescription or over-the-counter (OTC).

1.5 *Pharmaceutics* is the science of pharmacy.

1.6 Drug regulations were created to protect the public from drug misuse.

1.7 U.S. drug standards have become increasingly complex.

1.8 There are four stages of approval for therapeutic and biologic drugs.

1.9 Once criticized for being too slow, governmental agencies face new challenges for ensuring the safety of drugs.

1.10 Similar drug standards protect Canadian consumers.

1.11 A look forward in pharmacology: What will be the next challenge for the healthcare professional?

OBJECTIVES

After reading this chapter, the student should be able to:

1. Explain the interdisciplinary nature of pharmacology and give examples of subject area expertise needed to learn the discipline well.

2. Explain how the disciplines of therapeutics and pharmacology are interconnected.

3. Distinguish between therapeutic drugs and agents such as foods, household products, and cosmetics.

4. Compare and contrast traditional drugs, biologics, and natural alternative therapies.

5. Identify the advantages and disadvantages of prescription and over-the-counter (OTC) drugs.

6. Distinguish between pharmaceutics and pharmacology.

7. Discuss the history of U.S. standards, acts, and organizations leading to the requirement that drug safety must be proven before marketing.

8. Discuss the role of the U.S. Food and Drug Administration in determining whether or not drugs may be used for therapy.

9. Discuss the roles and responsibilities of branches within the FDA in overseeing traditional therapeutic drugs, biologics, and integrative therapies.

10. Identify four stages of approval for therapeutic and biologic drugs.

11. Discuss current challenges facing the FDA in approving new drugs for market.

12. Explain the role of Health Canada in the management of Canadian health, drug, and safety issues.

13. Describe the Canadian drug approval process and explain points of similarity to the United States' approval process.

14. Identify possible future challenges for healthcare providers working in the field of pharmacology.

PharMedia www.prenhall.com/holland

Additional interactive resources and activities for this chapter can be found on the Companion Website. For animations, audio glossary, and review access the accompanying CD-ROM in this book.

More drugs are being administered to consumers than ever before. According to the National Association of Chain Drug Stores, over 2.78 billion prescriptions were dispensed within the United States in 1998, and by 2005 the number of prescriptions is expected to reach 4 billion. Because of the volume of new drugs being made available for therapy, some experts are concerned that clients might be harmed if drugs are not thoroughly tested.

The purpose of this chapter is to introduce the subject of pharmacology and to emphasize the role of the government in ensuring drugs and natural alternatives are safe and effective for public use. The chapter also addresses the role that drug therapy has in fighting disease as governmental regulators, consumers, and healthcare professionals face new challenges in the years ahead.

1.1 Pharmacology is an integrated subject.

The word **pharmacology** is derived from two Greek words, *pharmakon,* which means "medicine," and *logos,* which means "study." Thus, *pharmacology* is defined as *"the study of medicine."*

pharmac = *drugs*
ology = *the study of*

Healthcare practitioners practice the discipline of pharmacology because it is the study of how drugs improve the health of the human body. If applied properly, drugs can dramatically improve our quality of life. If applied improperly, the consequences of drug action can be devastating.

The subject of pharmacology is an expansive topic ranging from a study of how drugs enter and travel throughout the body to the actual responses they produce. In order to learn the discipline well, students must master concepts from several interrelated areas including anatomy, physiology, chemistry, and **pathophysiology**. The useful application of drugs depends upon knowledge from at least these areas.

patho = *disease*
physio = *the nature of*
ology = *the study of*

Over 10,000 brand and generic varieties of drugs with many different names, interactions, side effects, and complicated mechanisms of action are currently available. Keeping up with the numbers of drugs is a huge challenge. Many drugs may be prescribed for more than one disease and most produce multiple effects in the body. Further complicating the study of pharmacology is the fact that drugs may elicit different responses depending on factors such as sex, age, health status, body mass, and genetics.

1.2 For healthcare professionals, the fields of pharmacology and therapeutics are connected.

It is obvious that a thorough knowledge of pharmacology is important to those health professionals who prescribe drugs on a daily basis. This group includes physicians, physician's assistants, dentists, and advanced nurse practitioners. Depending upon state or provincial law, other groups may also be permitted to prescribe medications. In this textbook, the group of occupations that is allowed to prescribe drugs will be referred to as *healthcare practitioners*.

A second group of occupations includes nursing, allied health, and community service employees. These occupations have in common direct contact with clients or healthcare practitioners. Examples of other occupations include certified nursing assistants, dental hygienists and assistants, pharmacy technicians, radiologic technologists, lab technicians, emergency medical technicians, paramedics, nutritionists, home healthcare workers, nursing home employees, mental health workers, medical office workers, and members of law enforcement. Persons in occupations such as these may be directly involved with drug administration as well as with issues related to drug education, management, and/or enforcement of drug laws. In this text, these occupations will be referred to as *healthcare providers*.

Some healthcare providers, such as nurses, may administer drugs on a daily basis while others, such as radiographers, may administer drugs occasionally. A strong knowledge of pharmacology is necessary in order to properly educate and advise clients regarding their healthcare needs. This knowledge is also essential in order to communicate effectively with healthcare practitioners, who rely heavily on nurses and allied health professionals to gather medical data from their clients and to follow up on results of therapy.

While the role of some healthcare providers is generally widely known, the roles of others in this group are less understood. In this text, many chapters will include a feature called *On the Job* that highlights the roles of various healthcare providers so that the importance of studying pharmacology may be more widely appreciated.

For healthcare providers studying pharmacology, it usually becomes apparent that the fields of pharmacology and therapeutics are connected. **Therapeutics** is the branch of medicine concerned with the treatment of disease and suffering. **Pharmacotherapeutics** is the use of drugs to treat disease.

1.3 Agents may be classified as traditional drugs, biologics, and natural alternatives.

Drugs are chemical agents that produce biological responses within the body. From a broader perspective, drugs may be considered a part of the body's normal activities, from the essential gases that we breathe to the foods that we eat. Because drugs are defined so broadly, it is necessary to clearly separate them from other substances such as foods, household products, and cosmetics. Many agents such as antiperspirants, sunscreens, toothpastes and shampoos might alter the body's normal activities, but they are not considered to be medically therapeutic, as are drugs.

Therapeutic drugs are sometimes classified on the basis of how they are produced, either chemically or naturally. Most traditional drugs are chemically-produced or synthesized in a laboratory. **Biologics** are agents naturally produced in animal cells, microorganisms, or by the body itself. **Natural alternative therapies** are herbs, natural extracts, vitamins, minerals, or dietary supplements. Table 1.1 contains a summary of characteristics associated with traditional drug therapies, biologics, and natural alternative therapies. Because drugs may be described in many ways, this text will limit its focus to agents used for therapy in a clinical or home setting. Traditional drugs and drug classes will be discussed more thoroughly in Chapter 2. Natural alternatives will be discussed more thoroughly in Chapter 26 . In addition, most chapters include a feature called *Natural Alternatives* that highlights a specific herbal therapy or dietary supplement.

1.4 Drugs are available by prescription or over-the-counter.

Legal drugs are obtained either by a prescription or over-the-counter (OTC). There are differences between the two methods of dispensing. In order to obtain prescription drugs, clients must obtain a physician's order authorizing the client to receive the drugs. The advantages to this are numerous. The practitioner has an opportunity to examine the client and determine a

TABLE 1.1	Characteristics of Traditional Drug Therapies, Biologics, and Natural/Alternative Therapies	
TRADITIONAL DRUG THERAPIES	**BIOLOGICS**	**NATURAL/ALTERNATIVE THERAPIES**
chemically-produced	naturally-produced	naturally-produced
synthesized in a laboratory	made by the body's cells	herbs
used routinely by health practitioners	associated with the bloodstream	vitamins
	hormones	minerals
	vaccines	extracts from a natural source
	animal products	
	made by microorganisms	
	used routinely by health practitioners	

specific diagnosis. The practitioner can maximize therapy by ordering the proper drug for the client's condition, controlling specifically the amount and frequency of the drug to be dispensed. The healthcare practitioner may give instructions on how to use the drug properly and what side effects to expect.

In some instances, the margin of safety observed after use of a specific drug over a longer period of time prompts regulators to change its status from prescription to OTC. In contrast to prescription drugs, OTC drugs do not require a physician's order. Clients may treat themselves safely if they carefully follow instructions included with the medication. If clients do not follow these guidelines, OTC drugs can have serious side effects.

Clients often prefer to take OTC medications for many reasons. They may obtain OTC drugs more easily than prescription drugs. They do not have to make an appointment with a physician, thereby saving time and money. Without training, however, choosing the proper medication for a specific problem may be very challenging. OTC drugs may react with foods, herbal products, and prescription or other OTC drugs. Clients may not be aware that some medications can impair their ability to function safely. Self-treatment is sometimes ineffective, and the potential for injury is much greater if the disease is allowed to progress.

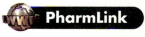

PharmLink

TAKING MEDICATION

1.5 *Pharmaceutics* is the science of pharmacy.

Pharmaceutics is the science of preparing and dispensing drugs and is a very important component of pharmacotherapy. Often, the general public confuses the science of pharmaceutics with pharmacology. Generally, consumers recognize the root *pharm* and assume that *pharmacology* is the same as *pharmacy*. Correctly, pharmaceutics is the science of pharmacy. To describe it simply, pharmaceutics involves the dispensation of a drug to a client after he or she has been examined by a licensed practitioner. Pharmacists are expert at cataloguing signs, symptoms, side effects, and drug interactions. They often act as drug advisors to clients, making sure that they receive the proper medication and educating then about undesirable symptoms or interactions.

Concept review 1.1

- Explain the meaning of this statement: "Pharmacotherapy involves the science of therapeutics and pharmaceutics."

1.6 Drug regulations were created to protect the public from drug misuse.

For many years, there were no standards or guidelines to protect the public from drug misuse. Clients could not be assured that available medicines were not a form of quackery. The archives

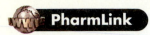

OLD FASHIONED REMEDIES

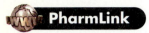

U.S. PHARMACOPOEIA

of drug regulatory agencies are filled with examples of early medicines including rattlesnake oil for rheumatism, epilepsy treatment for spasms, hysteria, and alcoholism, and fat reducers for a slender, healthy figure. (See PharmLink: Old Fashioned Remedies for these and other examples.) It became quite clear that drug regulations were needed to protect the public.

The first standards commonly used by pharmacists were early formularies, or lists of drugs and drug recipes. In 1820, the first comprehensive publication of drug standards called the *U.S. Pharmacopoeia (USP)* was established. (See the timeline in Figure 1.2.) A pharmacopoeia is a medical reference summary indicating standards of drug purity, strength, and directions for synthesis. In 1852, a national professional society of pharmacists—the American Pharmaceutical Association (APhA)—was founded. From 1852 until 1975, two major compendia maintained drug standards in the United States—the *U.S. Pharmacopoeia* and the *National Formulary (NF)* established by the APhA. All drug substances and products were covered in the USP; the NF focused on pharmaceutic ingredients. In 1975, the two organizations announced their union, creating a single publication named the *U.S. Pharmacopoeia–National Formulary (USP-NF)*. Official monographs and interim revision announcements for the USP-NF are published regularly. Today, the USP label can be found on many medication vials verifying the exact ingredients found within the container, as shown in Figure 1.1.

In the early 1900s, in order to protect the public, governing authorities began to develop and enforce tougher drug legislation. In 1902, the Biologics Control Act was passed to standardize the quality of serums and other blood-related products. The Pure Food and Drug Act of 1906 gave the government power to control the labeling of medicines. In 1912, the Sherley Amendment prohibited the sale of drugs labeled with false therapeutic claims intended to defraud the consumer.

FIGURE 1.1	

Examples of USP labels
SOURCE: Courtesy of Novartis Pharmaceuticals Corporation and Mallinckrodt Pharmaceuticals.

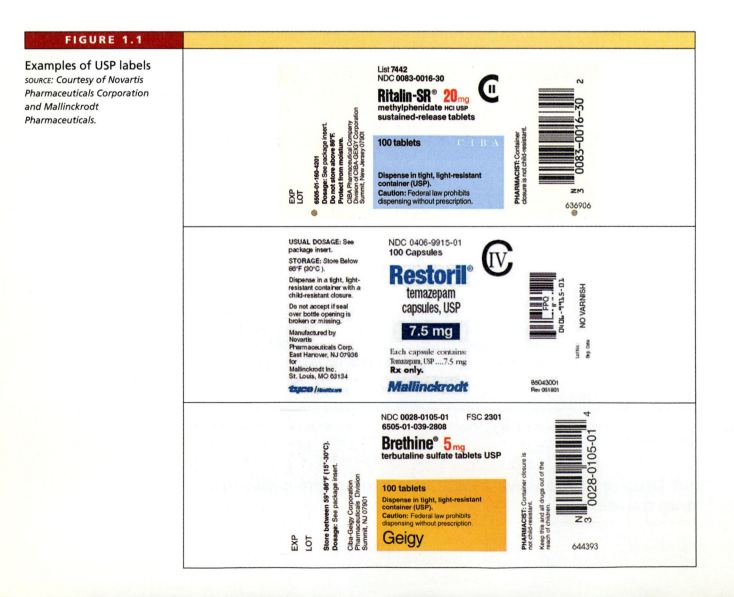

FIGURE 1.2	
TIMELINE	**REGULATORY ACTS, STANDARDS, AND ORGANIZATIONS**
1820	A group of physicians established the first comprehensive publication of drug standards called the **U.S. Pharmacopeia (USP)**.
1852	A group of pharmacists founded a national professional society called the **American Pharmaceutical Association (APhA)**. The APhA then established the **National Formulary (NF)**, a standardized publication focusing on pharmaceutical ingredients. The USP continued to catalogue all drug related substances and products.
1862	This was the beginning of the **Federal Bureau of Chemistry**, established under the administration of President Lincoln. Over the years and with added duties, it gradually became the Food and Drug Administration (FDA).
1902	Congress passed the **Biologics Control Act** to control the quality of serums and other blood-related products.
1906	**The Pure Food and Drug Act** gave the government power to control the labeling of medicines.
1912	**The Sherley Amendment** made medicines safer by prohibiting the sale of drugs labeled with false therapeutic claims.
1938	Congress passed the **Food, Drug, and Cosmetic Act**. It was the first law preventing the marketing of drugs not thoroughly tested. This law now provides for the requirement that drug companies must submit a New Drug Application (NDA) to the Food and Drug Administration (FDA) prior to marketing a new drug.
1944	Congress passed the **Public Health Service Act**, covering many health issues including biological products and the control of communicable diseases.
1975	The U.S. Pharmacopeia and National Formulary announced their union. The **USP-NF** became a single standardized publication.
1986	Congress passed the **Childhood Vaccine Act**. It authorized the FDA to acquire information about patients taking vaccines, to recall biologics, and to recommend civil penalties if guidelines regarding biologic use were not followed.
1988	The **FDA** was officially established as an agency of the **U.S. Department of Health and Human Services**.
1992	Congress passed the **Prescription Drug User Fee Act**. It required that non-generic drug and biologic manufacturers pay fees to be used for improvements in the drug review process.
1997	**The FDA Modernization Act** reauthorized the Prescription Drug User Fee Act. This act represents the largest reform effort of the drug review process since 1938.

A historical timeline of regulatory acts, standards, and organizations

In 1938, Congress passed the Food, Drug, and Cosmetic Act. This was the first law preventing the marketing of drugs that had not been thoroughly tested prior to marketing. According to the provisions of this law, drug companies were required to prove the safety and efficacy of any drug before it could be sold within the United States.

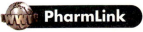

U.S. GOVERNMENTAL DRUG REGULATION

1.7 U.S. drug standards have become increasingly complex.

Much has changed in the regulation of drugs since 1938. In 1988, the Food and Drug Administration (FDA) was officially established as an agency of the U.S. Department of Health and Human Services. Today, the Center for Drug Evaluation and Research (CDER), a branch of the FDA, exercises powerful control over whether or not prescription drugs and OTC drugs may be used for therapy. The CDER states its mission as "facilitating the availability of safe effective drugs, keeping unsafe or ineffective drugs off the market, improving the health of Americans, and providing clear, easily understandable drug information for safe and effective use." Any pharmaceutical laboratory, whether private, public, or academic, must obtain FDA approval before marketing any drug.

Another branch of the FDA, the Center for Biologics Evaluation and Research (CBER), regulates the use of biologics including serums, vaccines, and products found in the bloodstream. One historical achievement involving biologics is the 1986 Childhood Vaccine Act. This act authorized the FDA to acquire information about patients taking vaccines, to recall biologics, and to recommend civil penalties if guidelines regarding biologics were not followed.

The FDA also oversees administration of herbal products and dietary supplements, but the Center for Food Safety and Applied Nutrition (CFSAN) regulates use of these substances. Herbal products and dietary supplements are regulated by the Dietary Supplement Health and Education Act of 1994. This Act does not provide the same degree of protection as the Food, Drug, and Cosmetic Acts of 1938. Herbal and dietary supplements may be marketed without prior approval from the FDA. This act is discussed in more detail in Chapter 26 🔗 .

1.8 There are four stages of approval for therapeutic and biologic drugs.

The amount of time spent in the review and approval process, for both prescription and OTC drugs, depends on several checkpoints along a well-developed and organized plan. Most therapeutic drugs and biologics are reviewed in four phases, which are summarized in Figure 1.3. These are:

1. Pre-clinical investigation
2. Clinical investigation
3. Submission of a New Drug Application (NDA) with review
4. Post-marketing surveillance

Pre-clinical investigation involves basic science research. Scientists perform many tests on cells grown in the laboratory (a process called *culture*) or studies are performed in animals to examine the effectiveness of a range of drug doses and to look for any adverse effects. Laboratory tests on cells and animals are important because they assist in predicting whether or not drugs will cause harm in humans. Because laboratory tests do not always reflect the way a human responds, pre-clinical investigation results are always inconclusive.

Clinical pharmacology is an area of medicine devoted to the evaluation of drugs used for human benefit. Clinical investigation, the second stage of drug approval, takes place in three different phases termed *clinical phase trials*. Clinical phase trials are the longest part of the drug approval process. Clinical pharmacologists perform tests on volunteers and large groups of selected clients with certain diseases. Both scientists and healthcare practitioners establish drug doses and try to identify adverse effects. Clinical investigators address concerns such as whether the drug worsens other medical conditions, interacts unsafely with existing medications, or affects one type of client more than others.

Clinical phase trials are an essential component of drug evaluations because of the potential variability of responses among clients. If a drug appears to be effective without serious side effects, approval for marketing may be accelerated, or the drug may be used for treatment immediately in special cases with careful monitoring. If the drug shows promise but precautions are noted, the process is delayed until concerns are addressed. In any case, a New Drug Application (NDA) must be submitted before a drug is allowed to proceed to the next stage of the approval process.

A review of the NDA is the third stage of drug approval. During this stage, clinical phase III trials and animal testing may continue depending on the results obtained from pre-clinical testing. If the NDA is approved, the process continues to the final stage. If the NDA is rejected, the process stops until noted concerns are addressed.

Post-marketing surveillance, the fourth stage of the drug approval process, takes place after clinical trials and the NDA review process have been completed. The purpose of Stage IV testing is to survey for any new harmful effects in a larger and more diverse population. Some adverse effects take longer to appear and are not identified until a drug is circulated to large numbers of clients. One example is the diabetes drug troglitazone (Rezulin), which was placed on the market in 1997. In 1998, Great Britain banned its use after at least one death and several cases of liver failure were reported in diabetic clients taking the drug. The FDA became aware of a number of cases in the U.S. where Rezulin was linked with liver failure. Consumer advocates also claimed the drug caused several cases of heart failure. Rezulin was recalled in March 2000 after health professionals asked the FDA to reconsider its risks.

The FDA holds annual public meetings to hear comments from clients and professional and pharmaceutical organizations regarding the effectiveness and safety of new drug therapies. If the

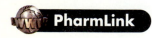

U.S. DRUG RECALLS

FIGURE 1.3

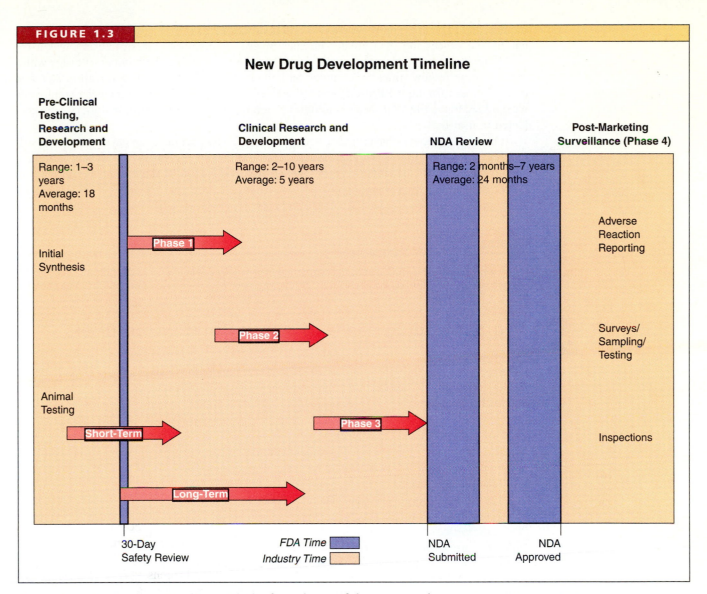

New Drug Development Timeline

| Pre-Clinical Testing, Research and Development | Clinical Research and Development | NDA Review | Post-Marketing Surveillance (Phase 4) |

Range: 1–3 years
Average: 18 months

Range: 2–10 years
Average: 5 years

Range: 2 months–7 years
Average: 24 months

Initial Synthesis

Adverse Reaction Reporting

Phase 1

Phase 2

Surveys/ Sampling/ Testing

Animal Testing

Short-Term

Phase 3

Inspections

Long-Term

30-Day Safety Review

FDA Time
Industry Time

NDA Submitted

NDA Approved

A new drug-development timeline, with the four phases of drug approval   *SOURCE: Pearson Education/PH College*

FDA discovers a serious problem, it will mandate that a drug be withdrawn from the market and its use discontinued. The FDA's ban of Rezulin is an ideal example of post-marketing surveillance in action.

1.9 Once criticized for being too slow, governmental agencies face new challenges for ensuring the safety of drugs.

The public once criticized the FDA and other regulatory agencies for being too slow in bringing new, potentially life-saving drugs to the consumer. In the early 1990s, because of pressures from organized consumer groups and various drug manufacturers, governmental officials began to examine how they could speed up the drug review process. Reasons for the delay in the FDA drug approval process included outdated guidelines, poor communication, and agency understaffing.

In 1992, FDA officials, members of Congress, and representatives from pharmaceutical companies negotiated the Prescription Drug User Fee Act on a five-year trial basis. This act required drug and biologic manufacturers to provide yearly product user fees. With this extra income, the FDA hired more employees and restructured its organization to more efficiently handle the processing of a greater number of drug applications. Restructuring was a resounding success. From 1992 to 1996, the FDA approved double the number of drugs while cutting some review times by as much as half. In 1997, the FDA Modernization Act was passed, reauthorizing the Prescription Drug User Fee Act. Nearly seven hundred employees were added to the FDA's drug and biologics program, and over $300 million dollars were collected in user fees.

One concern now is that drugs are being developed at a faster rate than risks can be assessed. Officials are calling for clients, pharmacists, allied health workers, nurses, physicians, hospitals, and pharmaceutical companies to work together so that risks can be minimized. Because of the higher numbers of drugs being approved for therapy, the potential for adverse drug-drug and drug-herbal interactions are greater than ever before.

Concept review 1.2

∎ Can you recall the major U.S. acts, standards, and organizations leading up to the present time? When was the FDA established? What current U.S. laws regulate how drugs are approved for marketing?

1.10 Similar drug standards protect Canadian consumers.

In Canada, the Health Protection Branch (HPB) serves under the auspices of the Department of Health and Welfare. The Health Protection Branch is tasked with protecting Canadians from the potential health hazards of marketed products, imported goods, and environmental agents. The Deputy Minister enforces regulations concerned with consumer protection issues such as the Food and Drugs Act and the Tobacco Act.

Health Canada is the federal department working in partnership with provincial and territorial governments. It also works with other federal departments to ensure proper management of health and safety issues.

The Health Products and Food Branch (HPFB) of Health Canada regulates the use of therapeutic substances through several national programs: the Therapeutic Products Programme (TPP), the Office of Natural Health Products, and the Food Directorate. The TPP covers drugs including pharmaceuticals, narcotic, controlled and restricted drugs, and biologics. Some natural health products and food-based products called *nutraceuticals* are also regulated. The Office of Natural Health Products limits its focus to natural substances, for example, homeopathic and herbal remedies. The Food Directorate regulates nutraceuticals.

The Food and Drugs Act is an important document in all aspects of health protection because it specifies that drugs cannot be marketed without a Notice of Compliance (NOC) and Drug Identification Number (DIN) from Health Canada. Amended guidelines date back to 1953, stating that the use of foods, drugs, cosmetics, and therapeutic devices must follow established guidelines. Any drug that does not comply with standards established by recognized pharmacopoeias and formularies in the United States, Europe, Great Britain, or France cannot be labeled, packaged, sold, or advertised in Canada.

The basic outline for how drugs are approved in Canada is provided in Table 1.2. There are many similarities between how drugs are regulated in Canada and the U.S. Both governments have realized a need to monitor natural products, minerals, vitamins, and herbs very carefully because the potential for adverse effects is high as well as with newly developed traditional drug therapies. Canadian drugs may share the same names as their counterparts in the United States, or they may have unique names. A listing of unique Canadian drug names and their U.S. equivalents are shown in Appendix B .

PharmLink

CANADIAN DRUG REGULATION

1.11 A look forward in pharmacology: What will be the next challenge for the healthcare professional?

Within the past one hundred years, the most significant challenges for health professionals involved the threat of diseases such as influenza, malaria, mumps, polio, smallpox, tuberculosis, Ebola, her-

TABLE 1.2	Steps of Approval for Drugs Marketed Within Canada
Step 1	Pre-clinical studies or experiments performed in culture, living tissue, and small animals are performed, followed by extensive clinical trials or testing done in humans.
Step 2	A drug company completes *a drug submission* to Health Canada. This report details important safety and effectiveness information including how the drug product will be produced and packaged, expected therapeutic benefits, and adverse reactions.
Step 3	A committee of drug experts including medical and drug scientists reviews the drug submission to identify potential benefits and drug risks.
Step 4	Health Canada reviews information about the drug product and passes on important details to health practitioners and consumers.
Step 5	Health Canada issues a Notice of Compliance (NOC) and Drug Identification Number (DIN). Both permit the manufacturer to market the drug product.
Step 6	Health Canada monitors the effectiveness and concerns of the drug after it has been marketed. This is done by regular inspection, notices, newsletters, and feedback from consumers and healthcare professionals.

pes, hepatitis, and autoimmune deficiency syndrome (AIDS). Some disorders have been successfully treated with drugs and biologics; others have not. Health professionals, governmental agencies and scientists recognize the importance of medications and treatments in combating these disorders. Drugs are the most powerful weapon we have against worldwide epidemics and diseases.

It is important that students entering the study of pharmacology realize the significant role that drugs play in controlling or eliminating disease outbreaks. One could imagine the devastation if laboratories and healthcare professionals were not able to identify, isolate, or treat the causes of these diseases. A major outbreak would allow precious little time to develop antidotes, and this could easily overwhelm healthcare resources.

The remaining chapters in this book present our current knowledge of how drugs treat disorders in many different areas. What kind of impact do you think drugs will make should major diseases re-emerge in the future? Further, what would be your role as a healthcare provider should this happen?

CHAPTER REVIEW

 Core Concepts Summary

1.1 **Pharmacology is an integrated subject.**

Pharmacology, the study of medicine, is a subject devoted to proper drug treatment and health of the human body. It is an expansive topic utilizing concepts from human biology, disease processes, and chemistry.

1.2 **For healthcare professionals, the fields of pharmacology and therapeutics are connected.**

Therapeutics is the science associated with the treatment of suffering and the prevention of disease.

Pharmacotherapeutics is the useful application of drugs for the purpose of fighting disease. The study of pharmacology is important to health professionals from many different areas.

1.3 **Agents may be classified as traditional drugs, biologics, and natural alternatives.**

Drugs are chemical agents used to treat disease by producing biological responses within the body. Therapeutic drugs are classified as substances produced chemically or naturally. Biologics are natural agents produced by animal cells on microorganisms. Alternative therapies include natural herbs, plant extracts, on dietary supplements.

1.4 Drugs are available by prescription or over-the-counter (OTC).

There are two major methods of dispensing drugs. Prescription drugs require a physician's order; OTC drugs do not. There are advantages and disadvantages to both dispensing methods.

1.5 *Pharmaceutics* is the science of pharmacy.

Pharmaceutics involves the successful dispensation of drugs for therapeutic purposes. Dispensing medication safely is a major challenge for healthcare practitioners and clients.

1.6 Drug regulations were created to protect the public from drug misuse.

The first drug laws were acts created by Congress to protect clients from wrongful therapeutic claims. These and other standards form the basis of modern drug regulation agencies and organizations such as the Food and Drug Administration, and publications such as the *U.S. Pharmacopoeia-National Formulary.*

1.7 U.S. drug standards have become increasingly complex.

The Food and Drug Administration, a branch of the U.S. Department of Health and Human Services, is the primary agency regulating drug safety. Three branches of the FDA control policies regarding drug therapies: the Center for Drug Evaluation and Research (CDER), the Center for Biologics Evaluation and Research (CBER), and the Center for Food Safety and Applied Nutrition (CFSAN).

1.8 There are four stages of approval for therapeutic and biologic drugs.

Drug approval involves four stages: pre-clinical investigation, clinical investigation, submission of a New Drug Application (NDA) with review, and post-marketing surveillance. Clinical phase trials must be completed before drugs are approved for public use.

1.9 Once criticized for being too slow, governmental agencies face new challenges for ensuring the safety of drugs.

FDA officials, members of Congress, and pharmaceutical company representatives negotiated the Prescription Drug User Fee Act and FDA Modernization Act. These acts have sped up the approval process and require drug and biologic manufacturers to provide yearly product user fees. The concern now is that drugs are being approved at a rate faster than risks can be assessed.

1.10 Similar drug standards protect Canadian consumers.

In Canada, the Health Protection Branch of the Department of Health and Welfare enforces regulations concerned with the Canadian Food and Drugs Act. The Health Products and Food Branch of Health Canada regulates the proper use of therapeutic drugs by issuing a Notice of Compliance (NOC) and Drug Identification Number (DIN) prior to drugs being marketed. Drugs in Canada are regulated in a fashion similar to that used in the United States.

1.11 A look forward in pharmacology: What will be the next challenge for the healthcare professional?

Drugs are among the most powerful weapons we have to combat diseases of epidemic proportion. The question is raised concerning the role that drugs and healthcare providers would play should a major epidemic emerge.

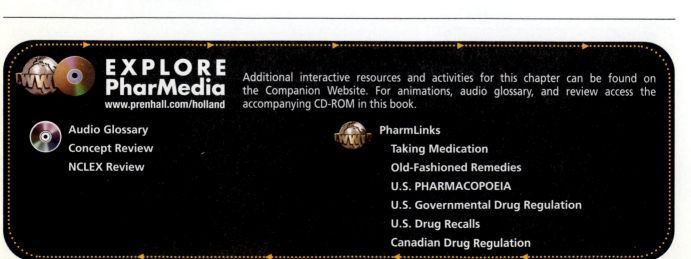

EXPLORE PharMedia
www.prenhall.com/holland

Additional interactive resources and activities for this chapter can be found on the Companion Website. For animations, audio glossary, and review access the accompanying CD-ROM in this book.

Audio Glossary
Concept Review
NCLEX Review

PharmLinks
  Taking Medication
  Old-Fashioned Remedies
  U.S. PHARMACOPOEIA
  U.S. Governmental Drug Regulation
  U.S. Drug Recalls
  Canadian Drug Regulation

2 Drug Classes, Schedules, and Categories

CORE CONCEPTS

2.1 Drugs may be organized by their therapeutic and pharmacological classification.

2.2 Drugs have more than one name.

2.3 Generic drugs are less expensive than brand name drugs, but they may differ in their bioavailability.

2.4 Drugs with a potential for abuse are categorized into schedules.

2.5 Drugs in Canada are also controlled for the protection of consumers.

2.6 All prescription drugs are classified according to safety in pregnancy categories in order to protect the unborn.

OBJECTIVES

After reading this chapter, the student should be able to:

1. Discuss the basis for placing drugs into therapeutic and pharmacological classes.

2. Explain the prototype approach to drug classification.

3. Describe what is meant by a drug's mechanism of action.

4. Distinguish between a drug's chemical name, generic name, and trade name.

5. Explain why generic drug names are preferred to other drug names.

6. Discuss why drugs are sometimes placed on a restrictive list and the controversy surrounding this issue.

7. Explain the meaning of the term *controlled substance.*

8. Explain the U.S. Controlled Substance Act of 1970 and the role of the U.S. Drug Enforcement Agency (DEA) in controlling drug abuse and misuse.

9. Identify the five drug schedules and examples of drugs at each level.

10. Explain how drugs are scheduled taking into account Parts III and IV of the Canadian Food and Drugs Act and the Narcotic Control Act.

11. Identify the five pregnancy categories and explain what each category represents.

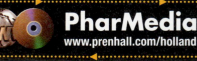

PharMedia
www.prenhall.com/holland

Additional interactive resources and activities for this chapter can be found on the Companion Website. For animations, audio glossary, and review access the accompanying CD-ROM in this book.

addiction (uh-DIK-shun): compulsive behavior that drives someone to use a drug repeated / *page 19*

bioavailability (BEYE-oh-ah-VALE-ah-BILL-ih-TEE): the ability of a drug to reach the bloodstream and its target tissues / *page 17*

chemical name: strict chemical nomenclature used for naming drugs established by the International Union of Pure and Applied Chemistry (IUPAC) / *page 17*

combination drug: drug product with more than one active generic ingredient / *page 18*

controlled substance: in the U.S., this is a drug whose use is restricted by the Comprehensive Drug Abuse Prevention and Control Act. In Canada, it is a drug subject to guidelines outlined in Part III, Schedule G of the Canadian Food and Drugs Act / *page 19–20*

generic (je-NARE-ik) **name**: nonproprietary name of a drug assigned by the government / *page 17*

mechanism of action: how a drug exerts its effects / *page 16*

pharmacological (FAR-mah-koh-LOJ-ik-ul) **classification**: method for organizing drugs on the basis of their mechanism of action / *page 15*

pregnancy category: system for grouping drugs based upon how safe they are for the unborn / *page 21*

prototype (PRO-toh-type) **drug**: an original, well-understood model drug from which other drugs in a pharmacological class have been developed / *page 16*

restricted drug: in Canada, a drug not intended for human use, covered in Part IV, Schedule H of the Canadian Food and Drugs Act / *page 20*

scheduled drug: in the U.S., a term describing a drug placed into one of five categories (I through V) based on its potential for misuse or abuse / *page 19*

teratogen (TER-ah-toh-jen): a chemical substance that harms a developing fetus or embryo / *page 21*

therapeutic (ther-ah-PEW-tik) **classification**: method for organizing drugs on the basis of their *therapeutic usefulness* / *page 15*

trade name: proprietary name of a drug assigned by the manufacturer; also called the *brand name* or *product name* / *page 17*

withdrawal: physical signs of discomfort associated with drug abuse / *page 19*

Understanding drug classes can be very challenging. There are many ways that drugs can be classified, from a strict chemical group name to a name provided by the manufacturer. Because of the large number of drugs available practitioners and consumers must have a system for identifying drugs and determining the limitations of their use. This chapter covers the various methods that drugs may be organized by therapeutic or pharmacological classification. This chapter also discusses drug schedules and pregnancy categories because these types of classification affect the routine use of many drugs.

2.1 Drugs may be organized by their therapeutic and pharmacological classification.

Medications may be classified in two major ways. Drugs may be organized on the basis of their *therapeutic usefulness*. This is referred to as a therapeutic classification. Drugs also may be categorized on the basis of *how they work pharmacologically*. This is referred to as a pharmacological classification. Both methods are widely used in studying pharmacology. Few practitioners make the distinction in a setting where the primary purpose of drug therapy is to improve the health of their clients.

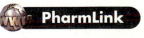

THERAPEUTIC DRUG CLASSES

Table 2.1 shows the use of therapeutic classification, using cardiac care as an example. The cardiovascular system is concerned with the proper functioning of the heart and blood vessels. Many different types of drugs affect cardiovascular function. Some drugs influence blood clotting while others lower blood cholesterol or prevent the onset of stroke. Drugs may be used to lower blood pressure, treat heart failure, correct abnormal heart rhythm, alleviate chest pain, and treat or prevent circulatory shock. Drugs that affect cardiac disorders may be placed in several therapeutic classes. For example, drugs that influence blood clotting are called *anticoagulants*. Medications that lower blood cholesterol are called *antihyperlipidemics*. Drugs that lower blood pressure are called *antihypertensives*.

A therapeutic classification need not be complicated. For example, it is appropriate to classify a medication simply as a *"drug used for stroke"* or *"a drug used for shock."* The key to therapeutic classification is to state clearly what a particular drug does clinically. A few examples of therapeutic classification are provided in Table 2.2.

TABLE 2.1	Organizing Drug Information by Therapeutic Classification

THERAPEUTIC FOCUS

Cardiac care / Drugs affecting cardiovascular function

THERAPEUTIC USEFULNESS	THERAPEUTIC CLASSIFICATION
influencing blood clotting	anticoagulants
lowering blood cholesterol	antihyperlipidemics
lowering blood pressure	antihypertensives
treating abnormal rhythm	antidysrhythmics
treating chest pain (angina)	antianginal drugs

A second way that drugs may be grouped is by pharmacological classification. Pharmacological classification addresses a drug's **mechanism of action**, or how a medication produces its effect in the body.

Table 2.3 shows various types of pharmacological classifications using high blood pressure (hypertension) as an example. A *diuretic* is a class of drug used to treat hypertension by lowering plasma volume. Lowering plasma volume is the mechanism of action by which diuretics work. *Calcium channel blockers* treat hypertension by limiting the force of heart contractions. Other drugs block components of a hormonal network called the *renin-angiotensin pathway,* thereby reducing hypertension. Notice that each example describes *how* hypertension may be controlled. A drug's pharmacological classification is more specific than a therapeutic classification and requires an understanding of human biochemical and physiological principles.

When studying a particular drug's mechanism of action, the information in a textbook or journal may be basic or quite advanced depending on the source of drug information. Although drugs may be described with varying degrees of complexity, it is recommended that students first become comfortable with the broad drug classes and then gradually move to more specific examples.

Prototype drugs are an excellent place to start. A **prototype drug** is the original, well-understood drug model from which other medications in a pharmacological class have been developed. By learning the prototype drug, students may then predict the actions and adverse effects of other drugs in the same class. For example, by knowing the effects of penicillin V, students can extend this knowledge to the other drugs in the penicillin antibiotic class. *Students should be aware, however, that in many cases, the original drug prototype is not the most widely used drug in its class.* As new drugs are developed, features such as antibiotic resistance, fewer side-effects, or a more focused sight of action might be factors that sway health practitioners away from using older drugs. Therefore, being familiar with the original drug prototypes and keeping up with newer and more popular drugs is an essential part of mastering the subject of pharmacology.

TABLE 2.2	Examples of Therapeutic Drug Classes*
anti-inflammatory drugs	antihypertensives
drugs that lower blood cholesterol	drugs for vomiting (emesis)
anti-psychotic drugs	anti-diarrheal drugs
anti-anxiety drugs	antacids
antidepressants	antibiotic drugs

*Note: While the names of some therapeutic categories may sound complicated, drug terminology will become more familiar as you begin to study drugs and drug classes. When studying this topic, always use a medical dictionary and reference drug guide.

TABLE 2.3	Organizing Drug Information by Pharmacological Classification

FOCUSING ON HOW A THERAPY MAY BE APPLIED

Therapy for high blood pressure may be achieved by:

MECHANISM OF ACTION	PHARMACOLOGICAL CLASSIFICATION
lowering plasma volume	diuretics
blocking heart calcium channels	calcium channel blockers
blocking hormonal activity	angiotensin converting enzyme inhibitors
blocking stress-related activity	sympatholytics
dilating peripheral blood vessels	vasodilators

Prototypes and other widely prescribed medications are featured as Drug Profiles beginning in Chapter 6 . These Drug Profiles highlight a representative drug in detail so that the student can apply this knowledge to other medications in the same class. Many of the Profile Drugs appear in the Top 200 Prescription Drug listing that is included on the Companion Website. A list of all the Profile Drugs contained in this text is included on the inside cover.

Concept review 2.1

■ What is the difference between a therapeutic classification and a pharmacological classification? What is a *prototype drug,* and how is it different from any other drug within a pharmacological class?

2.2 Drugs have more than one name.

One of the major difficulties in learning pharmacology is memorizing the names of the thousands of drugs. Adding to this difficulty is that drugs have multiple names. The three basic types of names are chemical, generic, and trade.

The first important description is a drug's chemical name. All drugs are named using strict nomenclature established by the International Union of Pure and Applied Chemistry (IUPAC). A drug has only one chemical name. Chemical names often convey a clear and concise meaning about the nature of a drug.

One drawback is that chemical names are almost always complicated and difficult to remember or pronounce. In only a few cases will health practitioners need to know chemical names. However, chemical names are often helpful because they provide information about a substance's physical and chemical properties, and they allow scientists and practitioners to predict drug bioavailability and action. Bioavailability refers to the ways that drugs become available to body tissues. This is discussed in more detail in Chapter 4 .

Sometimes drugs are classified by chemical group. Examples are antibiotics such as flouroquinolones and cephalosporins. Other examples include phenothiazines (antipsychotics), thiazides (diuretics), and benzodiazepines (sedative-hypnotics). Knowledge of terms such as these becomes invaluable as a student begins to learn and understand major drug groups.

Another important description is a drug's generic name. The generic name is given by the United States Adopted Name Council. Generic names are usually preferred and less complicated than any of the other naming methods. Many organizations, including the FDA, the U.S. *Pharmacopoeia,* and the World Health Organization, routinely describe a medication by its generic name. There is only one generic name for each drug and students generally must memorize it.

A drug's trade name or proprietary name is assigned by the company marketing the drug and identifies a medication by its slogan name. This is the same as a product name or brand name. The term *proprietary* suggests ownership. In the U.S., a drug developer is given exclusive rights to name and market a drug for 17 years after submission of a new drug application to the FDA. Because it takes several years for a drug to be approved, the amount of time spent in approval is

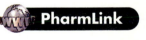

PharmLink

IUPAC

bio = biological
availability = free to
activate cellular targets

TABLE 2.4	Some Examples of Brand Name Products Containing Popular Generic Substances

GENERIC SUBSTANCE

Diphenhydramine	Ibuprofen	Aspirin

BRAND NAMES

Diphenhydramine	Ibuprofen	Aspirin
Allerdryl, Benadryl, Benahist, Bendylate, Caladryl, Compoz, Diahist, Diphenadril, Eldadryl, Fenylhist, Fynex, Hydramine, Hydril, Insomnal, Noradryl, Nordryl, Nytol, Tusstat, Wehydryl	Advil, Amersol, Apsifen, Brufen, Haltran, Medipren, Midol 200, Motrin, Neuvil, Novoprofen, Nuprin, Pamprin IB, Ruten, Trendar	Acetylsalicylic Acid, Anacin, Acuprin, Aspergum, Bayer, Bufferin, Ecotrin, Empirin, Excedrin, Maprin, Norgesic, Salatin, Salocol, Salsprin, Supac, Talwin, Triaphen-10, Vanquish, Verin, Zorprin

usually subtracted from the 17 years. For example, if it takes seven years for a drug to be approved, competing companies will not be allowed to market a generic equivalent drug for another 10 years. The rationale is that the developing company must be allowed sufficient time to recoup the millions of dollars in research and development from designing the new drug. After 17 years, competing companies may sell a generic equivalent drug, sometimes using a different name, which the FDA must approve.

Trade names are a challenge because there may be literally dozens of product names containing similar ingredients. Also, many products contain more than one active ingredient. Drugs with more than one active generic ingredient are called combination drugs. This poses a problem in trying to match one generic name with one product name. As an example, refer to Table 2.4 and consider the drug diphenhydramine (generic name), also called Benadryl (one of many trade names). Diphenhydramine is an antihistamine (pharmacological class). Low doses of diphenhydramine may be purchased OTC. Higher doses require a prescription. If you are looking for diphenhydramine, you may find it listed under many trade names such as Allerdryl and Compoz, provided alone or in combination with other active ingredients. Ibuprofen and aspirin are also examples of drugs with many different trade names. The rule of thumb is that the active ingredients in a medication are described by their generic name. When referring to a drug, the generic name is usually written in lower case while the trade name is capitalized.

Concept review 2.2

- What are the major differences between a chemical, generic, and trade name? Which name is most often used to describe the active ingredients within a drug product?

2.3 Generic drugs are less expensive than brand name drugs, but they may differ in their bioavailability.

Generally, generic drugs are less expensive than brand name drugs. In some states, pharmacists may routinely substitute a generic drug when the prescription calls for a brand name. In other states, the pharmacist must dispense drugs directly as written by a physician or else obtain approval before providing a generic substitute.

Those who market brand name drugs often lobby aggressively against laws that might restrict the routine use of certain brand name drugs. The lobbyists claim that allowing clients to switch between a brand name drug and its generic equivalent may be very risky. Consumers, on the other hand, argue that generic substitutions should always be permitted because of the higher prices brand name products impose on clients.

Another argument concerns differences in bioavailability between some brand name products and their generic equivalents. Drug formulations are not always identical. Some

TABLE 2.5	Negative Formulary List in Florida*
GENERIC NAME	**BRAND NAME EQUIVALENT**
digoxin	Lanoxin
digitoxin	Crystodigin
warfarin	Coumadin
conjugated estrogen	Premarin
quinidine gluconate	Quinaglute
dicumarol	Dicumarol
phenytoin	Dilantin
chlorpromazine	Thorazine
theophylline	TheoDur
levothyroxine sodium	Synthroid
pancrelipase	Pancrease

This list is current through April 2001.

brand name drugs have different inert ingredients, which may alter how quickly and the extent to which these drugs reach their target tissues. In addition, some generic medications may be prepared differently from brand name products. Many have active ingredients that are more tightly compressed than some brand name medications. These characteristics may also affect bioavailability.

In order to address this issue, some states have compiled a negative formularly list. In Florida, for example, drugs found on a negative drug formulary list must be dispensed exactly as written without allowing generic substitution. This list is shown in Table 2.5.

2.4 Drugs with a potential for abuse are categorized into schedules.

Some drugs are frequently abused or have a high potential for addiction. **Addiction** is a scientific term referring to the overwhelming feeling that drives someone to use a drug repeatedly. *Dependency* is a related term, often defined as a "physiological or psychological need for a substance." *Physical dependence* refers to an altered physical condition caused by the nervous system adapting to repeated drug use. In this case, when the drug is no longer available, the individual expresses physical signs of discomfort known as **withdrawal**. In contrast, when an individual is *psychologically dependent,* little or no sign of physical discomfort is observed when the drug is no longer available; however, the individual feels a need, a strong, compelling need to continue drug use. These concepts are discussed in more detail in Chapter 6 ⬤⬤ .

Drugs that cause dependency are restricted for use in situations of medical necessity, if at all. According to law, drugs that have a significant potential for abuse are placed into five categories called *schedules*. These **scheduled drugs** are classified according to their potential for abuse. Schedule I drugs have the highest potential for abuse, and Schedule V drugs have the lowest potential for abuse. Of the five schedules, Schedule I drugs have little to no therapeutic value or are intended for research purposes only. Drugs in the other four schedules may be dispensed only in cases where therapeutic value has been determined. Schedule V is the only category where some examples may be dispensed without a prescription. Table 2.6 shows the five drug schedules with examples. Not all drugs with an abuse potential are regulated or placed into schedules. Tobacco, alcohol, and caffeine are significant examples.

In the United States, **controlled substances** are drugs whose use is restricted by the Controlled Substances Act of 1970 and later revisions. The Control Substances Act is also called the Comprehensive Drug Abuse Prevention and Control Act. As mentioned in Chapter 1, the FDA Web site contains an excellent history of legislation leading to this act ⬤⬤ .

TABLE 2.6	Drug Schedules and Examples			
DRUG SCHEDULE	ABUSE POTENTIAL	DEPENDENCY POTENTIAL		EXAMPLES** (THERAPEUTIC USE)
		PHYSICAL	PSYCHOLOGICAL	
Schedule I	highest	high	high	heroin, LSD, marijuana, and methaqualone (limited or no therapeutic use)
Schedule II	high	high	high	morphine, PCP, cocaine, methadone, and methamphetamine (used therapeutically with prescription; some drugs no longer used)
Schedule III	moderate	moderate	high	anabolic steroids, codeine and hydrocodone with aspirin or Tylenol, and some barbiturates (used therapeutically with prescription)
Schedule IV	lower	lower	lower	Darvon, Talwin, Equanil, Valium, and Xanax (used therapeutically with prescription)
Schedule V	lowest	lowest	lowest	over-the-counter cough medicines with codeine (used therapeutically without prescription)

*These were obtained from the DEA Web site. For a more detailed list, further explanation of schedules, and information about the Controlled Substances Act, see our companion Web site.

2.5 Drugs in Canada are also controlled for the protection of consumers.

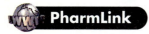

CANADIAN LAW AND DRUG CLASSIFICATION

In Canada, **controlled substances** are those drugs subject to guidelines outlined in Part III, Schedule G of the Canadian Food and Drugs Act. According to these guidelines, a practitioner or hospital may only provide these drugs to clients suffering from specific diseases or illnesses. Regulated drugs include amphetamines, barbiturates, methaqualone, and anabolic steroids. Controlled drugs must be labeled clearly with the letter "C" on the outside of the medication container.

Restricted drugs not intended for human use are covered in Part IV, Schedule H of the Canadian Food and Drugs Act. These are drugs used in the course of a chemical or analytical procedure for medical, laboratory, industrial, educational, or research purposes. They include hallucinogens such as LSD (lysergic acid diethylamide), MDMA (3,4-methylenedioxymethamphetamine; street name Ecstasy), and DOM (2,4-dimethoxy-5-methylamphetamine; street name STP).

Schedule F drugs are those drugs requiring a prescription for their sale. Examples are methylphenidate (Ritalin), diazepam (Valium), and chlordiazepoxide (Librium). Drugs such as morphine, heroin, cocaine, and cannabis are covered under the Narcotic Control Act and amended schedules. According to Canadian law, narcotic drugs must be labeled clearly with the letter "N" on the outside of the medication container. (In the context of law enforcement, the term *narcotic* refers to a larger group of drugs than in a health setting. This is discussed in Chapter 5 .

Concept review 2.3

■ Are controlled drugs described the same way in Canada as in the United States? What about restricted drugs?

2.6 All prescription drugs are classified according to safety in pregnancy categories in order to protect the unborn.

Often a major concern that pregnant women have is whether or not a drug will harm their developing baby. Pregnant clients should never take any prescribed, illegal, or OTC drug or any herbal or dietary supplement without the advice of their health care practitioner. Any substance that will harm a developing fetus or embryo is referred to as a teratogen.

In order to protect the unborn from the teratogenic effects of prescription drugs, the FDA has implemented a category system for classifying drugs based upon how safe they are for pregnant women. According to this system, drugs are placed into one of five pregnancy categories, labeled as A, B, C, D, and X. These labels appear within package inserts and identify levels of risk to the fetus. The levels are based on degrees to which a drug has been proven to cause birth defects in laboratory animals or in human beings. These categories are summarized in Table 2.7.

terato = *severe deformity*
gen = *something that produces*

TABLE 2.7	Categories of Safety in Pregnancy	
SAFETY CATEGORY	**EXPLANATION**	**EXAMPLES**
A Lowest Risk	Studies HAVE NOT shown a risk to women or to the fetus.	levothyroxine (Synthroid) thyroglobulin (Proloid) potassium chloride (K-Lor) potassium gluconate (Kaon Tablets) ferrous fumarate (Ferranol)
B	ANIMAL studies HAVE NOT shown a risk to the fetus or, if they have, studies in women have not confirmed this risk.	amoxicillin (Amoxil) insulin (Humulin R) fluoxetine (Prozac) loperamide (Imodium) penicillin V (Pen-Vee-K) rantidine (Zantac)
C	ANIMAL studies HAVE shown a risk to the fetus, but controlled studies have not been performed in women.	acyclovir (Zovirax) mineral oil (Fleet Mineral Oil) senna (Senokot) furosemide (Lasix) iron dextran (K-FeRON)
D	Use of this drug category MAY cause harm to the fetus, but it may provide benefit to the mother in a life-threatening situation or if a safer therapy is not available.	tetracycline (Achromycin) amitriptyline (Elavil) cortisone acetate (Cortistan) hydrochlorothiazide (HydroDiuril) warfarin (Coumadin)
X Highest Risk	Studies HAVE shown a significant risk to women and to the fetus.	iodinated glycerol (Organidin) castor oil (Purge) estrogen with progesterone (Ortho-Novum) dienestrol (DV) norethindrone (Norlutin) oxymetholone (Anadrol)

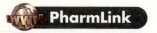

WOMEN'S HEALTH ISSUES

Consumers sometimes question whether or not the testing of laboratory animals is an effective way to predict harm to a developing human fetus or embryo. Results from animal testing are not always transferable to the human body. In fact, results from animal experimentation often vary from species to species. For this reason, consumers should always be cautious, even when there is reasonable assurance that a drug is extremely safe.

CHAPTER REVIEW

Core Concepts Summary

2.1 Drugs may be organized by their therapeutic and pharmacological classification.

Two common ways to classify drugs are by therapeutic classification and pharmacological classification. Therapeutic classes are based on a drug's clinical usefulness. Pharmacological classes are based on a drug's mechanism of action. Prototype drugs are used to compare drugs within the same classification.

2.2 Drugs have more than one name.

Drugs may be described by a chemical, generic, or trade name. There are advantages and disadvantages to each type of naming method.

2.3 Generic drugs are less expensive than brand name drugs, but they may differ in their bioavailability.

In most states, generic drugs may be substituted for brand name products if the prescribing practitioner does not object. When generic drugs are substituted, differences in bioavailability may affect the safety and effectiveness of drug therapy.

2.4 Drugs with a potential for abuse are categorized into schedules.

Drugs that have a high potential for abuse or dependency are placed into one of five schedules (Schedule I through Schedule V). Schedule I is the most restrictive category. Schedule V is the least restrictive category. The U.S. Drug Enforcement Agency (DEA) handles drug misuse.

2.5 Drugs in Canada are also controlled for the protection of consumers.

In Canada, drug use is controlled by schedules outlined in the Canadian Food and Drugs Act. Schedule G drugs are referred to as controlled drugs. Schedule H drugs are referred to as restricted drugs. Schedule F drugs require a prescription in order to be sold.

2.6 All prescription drugs are classified according to safety in pregnancy categories in order to protect the unborn.

All U.S. drugs are placed into one of five pregnancy categories, labeled as A, B, C, D, and X. Category A is the safest category. Category X is the most harmful.

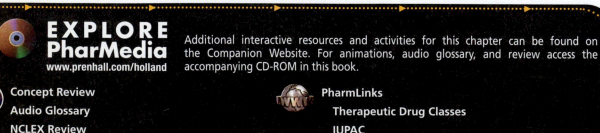

EXPLORE PharMedia
www.prenhall.com/holland

Additional interactive resources and activities for this chapter can be found on the Companion Website. For animations, audio glossary, and review access the accompanying CD-ROM in this book.

Concept Review
Audio Glossary
NCLEX Review

PharmLinks
Therapeutic Drug Classes
IUPAC
Canadian Law and Drug Classification
Women's Health Issues

3 Methods of Drug Delivery

CORE CONCEPTS

3.1 Drugs may be delivered by the enteral, parenteral, or topical routes.

3.2 The process of drug delivery involves three phases.

3.3 Physical properties of drugs influence how quickly they reach their target cells.

3.4 Drugs may be taken orally, sublingually, or rectally.

3.5 Drugs may be administered directly by injection into blood vessels.

3.6 Drugs may be injected into the skin.

3.7 Drugs may be injected directly into body cavities or joints.

3.8 Drugs may be applied directly to the surface of the skin.

3.9 Drugs may be applied to mucous membranes.

3.10 Drugs may be applied to the ears and the eyes.

OBJECTIVES

After reading this chapter, the student should be able to:

1. Compare and contrast the major routes of drug administration.

2. Discuss the three phases of drug delivery.

3. Name the four parts of the pharmacokinetic phase of drug delivery.

4. Identify the different physical compositions of drugs.

5. Explain why properties of viscosity and solubility are important in drug delivery.

6. Explain the difference between a drug mixture and a drug suspension.

7. Describe the importance of oral, sublingual, and rectal methods of drug delivery.

8. Identify different methods of parenteral drug delivery.

9. Discuss advantages and disadvantages of administering drugs directly into the bloodstream.

10. Describe the importance of topical drug delivery and give examples.

11. Explain why topical drug effects may be observed locally or systemically.

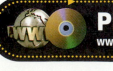

PharMedia
www.prenhall.com/holland

Additional interactive resources and activities for this chapter can be found on the Companion Website. For animations, audio glossary, and review access the accompanying CD-ROM in this book.

dissolution (di-so-LOO-shun): the dissolving process of solid drug preparations; the longer it takes for drugs to dissolve, the more delayed their onset of action / *page 28*

enteral (EN-tur-ul): the major route by which drugs enter the body through the digestive tract / *page 25*

epidural (EH-pee-DUR-ul): method of parenteral drug delivery where drugs are injected into the space overlying the dura mater / *page 33*

intra-arterial (IN-trah-ar-TEAR-ee-ul): method of parenteral drug delivery where drugs are injected into the arterial circulation / *page 31*

intradermal (IN-trah-DERM-ul): method of parenteral drug delivery where drugs are injected into the dermis of the skin; also called an *intracutaneous injection* / *page 31*

intramuscular (IN-trah-MUSK-lar): method of parenteral drug delivery where drugs are injected into layers of muscle beneath the skin / *page 31*

intraperitoneal (IN-trah-per-it-oh-NEE-ul): method of parenteral drug delivery where drugs are injected into the abdominal cavity / *page 33*

intrathecal (IN-trah-THEE-kul): method of parenteral drug delivery where drugs are injected into the spinal subarachnoid space / *page 32*

intravenous (IN-trah-VEE-nus): method of parenteral drug delivery where drugs are injected into the venous circulation / *page 29*

oral (OR-ul): method of enteral drug delivery in which drugs are swallowed, chewed, or allowed to slowly dissolve in the mouth / *page 28*

parenteral (pah-REN-tur-ul): the major route by which drugs enter the body by a way other than the digestive tract, usually by injection / *page 25*

rectal (REK-tul): method of enteral drug delivery where drugs are administered by way of the rectum / *page 28*

solubility (sol-yew-BIL-uh-tee): the ability to dissolve or mix / *page 28*

subcutaneous (sub-kew-TAY-nee-us): method of parenteral drug delivery where drugs are injected into the hypodermis of the skin / *page 31*

sublingual (sub-LIN-gwal): method of enteral drug delivery where drugs are placed under the tongue / *page 28*

topical (TOP-ik-ul): the route by which drugs are placed directly onto the skin and mucous membranes / *page 25*

transdermal (trans-DER-mul): method of drug delivery, usually by a patch, where drugs are absorbed across the layers of the skin for the purpose of entering the bloodstream / *page 35*

transmucosal (trans-mew-KOH-sul): method of topical drug delivery where drugs are applied directly to mucosal membranes, including the nasal and respiratory pathways and reproductive openings / *page 35*

viscosity (vis-KOS-uh-tee): the thickness of a liquid / *page 27*

There are many ways that drugs may be delivered to body tissues. Drugs may be swallowed, inhaled, injected, inserted, or rubbed onto the body's surface. The method of drug delivery depends upon the nature of the drug itself and how it is to be used. The different routes affect important aspects of pharmacology including how quickly the drug acts and how long its effects will last.

3.1 Drugs may be delivered by the enteral, parenteral, or topical routes.

CORE CONCEPTS

In general, all categories of drug delivery are associated with one of three major routes. The first major route is the digestive tract, or the **enteral** route. Drugs gaining access by this route enter the body either by the mouth, under the tongue, or into the rectum.

enteral = the digestive tract

The second major route is the **parenteral** method. By this method, drugs enter the body by a way *other than* the digestive tract, usually by injection directly into the cardiovascular circulation, the skin, or body cavities. If injected into the general circulation, drugs may be administered into veins or arteries. If injected through the skin, drugs may be administered into the dermis, beneath the dermis, or into muscles. If injected into a body cavity, drugs may be administered into spaces surrounding the spinal cord, abdominal organs, or into the joints.

par = beside
enteral = the digestive tract

The third major route of drug delivery is the **topical** route. Here drugs are placed directly onto the skin or associated membranes, such as the nasal and respiratory passages, the ears, the eyes, or the vagina. Table 3.1 summarizes some of the most widely utilized routes of drug administration.

top = placement
ical = related to

Concept review 3.1

■ It will be very important to remember the meanings of *enteral*, *parenteral*, and *topical*, as they will be used frequently. Use the root words to help you remember. What are the root words for *enteral*, *parenteral*, and *topical*?

TABLE 3.1	Examples of Drug Administration Routes
ROUTE	**DESCRIPTION**
Enteral	**by the digestive tract**
oral (PO)	by mouth
buccal	across membranes of the mouth (cheeks)
sublingual (SL)	under the tongue
rectal (PR)	by suppositories or enema
Parenteral	**by injection into the cardiovascular circulation**
intravenous (IV)	into the venous circulation
intra-arterial (IA)	into the arterial circulation (regional circulation)
intracoronary (IC)	into the coronary circulation
intradermal (ID)	into the dermis of the skin; intracutaneous
subcutaneous (SC)	under the skin; into the hypodermis
intramuscular (IM)	into the muscles
intraosseus	into the bone
intrathecal (IT)	into the spinal subarachnoid space
epidural	into the space overlying the dura mater
intraperitoneal (IP)	into the abdominal cavity
intrasynovial	into the joint
Topical	**by application onto the skin or associated membranes**
transcutaneous	across the skin
transdermal	across the dermis
transmucosal	across mucous membranes
ophthalmic	onto membranes of the eyes
otic	onto membranes of the deeper ear
vaginal	onto membranes of the vagina
intrauterine	onto membranes of the uterus lining

3.2 The process of drug delivery involves three phases.

The process of delivering drugs to the body's tissues involves three separate phases. These phases, which can also be thought of as steps, include the drug administration phase, the pharmacokinetic phase, and the pharmacodynamic phase. They are summarized in Figure 3.1.

This first phase, called *drug administration,* is sometimes referred to as the *pharmaceutical phase* because it is the means by which drugs are introduced into the body. Choices of drug delivery methods vary depending on the form of the medication, the speed with which drug action is needed, and the desired location of drug activity in the body.

In the second phase, drugs must move throughout the body to various targets. This is referred to as the *pharmacokinetic phase.* This phase deals with the absorption, distribution, metabolism, and excretion of drugs in the body.

In the third phase, drugs must produce a change or an effect at a specific target. This is called the *pharmacodynamic phase.* This phase usually involves interaction of a drug with its specific target, called a *receptor.* Pharmacokinetic and pharmacodynamic concepts are thoroughly covered in Chapter 4 ⊂⊃ .

FIGURE 3.1

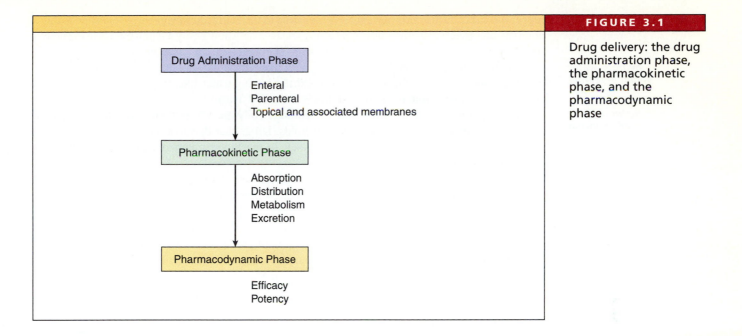

Drug delivery: the drug administration phase, the pharmacokinetic phase, and the pharmacodynamic phase

3.3 Physical properties of drugs influence how quickly they reach their target cells.

Before medications can produce a therapeutic effect, they must first travel to body tissues where they produce specific actions. The physical properties of a drug are important because they influence how the medication enters and moves throughout the body. The traditional delivery formulations are categorized as solid, liquid, or gas. These are summarized in Table 3.2.

Solid drugs are effective where there is a body opening. However, solids must dissolve before they can become active, and this slows down their onset of action. Tablets, capsules, suppositories, powders, and implantable devices are examples of vehicles for solid drugs. Tablets and capsules are the most common examples.

Liquid drugs move more quickly throughout the body, but in order to produce an effect they must first penetrate cellular membranes. Viscosity, the thickness of a liquid drug, is important because the

TABLE 3.2	Traditional Delivery Formulations	
SOLIDS	**LIQUIDS AND LIQUID-MIXTURES**	**GASES**
tablets	solutions	sprays
capsules	elixers	mists
suppositories	syrups	aerosols
powders	suspensions	inhalants
lozenges	emulsions	
pills	drops	
	creams	
	ointments	
	salves	
	gels	
	foams	

higher the viscosity, the more difficult it is for a drug to travel toward membranes. Solubility, a drug's ability to dissolve, is also important because it affects not only how easily a liquid travels to the body's membranes but also how easily it passes across membranes to reach its target tissue.

hydro = water
phobic = fearing

There is an expression that "like mixes with like," meaning that drugs having fat-like properties mix more easily in fats or lipids, while drugs having water-like properties mix more easily in water. Substances able to dissolve in lipids are called *hydrophobic.*

hydro = water
philic = loving

Hydrophobic drugs are better able to penetrate body membranes and reach their target tissues because membranes consist mostly of lipids. Drugs that dissolve more easily in water are called *hydrophilic.* Hydrophilic drugs mix well in the bloodstream but move less efficiently across body membranes.

Most *liquid solutions* are ideal for enteral and parenteral administration. *Liquid suspensions* are also widely used for topical application methods. Topical application methods include clear, paste-like, or frothy mixtures such as drops, creams, lotions, ointments, salves, gels, and foams.

The most favorable state for fast absorption is gaseous. Gaseous drugs are less compacted and are able to move more quickly toward an area of therapeutic interest and produce their actions in only a few seconds. Sprays, mists, aerosols, and inhalants are examples of gaseous delivery methods.

Concept review 3.2

■ What are the phases of drug delivery? Identify the different physical compositions of drugs. How quickly is each type of drug absorbed in the body?

3.4 Drugs may be taken orally, sublingually, or rectally.

Drugs swallowed, chewed, or allowed to slowly dissolve in the mouth are referred to as oral medications. Oral medications are found in many forms including tablets, capsules, powders, solutions, and suspensions. When a medication is prescribed for oral administration, it is ordered PO, which stands for the Latin term *per os,* meaning "by mouth." An advantage of taking a medication in liquid form is a relatively faster onset of action. Medications taken in tablet, capsule, or powder form take more time because they must dissolve before being absorbed.

The process of dissolving is referred to as dissolution. The longer the dissolution time, the more delayed the onset of action. To help with dissolution and to make the medication easier to swallow, water is usually taken in combination with a tablet or capsule. To reduce nausea and to remind clients to take their medication regularly, health practitioners often encourage clients to take some medications after a meal.

In some cases, drugs are placed under the tongue as shown in Figure 3.2. This is known as sublingual administration. Drugs administered sublingually are absorbed very quickly. They enter the bloodstream directly and avoid metabolic processes associated with the liver. The metabolism of drugs encountered by the liver after intestinal absorption is called the *first pass effect* and will be discussed in Chapter 4 ⬭ . One example of a popular sublingual medication is nitroglycerin. Nitroglycerin is absorbed very quickly across oral mucosal membranes and produces its effect within several minutes.

The rectal end of the digestive tract may also be used for drug delivery. Rectal administration is ideal for unconscious clients, those who are experiencing nausea or vomiting, or for infants who cannot swallow pills. Blood leaving the large intestine also does not travel directly to to the liver; therefore, enzymes in the liver are less active in breaking down drugs administered by this route. In addition, rectal drugs avoid all of the destructive enzymes normally encountered by the oral route, including enzymes of the mouth, stomach, and small intestine. Although the rectum has a considerably smaller surface area for drug absorption than the small intestine, it has a sufficient supply of blood vessels to produce a rapid onset of action. The rectal route often results in a faster onset of action than the oral route. Suppositories and enemas are examples of rectal administration.

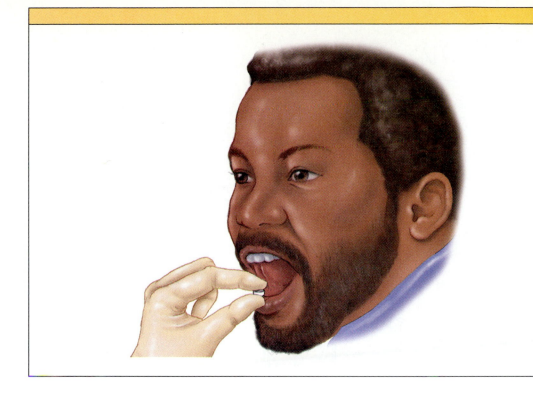

FIGURE 3.2

Sublingual drug administration *SOURCE: Pearson Education/PH College.*

3.5 Drugs may be administered directly by injection into blood vessels.

The most common method by which drugs are administered into the bloodstream is the **intravenous** (IV) route (see Figure 3.3). Drugs administered IV may be given as a *bolus* injection or by *infusion* IV. Bolus injections involve a single dose administered by means of a needle and syringe, usually over a short period of time. IV infusions involve a larger quantity of drug administered over a longer time by means of an IV line with a needle or catheter. An infusion pump with a flow regulator is usually used to regulate medication flow. An access needle and ports may provide quick delivery of IV drugs, as shown in Figure 3.3.

One advantage to IV administration is that pharmacological effects may be produced very quickly. Also, an exact concentration of drug may be administered, bypassing the destructive enzymes of the gastrointestinal tract and the metabolic processes of the liver. A major disadvantage

ON THE JOB

Nursing Assistants and Pharmacotherapy

Nursing assistants, although not directly involved with dispensing of medications, can assist the nurse or nurse practitioner in a healthcare setting. Oftentimes they can help to communicate to the nurse when the client is in need of pharmacotherapy. Medications may be ordered as p.r.n. (*pro re nata*), which means "whenever necessary." In this case, the nurse may deliver drugs to clients who are in discomfort. Nursing assistants may also report to the nurse any suspected adverse effects from the medication.

Nursing assistants can also help nurses give bedridden clients medications in an upright position (as with oral medications), or in face-down position (as with IM injections). In most cases, the nurse is extremely busy. Anything the nursing assistant can do in order ensure that the choice of drug delivery is the most effective is helpful. ■

FIGURE 3.3

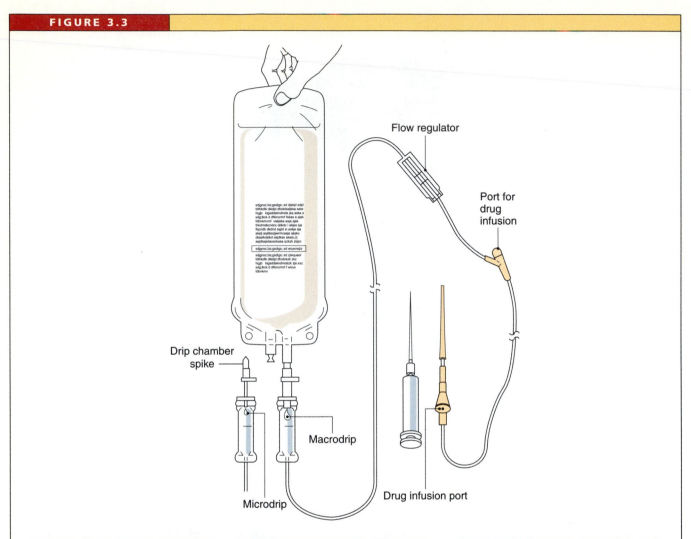

Flow regulator

Port for drug infusion

Drip chamber spike

Macrodrip

Microdrip

Drug infusion port

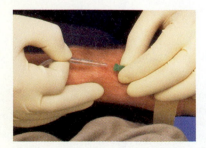

The constricting band is placed.

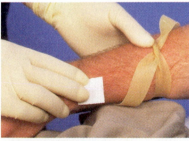

The venipuncture site is cleansed.

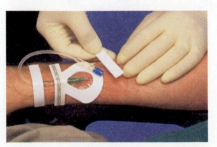

The intravenous cannula is inserted into the vein.

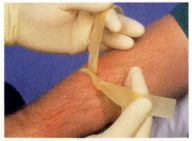

The IV tubing is connected.

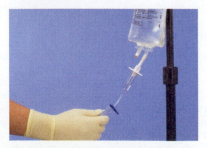

The IV is turned on and the flow is checked.

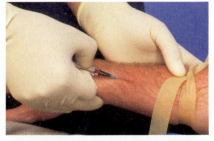

The site is secured.

Intravenous drug administration *SOURCE: Pearson Education/PH College.*

is that if excessive amounts of a drug are administered with the IV method, the process cannot easily be reversed. In addition, harmful effects may be produced if a clot forms within the blood vessel, or if air or microbes are introduced.

A less common method of parenteral administration that is performed only by experienced licensed practitioners is the intra-arterial (IA) route. Arteries are practical sites for injection when agents must reach body tissues directly. This route may be used to deliver high concentrations of anti-cancer drugs to tumors or to deliver opaque contrast media to diagnose disorders of the coronary arteries.

3.6 Drugs may be injected into the skin.

Injection into the skin delivers drugs directly to the bloodstream via blood vessels in the dermis. Thus, it is considered a parenteral route. Drugs may be injected intradermally, subcutaneously (SC or SUBQ), or intramuscularly (IM) (Figures 3.4, 3.5, and 3.6). The major difference between these methods is the depth of injection. The terms intradermal and subcutaneous refer to more superficial skin layers. The term intramuscular refers to layers of skeletal muscle beneath the skin. Refer to Figures 3.4, 3.5, and 3.6.

In order to fully understand each method, it is important to review some anatomy. There are three layers of the skin: the epidermis, the dermis, and the hypodermis. The middle layer of skin is the dermis. An intradermal injection is an injection made *directly into the dermis*. Because the dermis contains more blood vessels than the deeper subcutaneous layer, drugs are more easily ab-

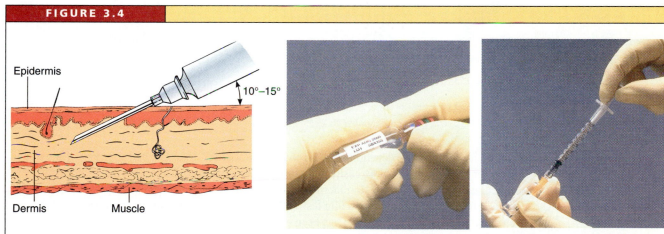

The medication is checked.

The medication is drawn.

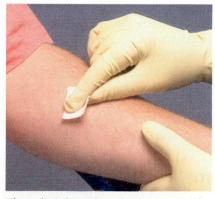

The administration site is prepared.

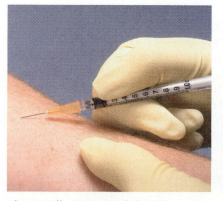

The needle is inserted, bevel up at 10°–15°.

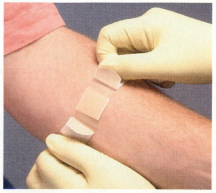

The needle is removed and the puncture site is covered with an adhesive bandage.

Intradermal drug administration   *SOURCE: Pearson Education/PH College.*

FIGURE 3.5

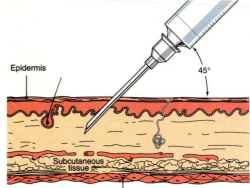

Epidermis

45°

Subcutaneous tissue

Muscle

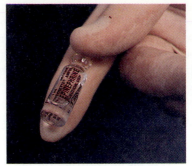

The medication is checked.

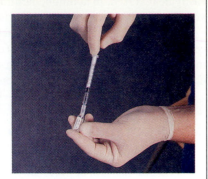

The medication is drawn.

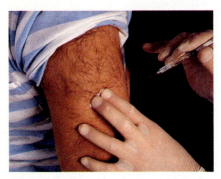

The administration site is prepared.

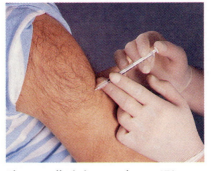

The needle is inserted at a 45° angle.

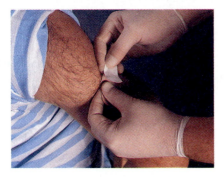

The needle is removed and the puncture site is covered with an adhesive bandage.

Subcutaneous drug administration   SOURCE: Pearson Education/PH College.

sorbed here. However, depending on the physical properties of an injected solution—for example, whether the drug mixes more easily in fat or water—drugs may also be absorbed within the deeper subcutaneous layer as well. Intradermal injections are sometimes given to test for allergic reactions. One example is the tuberculin test with purified protein derivative (ppd) that is used to determine whether or not the client has been exposed to tuberculosis.

Subcutaneous means "beneath the skin" and refers to the deepest of the skin layers. It is a region filled with fat cells called the *hypodermis*. Drugs may be administered directly to the hypodermis via a hypodermic needle or implant. A common example of an implant is the contraceptive Norplant.

Advantages to subcutaneous delivery are that practitioners may reliably predict the final drug concentration within the bloodstream, and drugs may be confined to a precise location. Drugs may also be administered to unconscious clients and children. The disadvantages to this approach include pain, swelling, tissue damage, and the potential for introducing microorganisms into the body. Only small amounts of medication can be administered SC without causing discomfort.

A faster onset of action occurs when drugs are administered intramuscularly (IM). This is because blood flow is greater in muscle tissue than in the more superficial skin layers. IM injections essentially have the same advantages and disadvantages as subcutaneous injections.

a = without
septic = infection

3.7 Drugs may be injected directly into body cavities or joints.

Drugs injected directly into body cavities may be administered intrathecally (IT), epidurally, intraperitoneally (IP), or into the joints. These routes of drug delivery are less common but nevertheless important in specific diseases or conditions.

An **intrathecal** injection is an injection made directly into the spinal subarachnoid space. This space is found in the dorsal spinal cavity beneath a protective sheath surrounding the spinal cord

FIGURE 3.6

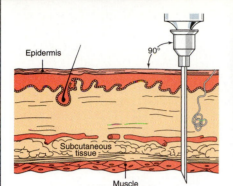

Epidermis

90°

Subcutaneous
tissue

Muscle

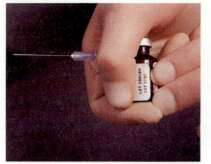

The medication is checked.

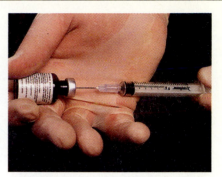

The medication is drawn.

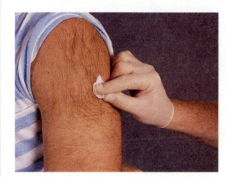

The administration site is prepared.

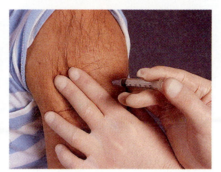

The needle is inserted at 90° angle.

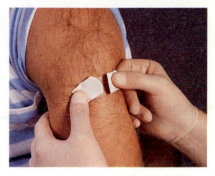

The needle is removed and the puncture site is covered with an adhesive bandage.

Intramuscular drug administration   *source: Pearson Education/PH College.*

called the *arachnoid mater.* It is an important site for the administration of spinal anesthetics or for drugs that might enter the cerebral spinal fluid.

An **epidural** injection is an injection made directly into a space overlying the dura mater. The dura mater is the most superficial of the three layers protecting the central nervous system, as shown in Figure 3.7 a-c.

An **intraperitoneal** (IP) injection is an injection made directly into the abdominal cavity. It represents a route by which drugs may enter the body when fast absorption is needed. This site is very important in veterinary medicine where many anesthetic drugs are administered to animals. It is rarely used in human clients.

Occasionally, drugs may be administered into joint spaces. Analgesics or anti-inflammatory drugs are examples of medications that might be administered directly by this method, for instance, in cases where there is severe athletic injury to a joint.

Concept review 3.3

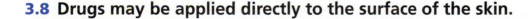

- Briefly outline the three routes of enteral drug delivery. Do the same for the methods of parenteral drug delivery. (For example, there are three major parenteral routes: into the bloodstream, into the skin, and into body cavities and joints.) Each major route has smaller, more specific routes that have been discussed. What are they?

3.8 Drugs may be applied directly to the surface of the skin.

Drugs placed directly on the surface of the skin are referred to as *topicals.* However, it is not necessary to strictly associate the term *topical* with the skin because topical drugs may also be applied to the nasal membranes, eyes, ears, and reproductive openings. One drawback to topical

FIGURE 3.7

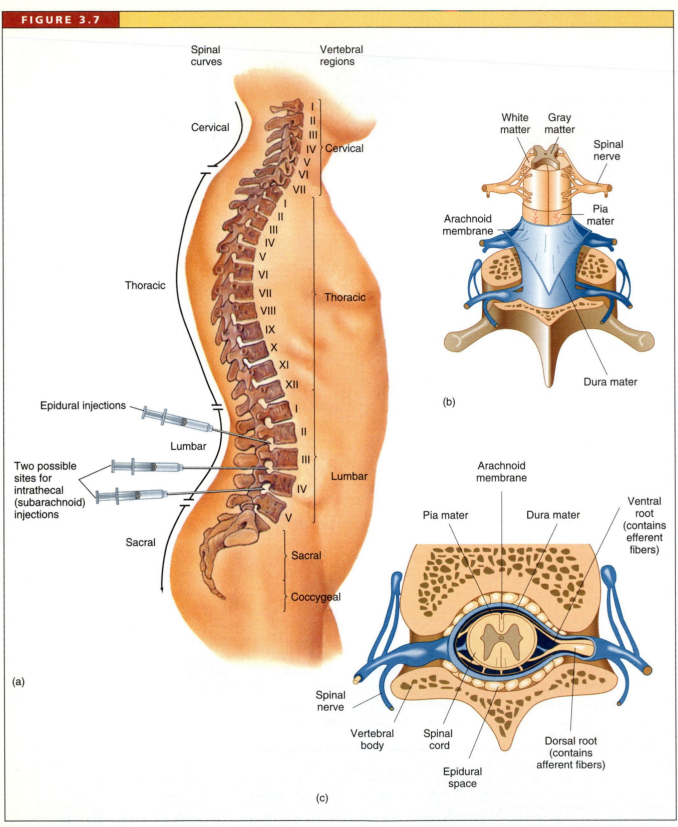

Spinal curves

Vertebral regions

Cervical

Thoracic

Epidural injections

Two possible sites for intrathecal (subarachnoid) injections

Lumbar

Sacral

I II III IV V VI VII ⟩ Cervical

I II III IV V VI VII VIII IX X XI XII ⟩ Thoracic

I II III IV V ⟩ Lumbar

Sacral

Coccygeal

(a)

White matter   Gray matter

Spinal nerve

Arachnoid membrane

Pia mater

Dura mater

(b)

Arachnoid membrane

Pia mater   Dura mater

Ventral root (contains efferent fibers)

Spinal nerve

Vertebral body   Spinal cord

Dorsal root (contains afferent fibers)

Epidural space

(c)

Intrathecal and epidural drug administration: (a) the vertebral column; (b) posterior view of the spinal cord showing the meningeal layers; (c) sectional view of the spinal cord   SOURCE: *Pearson Education/PH College.*

TABLE 3.3	Examples of Drugs Delivered by Transdermal Patches
THERAPEUTIC APPLICATION	**DRUG EXAMPLES**
smoking cessation	nicotine
chest pain and cardiovascular problems	nitroglycerin
nausea and vertigo	scopolamine
hormone replacement	estrogen
pain management	fentanyl

drug delivery is that surface areas may become irritated, dry, cracked, or infected with prolonged drug application.

Topical medications may produce effects *locally* or *systemically,* throughout the rest of the body. For a local effect, the key to drug action is to prevent medication from penetrating the skin barrier. Adverse effects may result if the drug is absorbed.

In some cases, it is desirable for the topically applied drug to be absorbed and reach the bloodstream. This is called a systemic effect. One popular method of delivering drugs safely and effectively into the bloodstream is by the transdermal patch. Applied to the skin, transdermal patches are useful when a drug must be delivered at a slow, steady rate. Many different kinds of drugs and drug mixtures are routinely administered with transdermal patches, and examples are given in Table 3.3.

3.9 Drugs may be applied to mucous membranes.

Openings connected with the skin are lined with mucous membranes that provide another surface for drug delivery. Mucous membranes line the surface of many organs including the digestive, respiratory, and reproductive tracts. Because digestive mucous membranes are associated with oral and rectal drug delivery, transmucosal drugs are generally agents delivered to the upper and lower respiratory tract and the reproductive openings. In this sense, inhalation may be considered a type of topical drug delivery because drugs must cross membranes lining the respiratory tract. Application of drugs to the vaginal mucosa may also be considered a form of topical medication delivery.

Transmucosal drugs, which may produce both local and systemic effects, are administered in many different forms including suppositories, sprays, mists, foams, aerosols, or volatile agents. Examples of transmucosal drugs are those used to treat asthma and vaginal infections.

3.10 Drugs may be applied to the ears and the eyes.

Drugs used for the ears and eyes are other examples of topical medications. The eyes represent body surface structures that must remain moist in order to function properly. Many topical medications for the eyes are designed to lubricate, prevent inflammation, or treat infections of the cornea. Other medications treat disorders such as glaucoma or are used to dilate pupils and relax eye structures during eye examinations. Ointments, salves, or drops are efficient delivery methods for these treatments.

The ears represent body surface structures that double as small conduction cavities. One common problem with the ear is the overproduction of earwax. Other common problems are the development of ear infections or accumulation of fluid. In order to effectively treat such problems, drugs must be able to penetrate the ear canal and middle ear. The most common form of drug used for ear disorders are drops because they can easily penetrate these sections of the ear.

Concept review 3.4

▪ Topical drugs delivery methods are subdivided on the basis of where drugs are placed onto the body surface. Names three general locations where topical drugs are applied.

CLIENT TEACHING

Clients need to know the following:

1. Some oral medications may be taken with food and water to reduce nausea, but you should always ask the practitioner or pharmacist which medication may be taken this way.

2. You should establish a routine for taking medicine, selecting a familiar time of the day, usually at an hourly interval. There are special organizers that you can use to properly sort medication times, days, and dosages.

3. It is important to follow the dosing times exactly. If a medication is missed, you should not try to "catch up" on the next scheduled dose. If you remember soon, it is appropriate to take the medicine. Otherwise, you should wait until the next scheduled dose. An exception would be if the next dose is not scheduled until the next day. For answers to specific questions, you should consult your practitioner.

4. You should store medications in a safe, dry place. If medications become old or outdated, they should be discarded.

5. You should take medication with the calibrated insert provided by the drug manufacturer. You should not rely on kitchen utensils to judge the exact recommended dose. ■

CHAPTER REVIEW

Core Concepts Summary

3.1 Drugs may be delivered by the enteral, parenteral, or topical routes.

The enteral route involves the mouth, the area under the tongue, and the rectum. Delivery by the parenteral route includes injection into the cardiovascular circulation, the skin, or body cavities. Topical delivery involves the skin's surface, the nasal and respiratory passages, ears, eyes, vagina, and the uterus.

3.2 The process of drug delivery involves three phases.

The three phases of drug delivery are drug administration (involving drug dispensing), the pharmacokinetic phase (involving drug movement throughout the body), and the pharmacodynamic phase (involving drug action).

3.3 Physical properties of drugs influence how quickly they reach their target cells.

Medications are dispensed in either solid, liquid, or gas form. Gaseous drugs reach their target tissues most quickly. Solid and liquid drugs are delivered at variable rates depending on how they are formulated.

3.4 Drugs may be taken orally, sublingually, or rectally.

Oral drugs are drugs taken by mouth, sublingual drugs are taken under the tongue, and rectal drugs are drugs taken by suppository. Oral drugs are metabolized by the first pass effect in the liver before entry into the bloodstream. Sublingual drugs and suppositories avoid the first pass effect.

3.5 Drugs may be administered directly by injection into blood vessels.

Drugs may be administered parenterally, which involves an injection directly into blood vessels, through the skin, or into various body cavities. Drugs administered directly into blood vessels may be given intravenously or intra-arterially. There are advantages and disadvantages to each type of delivery method.

3.6 Drugs may be injected into the skin.

Drugs administered through the skin may be given intradermally, subcutaneously, or intramuscularly. Absorption is variable with each type of drug delivery. Intramuscular injections generally have the fastest onset of action.

3.7 Drugs may be injected directly into body cavities or joints.

Drugs administered into body cavities may be given intrathecally, epidurally, intraperitoneally, or directly into joint spaces. Each type of delivery method is applied in very specific cases.

3.8 Drugs may be applied directly to the surface of the skin.

Medications applied to the surface of the body or to mucous membranes are referred to as topicals. Drugs applied to the skin may produce local or systemic effects. Transdermal patches allow safe and effective sustained release of certain drugs into the systemic circulation.

3.9 Drugs may be applied to mucous membranes.

Drugs applied to nasal and respiratory membranes are referred to as transmucosal drugs. Each type of respiratory therapy or procedure utilizes a slightly different method of drug delivery, distinguished mainly by the drug formulation. Drugs applied to reproductive openings may be administered as salves, creams, gels, soaps, foams, suppositories, or tablets.

3.10 Drugs may be applied to the ears and the eyes.

Ear and eye medications lubricate, treat infections, maintain proper physiological function, and support certain types of diagnostic tests.

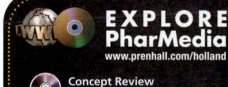

EXPLORE PharMedia
www.prenhall.com/holland

Concept Review
NCLEX Review
Audio Glossary

Additional interactive resources and activities for this chapter can be found on the Companion Website. For animations, audio glossary, and review access the accompanying CD-ROM in this book.

4 What Happens After a Drug Has Been Administered

CORE CONCEPTS

4.1 Pharmacokinetics focuses on how drugs are handled by the body.

4.2 Absorption is the first step in drug transport.

4.3 Distribution represents how drugs are transported throughout the body.

4.4 Metabolism is a process whereby drugs are made less or more active.

4.5 Excretion processes remove drugs from the body.

4.6 The rate of elimination and half-life characteristics influence drug responsiveness.

4.7 Pharmacodynamics focuses on how the body responds to drugs.

4.8 Drugs activate specific receptors in order to produce a response.

4.9 *Potency* and *efficacy* are terms used to describe the success of drug therapy.

OBJECTIVES

After reading this chapter, the student should be able to:

1. Identify the four major areas of pharmacokinetics.

2. Discuss the factors affecting drug absorption.

3. Describe how high molecular weight plasma proteins affect drug distribution.

4. Explain the significance of the blood-brain barrier, blood-placental barrier, and blood-testicular barrier to drug therapy.

5. Explain the importance of the first-pass effect.

6. Describe how metabolic enzymes differ in younger and in older clients, and explain the significance of this difference to drug therapy.

7. Explain how intermediate products of drug metabolism may produce more activity in the bloodstream.

8. Identify the major processes by which drugs can be eliminated from the body.

9. Explain how enterohepatic recirculation affects drug activity.

10. Explain how rate of elimination and plasma half-life ($t_{1/2}$) are related to the duration of drug action.

11. Discuss the importance of pharmacodynamics to drug therapy.

12. Explain the significance of the receptor theory to drug action.

13. Describe how antagonists affect drug action.

14. Compare and contrast the terms potency and efficacy.

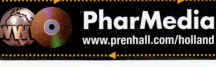

PharMedia
www.prenhall.com/holland

Additional interactive resources and activities for this chapter can be found on the Companion Website. For animations, audio glossary, and review access the accompanying CD-ROM in this book.

absorption (ab-SORP-shun): the process of moving a drug across body membranes / *page 40*

agonists (AG-on-ists): drugs that are capable of binding with receptors in order to induce a cellular response / *page 47*

antagonists (an-TAG-oh-nists): drugs that block the response of another drug / *page 47*

biotransformation (BEYE-oh-trans-for-MAY-shun): the metabolism or chemical conversion of drugs from one form to another that may result in increased or decreased activity / *page 42*

blood-brain barrier: an anatomical structure that prevents some substances from gaining access into the brain / *page 42*

blood-placental (pla-SEN-tal) **barrier**: an anatomical structure that prevents some substances from moving into the bloodstream of the fetus / *page 42*

blood-testicular (tes-TIK-u-lar) **barrier**: an anatomical structure that prevents some substances from entering male reproductive tissue / *page 42*

distribution (dis-tree-BU-shun): the process of transporting drugs through the body / *page 42*

efficacy (EFF-ik-ah-see): the effectiveness of a drug in producing a more intense response as its concentration is increased / *page 48*

enterohepatic (EN-ter-oh-HEE-pah-tik) **recirculation**: recycling of drugs and other substances by the circulation of bile through the intestine and liver / *page 43*

excretion (eks-KREE-shun): the process of removing substances from the body / *page 43*

first-pass effect: a mechanism whereby drugs are absorbed across the intestinal wall and enter into the hepatic portal circulation / *page 42*

half-life ($t_{1/2}$): the length of time required for a drug to decrease its concentration in the plasma by one-half of the original amount / *page 45*

metabolism (meh-TAHB-oh-liz-ehm): the sum total of all chemical reactions in the body / *page 42*

pharmacodynamics (FAR-mah-koh-deye-NAM-iks): the study of how the body responds to drugs and natural substances / *page 46*

pharmacokinetics (FAR-mah-koh-kee-NET-iks): the study of how drugs are handled by the body / *page 39*

potency (POH-ten-see): the power or strength of a drug at a specified concentration or dose / *page 47*

prodrugs: drugs that become more active after they are metabolized / *page 42*

rate of elimination (ee-lim-in-NAY-shun): the amount of drug removed from the body during a specified period of time / *page 44*

receptor (ree-SEP-tor): the structural component of a cell to which a drug binds in a dose-related manner in order to produce a response / *page 46*

receptor theory: a cellular mechanism by which most drugs produce their effects / *page 46*

Drugs do not affect all clients the same way. Whether a drug achieves or falls short of achieving a therapeutic response is an important concern to clients and healthcare professionals. Within a population, a dose of medication may produce a dramatic response in one client while having no effect in another.

Many situations may alter a drug's response. Clients sometimes take medications under conditions that interfere with drug activity. This interference is called a drug interaction. Well-known examples of food-drug interactions may occur when clients take their medication with food or beverages. Clients often take more than one medication at the same time. After drugs have been absorbed, the effectiveness of drug therapy may be altered by drug-drug interactions in the bloodstream.

In order to understand the impact that drug interactions have on drug safety and effectiveness, one must understand concepts from two important areas: pharmacokinetics and pharmacodynamics.

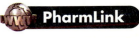

COUNCIL ON FAMILY HEALTH

4.1 Pharmacokinetics focuses on how drugs are handled by the body.

Pharmacokinetics is an essential subject in pharmacology. **Pharmacokinetics** describes how the body handles drugs. As the root words indicate, pharmacokinetics focuses on how drugs move within the body. Drug movement involves four processes: absorption, distribution, metabolism, and excretion, as shown in Figure 4.1. A thorough knowledge of pharmacokinetics enables the healthcare provider to understand the therapeutic effects of a drug, as well as to predict potential adverse effects of drug therapy.

pharmaco *= drug-related*
kinetics *= movement*

FIGURE 4.1

The four processes of
drug movement
(pharmacokinetics):
absorption, metabolism,
distribution, excretion

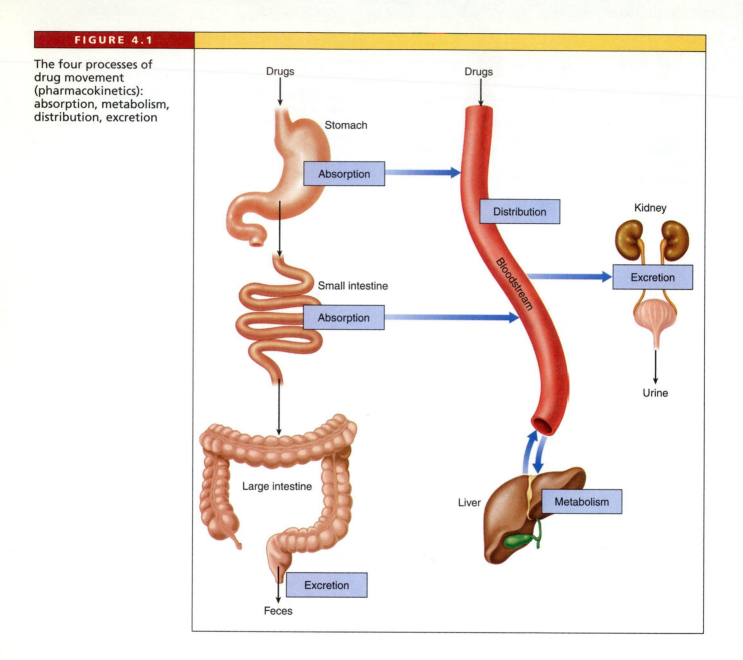

FIGURE 4.1

The four processes of drug movement (pharmacokinetics): absorption, metabolism, distribution, excretion

4.2 Absorption is the first step in drug transport.

Absorption is the first step in how the body handles a drug. Absorption is a process involving the movement of a substance from its site of administration across one or more body membranes. A drug may be absorbed locally and produce a biological effect at a site remote from where it was applied. Absorption may occur across the skin and associated mucous membranes, or drugs may move across membranes that line blood vessels. Ultimately most drugs move across many membranes to reach their target cells. Many basic science textbooks cover the ways that foods and drugs are absorbed. A comparison of general factors affecting drug absorption is shown in Table 4.1.

TABLE 4.1	Comparison of General Factors Affecting Absorption		

	ABSORPTION/DISTRIBUTION RATES		
DRUG CHARACTERISTICS	**FASTER**	**SLOWER**	
Size of drug particles			
Larger		✔	
Smaller	✔		
Physical state of drug particles			
Solid		✔	
Liquid	✔		
Gas (as with an inhalant)	✔ (faster than liquid)		
Properties of a drug			
Thickness of the drug mixture		✔	
Ability to mix with lipid	✔		
Ability to mix with water		✔	
Chemically charged (ionized)		✔	
Chemically neutral (non-ionized)	✔		
Dispensing temperature			
Warm	✔		
Room temperature	✔ (slower than warm temperatures)		
Cold		✔	
ABSENCE OR PRESENCE OF FOOD IN THE DIGESTIVE TRACT	**FASTER**	**SLOWER**	
Food absent	✔		
Food present		✔	
MEMBRANE CHARACTERISTICS	**FASTER**	**SLOWER**	
Thickness of membranes			
Thick (as across the skin)		✔	
Thin (as found in the lungs)	✔		
Surface area of membranes			
Large (as with the intestines)	✔		
Small (as within a minor body cavity)		✔	
How cellular membranes are connected			
Tightly connected (as with blood vessels in the brain)		✔	
Not tightly connected (as in the liver)	✔		
BLOODSTREAM FACTORS	**FASTER**	**SLOWER**	
Binding of a drug to plasma proteins			
Increased		✔	
Reduced	✔		
Body temperature			
Increased	✔		
Reduced		✔	

4.3 Distribution represents how drugs are transported throughout the body.

Distribution is the process by which drugs are transported after they have been absorbed or administered directly into the bloodstream. Between the site of drug administration and its target cells, there are many factors that affect drug movement. One important example is the binding that occurs between drugs and other substances already present in the bloodstream, such as plasma proteins. When a drug binds with a plasma protein such as albumin, the drug is held in the bloodstream and is unable to reach its target cells. Often a drug may be displaced from these proteins by a second drug, making the activity of the first drug more intense. The term *bioavailablity* is often used to describe how much of a drug will be available to produce a biological effect after administration.

Even if a drug is not bound by plasma proteins, it still may not be able to reach all body tissues. Three important organs contain anatomical barriers that prevent some drugs from gaining access. These are the brain, the placenta, and the testes. Even though these organs have a larger blood supply compared to most other organs in the body, usually only lipid-soluble substances may pass across these cellular barriers. These special barriers are called the **blood-brain barrier**, **blood-placental barrier**, and **blood-testicular barrier**.

Some drugs are able to cross the blood-brain barrier without difficulty. These include medications such as anti-anxiety drugs, sedatives (sleep-inducing), and psychoactive (or mind-altering) drugs. Other medications, such as many antibiotics and anti-cancer medications, are absorbed easily from the intestinal tract because of their water-soluble properties, but they do not easily cross into the brain.

The blood-placental barrier serves an important protective function because it regulates which substances pass from the mother's bloodstream to the fetus. However, many potentially damaging agents such as cocaine and alcohol and even some prescription or OTC medications are not prevented from crossing this barrier. This is an extremely important issue: all food items and therapeutic drugs should be evaluated to assess their adverse effects on prospective mothers and the unborn. Each prescription drug has been assigned a Pregnancy Category, as discussed in Chapter 2 ⬤▭⬤ .

The blood-testicular barrier exists between the blood supply and the male reproductive tissue. This often produces difficulty in treating disorders of the gonads, especially if the drugs are not lipid-soluble.

PharmLink

PREGNANCY

4.4 Metabolism is a process whereby drugs are made less or more active.

Metabolism is the next step in pharmacokinetics, involving the biochemical pathways and reactions that affect drugs, nutrients, vitamins, and minerals. Metabolism is a process that occurs in almost every cell, although the liver is the primary site. Similar reactions occur in other organs, such as the intestinal tract and the kidneys. Metabolism is often described as the sum total of all chemical reactions in the body. Individual chemical reactions are often referred to as **biotransformation** reactions.

Metabolism is important to drug therapy because metabolic reactions deactivate most drugs. There are instances, such as with **prodrugs**, where drugs are actually made more active after metabolism. Any drug or disease that affects metabolism has the potential to affect drug activity.

One important mechanism affecting metabolism and drug action is the **first–pass effect**. Substances absorbed across the intestinal wall enter blood vessels known as the *hepatic portal circulation,* which carries blood directly to the liver (see Figure 4.2). Drugs administered by the oral route are absorbed directly into the hepatic portal circulation. This is different than other areas in the body. Most veins lead directly back to the heart. Veins draining the upper digestive tract, however, take the nutrient-rich blood to the liver for metabolism first, before continuing on to the heart. Thus, drugs may be rendered inactive by metabolic reactions in the liver before they are distributed to the rest of the body and their target organs. In some cases, the first-pass effect can deactivate over 90% of an orally-administered drug before it can reach the general circulation.

bio = *biological*
transformation = *changing process*

pro = *before*
drug = *medication form*

ON THE JOB

Dental Hygienists and Anesthetics

In most cases in pharmacology, a drug must be absorbed in order to reach its target organ and produce a therapeutic effect. For the dental client receiving a local anesthetic, however, absorption into the general circulation is undesirable and may even be fatal.

Local anesthetics such as lidocaine used in dentistry are injected near the affected nerves, and the drug infiltrates through that area. A small amount of epinephrine is sometimes added to the injected mixture. The epinephrine causes vasoconstriction of the surrounding vessels, thus slowing the absorption of the lidocaine and prolonging its action on the local nerves. As long as the lidocaine remains local and enters the circulation very slowly, few adverse effects are observed. The dental hygienist, however, must observe the client for signs that lidocaine is entering the bloodstream too quickly. These signs may include initial stimulation of the central nervous system (excitement), followed by depression. Although rare, high levels may cause hypotension or cardiac arrest. ▪

Many clients differ with respect to how efficiently their metabolic enzymes function. Age, kidney and liver disease, genetics, and other factors may dramatically affect enzymatic activity. Some clients metabolize drugs very slowly; others metabolize drugs very quickly. Enzyme activity is generally reduced in very young and in elderly clients; therefore, pediatric and geriatric clients are usually more sensitive to medications than middle-aged clients. Drug doses to these age groups often are reduced to compensate for their physiological differences. Clients with liver disease usually receive much lower doses than normal because the liver is unable to deactivate the drug.

4.5 Excretion processes remove drugs from the body.

The last step of pharmacokinetics is excretion. Most substances that enter the body are removed by urination, exhalation, defecation, and/or sweating. Drugs are normally removed from the body by the kidneys, respiratory tract, bile, or glandular activity.

The main organ involved with excretion is the kidney. The major role of the kidneys is to remove all nonnatural and harmful agents in the bloodstream while maintaining a balance of the other natural substances. The majority of drugs are excreted by the kidneys. Damage to the kidneys can significantly prolong the duration of drug action and is a common cause of adverse reactions. Drugs that affect the kidney and the processes the kidney uses to remove substances from the body are presented in Chapter 27 ⬭ .

Drugs easily changed into a gaseous form are especially suited for excretion by the respiratory system. The rate of respiratory excretion is dependent on the many factors that affect gas exchange, including diffusion, gas solubility, and blood flow. The greater the blood flow into lung capillaries, the greater the excretion. In contrast to other methods of excretion, the lungs excrete most drugs in their original unmetabolized form.

Some drugs are excreted through the bile. However, most components of bile are circulated back to the liver by a process known as enterohepatic recirculation, as shown in Figure 4.3. Recirculating drugs are ultimately metabolized by the liver and excreted by the kidneys. The fraction of drugs that is not recirculated continues on its way to the feces. Elimination of drugs in this way may continue for several weeks after therapy has been discontinued and result in a prolonged duration of action.

Glands that produce body fluids such as saliva and sweat are less significant excretion mechanisms, with the exception of breast milk. Most agents secreted in the saliva or perspiration are substances eliminated naturally, such as urea or other waste products. Excretion into breast milk is more important because any drug capable of crossing these membranes may potentially affect the nursing infant. A nursing mother should always check with her physician before taking any type of prescription drug, OTC drug, or natural alternative therapy.

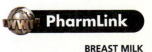

BREAST MILK

FIGURE 4.2

First-pass effect

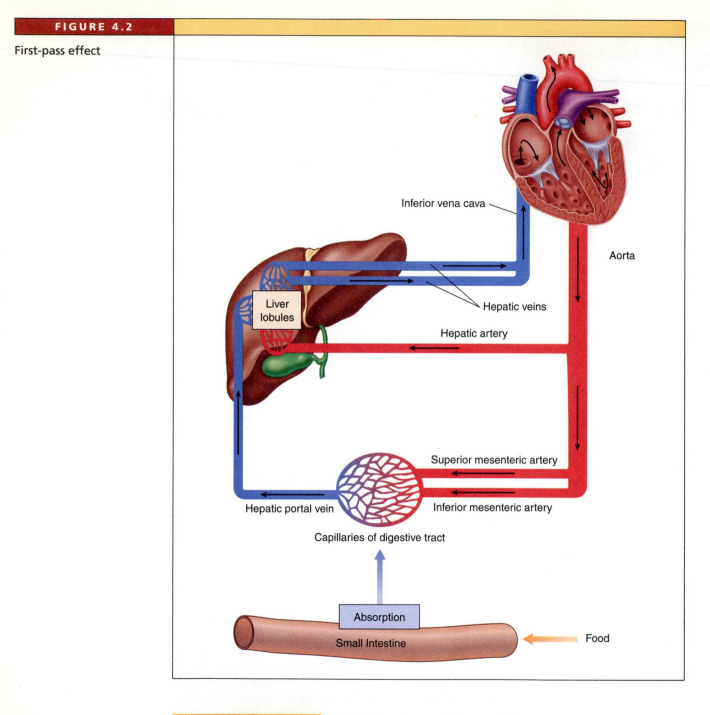

Inferior vena cava

Aorta

Hepatic veins

Liver lobules

Hepatic artery

Superior mesenteric artery

Hepatic portal vein

Inferior mesenteric artery

Capillaries of digestive tract

Absorption

Small Intestine

Food

Concept review 4.1

■ What does the term *pharmacokinetics* mean? Can you describe the four major parts of pharmacokinetics?

4.6 The rate of elimination and half-life characteristics influence drug responsiveness.

Elimination, which is another term for *excretion,* is often measured so that dosages of drugs can be determined more accurately. The term rate of elimination refers to the amount of drug removed per unit of time from the body by normal physiological processes. The rate of elimination is helpful in determining how long a particular drug will remain in the bloodstream and is thus an indicator of how long a drug will produce its effect.

FIGURE 4.3

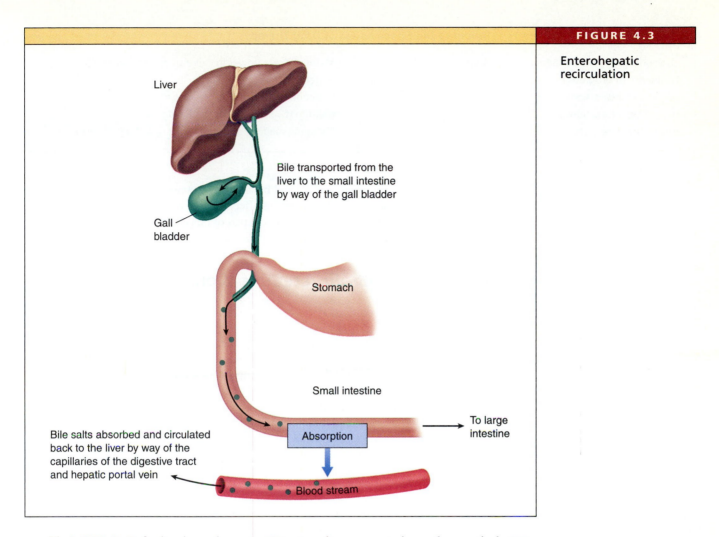

Liver

Bile transported from the
liver to the small intestine
by way of the gall bladder

Gall
bladder

Stomach

Small intestine

To large
intestine

Bile salts absorbed and circulated
back to the liver by way of the
capillaries of the digestive tract
and hepatic portal vein

Absorption

Blood stream

The **half-life (t$_{1/2}$)** of a drug is another measurement used to ensure maximum therapeutic dosages. Half-life is defined as the length of time required for a drug to decrease concentration in the plasma by one-half. It is another indicator of how long a drug will produce its effect in the body. The larger the half-life value, the longer it takes for a drug to be eliminated. For example, a drug with a half-life of 10 hours will take longer to be eliminated from the body than a drug with a half-life of five hours. Drugs with longer half-lives may be given less frequently, for example, once per day.

Whenever a client has a renal or hepatic disease, the plasma half-life of a drug will increase. This reflects its important relationship to two processes that have already been discussed: metabolism and excretion. Some drugs have a half-life of just a few minutes, while others have a half-life of several hours or days.

Concept review 4.2

▪ Why are rate of elimination and half-life (t$_{1/2}$) important to the healthcare practitioner?

4.7 Pharmacodynamics focuses on how the body responds to drugs.

As discussed earlier, many variables influence the effectiveness of drug therapy, such as rate of administration, frequency of drug dosing, and a changing medical condition. Some of these factors are summarized in Table 4.2.

Successful pharmacotherapy depends on the impact of these variables as well as how effectively the body responds to drugs at specific target locations. This leads to another important core area of pharmacology: the field of pharmacodynamics. The field of pharmacodynamics is complex,

TABLE 4.2	Factors That Influence the Effectiveness of Drug Therapy	
Concentration (dose) of administered drug		Metabolic rate (lower in children and the elderly)
Frequency of drug dosing		Genetics
Food-drug interactions		Excretion rate (rate of elimination)
Drug-drug interactions		Half-life ($t_{1/2}$) of administered drug
Absorption rate (refer to Feature 4.1)		Changing medical condition (liver or kidney disease)

pharmaco = *drug-related*

dynamics = *power*

requiring extensive knowledge of physiology and biochemistry. **Pharmacodynamics** deals with the mechanisms of drug action, or how the drug exerts its effects. As the root words suggest, drugs have a powerful influence on body processes. The remaining part of this chapter will be devoted to a few basic pharmacodynamic principles.

4.8 Drugs activate specific receptors in order to produce a response.

Successful pharmacotherapy is based on the principle that, in order to treat a disorder, a drug must interact with specific receptors in its target tissue. The **receptor theory** is a classic theory referring to the cellular mechanism by which most drugs cause change. A **receptor** is any structural component of a cell to which a drug binds in a dose-related manner. The receptor is often depicted as a three-dimensional shaped protein connected with the cell's plasma membrane as shown in Figure 4.4. The drug or natural body substance attaches to its receptor much like a lock and key. Other receptors are not associated with the plasma membrane and involve drug interaction with sites inside the cytoplasm or nucleus. Some drug actions are not linked to a receptor, but are connected directly with cell function such as changing the membrane excitability or stability of a nerve or muscle cell.

FIGURE 4.4	

Cellular receptors

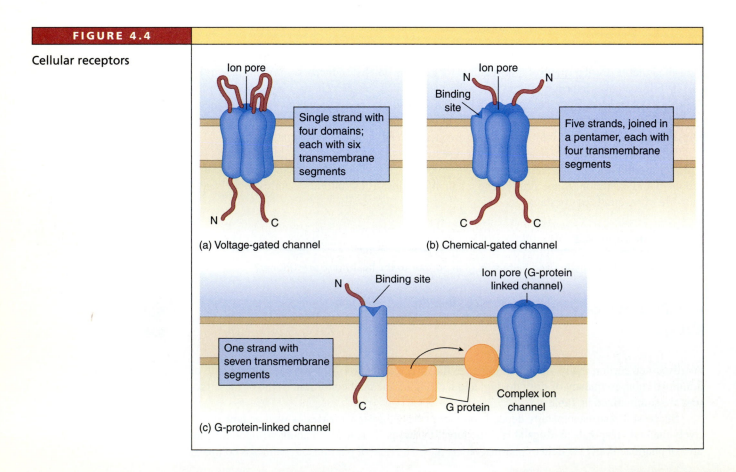

(a) Voltage-gated channel

Ion pore

Single strand with four domains; each with six transmembrane segments

N   C

(b) Chemical-gated channel

Ion pore

N   N

Binding site

Five strands, joined in a pentamer, each with four transmembrane segments

C   C

(c) G-protein-linked channel

N   Binding site

Ion pore (G-protein linked channel)

One strand with seven transmembrane segments

C   G protein   Complex ion channel

Two important terms, *agonist* and *antagonist,* are used to describe drug action at the receptor. Agonists are drugs capable of binding with receptors and inducing a cellular response; these are *facilitators* of cellular action. Whenever they are present in the bloodstream, agonists induce the cell to respond, resulting in a therapeutic action. Antagonists are drugs that inhibit or block the responses of agonists. Antagonists are sometimes called *blockers.*

ant = against
agonist = activator

4.9 *Potency* and *efficacy* are terms used to describe the success of drug therapy.

Potency refers to a drug's strength at a certain concentration or dose. As shown in Figure 4.5a, dose-response curves are used to compare potencies of different drugs. If a drug has a higher potency, it means that this medication, if taken in the same dose as another similarly acting drug, will produce a more intense effect. A higher potency also means that a much smaller dose of this medication will be required to produce the same effect as another drug, as shown by the shifting to the left of the dose-response curve.

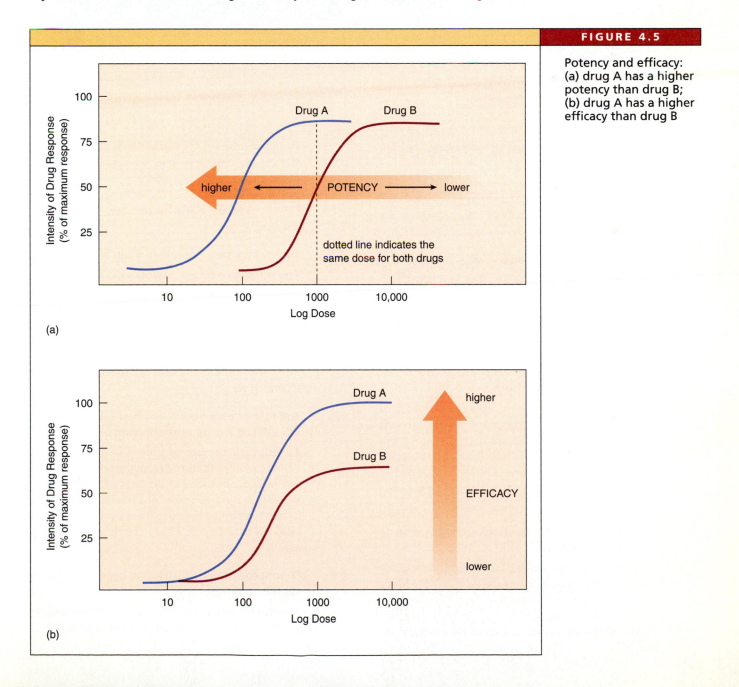

FIGURE 4.5

Potency and efficacy: (a) drug A has a higher potency than drug B; (b) drug A has a higher efficacy than drug B

Another core concept is efficacy. Efficacy refers to the ability of a drug to produce a more intense response as the concentration is increased. As an example, consider Figure 4.5b. If the doses of two similarly acting drugs are increased, they will both produce a more intense effect, but one drug will have a maximum intensity that is lower than the other drug. The drug reaching a lower maximum intensity compared to another drug is said to have a lower efficacy. In pharmacotherapeutics it is generally more important to have a drug with higher efficacy, than one with higher potency.

Concept review 4.3

- What does the term *pharmacodynamics* mean? Identify the importance of receptors, agonists, and antagonists in how they influence drug action. What is the difference between a drug's potency and its efficacy?

CHAPTER REVIEW

Core Concepts Summary

4.1   Pharmacokinetics focuses on how drugs are handled by the body.

Pharmacokinetics is an area of pharmacology dealing with how drugs move throughout the body. There are four components of drug transport: absorption, distribution, metabolism, and excretion.

4.2   Absorption is the first step in drug transport.

Absorption represents the first step in pharmacokinetics. It involves movement of a drug from its site of administration across body membranes. Drugs cross many membranes before reaching target organs. Drug absorption is affected by many factors.

4.3   Distribution represents how drugs are transported throughout the body.

Distribution begins after absorption and continues until drug action. Drugs bound to plasma proteins may be isolated in the plasma and prevented from reaching their target cells. The blood-brain barrier, blood-placental barrier, and blood-testicular barrier all represent areas in the body where drug distribution may be limited.

4.4   Metabolism is a process whereby drugs are made less or more active.

Metabolic processes take place in the liver and occur to a lesser extent in organs such as the kidney and cells of the gastrointestinal tract. The first-pass effect is an important phenomenon because many drugs absorbed across intestinal membranes are routed directly to the liver. Metabolic liver enzymes are usually less active in younger and in older clients; therefore, drug effects will most likely be enhanced in these age groups. Prodrugs are agents converted to an active form when metabolically changed.

4.5   Excretion processes remove drugs from the body.

The kidneys, lungs, sweat glands, mammary glands, and gall bladder are the major routes by which drugs are eliminated from the body. The main organ involved with excretion is the kidneys. The enterohepatic recirculation is a unique type of mechanism responsible for recirculating bile back into the bloodstream from the gastrointestinal tract.

4.6   The rate of elimination and half-life characteristics influence drug responsiveness.

The elimination rate of a drug is defined as the amount of drug removed from the body by normal physiological processes per unit of time. Plasma half-life is the amount of time it takes for the body to remove half of the drug from the general circulation. These factors affect the duration of drug action.

4.7   Pharmacodynamics focuses on how the body responds to drugs.

Pharmacodynamics is an area of pharmacology concerned with how drugs produce a response or change within the body. Successful drug therapy depends on the effectiveness of these changes.

4.8 Drugs activate specific receptors in order to produce a response.

Generally, the response of a drug begins when the agent encounters at the receptor of its target cell. The receptor theory states that most responses in the body are caused by interactions of drugs with specific receptors. Receptors may be located on the plasma cell membrane, or they be found in the cytoplasm or nucleus.

4.9 Potency and efficacy are terms used to describe the success of drug therapy.

Potency relates to the concentration or amount of drug required to produce a maximum response. Efficacy refers to the magnitude of maximal response comparable with another drug.

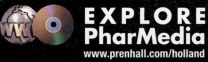

EXPLORE
PharMedia
www.prenhall.com/holland

Additional interactive resources and activities for this chapter can be found on the Companion Website. For animations, audio glossary, and review access the accompanying CD-ROM in this book.

Concept Review
NCLEX Review
Audio Glossary

 PharmLinks
Council on Family Health
Pregnancy
Breast milk

5 Substance Abuse

CORE CONCEPTS

5.1 A wide variety of different substances may be abused by individuals.

5.2 Addiction has both neurobiological and psychosocial components.

5.3 Physical and psychological dependence result in continued drug-seeking behavior.

5.4 Withdrawal results when an abused substance is no longer available.

5.5 Tolerance occurs when higher and higher doses of a drug are needed to achieve the same initial response.

5.6 Ethyl alcohol is one of the most commonly abused drugs.

5.7 Nicotine is a powerful and highly addictive cardiovascular and CNS stimulant.

5.8 Marijuana produces less physical dependence and tolerance than most other drugs of abuse.

5.9 Hallucinogens cause an altered state of thought and perception similar to that found in dreams.

5.10 CNS stimulants increase the activity of the central nervous system.

5.11 CNS depressants decrease the activity of the central nervous system.

OBJECTIVES

After reading this chapter, the student should be able to:

1. Discuss the underlying causes of addiction.

2. Compare and contrast psychological and physical dependence.

3. Compare and contrast classic and conditioned withdrawal.

4. Explain the significance of drug tolerance to pharmacology.

5. Explain the major characteristics of abuse, dependence, and tolerance resulting from the following drugs and drug classes.
   a. alcohol
   b. nicotine
   c. marijuana
   d. hallucinogens
   e. CNS stimulants
   f. CNS depressants
   g. narcotics/opioids

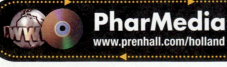

PharMedia
www.prenhall.com/holland

Additional interactive resources and activities for this chapter can be found on the Companion Website. For animations, audio glossary, and review access the accompanying CD-ROM in this book.

addiction (ah-DIK-shun): the continued use of a substance despite its negative health and social consequences / *page 52*

attention deficit disorder (ADD): difficulty focusing attention on a task for sufficient lengths of time / *page 60*

cirrhosis (sir-OH-sis): a chronic disease, often seen in alcoholics, in which the liver fails to perform its normal functions / *page 56*

classic withdrawal (KLAS-ik with-DRAW-ul): unpleasant symptoms experienced when a physically dependent client discontinues the use of an abused drug / *page 54*

conditioned withdrawal (kon-DISH-und with-DRAW-ul): a theory that states that environment and social contacts contribute to relapse after an addict is no longer abusing a substance / *page 55*

designer drugs (de-ZEYE-ner drugs): drugs that are produced in a laboratory and are intended to mimic the effects of other psychoactive controlled substances / *page 59*

opioid (OH-pee-oyd): substance obtained from the unripe seeds of the poppy plant / *page 62*

physical dependence (FIZ-ee-kul dee-PEN-dens): the condition of experiencing unpleasant withdrawal symptoms when a substance is discontinued / *page 54*

psychodelics (seye-koh-DEL-iks): substances that alter perception and reality / *page 57*

psychological dependence (seye-koh-LOJ-ee-kul dee-PEN-dens): an unpleasant, intense craving for a drug after it has been withdrawn / *page 54*

reticular formation (ree-TIK-you-lur): portion of the brain affecting awareness and wakefulness / *page 60*

substance abuse: the use, by self-administration, of a drug that does not conform to the medical or social norms within the client's given culture or society / *page 51*

tetrahydrocannabinol (THC)(TEH-trah-HEYE-droh-cah-NAB-in-ol): the active chemical in marijuana / *page 57*

tolerance (TOL-er-anse): the process of adapting to a drug over a period of time, and subsequently requiring higher doses to achieve the same effect / *page 55*

Substance abuse is the use of a drug, by self-administration, that does not conform to the medical or social norms within the client's given culture or society. Throughout history, individuals have consumed both natural substances and therapeutic drugs to increase performance, assist with relaxation, alter psychological state, or to simply "fit in with the crowd." Societal attitudes about substance abuse vary from acceptance and understanding to stigma associated with the problems of abuse. Substance abuse has a tremendous economic, social, and public health impact.

Fast Facts Substance Abuse in the United States

- Twenty-eight million Americans have used illicit drugs at least once.
- During the 2000–2001 school year, 25% of high school students used an illegal drug on a monthly or more frequent basis.
- An estimated 2.4 million Americans have used heroin during their lives.
- About one in five Americans has lived with an alcoholic while growing up. Children of alcoholic parents are four times more likely to become alcoholics than children of non-alcoholic parents.
- Alcohol is an important factor in 68% of manslaughters, 54% of murders, 48% of robberies, and 44% of burglaries.
- Among youth between the ages of 12–17, 7.2 million drank alcohol at least once in the past year. Girls are as likely as boys to drink alcohol.
- Barbiturate overdose is a factor in almost one-third of all drug-related deaths.
- In 1999, 22% of eighth graders and almost 50% of twelfth graders reported using marijuana. These are almost double the percentages reported in the early 1990s.
- In 1999, 9.8% of high school seniors reported using cocaine, up from 5.9% in 1994.
- In 1998, 1.7 million Americans were currently using cocaine on a monthly basis; about 437,000 used crack cocaine.
- Approximately 70% of the cocaine entering the United States comes from Columbia and passes through south Florida.
- In 1997, 21% of eighth graders and 16% of twelfth graders reported using volatile inhalants.
- In 1998, 28% of all Americans were cigarette smokers, including 18% of those between the ages of 12–18.
- In 1999, 44% of eighth graders and 65% of twelfth graders reported they had tried smoking cigarettes. Thirteen percent of the twelfth graders consumed one pack or more each day.

- In 2000, 11% of twelfth graders reported using ecstasy (MDMA).
- LSD is one of the most potent drugs known, with only 25–150 micrograms constituting a dose. In 1997, almost 14% of twelfth graders reported using LSD.

5.1 A wide variety of different substances may be abused by individuals.

Abused substances come from a wide variety of chemical classes and are taken by many different routes. Although the general public associates substance abuse with illegal drugs, this is not necessarily the case: alcohol and nicotine, both legal substances, are the two most commonly abused drugs. Marijuana is the most frequently abused illegal drug. Other illegal substances that are frequently abused include volatile inhalants such as aerosols and paint thinners, narcotics and hallucinogens such as lysergic acid diethylamide (LSD), phencyclidine hydrochloride (PCP), and psilocybin, a compound extracted from mushrooms.

Several drugs once used for therapeutic purposes are now considered illegal. Cocaine was once widely used as a local anesthetic, but today nearly all the cocaine acquired by users is obtained illegally. LSD is now illegal, although in the 1940s and 1950s, it was used in psychotherapy. Phencyclidine was popular back in the early 1960s as an anesthetic, but was withdrawn from the market in 1965 because of reports of hallucinations, delusions, and anxiety after recovery from anesthesia. Many amphetamines once used for bronchodilation were discontinued in the 1980s after psychotic episodes were reported in some clients. Commonly abused drugs are shown in Table 5.1, categorized by drug group.

5.2 Addiction has both neurobiological and psychosocial components.

addict = *given over*

Addiction is an overwhelming feeling that drives someone to repeat drug-taking behavior, despite serious health and social consequences. People view addiction differently. Some link it with emotional instability while others think of it as a genetic problem or mental illness. Most healthcare providers have come to recognize addiction as a neurobiological problem linked closely to the client's psychological state and social setting. Attempts to predict a client's addictive tendency using psychological profiles or genetic markers have largely been unsuccessful. Addiction is not only a problem for the client, but for society as well because of its negative influence on public health, safety, productivity, and financial resources.

In the case of prescription drugs, addiction may begin with the client's medical need for the treatment of an illness. This may occur when narcotic analgesics are prescribed for pain relief or when sedatives are prescribed for sleep disorders. These drugs may result in a favorable experience, such as pain relief or sleep, and clients will want to repeat these positive experiences. So the theory that addiction results from reward and positive reinforcement may be valid. Simply stated, some people take drugs because they like the state of mind the drug produces.

It is a common misunderstanding, even among some healthcare providers, that the therapeutic use of narcotics and sedatives creates large numbers of addicted clients. In fact, prescription drugs rarely cause addiction when used according to accepted medical protocols. The risk of addiction is a function of the drug dose and the length of therapy. Because of this, drugs having a potential for addiction are usually prescribed at the lowest effective dose and for the shortest time necessary to correct the medical problem. As discussed in Chapters 1 and 2, numerous laws have also been passed in an attempt to limit drug abuse and addiction ⚭.

TABLE 5.1	Classifications of Abused and Misused Substances		
	NATURAL SUBSTANCES	**DRUGS USED IN TRADITIONAL THERAPIES**	
LEGAL SUBSTANCES WITHOUT PRESCRIPTION		Presently	Discontinued
(some substances may be found in OTC or prescription products)			
CNS Depressants			
Alcohol (ethyl alcohol)	X	X	
Volatile inhalants (aerosols, paint thinners, glue)			
CNS Stimulants			
Tobacco (nicotine)	X		
Caffeine	X	X	
LEGAL SUBSTANCES WITH PRESCRIPTION			
CNS Depressants			
Barbiturates		X	
Benzodiazepines		X	
Opioids			
Opium (morphine)	X	X	
Synthetic opioids		X	
CNS Stimulants			
Amphetamines		X	
Dextroamphetamines		X	
Methamphetamines		X	
Methylphenidate (Ritalin)		X	
Hallucinogens			
Ketamine		X	
ILLEGAL SUBSTANCES			
Cannabis (Marijuana)	X		
CNS Depressants			
Opioids			
Heroin			X
CNS Stimulants			
Cocaine	X		
Some methamphetamines			
Hallucinogens			
Lysergic acid diethylamide (LSD)			X
Mushrooms (psilocybin)	X		
Peyote cactus (mescaline)	X		
Phencyclidine hydrochloride (PCP)			X
Methoxy-methylenedioxy-methamphetamine (MDMA)			
Dimethoxy-methyl-amphetamine (DOM)			
Methylenedioxy-methamphetamine (MDA)			X

5.3 Physical and psychological dependence result in continued drug-seeking behavior.

Whether or not a drug is addictive is related to how easily an individual can stop taking the drug on a repetitive basis. Whenever a person has an overwhelming desire to take a drug and cannot stop, he or she is described as *dependent*. Dependence is classified in two categories: physical dependence and psychological dependence.

Physical dependence refers to an altered physical condition caused by the nervous system adapting to repeated drug use. Over time, the body's cells are tricked into believing that they are normal in the presence of the drug. With physical dependence, uncomfortable symptoms known as *withdrawal* result when the drug is discontinued. Narcotics, such as morphine and heroin, may produce physical dependence relatively quickly with repeated doses, particularly when taken IV. Alcohol, CNS depressants, some stimulants, and nicotine are examples of substances that may produce physical dependence relatively easily with extended use.

In contrast, psychological dependence produces no signs of physical discomfort after the drug is discontinued. The user, however, has an intense desire to continue drug use despite negative economic, physical, or social consequences. This intense craving may be associated with the client's home environment or social contacts. Strong psychological craving for a drug is often responsible for relapses during substance abuse therapy and the client's return to drug-seeking behavior. Psychological dependence usually requires relatively high doses of a drug taken over a prolonged period, such as with marijuana and antianxiety drugs. However, psychological dependence may develop quickly—perhaps after only one use—with crack, a potent, inexpensive form of cocaine.

5.4 Withdrawal results when an abused substance is no longer available.

Once a client becomes physically dependent and the substance is discontinued, classic withdrawal symptoms will occur. Withdrawal may be particularly severe for clients physically dependent on alcohol and sedatives. Because of the severity of the symptoms, the process of withdrawal from these substances is best accomplished in the controlled environment of a substance abuse treatment facility. Examples of the types of withdrawal symptoms experienced with the different abused substances are shown in Table 5.2.

Prescription drugs may be used to reduce the severity of the symptoms associated with the withdrawal process. For example, alcohol withdrawal may be treated with chlordiazepoxide (Librium), and opioid withdrawal may be treated with methadone (Dolophine). Withdrawal from chronic use of CNS stimulants, hallucinogens, marijuana, and inhalants may be treated with lorazepam (Ativan). Symptoms of nicotine withdrawal may be relieved by using nicotine in the

---

ON THE JOB

Physical Therapists Taking Notice of Clients with Drug Abuse

You might think that healthcare professionals who are not directly involved in the dispensing of medications have no opportunity to observe cases of drug or substance abuse. But what about physical therapists or physical therapist assistants working with clients who have musculoskeletal disorders? Suppose a client has been experiencing moderate pain for a time, and despite attempts of the treatment team to control the pain, the situation has become progressively worse. In cases of abuse, therapists might be in an excellent position to notice if a client is becoming dependent on pain medication. Many opioids, for example, have a high potential for both physical and psychological dependence, as well as tolerance. Small doses can cause addiction over an extended period of time, and withdrawal signs are particularly noticeable. Healthcare providers are in an ideal position to recognize if a client is experiencing watery eyes, running nose, chills, tremors, or nausea. ■

TABLE 5.2	Withdrawal Symptoms of Selected Drugs of Abuse
Narcotic analgesics/Opioids	excessive sweating, restlessness, dilated pupils, agitation, goosebumps, tremor, violent yawning, increased heart rate and blood pressure, nausea/vomiting, abdominal cramps and pain, muscle spasms with kicking movements, weight loss
Barbiturates and other sedative-hypnotics	insomnia, anxiety, weakness, abdominal cramps, tremor, anorexia, seizures, hallucinations, delirium
Benzodiazepines	insomnia, restlessness, abdominal pain, nausea, sensitivity to light and sound, headache, fatigue, muscle twitches
Alcohol	tremors, fatigue, anxiety, abdominal cramping, hallucinations, confusion, seizures, delirium
Cocaine and amphetamines	mental depression, anxiety, extreme fatigue, hunger
Nicotine	irritability, anxiety, restlessness, headaches, increased appetite, insomnia, inability to concentrate, decrease in heart rate and blood pressure
Marijuana	irritability, restlessness, insomnia, tremor, chills, weight loss
Hallucinogens	rarely observed; dependent upon specific drug

form of Habitrol, Nicoderm, or Nicorette. Bupropion (Zyban, Wellbutrin), an antidepressant, is also prescribed with transdermal nicotine in some smoking cessation programs.

Another type of withdrawal is called **conditioned withdrawal**. With chronic substance abuse, clients will often associate their conditions and surroundings, including the company of other users, with the taking of the drug. Users tend to revert back to drug-seeking behavior when they return to the company of other substance abusers. Substance abuse counselors often encourage users to refrain from associating with their past social contacts or relationships with other drug users, other than in self-help groups, to lessen the possibility of relapse.

5.5 Tolerance occurs when higher and higher doses of a drug are needed to achieve the same initial response.

Tolerance is a condition whereby an individual adapts to a drug over a period of time, such that higher and higher doses of the drug are required in order to produce the same initial effect. For example, a client may find that 2 mg of a sedative is effective in inducing sleep. After taking the drug for several months, the client notices that it takes 4 or perhaps 6 mg to fall asleep. Development of drug tolerance is common for drugs that affect the nervous system.

The terms *immunity* and *resistance* are often confused with tolerance. These terms more correctly refer to the immune system and infections and should not be used interchangeably with

NATURAL ALTERNATIVES

Herbal Stimulants

Recovering from addiction may be a difficult experience. Some claim that discretionary use of some herbal stimulants may ease the symptoms associated with recovery. Examples include kola, damiana, Asiatic and Siberian ginseng, and gotu kola. These agents are thought to stimulate the central nervous system, providing just enough effect to reduce tension and the stresses associated with drug craving. ■

tolerance. For example, microorganisms may become resistant to the effects of an antibiotic: they do not become tolerant. Clients may become tolerant to the effects of pain relievers: they do not become resistant.

Tolerance does not develop at the same rate for all actions of a drug. For example, clients usually develop tolerance to the nausea and vomiting produced by narcotic analgesics after only a few doses. Tolerance to the mood-altering effects of these drugs and to their ability to reduce pain develops more slowly, but eventually may be complete. Tolerance never develops to the drug's ability to constrict the pupils. Clients will often endure annoying side effects of drugs, such as the sedation caused by antihistamines, if they know that tolerance to these effects will develop quickly.

Concept review 5.1

▪ What is the difference between physical dependence and psychological dependence? How do clients know when they are physically dependent on a substance?

5.6 Ethyl alcohol is one of the most commonly abused drugs.

One of the most commonly abused drugs is ethyl alcohol, commonly referred to as *alcohol,* which is the pharmacologically active agent in beer, wine, and liquor. The economic, social, and health consequences of alcohol abuse are staggering. Curiously, however, small quantities of alcohol consumed on a daily basis have been found to reduce the risk of stroke and heart attack.

Alcohol is considered a central nervous system (CNS) depressant because it has the ability to slow the region of the brain responsible for alertness and wakefulness. Effects of alcohol include sedation, relaxation, blurred memory, loss of motor coordination, reduced judgment, and decreased inhibition. Alcohol also increases blood flow to certain areas of the skin, causing a flushed face, pink cheeks, or red nose.

Perhaps the most serious concern among the public is alcohol's ability to impair coordination and judgment, particularly when the user drives a vehicle or operates machinery. Alcohol easily crosses the blood-brain barrier so its effects are observed quickly, within five to thirty minutes after consumption. Alcohol should never be combined with other CNS depressants because their effects are cumulative and profound sedation or coma may result.

Absorption across membranes of the gastrointestinal tract may be slowed by the presence of food. Therefore, if an individual is combining food with alcohol, the onset of action may be delayed. Effects of alcohol in the body are directly related to the amount of alcohol consumed. Acute overdoses of alcohol produce vomiting, severe hypotension, respiratory failure, and coma. Death due to alcohol poisoning is not uncommon.

Chronic alcohol consumption produces both psychological and physiological dependence and results in a large number of adverse health effects. The organ most affected by chronic alcohol abuse is the liver, which is responsible for metabolizing and detoxifying alcohol. Alcoholism is a common cause of cirrhosis, a debilitating and often fatal failure of the liver to perform its vital functions. Liver failure results in abnormalities in blood clotting and nutritional deficiencies, and makes the client very sensitive to the effects of drugs. Drug doses for clients with alcoholism are lower than normal doses and the patient is more susceptible to adverse drug effects and drug interactions.

cirr = orange/yellow
osis = condition

Alcohol withdrawal is severe and may be life-threatening. The use of anticonvulsants in the treatment of alcohol withdrawal is discussed in Chapter 8 ⬚. Long-term treatment for alcohol abuse includes behavioral counseling and self-help groups such as Alcoholics Anonymous. Disulfiram (Antabuse) may be given to discourage relapses. If alcohol is consumed while taking disulfiram, the client becomes violently ill with headache, shortness of breath, nausea, vomiting and other unpleasant symptoms.

5.7 Nicotine is a powerful and highly addictive cardiovascular and CNS stimulant.

The most common method by which nicotine enters the body is through the inhalation of cigarette, pipe, or cigar smoke. Tobacco smoke contains over 1,000 chemicals, a significant number of which are carcinogens. The primary addictive drug present in cigarette smoke is nicotine. Effects of inhaled nicotine may last anywhere from 30 minutes to several hours.

Nicotine affects many body systems including the nervous, cardiovascular, and endocrine systems. Nicotine stimulates the CNS directly, causing symptoms ranging from increased alertness and ability to focus, to feelings of relaxation or light-headedness. The cardiovascular effects of nicotine include an accelerated heart rate and increased blood pressure, caused by activation of nicotinic receptors located throughout the autonomic nervous system (Chapter 6 ⬭). These cardiovascular effects can be particularly serious in clients taking oral contraceptives: the risk of a fatal heart attack is five times greater in smokers than in non-smokers. Muscular tremors may occur with moderate doses of nicotine and convulsions may result from very high doses. Nicotine affects the endocrine system by increasing metabolism, leading to weight loss. Nicotine also reduces appetite. Chronic use leads to emphysema, chronic obstructive pulmonary disease (COPD), and lung cancer.

Both psychological and physical dependence occur relatively quickly with nicotine. Once started on tobacco, clients tend to continue their drug use for many years, despite overwhelming medical evidence that the quality and quantity of their life will be adversely affected. Discontinuation results in agitation, weight gain, anxiety, headache, and an extreme craving for the drug. Although nicotine patches and gum assist clients in dealing with the unpleasant withdrawal symptoms, only 25% of clients who attempt to stop smoking remain tobacco-free one year later.

Concept review 5.2

- Name three legal substances abused more often than illegal drugs. Are these natural or synthetic substances?

5.8 Marijuana produces less physical dependence and tolerance than most other drugs of abuse.

Marijuana, also known as grass, pot, weed, reefer, or dope, is a natural product obtained from the plant *Cannabis sativa,* which thrives in tropical climates. The active ingredient in marijuana is **tetrahydrocannabinol (THC)**. THC slows motor activity, decreases coordination, and causes disconnected thoughts, feelings of paranoia, and euphoria. It increases thirst and craving for food, particularly chocolate and other candies. One hallmark symptom of marijuana use is red or bloodshot eyes, caused by dilation of blood vessels. THC accumulates in reproductive tissues, particularly the gonads.

eu = healthy or well
phoria = bearing
para = beside
noia = mind

When inhaled, marijuana produces effects that occur within minutes and last up to 24 hours. Because marijuana smoke is often inhaled more deeply and held within the lungs for a longer period of time than cigarette smoke, marijuana smoke introduces four times more particulates (tar) into the lungs than does tobacco smoke. Smoking marijuana on a daily basis may increase the risk of lung cancer and other respiratory disorders. Chronic use is associated with a lack of motivation in achieving or pursuing life goals.

Unlike most drugs of abuse, marijuana produces very little physical dependence or tolerance. Withdrawal symptoms are mild, if they are experienced at all. Metabolites of THC, however, remain in the body for months to years, allowing laboratory specialists to easily determine whether someone has used marijuana. For several days after use, THC can also be detected in the urine. Some groups advocate legalization of marijuana for nausea relief and appetite stimulation in clients with cancer. Despite numerous attempts to demonstrate therapeutic applications for marijuana, results have been controversial.

5.9 Hallucinogens cause an altered state of thought and perception similar to that found in dreams.

Hallucinogens are a diverse class of chemicals that have in common the ability to produce an altered, dream-like state of consciousness. Sometimes called **psychodelics**, the prototype agent for

FIGURE 5.1

Comparison of the
chemical structures of
psilocybin and LSD.
Psilocybin is derived
from a mushroom,
shown in the photo in
(a) an LSD "blot" is
shown in photo (b)
*SOURCE: Pearson Education/PH
College.*

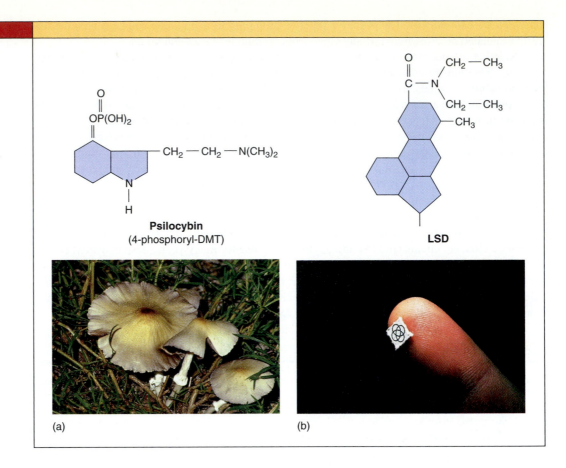

Psilocybin
(4-phosphoryl-DMT)

LSD

(a)

(b)

this class is lysergic acid diethylamide (LSD). The chemical similarities between several hallucinogenic drugs are shown in Figures 5.1 and 5.2. All hallucinogens are Schedule I drugs and have no therapeutic applications.

Drugs of abuse normally produce predictable sets of symptoms in every user. Drug effects from hallucinogens, however, are highly variable and dependent upon the mood and expectations of the user and the surrounding environment in which the drug is used. Two clients taking the same

FIGURE 5.2

The chemical structure
of mescaline, derived
from the peyote plant
(shown in photo)
*SOURCE: Pearson Education/PH
College.*

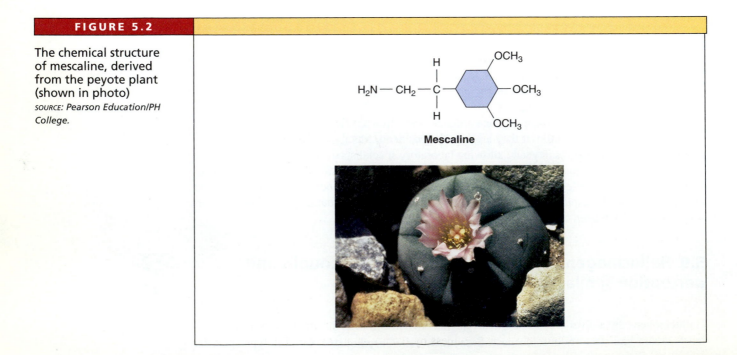

Mescaline

drug will report completely different symptoms and the same client may report different symptoms with each use. Users who take LSD or psilocybin (also called magic mushrooms, or shrooms) may experience symptoms such as laughter, visions, religious revelations, and deep personal insights. Common occurrences are hallucinations and after-images being projected onto people as they move. Users also report extremely bright lights and vivid colors. Some users hear voices; others report smells. Many experience a profound sense of truth and deep, directed thoughts. Unpleasant experiences can be terrifying and may include anxiety, confusion, severe depression, and paranoia.

LSD (also called acid, the beast, blotter acid, and California sunshine) is derived from a fungus that grows on rye and other grains. LSD is almost always administered orally and can be manufactured in capsule, tablet, or liquid form. A common and inexpensive method for distributing LSD is to place drops of the drug on paper that often contains the images of cartoon characters or graphics related to the drug culture (see Figure 5.1B). After drying, the paper containing the LSD is ingested to produce the drug's effects.

LSD is distributed to the brain and throughout the body immediately after use. Effects can be felt within an hour, and may last from six to twelve hours. Within 20 minutes after use, all traces of LSD are gone from the brain. It affects the central and autonomic nervous systems, increasing blood pressure, elevating body temperature, dilating pupils, and increasing the heart rate. Repeated use may cause impaired memory and inability to reason. In extreme cases, clients may develop psychoses. One common adverse effect is flashbacks, in which the user experiences the effects of the drug again, sometimes weeks, months, or years after the drug was initially taken. While tolerance is observed, little or no dependence occurs with many of the hallucinogens.

A number of other hallucinogens are abused. These include the following:

- Mescaline: found in the peyote cactus of Mexico and Central America.
- MDMA (3,4–methylenedioxymethamphetamine, XTC, or ecstasy): an amphetamine originally synthesized for legitimate research purposes, but has since been classified as a **designer drug** due to its illegal use.
- DOM (2,5 dimethoxy-4-methylamphetamine): a recreational drug often linked with rave parties as a drug of choice having the name STP.
- MDA (3.4-methylenedioxyamphetamine): called the love drug due to a belief that it enhances sexual desires.
- Phenylcyclohexylpiperadine (PCP; angel dust, or phencyclidine): produces a trance like state that may last for days and result in severe brain damage.
- Ketamine (date rape drug or special coke): produces unconsciousness and amnesia. Administered in conjunction with diazepam (Valium), ketamine's primary legal use is as an anesthetic.

Concept review 5.3

- In examining and interviewing a client, how could you determine whether he/she is under the influence of marijuana or hallucinogens?

5.10 CNS stimulants increase the activity of the central nervous system.

The stimulants include a diverse family of drugs known for their ability to increase the activity of the CNS. Examples of stimulants include the following.

- amphetamine, dextroamphetamine, methamphetamine
- cocaine
- methylphenidate
- caffeine

Stimulants have effects similar to the neurotransmitter norepinephrine (Chapter 6 ⬭). Norepinephrine affects awareness and wakefulness by activating neurons in a part of the brain called the reticular formation. High doses of amphetamines give the user a feeling of self-confidence, euphoria, alertness, and empowerment. But just as short-term use induces favorable feelings, long-term use often results in feelings of restlessness, anxiety, and fits of rage, especially when the user is coming down from a high induced by the drug.

Most stimulants affect cardiovascular and respiratory activity, resulting in elevated blood pressure and an increased breathing rate. Other symptoms include dilated pupils, sweating, and tremors. Overdoses of some stimulants lead to seizures and cardiac arrest.

Amphetamines and dextroamphetamines were once prescribed for depression, obesity, drowsiness, and congestion. Due to the development of safer medications, the current therapeutic uses of these drugs are extremely limited. Dextroamphetamine (Dexedrine) may be used for short-term weight loss when all other attempts to reduce weight have been exhausted, and to treat a rare disease called *narcolepsy,* which causes clients to fall asleep unexpectedly.

narco = numbness or stupor
lepsy = seizure

Methamphetamine, commonly called "crank" or "ice," is often used as a recreational drug for users who like the euphoric rush that it gives them. Methamphetamine usually is administered in powder or crystal form, but it may also be smoked. Methamphetamine is a Schedule II drug marketed under the trade name Desoxyn, although most abusers obtain it from illegal sources.

Cocaine is a Schedule II drug that produces effects similar to the amphetamines. Routes of administration include snorting, smoking, and injecting. In small doses, cocaine produces feelings of intense euphoria, a decrease in hunger and pain, illusions of physical strength, and increased sensory perception. Larger doses will increase these effects and also cause rapid heartbeat, sweating, dilation of the pupils, and an elevated body temperature. After the feelings of euphoria diminish, the user may be left with a sense of irritability, insomnia, depression, and extreme distrust. Some users report the sensation that insects are crawling under the skin. Users who snort cocaine develop a runny nose, a crusty redness around the nostrils, and deterioration of the nasal cartilage. Overdose can result in disturbances in cardiac rhythm, convulsions, stroke, or death due to respiratory arrest. Withdrawal symptoms from amphetamines and cocaine are much less intense than those from alcohol or CNS depressant abuse.

Methylphenidate (Ritalin) is a CNS stimulant widely prescribed for children diagnosed with attention deficit disorder (ADD) or attention deficit hyperactive disorder (ADHD). Ritalin has a calming effect in children who are inattentive or hyperactive. Ritalin stimulates the alertness center in the brain and the child is able to focus on tasks for longer periods of time. The use of methylphenidate in the treatment of ADD is discussed in Chapter 9 ▭ .

Ritalin is sometimes abused by adolescents and adults who are seeking euphoria without the difficulty associated with obtaining other amphetamine-like drugs. Tablets are sometimes crushed and used intranasally. Ritalin is sometimes mixed with heroin, a combination called a "speedball."

Caffeine is a natural substance found in the seeds, leaves, or fruits of more than 63 plant species throughout the world. Caffeine is commonly consumed in chocolate, coffee, tea, soft drinks, and ice cream. Caffeine is sometimes added to OTC pain relievers and stimulants because it has been shown to increase the effectiveness of these medications. Because it is soluble in water, caffeine travels to almost all parts of the body after ingestion. Several hours are needed for the body to metabolize and eliminate the drug. Caffeine has a diuretic effect, causing an individual to urinate more frequently.

Effects of caffeine include increased mental alertness, restlessness, nervousness, irritability, and insomnia. Other effects include dilation of the respiratory passages, increased blood pressure, increased production of stomach acid, and changes in blood sugar levels. Repeated use of caffeine may result in physical dependence and tolerance. Withdrawal symptoms include severe headaches, fatigue, depression, and impaired performance of daily activities. Types of beverages and OTC preparations with the relative amount of caffeine in each are summarized in Table 5.3.

Concept review 5.4

■ Identify three groups of stimulants discussed in this section and give examples for each group. Identify three major systems in the body affected by stimulants.

TABLE 5.3	Caffeine Content of Common Foods and Beverages	
OVER-THE-COUNTER DRUGS	**SERVING SIZE**	**CAFFEINE (MG)**
NoDoz, maximum strength; Vivarin	1 tablet	200
Excedrin	2 tablets	130
NoDoz, regular strength	1 tablet	100
Anacin (also available in caffeine-free formulation)	2 tablets	64
COFFEES		
Coffee, brewed and instant	8 ounces	95–135
Coffee, decaffeinated	8 ounces	5
TEAS		
Tea, leaf or bag	8 ounces	50
Tea, green	8 ounces	30
Tea, instant	8 ounces	15
SOFT DRINKS		
Mountain Dew	12 ounces	55.5
Diet Coke	12 ounces	46.5
Coca-Cola Classic	12 ounces	34.5
Pepsi-Cola	12 ounces	37.5
FROZEN DESSERTS AND YOGURTS		
Starbucks Coffee Ice Cream, assorted flavors	1 cup	40–60
Dannon Coffee Yogurt	8 ounces	45
CHOCOLATES AND CANDIES		
Hershey's special dark chocolate bar	1 bar (1.5 ounces)	31
Hershey bar (milk chocolate)	1 bar (1.5 ounces)	10
Cocoa or hot chocolate	8 ounces	5

5.11 CNS depressants decrease the activity of the central nervous system.

CNS depressants form a group of drugs that cause sedation or relaxation. Drugs in this class include barbiturates, non-barbiturate sedative-hypnotics, benzodiazepines, and opioids. Although the majority of the drugs in this group are legal, many are controlled due to their abuse potential. Alcohol is also classified as a CNS depressant, as discussed in Section 5.6.

Barbiturates, commonly referred to as sedatives or tranquilizers, are primarily prescribed for sleep disorders and certain forms of epilepsy. Physical dependence, psychological dependence, and tolerance develop when these drugs are taken for extended periods at high doses. Often clients abuse these drugs by faking prescriptions or by sharing their medication with friends. They are commonly combined with other drugs of abuse, such as stimulants or alcohol. Addicts often alternate between amphetamines, which keep them awake for several days, and barbiturates, which are then needed in order to relax and fall sleep.

Many CNS depressants have a long duration of effect in the body. Onset of action may be within 30 minutes, and effects last up to an entire day, depending on the specific drug. Clients may appear dull or apathetic. Effects of higher doses resemble those of alcohol intoxication, including slurred speech and motor incoordination. Four commonly abused barbiturates are pentobarbital

(Nembutral), amobarbital (Amytal), secobarbital (Seconal), and a combination of secobarbital and amobarbital (Tuinal). The use of the barbiturates in treating sleep disorders is discussed in Chapter 7, and their use in epilepsy is presented in Chapter 8 .

Overdoses of barbiturates and non-barbiturate sedative-hypnotics are extremely dangerous. These drugs suppress the respiratory centers in the brain and the user may stop breathing or, in some cases, lapse into coma. Death is not uncommon. Withdrawal symptoms from these drugs resemble those of alcohol withdrawal and may be life-threatening.

anxio = anxiety/
restlessness
lytic = destruction

Benzodiazepines, referred to as *anxiolytics,* are used therapeutically for clients experiencing anxiety or panic attacks (Chapter 7). Benzodiazepines are also used to prevent seizures (Chapter 8) and as muscle relaxants (Chapter 30). Popular benzodiadepines include alprazolam (Xanax), diazepam (Valium), and flurazepam (Dalmane).

Individuals abusing benzodiazepines may act detached, sleepy, or disoriented. Often, clients will appear carefree and without worry. Benzodiazepines are much safer than barbiturates: death due to overdose is rare, even with extremely high doses. An individual usually will become sedated and sleep for a long period of time. Withdrawal symptoms are less severe than with barbiturates.

Opioids, also known as narcotics, are prescribed for severe pain, persistent cough, and diarrhea. The opioids include natural substances obtained from the unripe seeds of the poppy plant such as opium, morphine, and codeine, and synthetic drugs such as propoxyphene (Darvon), meperidine (Demerol), oxycodone (OxyContin), fentanyl (Duragesic, Sublimaze), methadone (Dolophine), and heroin. The therapeutic effects of the opioids are discussed in detail in Chapter 11 .

Oral opioids produce effects within 30 minutes and that may last over a day. Parenteral forms produce immediate effects, including the brief, intense rush of euphoria sought by heroin addicts. Individuals experience a range of emotions, from extreme pleasure to slowed body activities and profound sedation. Physiological symptoms include constricted pupils, an increase in the pain threshold or analgesia, and respiratory depression.

Addiction to opioids can occur rapidly and withdrawal can produce very intense and unpleasant symptoms, as listed in Table 5.2. While extremely unpleasant, withdrawal from opioids is not life threatening, compared to barbiturate withdrawal. Methadone is a narcotic sometimes used to treat opioid addiction. Although methadone has addictive properties of its own, it does not produce euphoria to the degree that other narcotics do, and its effects are longer lasting. Heroin addicts are switched to methadone in order to prevent the unpleasant withdrawal symptoms and to discourage erratic dosages of illegal drugs. Clients sometimes remain on methadone maintenance the remainder of their lives. Withdrawal from methadone is more prolonged than with heroin or morphine, but the symptoms are less intense.

CLIENT TEACHING

Clients taking medications with abuse potential need to know the following:

1. Limit alcoholic beverage intake to two drinks per day for men or one drink per day for women.
2. If you have liver disease, gastric reflux, peptic ulcers, or are pregnant, avoid alcohol use entirely.
3. Consuming more than one alcoholic drink per hour will usually result in blood alcohol levels above the legal limit for operating a vehicle.
4. If taking methylphenidate (Ritalin), avoid sources of caffeine such as OTC drugs with caffeine, chocolate, coffee, and tea.
5. Always take methylphenidate (Ritalin) at least six hours prior to sleep in order to avoid insomnia.
6. Never take more CNS depressant medication than prescribed by your healthcare practitioner. If the prescribed dose is not providing sufficient relief, you should notify your physician, as you may have developed tolerance.
7. Never combine CNS depressants (including alcohol) unless advised to do so by your physician.
8. If you smoke tobacco, remember that your second-hand smoke is dangerous, particularly to children and pregnant individuals. ■

Concept review 5.5

■ Compare barbiturates and benzodiazepines, relative to their potential for causing death due to overdose.

CHAPTER REVIEW

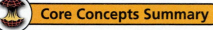 **Core Concepts Summary**

5.1 **A wide variety of different substances may be abused by individuals.**

Abused substances come from many different chemical classes. Some abused substances, such as alcohol and nicotine, are available without a prescription. Others, such as barbiturates, benzodiazepines, and most opioids, have legitimate medical uses. Still others, such as LSD and heroin, are illegal, having no current medical applications.

5.2 **Addiction has both neurobiological and psychosocial components.**

Addiction is an overwhelming feeling that causes someone to continue taking drugs. Although ideas have changed about addiction over the years, healthcare providers now recognize it as a neurobiological problem interacting with the client's psychological state and social setting.

5.3 **Physical and psychological dependence result in continued drug-seeking behavior.**

Dependence is an overwhelming need to take drug on a continuous basis. Physical dependence occurs when the client exhibits signs of withdrawal after the drug is discontinued. Psychological dependence is an intense craving for drug use.

5.4 **Withdrawal results when an abused substance is no longer available.**

When an abused drug is discontinued, clients may experience uncomfortable physical symptoms known as withdrawal. Symptoms vary depending upon the specific drug of abuse, and range from mild to life threatening.

5.5 **Tolerance occurs when higher and higher doses of a drug are needed to achieve the same initial response.**

Tolerance occurs over a period of time when clients adapt to continued drug use and require higher doses in order to produce the same initial effect.

5.6 **Ethyl alcohol is one of the most commonly abused drugs.**

Alcohol abuse results in extreme social, economic, and health consequences. Acute doses may cause coma or death. Chronic abuse leads to liver cirrhosis and many other health problems.

5.7 **Nicotine is a powerful and highly addictive cardiovascular and CNS stimulant.**

Nicotine exerts profound effects upon the cardiovascular and nervous systems. Chronic use may severely affect the lungs and the cardiovascular system.

5.8 **Marijuana produces less physical dependence and tolerance than most other drugs of abuse.**

Although marijuana produces little dependence or tolerance, long-term abuse can lead to lung damage and lack of ambition. Therapeutic uses for the drug remain controversial.

5.9 **Hallucinogens cause an altered state of thought and perception similar to that found in dreams.**

Hallucinogens produce an altered, dream-like state of consciousness in which the user is out of touch with reality. Effects of the drugs are highly variable among users and little dependence occurs.

5.10 **CNS stimulants increase the activity of the central nervous system.**

Amphetamines, cocaine, methylphenidate, and caffeine increase alertness by stimulating the CNS. Medical uses of these drugs—with the exception of methylphenidate—are extremely limited. Many of the stimulants readily produce physical and psychological dependence. Methylphenidate is widely used for attention deficit disorder in children.

5.11 **CNS depressants decrease the activity of the central nervous system.**

Commonly abused CNS depressants include barbiturates, non-barbiturate sedative-hypnotics, benzodiazepines, and opioids. All the CNS depressants can produce dependence and tolerance. Withdrawal symptoms from barbiturates can be especially severe.

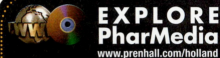

EXPLORE PharMedia
www.prenhall.com/holland

Additional interactive resources and activities for this chapter can be found on the Companion Website. For animations, audio glossary, and review access the accompanying CD-ROM in this book.

Audio Glossary
Concept Review
NCLEX Review

2

THE NERVOUS SYSTEM

6 Drugs for Disorders Associated with the Autonomic Nervous System

CORE CONCEPTS

6.1 The peripheral nervous system is divided into somatic and autonomic components.

6.2 The autonomic nervous system has sympathetic and parasympathetic branches.

6.3 Synapses are common sites of drug action.

6.4 Acetylcholine and norepinephrine are the two primary neurotransmitters in the autonomic nervous system.

Autonomic Drugs

6.5 Autonomic drugs are classified by which receptors they stimulate or block.

Parasympathomimetics

6.6 Parasympathomimetics have few therapeutic uses because of their numerous side effects.

Anticholinergics

6.7 Anticholinergics are used to dry secretions, treat asthma, and prevent motion sickness.

Sympathomimetics

6.8 Sympathomimetics are primarily used for their effects on the heart, bronchial tree, and nasal passages.

Adrenergic-Blockers

6.9 Adrenergic-blockers are primarily used for hypertension and are the most widely prescribed class of autonomic drugs.

OBJECTIVES

After reading this chapter, the student should be able to:

1. Identify the two primary divisions of the nervous system.

2. Identify the three primary functions of the nervous system.

3. Compare and contrast the actions of the sympathetic and parasympathetic nervous systems.

4. Describe the three parts of a synapse.

5. Identify the neurotransmitters important to the autonomic nervous system and the types of nerves with which they are associated.

6. Compare and contrast nicotinic and muscarinic receptors.

7. Compare and contrast the types of effects when a drug stimulates $alpha_1$, $alpha_2$, $beta_1$, or $beta_2$-adrenergic receptors.

8. For each of the following classes, explain the mechanism of drug action, primary actions, and important adverse effects.
   a. parasympathomimetics
   b. anticholinergics
   c. sympathomimetics
   d. adrenergic-blockers

PharMedia
www.prenhall.com/holland

Additional interactive resources and activities for this chapter can be found on the Companion Website. For animations, audio glossary, and review access the accompanying CD-ROM in this book.

acetylcholine (ah-SEET-ul-KOH-leen): primary neurotransmitter of the parasympathetic nervous system; also present at somatic neuromuscular junctions and at sympathetic preganglionic nerves / *page 69*

adrenergic (add-rah-NUR-jik): a term relating to nerves that release norepinephrine or epinephrine / *page 70*

adrenergic-agonist (add-rah-NUR-jik AG-un-ist): another name for a sympathomimetic drug / *page 72*

adrenergic-blocker: drug that blocks the actions of the sympathetic nervous system / *page 73*

alpha-receptor: type of subreceptor found in the sympathetic nervous system / *page 72*

anticholinergic: drug that inhibits the action of acetylcholine at its receptor / *page 73*

autonomic nervous system: portion of the peripheral nervous system that gives involuntary control over smooth muscle, cardiac muscle, and glands / *page 68*

beta-receptor: type of subreceptor found in the sympathetic nervous system / *page 72*

central nervous system (CNS): division of the nervous system consisting of the brain and spinal cord / *page 68*

cholinergic (kol-in-UR-jik): a term relating to nerves that release acetylcholine / *page 70*

cholinergic-agonist: another name for a parasympathomimetic drug / *page 72*

cholinergic-blocker: drug that blocks the actions of the parasympathetic nervous system / *page 73*

fight-or-flight response: signs and symptoms produced when the sympathetic nervous system is activated / *page 69*

ganglion (GANG-lee-on): a collection of neuron cell bodies located outside the CNS / *page 70*

muscarinic (MUS-kah-RIN-ik): type of cholinergic-receptor found in smooth muscle, cardiac muscle, and glands / *page 72*

myasthenia gravis (MEYE-ahs-THEE-nee-uh GRAV-us): disease characterized by a destruction of nicotinic receptors on skeletal muscles / *page 73*

mydriasis (meye-DRY-uh-sis): dilation of the pupil / *page 75*

neuron (NYOUR-on): cell that is the functional unit of the nervous system / *page 69*

neurotransmitter (NYOUR-oh-TRANS-mitt-ur): a chemical mediator that is released by nerves at synapses and neuromuscular junctions / *page 69*

nicotinic (NIK-oh-TIN-ik): type of cholinergic-receptor found in ganglia of both the sympathetic and parasympathetic nervous systems / *page 72*

norepinephrine (nor-EH-pin-NEF-rin): primary neurotransmitter in the sympathetic nervous system / *page 69*

parasympathetic nervous system (PAIR-ah-SIM-pah-THET-ik): portion of the autonomic system that is active during periods of rest and which produces the rest or relaxation response / *page 69*

parasympathomimetics (PAIR-ah-SIM-path-oh-mah-MET-ik): drugs that mimic the actions of the parasympathetic nervous system / *page 72*

peripheral nervous system (per-IF-urr-ul): division of the nervous system containing all nervous tissue outside the CNS, including the autonomic nervous system / *page 68*

postsynaptic nerve (POST-sin-AP-tik): nerve in the synapse that has receptors for the neurotransmitter / *page 69*

presynaptic nerve (PRE-sin-AP-tik): nerve that releases the neurotransmitter into the synaptic cleft / *page 69*

rest-or-relaxation response: signs and symptoms produced when the parasympathetic nervous system is activated / *page 69*

somatic nervous system (soh-MAT-ik): consists of nerves that provide voluntary control over skeletal muscle / *page 68*

sympathetic nervous system (SIM-pah-THET-ik): portion of the autonomic system that is active during periods of stress and which produces the fight-or-flight response / *page 69*

sympathomimetic (sim-PATH-oh-mih-MET-ik): drug that stimulates or mimics the sympathetic nervous system / *page 72*

synapse (SIN-aps): junction between two neurons consisting of a presynaptic nerve, a synaptic cleft, and a postsynaptic nerve / *page 69*

synaptic cleft (sin-AP-tik kleft): physical space between two neurons that must be crossed by the neurotransmitter / *page 69*

Neuropharmacology represents one of the largest, most complicated, and least understood branches of pharmacology. Nervous system medications are used to treat a large and diverse set of conditions, including pain, anxiety, depression, schizophrenia, insomnia, and convulsions. Through their effects on nerves, medications are also used to treat many disorders that are considered diseases of other organ systems. Examples include abnormalities in heart rate and rhythm, high and low blood pressure, pressure within the eyeball, asthma, and even a runny nose.

The study of nervous system pharmacology extends over the next seven chapters of this text. Traditionally, the study of neuropharmacology begins with the autonomic nervous system. A firm grasp of autonomic pharmacology is necessary in order to understand cardiovascular and respiratory pharmacology.

6.1 The peripheral nervous system is divided into somatic and autonomic components.

The nervous system has two major divisions: the central nervous system (CNS) and the peripheral nervous system. The CNS is made up of the brain and spinal cord. The peripheral nervous system consists of all nervous tissue outside the CNS. The basic functions of the nervous system are to:

- recognize changes in the internal and external environments
- process and integrate the environmental changes that are perceived
- react to the environmental changes by producing an action or response

Figure 6.1 shows the fundamental structural divisions of the peripheral nervous system. Nerves in the peripheral nervous system either recognize changes to the environment (sensory division) or respond to these changes by moving muscles or secreting chemicals (motor division). The somatic nervous system consists of nerves that provide voluntary control over skeletal muscle. Nerves of the autonomic nervous system, on the other hand, give involuntary control over

FIGURE 6.1

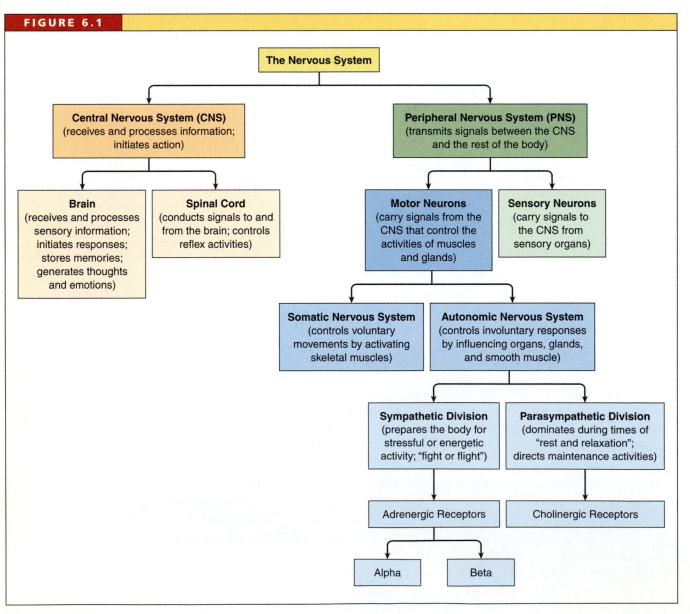

Functional divisions of the periphral nervous system

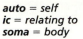

smooth muscle, cardiac muscle, and glands. Organs and tissues regulated by nerves from the autonomic nervous system include the heart, digestive tract, respiratory tract, reproductive tracts, arteries, salivary glands, and portions of the eye. While only a few drugs directly affect skeletal muscle, a large number of drugs affect autonomic nerves.

auto = self
ic = relating to
soma = body

6.2 The autonomic nervous system has sympathetic and parasympathetic branches.

The autonomic nervous system has two subcomponents called the *sympathetic nervous system* and the *parasympathetic nervous system*. With a few exceptions, organs and glands receive nerves from both branches of the autonomic nervous system.

The sympathetic nervous system is activated under conditions of stress, and produces a set of actions called the fight-or-flight response. On the other hand, the parasympathetic nervous system is activated under non-stressful conditions and produces symptoms called the rest-and-relaxation response. Most of the actions of the sympathetic branch are opposite to those of the parasympathetic branch. For example, activation of sympathetic nerves increases the heart rate while parasympathetic nerves decrease heart rate. The major actions of the two branches are shown in Figure 6.2. It is essential that the student learn these actions early in the study of pharmacology because knowledge of autonomic effects is used to predict the actions and side effects of many drugs.

Concept review 6.1

■ How would a person who is entering a fight benefit from the sympathetic effects of bronchodilation, slowed GI motility, and pupil dilation?

6.3 Synapses are common sites of drug action.

The basic functional cell of the nervous system is the neuron. In order for information to be transmitted throughout the nervous system, neurons must communicate with each other and with muscles and glands. As a nervous impulse travels along a nerve, it encounters a structure at the end of the nerve called a synapse. The synapse contains a physical space called the synaptic cleft, which must be bridged in order for the impulse to reach the next nerve. The nerve generating the original impulse is called the presynaptic nerve. The nerve on the other side of the synapse, waiting to receive the impulse, is called the postsynaptic nerve. The basic structure of a synapse is shown in Figure 6.3a.

pre = before
synaptic = relating to the synapse
post = after

The physical space of the synaptic cleft is bridged by chemicals called neurotransmitters. Neurotransmitters are released into the synaptic cleft when a nervous impulse reaches the end of a presynaptic nerve. The neurotransmitter travels across the synaptic cleft to reach receptors on the postsynaptic nerve, which then regenerates the impulse. This process is illustrated in Figures 6.3b and 6.3c. There are many different types of neurotransmitters located throughout the nervous system, each connected with particular functions. *Many drugs are identical or have the same general structure as neurotransmitters.* Drugs are used to affect autonomic functions by either blocking or enhancing the activity of these neurotransmitters.

6.4 Acetylcholine and norepinephrine are the two primary neurotransmitters in the autonomic nervous system.

The two primary neurotransmitters of the autonomic nervous system are norepinephrine (NE) and acetylcholine (Ach). In the sympathetic nervous system, NE is released at the junction of the postsynaptic nerve and the organ or gland to be acted upon. For example, sympathetic nerves in the heart release norepinephrine on cardiac muscle, which stimulates the heart to contract faster and

FIGURE 6.2

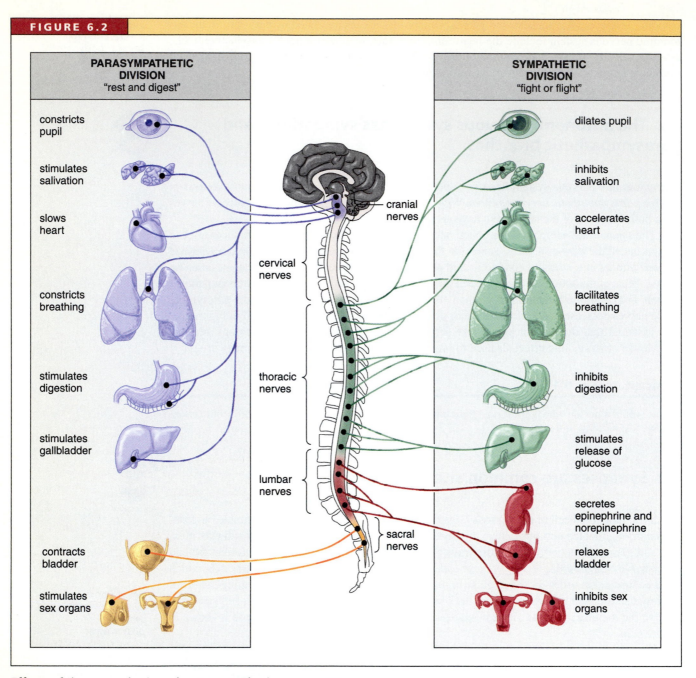

PARASYMPATHETIC DIVISION
"rest and digest"

constricts pupil

stimulates salivation

slows heart

constricts breathing

stimulates digestion

stimulates gallbladder

contracts bladder

stimulates sex organs

cranial nerves

cervical nerves

thoracic nerves

lumbar nerves

sacral nerves

SYMPATHETIC DIVISION
"fight or flight"

dilates pupil

inhibits salivation

accelerates heart

facilitates breathing

inhibits digestion

stimulates release of glucose

secretes epinephrine and norepinephrine

relaxes bladder

inhibits sex organs

Effects of the sympathetic and parasympathetic nervous systems   *source: Pearson Education IPH College.*

adren = adrenal gland
(adrenaline)
ic = relating to
choline = acetylcholine

with greater force. Sympathetic nerves also release NE on the smooth muscle lining the digestive tract, and its action is to slow contractions or motility. Sympathetic nerves are sometimes called adrenergic. This term comes from the word *adrenaline,* which is a chemical closely related to NE.

The physiology of acetylcholine is more complicated because it is released in several different locations. When released at the ends of parasympathetic nerves, it produces the opposite effects of NE, such as slowing the heart and increasing the motility of the digestive tract. Acetylcholine is also the neurotransmitter released at the end of all presynaptic nerves at sites called ganglia, which are collections of neuron cell bodies located outside of the spinal cord. In addition, acetylcholine is also a neurotransmitter of sympathetic neurons that activate sweat glands, a unique exception where Ach is associated with sympathetic activity rather than parasympathetic activity. Nerves releasing acetylcholine are often called cholinergic. The sites of acetylcholine and norepinephrine action are shown in Figure 6.4.

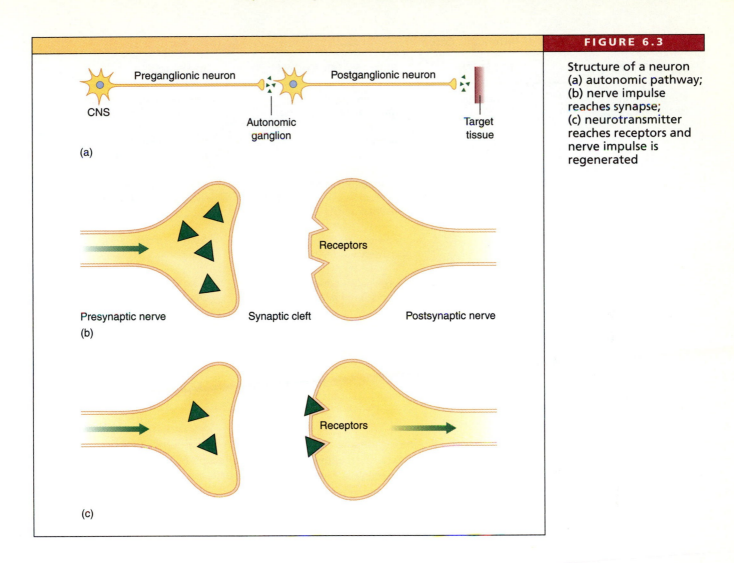

FIGURE 6.3

Structure of a neuron (a) autonomic pathway; (b) nerve impulse reaches synapse; (c) neurotransmitter reaches receptors and nerve impulse is regenerated

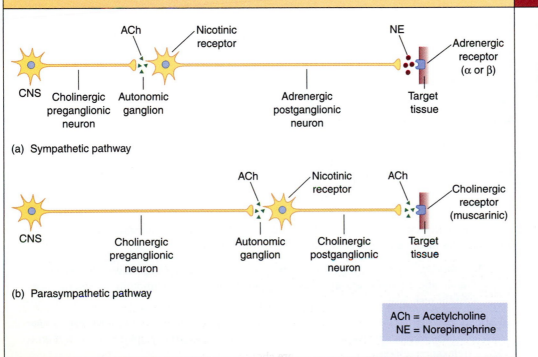

FIGURE 6.4

Receptors in the Autonomic Nervous System: (a) sympathetic pathways; (b) parasympathetic pathways

TABLE 6.1	Types of Autonomic Receptors		
NEUROTRANSMITTER	**RECEPTOR**	**PRIMARY LOCATIONS**	**RESPONSES**
acetylcholine (cholinergic)	muscarinic	parasympathetic target: organs other than the heart	stimulation of smooth muscle and gland secretions
		heart	decreased heart rate and force of contraction
	nicotinic	postganglionic neurons and neuromuscular junctions of skeletal muscle	stimulation of smooth muscle and gland secretions
norepinephrine (adrenergic)	alpha$_1$	all sympathetic target organs except the heart	constrict blood vessels, dilate pupils
	alpha$_2$	presynaptic adrenergic nerve terminals	inhibit release of norepinephrine
	beta$_1$	heart and kidneys	increased heart rate and force of contraction; release of renin
	beta$_2$	all sympathetic target organs except the heart	inhibition of smooth muscle

Because acetylcholine can stimulate receptors in both the ganglia and at the organ level, different names are assigned to these receptors. Acetylcholine receptors in the ganglia and in skeletal muscle are called nicotinic receptors, named after nicotine, the agent found in tobacco products. Acetylcholine receptors at the end of postsynaptic nerves in the parasympathetic nervous system are called muscarinic receptors, named after an extract of the mushroom *Amanita muscaria*. Nicotinic and muscarinic receptors are indicated in Figure 6.4.

Norepinephrine receptors are of two basic subtypes, alpha (α) and beta (β). *Alpha* and *beta* are Greek letters commonly used in the naming of chemical and scientific compounds. These receptors are further subdivided into beta$_1$, beta$_2$, alpha$_1$, and alpha$_2$. Drugs may be selective and affect only one type of NE receptor, or may affect all of them. The type of response depends on the specific type of receptor that is activated. Drugs may also affect one type of receptor at low doses and begin to affect other receptor subtypes as the dose is increased. Table 6.1 summarizes a list of receptors and expected responses once neurotransmitters are released.

AUTONOMIC DRUGS

6.5 Autonomic drugs are classified by which receptors they stimulate or block.

Given the opposite actions of the sympathetic and parasympathetic nervous systems, autonomic drugs are classified based upon one of four possible actions.

1. *Stimulation of the sympathetic nervous system.* These drugs are called sympathomimetics or adrenergic-agonists and produce the classic symptoms of the fight-or-flight response.

2. *Stimulation of the parasympathetic nervous system.* These drugs are called parasympathomimetics or cholinergic-agonists and produce the classic symptoms of the rest-and-relaxation response.

3. *Inhibition of the sympathetic nervous system.* These drugs are called **adrenergic-blockers** and produce actions opposite to those of the sympathomimetics.

4. *Inhibition of the parasympathetic nervous system.* These drugs are called **anticholinergics** or **cholinergic-blockers** and produce actions opposite to those of the parasympathomimetics.

Students beginning their study of pharmacology often have difficulty understanding the terminology and actions of autonomic drugs. Upon examining the four drug classes, however, it is evident that only one group need be learned because the others are logical extensions of the first. If the fight-or-flight symptoms of the sympathomimetics are learned, the other three groups are either the same or opposite. For example, both the sympathomimetics and the cholinergic-blockers increase heart rate and dilate the pupil. The other two groups, the parasympathomimetics and the adrenergic-blockers, have the opposite effects of slowing heart rate and constricting the pupils. It should be emphasized again that mastering the actions and terminology of autonomic drugs early in the study of pharmacology will reap rewards later in the course when these drugs are applied to various systems.

PARASYMPATHOMIMETICS

Parasympathomimetics are drugs that stimulate the parasympathetic nervous system. These drugs induce the rest-and-relaxation response.

6.6 Parasympathomimetics have few therapeutic uses because of their numerous side effects.

Only a handful of parasympathomimetics have therapeutic application, primarily because of their potential to adversely slow the heart rate and constrict the respiratory passages. Some of the parasympathomimetics having therapeutic use are shown in Table 6.2. This class of agents also includes organophosphate insecticides such as Malathion and toxic nerve gasses such as Sarin. Acute poisoning with these agents will result in intense stimulation of the parasympathetic nervous system, which may become fatal if untreated.

Several drugs in this class are not used for their parasympathetic action, but instead for their effects on acetylcholine receptors in skeletal muscle or in the CNS. **Myasthenia gravis** is a disease characterized by destruction of nicotinic receptors on skeletal muscles. Administration of pyridostigmine (Mestinon) or neostigmine (Prostigmin) will stimulate skeletal muscle contraction and help to reverse the severe muscle weakness characteristic of this disease. In addition, tacrine (Gognex) is useful in treating Alzheimer's disease because of its ability to increase the amount of acetylcholine in receptors in the CNS.

ON THE JOB

Ophthalmic Medical Technicians and Technologists

Ophthalmic technicians assist with examinations and treatments of the eye, under the supervision of an ophthamologist or other licensed practitioner. Technicians may administer diagnostic tests, take optical measurements, assist with the fitting of contact lenses, and sterilize and maintain optical instruments. In most states, ophthalmic technicians may also administer topical ophthalmic medications. Ophthalmic technician programs are generally one year in length, whereas ophthalmic technologist programs are often two years.

A strong knowledge of ocular medications, many of which are autonomic agents, is critical to patient safety. Autonomic drugs are used to dilate the pupil so that the ophthamologist can diagnose and treat eye disorders. Giving the incorrect drug can worsen glaucoma. Because these drugs commonly cause blurred vision and sensitivity to light, the ophthalmic technician plays an essential role in educating clients not to operate machinery and to limit exposure to bright light following examinations. ▪

DRUG PROFILE:
Bethanechol (Urecholine)

Actions:

Bethanechol is a direct-acting parasympathomimetic that interacts with acetylcholine receptors to cause actions typical of parasympathetic stimulation. Its effects are most noted in the digestive and urinary tracts, where it will stimulate smooth muscle contraction. These actions are particularly useful in stimulating the GI and urinary tracts to return to normal functioning following general anesthesia.

Adverse Effects:

The side effects of bethanechol are predicted from its parasympathetic actions. Symptoms include increased salivation, sweating, abdominal cramping, and hypotension that could lead to fainting. It should not be given to clients with suspected urinary or intestinal obstruction or those with active asthma.

TABLE 6.2	Selected Parasympathomimetics
DRUG	**PRIMARY USE**
bethanechol (Urecholine and others)	increase urination
neostigmine (Prostigmin)	myasthenia gravis, increase urination
physostigmine (Antilirum)	overdoses due to drugs with anticholinergic effects, glaucoma
pilocarpine (Isopto-Carpine)	glaucoma
pilocarpine (Salagen)	management of dry mouth due to radiation therapy of head/neck cancer
pyridostigmine (Mestinon)	myasthenia gravis
tacrine (Gognex)	Alzheimer's disease

ANTICHOLINERGICS

Anticholinergics are drugs that inhibit the parasympathetic branch. They induce symptoms of the fight-or-flight response.

6.7 Anticholinergics are used to dry secretions, treat asthma, and prevent motion sickness.

Although the term *anticholinergic* is commonly used, a better term for this class of drugs would be *muscarinic blockers*, as this more accurately describes the location of their action. Most therapeutic uses of the anticholinergics are predictable extensions of their autonomic actions: dilation of the pupil, increase in heart rate, drying of secretions, and dilation of the bronchi. Anticholinergics have been widely used in medicine for many disorders. A relatively high incidence of side effects and the development of safer, and sometimes more effective, medications has limited the current use of anticholinergics. For example, anticholinergics were once drugs of choice in treating peptic ulcers, but have been replaced by proton-pump inhibitors and H_2-receptor blockers (Chapter 25 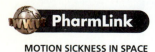). Two important side effects that limit their usefulness include tachycardia, or fast heart rate, and the tendency to cause urinary retention in men with prostate disorders. Some of the more common anticholinergics and their therapeutic applications are shown in Table 6.3.

PharmLink

MOTION SICKNESS IN SPACE

DRUG PROFILE:
Atropine

Actions:

Atropine is a natural product found in the deadly nightshade plant, or Atropa belladonna. By blocking acetylcholine (muscarinic) receptors, atropine induces symptoms of the fight-or-flight response. Most prominent are increased heart rate, bronchodilation, decreased motility in the GI tract, **mydriasis** (pupil dilation), and decreased secretions from glands. Over history, atropine has been used for a variety of purposes, although its use has declined because of the development of safer, more effective medications. Atropine is used to treat hyper-motility diseases of the GI tract such as irritable bowel syndrome, to suppress secretions during surgical procedures, to increase the heart rate in clients with bradycardia, to dilate the pupil during eye examinations, and to cause bronchodilation in clients with asthma.

Adverse Effects:

The adverse side effects of atropine limit the therapeutic usefulness of this drug and are predictable extensions of its autonomic actions. Expected side effects include dry mouth, constipation, urinary retention, and an increased heart rate. Atropine is usually contraindicated in clients with glaucoma because the drug may increase pressure within the eyeball.

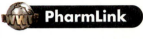

PharmLink

HISTORICAL USE OF
BELLADONNA

TABLE 6.3	Selected Anticholinergics
DRUG	**PRIMARY USE**
Pr atropine	produce a dry field prior to anesthesia, increase heart rate, dilate pupils
benztropine (Cogentin)	Parkinson's disease (central effect)
cyclopentolate (Cyclogyl)	dilate pupils
dicyclomine (Bentyl and others)	irritable bowel syndrome
glycopyrrolate (Robinul)	produce a dry field prior to anesthesia, peptic ulcers
ipratropium (Atrovent)	asthma
oxybutynin (Ditropan)	urinary bladder urgency and incontinence
propantheline (Pro-banthine)	irritable bowel syndrome, peptic ulcer
scopolamine (Hyoscine, Transderm-Scop)	motion sickness (central effect), irritable bowel syndrome, adjunct to anesthesia
trihexpheidyl (Artane and others)	Parkinson's disease (central effect)

Some of the anticholinergics are used for their effects on the CNS, rather than the autonomic nervous system. Examples include scopolamine (Hyoscine), which is used for sedation and motion sickness (Chapter 25), and benztropine (Cogentin), which is prescribed for Parkinson's disease (Chapter 10).

SYMPATHOMIMETICS

Sympathomimetics, or adrenergic-agonists, stimulate the sympathetic nervous system. They will produce symptoms characteristic of the fight-or-flight response.

6.8 Sympathomimetics are primarily used for their effects on the heart, bronchial tree, and nasal passages.

The sympathomimetics produce many of the same symptoms as the anticholinergics. However, because the sympathetic nervous system has alpha and beta-subreceptors, the actions of many of the sympathomimetics are more specific and have wider therapeutic application.

Although most effects of sympathomimetics are very predictable based on their autonomic actions, their primary effects depend upon which adrenergic-subreceptors are stimulated. Drugs such as phenylephrine (Neo-Synephrine) stimulate $alpha_1$-receptors and are often used to dry nasal secretions, whereas $alpha_2$-agonists such as clonidine (Catapres) are used to treat hypertension. Because $beta_1$-receptors are predominant in the heart, $beta_1$-agonists such as dobutamine (Dobutrex) are used to stimulate the heart rate and increase its strength of contraction. $Beta_2$-agonists such as albuterol (Proventil) cause bronchodilation and are useful in the treatment of asthma.

Some sympathomimetics are nonselective, stimulating more than one type of adrenergic-receptor. For example, epinephrine stimulates all four types of adrenergic-receptors and is used for cardiac arrest and asthma. Pseudoephedrine (Sudafed and others) stimulates both $alpha_1$ and $beta_2$-receptors and is used orally as a nasal decongestant. Isoproterenol (Isuprel) stimulates both $beta_1$ and $beta_2$-receptors and is used to increase the rate, force, and conduction speed of the heart,

TABLE 6.4	Selected Sympathomimetics	
DRUG	**PRIMARY RECEPTOR SUBTYPE**	**PRIMARY USE**
albuterol (Proventil, Ventilin, Provax)	$beta_2$	asthma
clonidine (Catapres)	$alpha_2$ (in CNS)	hypertension
dobutamine (Dobutrex)	$beta_1$	cardiac stimulant
dopamine (Intropin)	$alpha_1$ and $beta_1$	shock
epinephrine (Adrenalin, Primatene, Bronkaid)	alpha and beta	asthma, cardiac arrest
isoproterenol (Isuprel)	$beta_1$ and $beta_2$	asthma, dysrhythmias, heart failure
metaproterenol (Alupent)	$beta_2$	asthma
metaraminol (Aramine)	$alpha_1$ and $beta_1$	shock
methyldopa	$alpha_2$ (in CNS)	hypertension
norepinephrine (Levarterenol, Levophed)	$alpha_1$ and $beta_1$	shock
oxymetazoline (Afrin and others)	alpha	nasal congestion
phenylephrine (Neo-Synephrine)	alpha	nasal congestion
pseudoephedrine (Sudafed, Afrin, and others)	alpha and beta	nasal congestion
ritodrine (Yutopar)	$beta_2$	slow uterine contractions
salmeterol (Serevent)	$beta_2$	decongestant
terbutaline (Brethine and others)	$beta_2$	asthma

NATURAL ALTERNATIVES

Ma Huang or Ephedra as a Sympathomimetic

Ephedra is an herb that has been used in traditional Chinese medicine since antiquity. The primary plant species that contains ephedra is *Ephedra sinica*, also known as Ma Huang. Two active substances in Ma Huang are ephedrine and pseudoephedrine, both of which are available in OTC and prescription formulations. Dietary supplements of ephedra are usually standardized to contain 6–8% ephedrine alkaloids.

Ephedrine and pseudoephedrine are sympathomimetics and their actions are typical of sympathetic nervous system stimulation. The decongestant action of ephedra may benefit clients with allergies or the common cold. The bronchodilation effect may benefit those with asthma or chronic pulmonary disease. Many formulations of ephedra are marketed for use as energy enhancers and weight loss products. Some of these products combine ephedra with caffeine. As a sympathomimetic, ephedra can have adverse effects on the cardiovascular system, such as increased blood pressure and rapid heart rate. Clients with hypertension, diabetes mellitus, heart disease, or enlarged prostate should not take ephedra without seeking medical advice. ■

and occasionally for asthma. The non-selective drugs generally cause more autonomic-related side effects.

Some of the more commonly used sympathomimetics are shown in Table 6.4. Most drugs in this class are presented in other chapters of this text. For profiles of drugs in this class, see epinephrine (Adrenalin) and norepinephrine (Levophed) in Chapter 18, oxymetazoline (Afrin) in Chapter 20, and salmeterol (Serevent) in Chapter 24 ⬤▭.

Concept review 6.2

■ Why do the sympathomimetics produce many of the same symptoms as the anticholinergics?

ADRENERGIC-BLOCKERS

Adrenergic-blockers inhibit the sympathetic nervous system. These agents produce many of the same rest-and-relaxation symptoms as the parasympathomimetics, but they are more widely used.

6.9 Adrenergic-blockers are primarily used for hypertension and are the most widely prescribed class of autonomic drugs.

Because the sympathetic nervous system has alpha and beta-subreceptors, the actions of adrenergic-blockers are specific and have wide therapeutic application. In fact, they are the most widely prescribed class of autonomic drugs. Some of the adrenergic-blockers are shown in Table 6.5.

Alpha-adrenergic-blockers, or simply *alpha-blockers,* are primarily used for their effects on vascular smooth muscle. By relaxing vascular smooth muscle in small arteries, alpha$_1$-blockers such as doxazosin (Cardura) cause vasodilation which results in decreased blood pressure. Their primary use is in the treatment of hypertension, either alone or in combination with other agents.

Some drugs in this class selectively block beta$_1$-receptors. Because beta$_1$-receptors are only present in the heart, the effects of drugs such as atenolol (Tenormin) are often called *cardioselective.* By slowing the heart rate, they lower blood pressure, which is their primary use.

Some beta-blockers, such as propranolol (Inderal), are non-selective, blocking both beta$_1$ and beta$_2$-receptors. The non-selective beta-blockers are used to treat hypertension, angina, and cardiac rhythm abnormalities. Their non-selective actions generally result in more side effects than the selective beta-blockers. Profiles of adrenergic-blockers can be found for doxazosin (Cardura) in Chapter 14, propranolol (Inderal) in Chapter 16, and atenolol (Tenormin) and metoprolol (Lopressor) in Chapter 17 ⬤▭.

TABLE 6.5	Selected Adrenergic-Blockers	
DRUG	**PRIMARY RECEPTOR SUBTYPE**	**PRIMARY USE**
acebutolol (Sectral)	beta$_1$	hypertension, dysrhythmias, angina
atenolol (Tenormin)	beta$_1$	hypertension and angina
carteolol (Cartrol)	beta$_1$ and beta$_2$	hypertension and glaucoma
carvedilol (Coreg)	alpha$_1$, beta$_1$, and beta$_2$	hypertension
doxazocin (Cardura)	alpha$_1$	hypertension
esmolol (Brevibloc)	beta$_1$	hypertension and dysrhythmias
metoprolol (Lopressor)	beta$_1$	hypertension
nadolol (Corgard)	beta$_1$ and beta$_2$	hypertension
phentolamine (Regitine)	alpha	severe hypertension
prazosin (Minipress)	alpha$_1$	hypertension
propranolol (Inderal)	beta$_1$ and beta$_2$	dysrhythmias, hypertension, migranes, angina
sotalol (Betapace)	beta$_1$ and beta$_2$	dysrhythmias
terazosin (Hytrin)	alpha$_1$	hypertension
timolol (Blocadren, Timoptic)	beta$_1$ and beta$_2$	hypertension, angina, glaucoma

CLIENT TEACHING

Clients treated with autonomic medications need to know the following:

1. If you are taking prescription autonomic medications, do not take any OTC cold, cough, or sinus drugs without seeking medical advice because these likely contain autonomic agents.

2. Some of the most significant side effects of autonomic drugs relate to the cardiovascular system. Report any palpitations, shortness of breath, chest pain, or large changes in blood pressure immediately to your healthcare provider.

3. Be sure to notify your healthcare provider if you have thyroid disease, diabetes mellitus, dysrhythmias, or hypertension before taking autonomic drugs. These medications have the potential to cause serious side effects in clients with these conditions.

4. Do not discontinue the use of beta-blockers abruptly, as this can result in chest pain or rebound hypertension.

5. Many of the autonomics affect blood pressure. Move slowly when changing from a supine to an upright position to avoid dizziness and perhaps fainting.

6. If you experience a significant change in bowel habits or abdominal cramping after taking autonomic drugs, notify your healthcare provider.

7. Inform your healthcare provider before taking anticholinergic drugs if you have difficulty urinating or have been diagnosed with benign prostatic hypertrophy (BPH).

8. If you experience dry mouth when taking autonomic drugs, chew gum or suck on hard candies. Proper oral hygiene is important to avoid dental caries.

9. Alpha-blockers can sometimes cause impotence as a side effect. If you are having difficulties with ejaculation, notify your healthcare provider so that other drug options may be explored. ■

Concept review 6.3

■ Both parasympathomimetics and adrenergic-blockers produce similar actions. Why are the adrenergic-blockers used to treat hypertension, but the parasympathomimetics not used for this purpose?

CHAPTER REVIEW

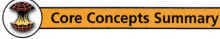 **Core Concepts Summary**

6.1 The peripheral nervous system is divided into somatic and autonomic components.

The peripheral nervous system consists of all nerves lying outside the brain and spinal cord. It consists of a voluntary portion (somatic) and an involuntary portion (autonomic).

6.2 The autonomic nervous system has sympathetic and parasympathetic branches.

Stimulation of sympathetic nerves causes symptoms of the fight-or-flight response. Stimulation of parasympathetic nerves induces the rest-and-relaxation response. With few exceptions, the actions of the two divisions are opposite of each other.

6.3 Synapses are common sites of drug action.

Synapses consist of a presynaptic nerve and a postsynaptic nerve with a physical space between them called the synaptic cleft. Neurotransmitters cross this synaptic cleft to regenerate the nerve impulse.

6.4 Acetylcholine and norepinephrine are the two primary neurotransmitters in the autonomic nervous system.

Acetylcholine is the neurotransmitter at the end of all presynaptic nerves (ganglia), at sweat glands, and in skeletal muscle. Ach receptors may be nicotinic or muscarinic. Norepinephrine is the neurotransmitter at the organ level in the sympathetic nervous system. NE receptors may be alpha or beta subtypes.

6.5 Autonomic drugs are classified by which receptors they stimulate or block.

Sympathomimetics stimulate sympathetic nerves and parasympathomimetics primarily stimulate parasympathetic nerves. Adrenergic-blockers inhibit the sympathetic division, whereas cholinergic-blockers mostly inhibit the parasympathetic branch.

6.6 Parasympathomimetics have few therapeutic uses because of their numerous side effects.

Parasympathomimetics are used to stimulate the urinary or digestive tracts following general anesthesia. Some are used for their effects at acetylcholine receptors in skeletal muscle for the treatment of myasthenia gravis.

6.7 Anticholinergics are used to dry secretions, treat asthma, and prevent motion sickness.

The use of cholinergic-blockers has declined due to their numerous side effects. They are used to dry secretions, to dilate the bronchi, and to dilate the pupil.

6.8 Sympathomimetics are primarily used for their effects on the heart, bronchial tree, and nasal passages.

Sympathomimetics may stimulate one or several subtypes of adrenergic-receptors. Uses include increasing the heart rate, dilating the bronchi, and drying excess secretions caused by colds.

6.9 Adrenergic-blockers are primarily used for hypertension and are the most widely prescribed class of autonomic drugs.

Adrenergic-blockers comprise the most commonly prescribed autonomic medications. They may be selective for only one receptor subtype, such as the beta$_1$-blockers, or inhibit several subtypes. Hypertension is their primary indication.

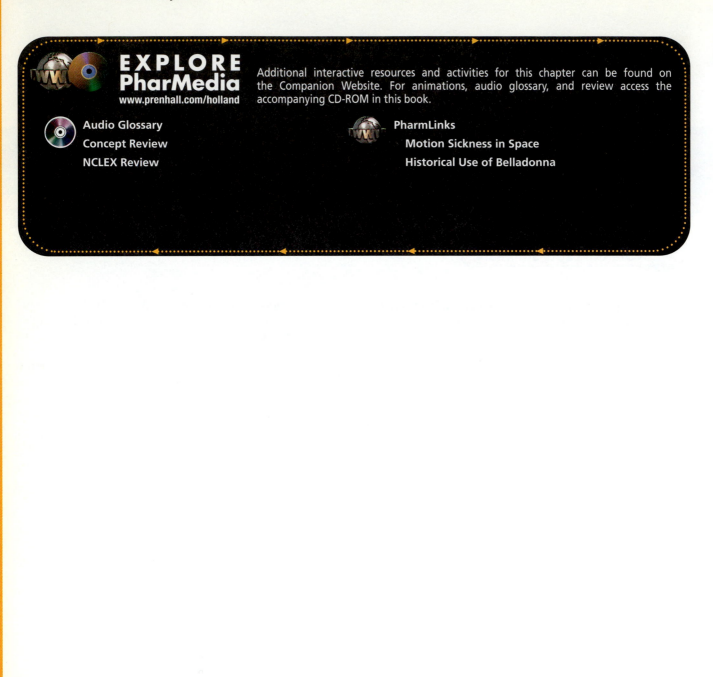

EXPLORE PharMedia
www.prenhall.com/holland

Additional interactive resources and activities for this chapter can be found on the Companion Website. For animations, audio glossary, and review access the accompanying CD-ROM in this book.

Audio Glossary
Concept Review
NCLEX Review

PharmLinks
    Motion Sickness in Space
    Historical Use of Belladonna

7 Drugs for Anxiety, Daytime Sedation, and Insomnia

CORE CONCEPTS

ANXIETY

7.1 The two major classifications of anxiety are generalized disorder and panic disorder.

7.2 Specific regions of the brain are responsible for anxiety and wakefulness.

CNS Depressants

7.3 Central nervous system (CNS) depressants are used to treat anxiety and restlessness.

Benzodiazepines

7.4 Benzodiazepines are drugs of choice for anxiety.

INSOMNIA

7.5 Insomnia, an inability to experience normal sleep, has more than one cause.

7.6 The electroencephalogram is used to diagnose sleep and seizure disorders.

7.7 Benzodiazepines may be prescribed for certain types of sleep disorders.

Barbiturates

7.8 Barbiturates are used for the short-term therapy of severe insomnia.

OBJECTIVES

After reading this chapter, the student should be able to:

1. Describe the major categories of anxiety and explain differences in how they might be treated pharmacologically.

2. Identify the two primary regions of the brain affected by stress and tension.

3. Compare and contrast the terms sedative, hypnotic, and anxiolytic.

4. Describe the different types of insomnia and explain their possible causes.

5. Explain why knowledge of sleep stages is important in drug therapy, and explain how sleep stages are measured.

6. For each of the following classes, know representative drugs, explain the mechanisms of drug action, primary actions, and important adverse effects.
   a. benzodiazepines
   b. barbiturates
   c. non-barbiturate CNS depressants

7. Categorize drugs used for anxiety and sedation based on their classification and mechanism of action.

PharMedia
www.prenhall.com/holland

Additional interactive resources and activities for this chapter can be found on the Companion Website. For animations, audio glossary, and review access the accompanying CD-ROM in this book.

More clients routinely experience nervousness and tension than any other symptom. Most healthcare providers agree that even though drugs are not the cure for this problem, they can help on a short-term basis to calm clients who are apprehensive or have difficulty falling asleep. This chapter deals with the various classes of drugs that treat anxiety, cause sedation, or help clients to sleep.

ANXIETY

Anxiety is a state of apprehension or dread and autonomic nervous system stimulation resulting from exposure to an unidentified threat.

7.1 The two major classifications of anxiety are generalized anxiety disorder and panic disorder.

According to the *International Classification of Diseases,* 10th revision (ICD-10), anxiety is a state of "apprehension, tension, or uneasiness that stems from the anticipation of danger, the source of which is largely unknown or unrecognized." There are two primary categories of anxiety. The two major types are referred to as *generalized anxiety,* and *panic disorder.* Other serious anxiety disorders include specific phobias, obsessive-compulsive disorder, and post-traumatic stress disorder. These disorders differ from generalized anxiety and panic attack because they often require more extensive behavioral therapy.

Generalized anxiety is characterized as difficult to control, excessive anxiety that lasts six months or more and interferes with normal day-to-day functions or causes considerable distress. Panic disorder, on the other hand, is characterized by episodes of immediate and intense apprehension, fearfulness, or terror associated with dread of future attacks and changes in behavior to avoid them. When a panic attack occurs, it is usually over within ten minutes, although it may be described by a client as seemingly endless.

TABLE 7.1	Common Phobias That Might Involve Anxiety Symptoms
acrophobia	fear of heights
agoraphobia	fear of leaving a familiar setting such as one's home
ailurophobia	fear of cats
algophobia	fear of pain
arachnophobia	fear of spiders
claustrophobia	fear of closed spaces
mysophobia	fear of dirt or germs
panophobia	fear of a wide variety of different situations, objects, or activities

phobia = fear

Phobias are fearful feelings attached to specific situations or objects that compel a client to avoid the fearful stimulus. Table 7.1 includes a list of common phobias. Obsessive-compulsive disorder involves recurrent, intrusive impulses or thoughts and repetitive behaviors aimed at reducing the distress associated with them. Post-traumatic stress disorder is a type of anxiety that develops in response to the threat or experience of severe injury or death. War, physical or sexual abuse, natural disasters, and murder may lead to a sense of helplessness and re-experiencing of the traumatic event.

anxio = anxiety
lytic = to dissolve away; break

In all of these cases, anxiolytics, or drugs having the ability to relieve anxiety, might be indicated; however, most of the anxiolytic drugs mentioned in this chapter are meant to address anxiety on a short term basis. Longer-term pharmacotherapy for phobias, obsessive-compulsive and post-traumatic stress disorders may include mood disorder drugs (Chapter 9 ⊂⊃).

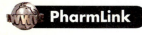

STRATEGIES FOR REDUCING STRESS

It is more productive to discover and to address the cause of anxiety rather than to disconnect from the symptoms through the use of drugs. When anxiety becomes severe enough to interfere with daily activities of life, drug therapy may be used while the client develops coping strategies to deal with the underlying causes.

Fast Facts Anxiety Disorders

- About 19,000,000 Americans experience anxiety every year.
- Other illnesses commonly co-exist with anxiety, including depression, eating disorders, and substance abuse.
- The top five causes of anxiety (listed in order) between the ages of 18–54 are:
  phobia (most common)
  post-traumatic stress
  generalied anxiety
  obsessive-compulsive feelings
  panic
- For details, see the National Institute of Mental Health Web site: http://www.nimh.nih.gov/anxiety/adfacts.cfm).

Concept review 7.1

- What does the term *anxiolytic* mean? For what kinds of disorders might anxiolytic drugs be used?

7.2 Specific regions of the brain are responsible for anxiety and wakefulness.

It is important to understand how anxiety might develop in relation to brain anatomy (see Figure 7.1). Neural systems associated with anxiety and restlessness include the limbic system and the reticular activating system.

ON THE JOB

Mental Health Nursing

A mental health nurse working for a large organization or counseling service is in a position to en-counter many clients who are restless and worried. Being familiar with how stress affects an individ-ual is of foremost importance in such a job because an understanding of stress factors will often dictate how problems should be treated. Medication is a short-term solution to anxiety and restlessness. Sometimes all clients need is a little bit of help until they can develop coping skills sufficiently to deal with a problem (or to remove themselves from a problem). Anxiolytics and sleep medication often pro-vide that extra help needed to cope. Of course, connected with this is always the possibility for drug abuse: some clients rely too strongly on medication and see it as a long-term solution rather than a short-term one. The mental health nurse often has to become a counselor and relay the important message that medication is meant to help solve a problem—not create another problem. ▪

The **limbic system** is a region in the middle of the brain responsible for emotional expression, learn-ing, and memory. Its physical relationship to the hypothalamus is shown in Figure 7.2a. The hypo-thalamus is an important center responsible for unconscious responses to extreme stress such as high blood pressure, elevated breathing rate, and dilated pupils. These are responses associated with the fight-or-flight response of the autonomic nervous system as discussed in Chapter 6. The hypothala-mus's many functions related to the endocrine system are also discussed in Chapter 28 ▭▭ .

Signals routed through the limbic system ultimately connect with the hypothalamus. Emo-tional states associated with this connection include anxiety, fear, anger, aggression, remorse, de-pression, sexual drive, and euphoria.

The hypothalamus also connects with the **reticular formation**, a network of neurons found along the entire length of the brain stem, as shown in Figure 7.2b. Stimulation of the reticular for-mation causes heightened alertness and arousal, while inhibition of the reticular formation causes general drowsiness and the induction of sleep.

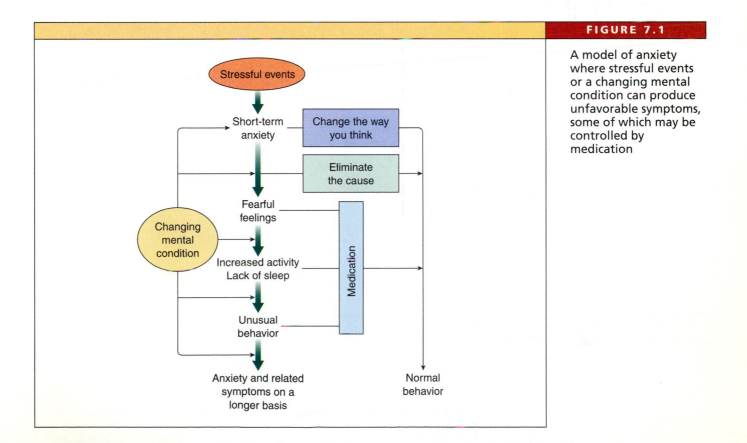

FIGURE 7.1

A model of anxiety where stressful events or a changing mental condition can produce unfavorable symptoms, some of which may be controlled by medication

FIGURE 7.2

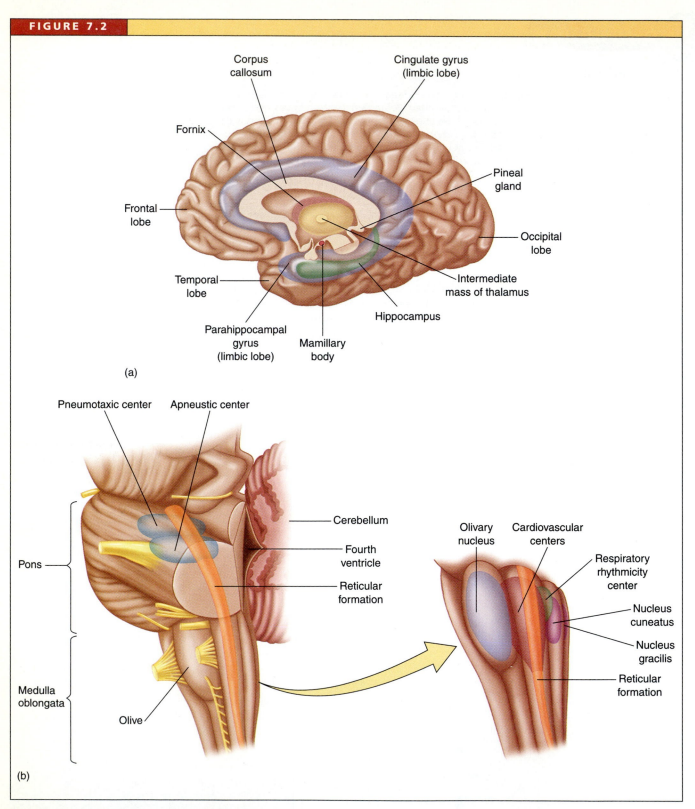

(a)

(b)

Two regions of the brain are strongly associated with anxiety, expressions of emotion, and a restless state: a) the limbic system and b) the reticular formation, a nucleus where nervous signals ascend to higher centers of the brain; this entire neural network is called the reticular activating system

The larger area in which the reticular formation is found is called the reticular activating system (RAS). This structure projects from the brain stem to the thalamus. The reticular activating system is responsible for sleeping and wakefulness and performs an alerting function for the cerebral cortex. It also helps a client to focus attention on individual tasks by transmitting information to higher brain centers.

If signals are prevented from passing through the RAS, no emotional signals are sent to the brain, resulting in a reduction in the general activity of the brain. If signals coming from the hypothalamus are allowed to proceed, then those signals are further routed through the RAS and on to higher brain centers. This is the neural mechanism thought to be responsible for emotions such as anxiety and fear. It is also the mechanism associated with restlessness and an interrupted sleeping pattern.

CENTRAL NERVOUS SYSTEM DEPRESSANTS

CNS depressants are drugs used to calm clients experiencing anxiety. These drugs are classified as benzodiazepines, barbiturates, and non-barbiturate CNS depressants.

7.3 Central nervous system (CNS) depressants are used to treat anxiety and restlessness.

CNS depressants are drugs used to calm clients suffering from anxiety and restlessness. The three major classes of drugs used to treat anxiety are the benzodiazepines, barbiturates, and non-barbiturate CNS depressants.

Some drugs that depress the central nervous system are also called sedatives because of their ability to sedate or relax a client. Hypnotics are CNS depressant drugs prescribed to help clients sleep. Thus, the term sedative-hypnotic is often used to describe a class of drugs with the ability to produce a calming effect at lower doses while causing sleep at higher doses. The term tranquilizer is sometimes used to describe a drug that produces a calm or tranquil feeling.

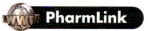

NATIONAL INSTITUTE OF MENTAL HEALTH

Concept review 7.2

▪ Describe what each of following terms means in relation to anxiety and alertness: *CNS depressants, sedatives, hypnotics, sedative-hypnotics* and *tranquilizers.*

BENZODIAZEPINES

The benzodiazepines are widely-prescribed drugs that treat anxiety and insomnia. The term *benzodiazepine* partly comes from the root word *benzo,* having to do with aromatic compounds. In chemistry, an aromatic compound is a class of chemicals having a ring structure attached to different atoms or another carbon ring. Two nitrogen atoms are incorporated into the ring structure, the reason for the *diazepine* name.

benzo = aromatic or ring structure
di = two
azepine = nitrogen-containing

7.4 Benzodiazepines are drugs of choice for anxiety.

Barbiturates (Section 7.9) were once commonly prescribed for anxiety. However, benzodiazepines are now drugs of choice for anxiety because of their greater margin of safety. The first benzodiazepines—chlordiazepoxide (Librium) and diazepam (Valium)—were introduced in the1960s. Because of their abuse potential, they are classified as Schedule IV drugs. They are also prescribed for seizure activity and alcohol withdrawal symptoms (Chapter 8), central muscle relaxation (Chapter 30), and as induction agents in general anesthesia (Chapter 12 ⌼).

DRUG PROFILE:
Diazepam (Valium)

Actions:

Diazepam produces its effects by suppressing neuronal activity in the limbic system and subsequent impulses that might be transmitted to the reticular activating system. Effects of this drug are calming without strong sedation and skeletal muscle relaxation. Maximum therapeutic effects may take from one to two weeks. Tolerance usually develops after about four weeks.

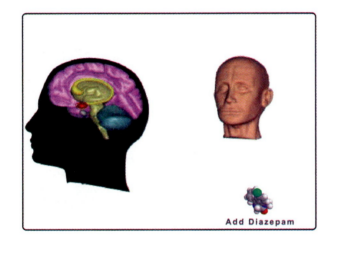

Add Diazepam

Adverse Effects:

Diazepam should not be taken with alcohol because of their combined sedative effects. Other drugs interactions include cimetidine (potentiates diazepam's action), levodopa (decreases diazepam's action), and phenytoin (diazepam increases the levels of this drug in the bloodstream). Smoking increases the metabolism of diazepam, thus lowering its effectiveness. When given IV, diazepam may cause hypotension, muscular weakness, tachycardia, and respiratory depression. Because of diazepam's potential for psychological dependence (chapter 6), long-term therapy should be discouraged, especially in clients who have a history of substance abuse.

Mechanism in Action:

The many therapeutic uses of diazepham include antianxiety and antiseizure activity, sedation, and skeletal muscle relaxation. These effects are produced by activation of gamma aminobutyric acid (GABA) receptors located throughout the central nervous system. When GABA receptors are activated, negatively charged chloride ions rush into the neuron and lower its negative charge. This inhibits action potentials.

Benzodiazepines act by binding to the gamma amino butyric acid (GABA) receptor-chloride channel molecule. These drugs intensify the effect of GABA, which is a natural inhibitory neurotransmitter found throughout the brain. Almost all of the benzodiazepines have the same action and adverse effects and differ only in their onset and duration of action.

Concept review 7.3

■ What is the major drug class used to treat generalized anxiety disorder and panic disorder? Name popular drugs within this class.

INSOMNIA

Insomnia is a condition characterized by a client's inability to fall asleep or remain asleep. Pharmacotherapy may be indicated if the sleeplessness interferes with normal daily activities.

TABLE 7.2	Drugs for Generalized Anxiety and/or Panic Attack	
DRUG	**ROUTE AND ADULT DOSE**	**REMARKS**
Pr diazepam (Valium)	PO; 2–10 mg bid; IM/IV; 2–10 mg, repeat if needed in 3–4 hrs.	For generalized anxiety, mild anxiety experienced before a medical procedure, and short-term treatment of anxiety symptoms.
alprazolam (Xanax)	For anxiety: PO 0.25–0.5 mg tid. For panic attacks: PO 1–2 mg tid.	For short-term treatment of anxiety symptoms and panic attack.
buspirone hydrochloride (Buspar)	PO; 7.5–15 mg in divided doses; may increase by 5 mg/day every 2–3 days if needed (max 60 mg/day).	Unrelated to benzodiazepines or barbiturates; used for short-term treatment of anxiety symptoms and management of major disorders associated with anxiety; acts by binding to brain dopamine and serotonin receptors.
chlordiazepoxide hydrochloride (Librium)	Mild anxiety: PO 5–10 mg tid or qid; IM/IV 50–100 mg 1 hr before a medical procedure. Severe anxiety: PO 20–25 mg tid or qid; IM/IV 50–100 mg followed by 25–50 mg tid or qid.	The first benzodiazepine made available to the public; for mild anxiety, tension experienced before a medical procedure, and severe anxiety.
clonazepam (Klonopin)	PO; 1–2 mg/day in divided doses (max 4 mg/day).	This medication is more popular as an anti-seizure medication; its unlabeled use is treatment for panic disorder.
clorazepate dipotassium (Tranxene)	PO; 15 mg/day at hs (may increase to 60 mg/day in divided doses).	For short-term treatment of anxiety symptoms.
halazepam (Paxipam)	PO; 20–40 mg tid or qid.	For short-term treatment of anxiety symptoms and management of anxiety disorders.
lorazepam (Ativan)	PO; 2–6 mg/day in divided doses (max 10 mg/day).	For anxiety disorders and short-term relief of anxiety symptoms; often used to reduce anxiety in preoperative clients.
oxazepam (Serax)	PO; 10–30 mg tid or qid.	For the management of anxiety and a wide range of emotional disturbances.

7.5 Insomnia, an inability to experience normal sleep, has more than one cause.

Another disorder sometimes connected with anxiety is insomnia. There are several major types of insomnia. Short-term or behavioral insomnia may be attributed to stress caused by a hectic lifestyle. When stress interrupts normal sleeping patterns, clients cannot sleep because their minds are too active. Worry about work, marriage, children, or health is a common reason for short-term loss of sleep.

TABLE 7.3	Suggestions for Reestablishing a Healthful Sleep Regimen

1. Establish regular times for going to bed and rising. Turn the clock face away from your view. Select and play one piece of music to signal that it is time to sleep, perhaps a favorite song. Avoid checking the time during night awakenings.

2. Avoid napping. Fill your day with activities you consider worthwhile.

3. Limit stimulants such as caffeine, chocolate, nicotine, and amphetamines, or limit stimulant use to the first part of your day.

4. Practice alcohol moderation or abstinence. Avoid alcohol intake close to bedtime.

5. Exercise at least three times a week a minimum of two to three hours before bedtime. Eat a moderate dinner. Avoid large, high fat snacks near bedtime.

6. Develop a comfortable sleep environment: cool, dark, at an acceptable noise level, private, and with comfortable bedding. If possible, redecorate the bedroom to project a relaxing atmosphere.

7. Plan for the next day, and then consciously decide to set your concerns aside. Learn and practice stress reduction and relaxation techniques.

8. Obtain treatment for sleep apnea, depression, anxiety, and pain if these are underlying causes for your sleep disturbance.

9. Limit sedatives and hypnotics to short-term use for insomnia.

10. Discuss with your healthcare practitioner sleep problems while on these medications: amphetamines, antidepressants, antihypertensives, antimetabolites, beta-blockers, bronchodilators, decongestants, thyroid hormones, and hypnotics.

11. Consult your healthcare practitioner before taking supplements for insomnia. Chamomile, hawthorn, kava-kava, lemon balm, melatonin, and valerian are often advertised for their calming or sleep-inducing effects.

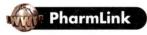

PharmLink

NATIONAL CENTER ON SLEEP
DISORDERS RESEARCH

Foods or beverages containing stimulants such as caffeine may interrupt sleep. Clients may also find that the use of tobacco products makes them restless and edgy. Stressful conditions such as too much light, uncomfortable room temperature, snoring, sleep apnea, and recurring nightmares also interfere with sleep. Suggestions for reestablishing a healthful sleep regimen are provided in Table 7.3.

Long-term insomnia may be caused by psychiatric disorders, chronic pain, and medication side-effects. In these cases, healthcare practitioners may prescribe a short course of hypnotics while helping clients address the underlying psychological and physiological concerns.

Long-term use of sleeping medications is likely to worsen insomnia and may cause physical or psychological dependence. Older clients, who more often use hypnotics, are also more inclined to experience medication-related problems. Some clients may experience a phenomenon referred to as rebound insomnia when hypnotic medication is discontinued abruptly or after its being taken for a long time: sleeplessness and symptoms of anxiety become markedly worse.

Fast Facts Insomnia

- One-third of the world's population has trouble sleeping during part of the year.
- Insomnia is more common in women than in men.
- Clients older than 65 sleep less than any other age group.
- Only about 70% of people with insomnia ever report this problem to their practitioner.
- People buy OTC sleep medications and combination drugs with sleep additives more than any other drug category. Trade name products include Anacin P. M., Exedrin P. M., Nytol, Quiet World, Sleep-Fez, Sominex, Tylenol P. M., and Unisom.
- As a natural alternative for sleep, some clients take melatonin, kava kava, or valerian.

Concept review 7.4

- Why might a client not be able to enjoy normal sleep? Why is long-term drug therapy for lack of sleep not a good idea?

7.6 The electroencephalogram is used to diagnose sleep and seizure disorders.

Health professionals often assist with or perform a procedure called the electroencephalogram (EEG), a tool for the diagnosis of many disorders, including insomnia, seizure activity, depression, and dementia. Four types of brainwaves—alpha, beta, delta, and theta—are identified on the basis of their shape, frequencies, and height on a graph. Brainwaves give the health practitioner an idea of how brain activity changes during various stages of sleep and consciousness. For example, alpha waves indicate an awake but drowsy client. Beta waves indicate an alert client whose mind is active.

With the EEG, researchers have identified two types of sleep: REM (rapid eye movement) sleep and non-REM (rapid eye movement) sleep. REM sleep is often called *paradoxical sleep* because this stage has a brain wave pattern similar to when clients are drowsy but awake. This is the stage when dreaming occurs. Clients with normal sleep patterns move from REM to non-REM sleep about every 90 minutes. Lack of adequate amounts of REM sleep may result in serious consequences such as sleep debt, impaired judgment, depression, and slowed reaction time.

Non-REM sleep, identified on the basis of a range of EEG recordings, is divided into four different stages. The following are the stages of REM and non-REM sleep.

- Non-REM Stage 1—At the onset of sleep, the client is in a stage of drowsiness for about one to seven minutes and may easily be awakened. This stage lasts for about 4–5% of total sleep time.

- Non-REM Stage 2—Client can still be easily awakened. Comprises the greatest amount of total sleep time, 45–55%.

- Non-REM Stage 3—Client may move into or out of a deeper sleep. Heart rate and blood pressure fall; gastrointestinal activity rises. This stage lasts for about 4–6% of total sleep time.

- Non-REM Stage 4—The deepest stage of sleep; lasts a little longer than Stage 1 or Stage 3 sleep, about 12–15%. This is the stage during which nightmares and sleep-walking occur in children. Heart rate and blood pressure remain low; gastrointestinal activity remains high.

- REM sleep—Characterized by eye movement and a loss of muscle tone. Eye movement occurs in bursts of activity (hence, rapid) and dreaming takes place. The mind is very active and resembles a normal waking state.

7.7 Benzodiazepines may be prescribed for certain types of sleep disorders.

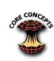

Because of their relative safety in higher doses, benzodiazepines are drugs of choice for short-term insomnia caused by anxiety. These drugs shorten the amount of time it takes for a client to fall asleep and reduce the frequency of interrupted sleep. Although most benzodiazepines increase total sleep time, some reduce stage four sleep. Some drugs in this class affect REM. In general, a different group of benzodiazepines from those drugs used to treat general anxiety and panic disorder are used to treat short-term insomnia. These are summarized in Table 7.4.

BARBITURATES

Barbiturates are drugs derived from barbituric acid; they act as CNS depressants and are used for their sedative, hypnotic, and anti-seizure effects.

7.8 Barbiturates are used for the short-term therapy of severe insomnia.

At low to medium doses, barbiturates reduce anxiety and cause drowsiness. At higher doses, they promote sleep, presumably by inhibiting brain impulses traveling through areas of the limbic system and the reticular activating system. Depending on the method of drug delivery, barbiturates

TABLE 7.4	Benzodiazepines for Short-Term Treatment of Insomnia	
DRUG	**ROUTE AND ADULT DOSE**	**REMARKS**
estazolam (ProSom)	PO; 1 mg at hs, may increase to 2 mg if necessary.	For short-term management of insomnia; reduces sleep stages 3 and 4 and REM sleep.
flurazepam (Dalmane)	PO; 15–30 mg at hs.	Induces sleep and increases total sleep time; reduces stage 4 sleep, the deepest sleep stage.
quazepam (Doral)	PO; 7.5–15 mg at hs.	Induces sleep, but significantly increases total sleep time; REM sleep remains unchanged.
temazepam (Restoril)	PO; 7.5–30 mg at hs.	Improves sleep parameters such as night and early morning awakenings; does NOT induce sleep; produces minimal change in REM sleep pattern.
triazolam (Halcion)	PO; 0.125–0.25 mg at hs; max 0.5 mg/day.	Improves parameters such as sleep time, night awakenings, and induces sleep.

may also induce anesthesia (Chapter 12 ⚬⚬). Therapy with barbiturates should be short-term because of the risk of psychological and physical dependence.

Like benzodiazepines, barbiturates act by binding to GABA receptor-chloride channel molecules, intensifying the effect of GABA throughout the brain. Barbiturates of importance for daytime sedation and insomnia are listed in Table 7.5. The anti-convulsant actions of barbiturates are discussed in Chapter 8 ⚬⚬ .

Non-barbiturate CNS depressants may also be used to treat insomnia. These agents, like barbiturates, are especially dangerous if administered in high doses. Respiratory depression occurs with overdose, and this can be fatal. They offer no particular advantage over the barbiturates and

DRUG PROFILE:
Secobarbital (Seconal)

Actions:

Although secobarbital acts by the same mechanism as diazepam (Valium), effects are slightly different. Secobarbital is used for preoperative sedation, to induce sleep, for convulsions, and as an adjunct in spinal anesthesia. This drug may also be used to calm clients who are extremely agitated. Absorption is rapid from 15 to 30 minutes when taken orally. Effects may begin as soon as one to three minutes after administration. When given by the oral route, effects last from one to four hours; IV effects last around 15 minutes.

Adverse Effects:

Like other barbiturates, secobarbital stimulates liver enzymes thereby increasing its own metabolism and reducing it own effectiveness with subsequent doses. It also reduces the effectiveness of related drugs with repeated use. This drug should be avoided during pregnancy, as it has a Category D classification. It causes extreme drowsiness, impaired judgment, respiratory depression, and hypotension when administered in higher doses. Close monitoring helps to prevent fatal respiratory depression due to overdose. It is not compatible with alcohol or some antidepressants (MAO inhibitors). Secobarbital may also produce irritability or restlessness in some clients, especially children, the elderly, and clients with pain. Long-term therapy may result in nutritional deficiencies; therefore, levels of folate (B$_9$) and vitamin D should be monitored. There is also a risk of dependence with long-term use. Secobarbital is a Schedule III drug. Withdrawal symptoms may be severe, as discussed in Chapter 6.

TABLE 7.5	Barbiturates for Daytime Sedation or Short-Term Treatment of Insomnia	
DRUG	**ROUTE AND ADULT DOSE**	**REMARKS**
Short Acting		
pentobarbital sodium (Nembutal)	Sedation: PO; 20–30 mg bid; qid. To induce sleep: PO; 120–200 mg. IM; 150–200 mg.	For daytime sedation; given prior to manipulative or diagnostic procedures; induces sleep.
Pr secobarbital (Seconal)	Sedation: PO; 100–300 mg/day in 3 divided doses. To induce sleep: PO/IM; 100–200 mg.	For sedation; may be used to induce sleep.
Intermediate Acting		
aprobarbital (Alurate)	Sedative: PO; 40 mg tid. Insomnia: PO; 40–160 mg.	For daytime sedation and short-term relief of insomnia; clients should not take this drug more than two weeks.
butabarbital sodium (Butisol)	PO; 50–100 mg at hs. Sedative: PO; 15–30 mg tid or qid.	For relief of anxiety; for short-term treatment of insomnia.
Longer Acting		
amobarbital (Amytal)	Sedative: PO; 30–50 mg bid or tid. Insomnia: PO/IM; 65–200 mg (max 500 mg).	For daytime sedation in cases where a client is agitated; also for short-term relief of insomnia.
phenobarbital (Luminal)	PO; 30–120 mg/day. IV/IM; 100–200 mg/day.	For sedation in cases when a client is extremely anxious.

should only be used short-term. CNS depressants of importance for sedation and treatment of insomnia are listed in Table 7.6.

Concept review 7.5

- Identify the two major drug classes used for daytime sedation and insomnia. Why are CNS depressants especially dangerous if administered in high doses?

TABLE 7.6	Other CNS Depressants for Daytime Sedation or Short-Term Treatment of Insomnia	
DRUG	**ROUTE AND ADULTS DOSE**	**REMARKS**
zolpidem (Ambien)	PO; 5–10 mg at hs.	Benzodiazepine-like drug for short-term treatment of insomnia preserves deep sleep. Limit use to 7 to 10 days.
ethchlorvynol (Placidyl)	Sedation: PO; 200 mg bid or tid. To induce sleep: PO; 500 mg–1 g at hs.	For short-term treatment of insomnia; clients should avoid taking this drug more than one week.
meprobamate (Equanil)	Sedation: PO; 1.2–1.6 g/day in 3–4 divided doses (max 2.4 g/day). To induce sleep: PO 400–800 mg.	For anxiety and tension in extremely agitated clients; promotes sleep.
paraldehyde (Paracetaldehyde)	Sedation: PO; 5–10 ml prn. To induce sleep: 10–30 ml prn. Oral doses must be diluted before they are administered.	For clients who are extremely anxious and agitated; often used for anxiety in cases of alcohol withdrawal.
chloral hydrate (Noctec)	Sedation: PO or by suppositories; 250 mg tid after meals. To induce sleep: PO; 500 mg–1 g 15–30 min before hs.	For general sedation and for short-term management of insomania, especially in the young and elderly.

NATURAL ALTERNATIVES

Valerian

Valerian root (*Valeriana officinalis*) is a popular herbal product found in Europe and North America. It is an herbal choice for nervous tension and anxiety. It is purported to promote rest without affecting REM sleep and has a reputation for calming an individual without causing side-effects or discomfort. Its name comes from the Latin *valere,* which means "to be well." One thing that is *not well* however, is its pungent odor, though many clients still claim that the smell is well worth the benefits. Valerian also is purported to reduce pain and headaches without the worry of dependency. There is no drug hangover as is sometimes experienced with tranquilizers and sedatives. It is available as a tincture (alcohol mixture), tea, or extract. Sometimes it is placed in juice and consumed immediately before taking a nap or going to bed. ■

CLIENT TEACHING

Clients taking anxiolytics and CNS depressants need to know the following:

1. It is important to avoid stimulants such as coffee, tea, and chocolate because they counteract anxiolytics and sedatives and increase the symptoms of anxiety.
2. Exercise, progressive muscle relaxation, and slow, deep breathing can assist with anxiety relief.
3. Alcohol and other CNS depressants can increase the effects of anxiolytics. They should be avoided to decrease the risk of accidental depressant overdose and death.
4. Store your anxiolytics and sedatives in a secure place to avoid accidental ingestion by children and animals. ■

CHAPTER REVIEW

Core Concepts Summary

7.1 The two major classifications of anxiety are generalized anxiety disorder and panic disorder.

Drug therapy is useful in at least five types of anxiety disorders: generalized anxiety, panic disorder, phobias, obsessive-compulsive disorder, and post-traumatic stress disorder.

7.2 Regions of the brain are responsible for anxiety and wakefulness.

Two important brain regions underlie anxiety and restlessness: the limbic system and the reticular activating system. Neural impulses transferred between these two areas of the brain are responsible for anxiety, fear, restlessness, and an interrupted sleeping pattern.

7.3 Central nervous system (CNS) depressants are used to treat anxiety and restlessness.

Sedatives, sedative-hypnotics, and CNS depressants are terms used to describe benzodiazepines, barbiturates, and other drugs. These agents suppress impulses traveling through the limbic and reticular activating systems, thereby reducing symptoms of stress, producing drowsiness, and promoting sleep.

7.4 Benzodiazepines are drugs of choice for anxiety.

Benzodiazepines are preferred over any other drug class to treat anxiety and panic attack. Diazepam, the prototype benzodiazepine, produces its effects by binding with the GABA receptor-chloride channel molecule, a natural receptor found throughout the entire brain.

7.5 Insomnia, an inability to experience normal sleep, has more than one cause.

There are many reasons why a client might experience sleepnessness. Stress is one factor in short-term insomnia. Others include caffeine, nicotine, room temperature, light, snoring, and sleep apnea. In long-term insomnia, psychological and physiological factors may be involved.

7.6 The electroencephalogram is used to diagnose sleep and seizure disorders.

The EEG is a diagnostic procedure used to examine brainwave patterns in clients with disorders such as insomnia and seizure activity. With this procedure, two types of sleep may be identified: non-REM and REM sleep.

7.7 Benzodiazepines may be prescribed for certain types of sleep disorders.

Benzodiazepines are also the drug of choice for insomnia. Several drugs are used, which generally differ from the ones used to treat anxiety.

7.8 Barbiturates are used for the short-term therapy of severe insomnia.

Barbiturates are the primary class of CNS depressants used to treat insomnia. Secobarbital, the prototype drug, produces its effects by the same mechanism as diazepam. This drug and other CNS depressants must be used cautiously to prevent accidental overdose, respiratory depression, and death.

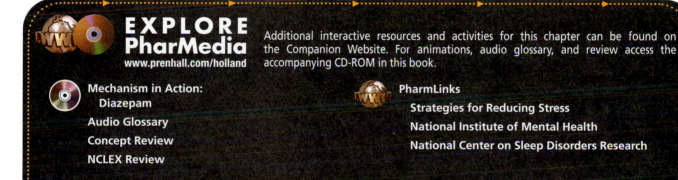

EXPLORE PharMedia
www.prenhall.com/holland

Additional interactive resources and activities for this chapter can be found on the Companion Website. For animations, audio glossary, and review access the accompanying CD-ROM in this book.

Mechanism in Action:
   Diazepam
Audio Glossary
Concept Review
NCLEX Review

PharmLinks
   Strategies for Reducing Stress
   National Institute of Mental Health
   National Center on Sleep Disorders Research

8 Drugs for Seizures

CORE CONCEPTS

SEIZURES

8.1 Seizures and convulsions are symptoms of epilepsy.

8.2 Signs of seizures are easy to recognize.

Anti-seizure Drugs

8.3 Anti-seizure drugs may be grouped within three pharmacological categories.

Drugs with GABA Action

8.4 By increasing the action of the inhibitory neurotransmitter GABA, abnormal neuronal activity can be suppressed.

Phenytoin and Phenytoin-like Drugs (Hydantoins)

8.5 Phenytoin and phenytoin-like drugs delay sodium influx into neurons.

Succinimides

8.6 Succinimides act by delaying calcium influx into neurons.

8.7 Some types of seizures are controlled by a preferred group of drugs.

8.8 Some anti-seizure drugs also control symptoms of alcohol withdrawal.

OBJECTIVES

After reading this chapter, the student should be able to:

1. Compare and contrast the terms epilepsy, seizures, and convulsions.

2. Identify the two major types of seizures.

3. Recognize signs and symptoms of specific types of seizures.

4. Explain the goal of anti-seizure medication with respect to neuronal activity.

5. Name and explain three major pharmacological categories of drugs used to control seizures.

6. For each of the following chemical classes, know representative drug examples, explain their mechanisms of action, primary actions, and important adverse effects.
   a. benzodiazepines
   b. barbiturates
   c. phenytoin and phenytoin-like drugs
   d. succinimides

7. Explain why anti-seizure medication is helpful in treating symptoms of alcohol withdrawal.

8. Categorize anti-seizure drugs based on their classification and mechanism of action.

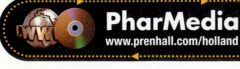

PharMedia
www.prenhall.com/holland

Additional interactive resources and activities for this chapter can be found on the Companion Website. For animations, audio glossary, and review access the accompanying CD-ROM in this book.

Epilepsy is a common disorder of the central nervous system characterized by symptoms of blackout, fainting spells, apparent clumsiness, temporary loss of memory, and/or irregular seizure activity. Over two million Americans have epilepsy, and except for when these symptoms are expressed, most of the time it appears that their health is not challenged.

Alcohol dependence is another common nervous system disorder. You may wonder what the topics of epilepsy and alcohol dependence have in common. The answer is the potential for seizures. Seizures do not occur as much when clients begin to drink as after they have been drinking for many years and try to quit. This chapter covers the very important medications used to prevent and treat seizures.

PharmLink

THE EPILEPSY FOUNDATION
OF AMERICA (EFA)

NATIONAL INSTITUTE OF
NEUROLOGICAL DISORDERS
AND STROKE

EPILEPSY CANADA

Fast Facts   Disorders Associated with Seizures

Epilepsy

- Close to 1,500,000 Americans have epilepsy.
- Most clients are under the age of 45.

Alcohol withdrawal

- About 10% of clients with alcohol dependency have problems with seizures.
- Among 400,000 adult alcoholics going to the emergency room with withdrawal complaints, 60% have seizures within six hours after arrival.

SEIZURES

Seizures are a symptom of epilepsy related to abnormal electrical activity of the brain. Seizures may cause a blank stare, a loss of consciousness, jerking body movements, or a period of general confusion for the client.

8.1 Seizures and convulsions are symptoms of epilepsy.

Seizures are caused by abnormal or uncontrollable neuronal discharges within the brain. Figure 8.1 is an example of EEG recordings for two types of seizures compared to a normal EEG recording.

FIGURE 8.1

EEG recordings showing the differences between normal, absence seizure, and generalized tonic-clonic seizure tracings

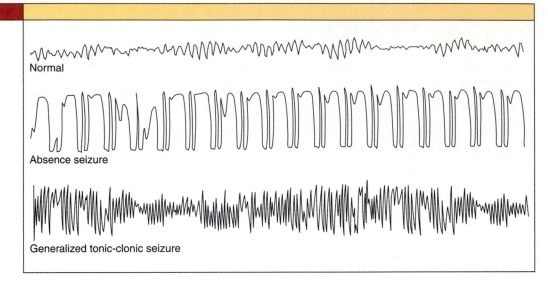

Normal

Absence seizure

Generalized tonic-clonic seizure

It is likely that seizures develop from neuronal damage or injury, although in many cases the source of injury is not known. Known causes of seizures are head trauma, extreme fever, heat exhaustion, brain tumor, infections, and stroke. Extreme metabolic shifts in the bloodstream such as lowered glucose levels or high protein levels, as seen in some pregnancies, may also cause seizures.

Some mood disorder, anti-psychotic, and local anesthetic medications given in high doses may cause seizures. Seizures may also occur from drug abuse, as with cocaine, or in situations where clients are withdrawing from alcohol or sedative-hypnotic medication.

People often confuse the term *seizure* with **convulsions**; however, convulsive symptoms are different. Convulsions are uncontrolled muscle contractions that may accompany major seizures. They are specific to only certain types of seizures and appear in cases where the brain is bombarded by electrical impulses resulting in extreme muscle tension and jerking body movements. The presence of convulsions usually indicates a more serious type of seizure.

8.2 Signs of seizures are easy to recognize.

foci = *plural of focus; a starting point*

There are two major types of seizures: **partial seizures** and **generalized seizures**. These are distinguished from each other on the basis of where neuronal impulses start and stop. Partial seizures generally start on one side of the brain and travel only a short distance before they stop. Generalized seizures, as the name suggests, are not localized to one area of the brain, but travel throughout the entire brain on both sides. Practitioners sometimes describe the areas where abnormal electrical activity start as *abnormal foci*.

Types of partial or generalized seizures may be recognized based on symptoms observed during a seizure episode. Some symptoms are very subtle and reflect the simple nature of neuronal misfiring; others are more complex. In some cases, death may result if a client undergoing seizures does not receive prompt medical attention.

The classification of seizures can be complicated; however, many signs are easy to recognize. Types of partial and generalized seizures are discussed below with their signs. Two common types of partial seizures are *simple* and *complex* seizures. Complex seizures are also called *psychomotor* or *temporal lobe* seizures because of the types of symptoms they produce or the area of the brain where abnormal neuronal activity occurs.

Simple Partial Seizures

Clients with simple partial seizures may feel for a brief moment that their precise location is vague. Often clients will hear and see things that are not there. Some clients may smell and taste things or have an upset stomach. Other clients may become emotional and experience a sense of joy, sorrow, or grief. Parts of the body such as the arms, legs, or face may start twitching in movements that travel throughout the rest of the body. Symptoms may not be very dramatic and may occur without any loss of consciousness.

Complex Partial Seizures (Psychomotor or Temporal Lobe Seizures)

Complex partial seizures usually start with a blank stare. Clients then start to chew or swallow repetitively. Some clients fumble with clothing or may wander around the room taking off their clothes. Most clients become disoriented and will not pay attention to verbal commands. Clients may look and act as if they have a psychiatric illness. After a seizure episode, clients do not remember what happened.

Absence Seizures (Petit Mal Seizures)

This type of generalized seizure most often occurs in children. Clients develop a blank stare without having any twitching facial or body movements. Seizures may last for only a few seconds. Clients then quickly recover and engage in normal activities.

Atonic Seizures (drop attacks)

These generalized seizures are called *drop attacks* because clients often stumble and fall for no apparent reason. Episodes are very brief, lasting only a matter of seconds. After these seizures, clients return to normal activities without difficulty.

a = *without*
tonic = *tension*

Myoclonic Seizures

These generalized seizures are marked by large, obvious body movements. Major muscle groups contract quickly, making a jerking motion. Clients appear unsteady and clumsy. They may fall from a sitting position or drop whatever they are holding.

myo = *muscle*
clonic = *jerking motion*

Generalized Tonic-Clonic Seizures (Grand Mal Seizures)

Generalized tonic-clonic seizures, also called *grand mal* seizures, are the most dangerous form of epilepsy. In adults, these seizures may be preceded by an *aura,* a warning that some clients describe as a spiritual feeling, a flash of light, or a special noise. Muscles then become tense, and rhythmic jerking motions develop, known as convulsions. Clients will often cry out or lose bladder or bowel control. Some clients may have difficulty breathing and turn pale or blue. After this kind of seizure, clients are momentarily disoriented and take several minutes to regain their composure. Some fall asleep after an episode.

A common type of tonic-clonic seizure in children is *febrile seizures.* This type of seizure is brought on by elevated fever, and usually occurs from ages three months to five years. As many as five percent of all children have febrile seizures. Episodes usually last up to several minutes, but shorter seizures are not uncommon. Preventing the onset of fever is the best way to control these seizures.

febrile = *fever*

Status Epilepticus

Status epilepticus is a medical emergency brought on by repeated generalized seizures and convulsions. Muscle spasms may block the airway, depriving the brain of oxygen. Other medical complications may occur, such as a severe lowering of blood pressure or an irregular heartbeat. Medical treatment involves the IV administration of anti-seizure medication. Steps must also be taken to keep the airway open.

status = *state of*
epilepticus = *seizure activity*

Concept review 8.1

▪ What is epilepsy? What is the difference between a seizure and a convulsion? Which drugs or abused substances may produce seizures? Name and identify signs of the more common types of seizures.

ANTI-SEIZURE DRUGS

Anti-seizure drugs are medications given to prevent or terminate seizures. These drugs produce their effects by inhibiting the neurotransmitter GABA, inhibiting the influx of sodium, or by delaying calcium entry into neurons.

8.3 Anti-seizure drugs may be grouped within three pharmacological categories.

In order to understand how anti-seizure drugs produce their effects, it is important to understand factors that control how neurons fire. Nutrients and ions must be delicately balanced across cell membranes before neurons will function properly. The concentration of ions such as sodium, potassium, calcium, and chloride are critical because these influence the rate and extent of neuronal activity. Nutrients such as glucose and protein also influence the rate of neuronal firing. This is very important in conditions such as diabetes and pregnancy. For example, pre-eclampsia and eclampsia are common ailments observed during pregnancy or childbirth that are characterized by the presence of seizures, some of which may be life threatening.

In a resting state, neurons are surrounded by a higher concentration of sodium, calcium, and chloride ions. Potassium levels are higher inside the cell. An influx of sodium or calcium ions into the neuron *enhances* neuronal activity, while an influx of chloride ion *suppresses* neuronal activity. Abnormal ion fluxes are the scientific basis for explaining how seizures occur at the cellular level. This is fundamental because anti-seizure drug therapy centers on controlling the movement of ions across neuronal membranes.

The goal of anti-seizure medication is to suppress neuronal activity just enough to prevent abnormal or repetitive firing. To this end, there are three mechanisms by which anti-seizure medications act. The three pharmacological categories are presented here.

- ■ drugs that stimulate an influx of chloride ion, an effect associated with the neurotransmitter GABA (drugs with GABA action)
- ■ drugs that delay an influx of sodium (phenytoin and phenytoin-like drugs)
- ■ drugs that delay an influx of calcium (succinimides)

Within three major pharmacological categories are four major *chemical categories* of anti-seizure medication: these are benzodiazepines, barbiturates, hydantoins, and succinimides. A fifth category is made up of a diverse set of drugs that are more difficult to compare chemically. These examples have been placed in a category labeled as "Miscellaneous." Table 8.1 summarizes the different classifications of anti-seizure medications. Some drugs are listed in two locations because they act by two different mechanisms.

DRUGS WITH GABA ACTION

Drugs with GABA action are drugs with an ability to mimic effects of the inhibitory neurotransmitter GABA. Benzodiazepines, barbiturates, and other miscellaneous drugs reduce seizure activity by intensifying GABA action.

8.4 By increasing the action of the inhibitory neurotransmitter GABA, abnormal neuronal activity can be suppressed.

Drugs that stimulate an influx of chloride ion interact with the GABA receptor-chloride channel molecule. A model of this receptor is shown in Figure 8.2. Whenever this receptor molecule is stimulated, chloride ions move into the cell, and this suppresses the ability of neurons to fire.

TABLE 8.1	Three Major Pharmacological Drug Classes Used to Control Seizures

DRUGS THAT STIMULATE AN INFLUX OF CHLORIDE ION (THROUGH INTERACTION WITH THE GABA RECEPTOR)

Benzodiazepines	Barbiturates	Miscellaneous
clonazepam (Klonopin)	amobarbital (Amytal)	gabapentin (Neurontin)
clorazepate (Tranxene)	pentobarbital (Nembutal)	primidone (Mysoline)
diazepam (Valium)	phenobarbital (Luminal)	tiagabine (Gabitril)
lorazepam (Ativan)	secobarbital (Seconal)	topiramate (Topamax)

DRUGS THAT DELAY AN INFLUX OF SODIUM

Hydantoins	Miscellaneous
phenytoin (Dilantin)	carbamazepine (Tegretol)
fosphenytoin (Cerebyx)	divalproex (Depakote)
	felbamate (Felbatol)
	lamotrigine (Lamictal)
	valproic acid (Depakene)
	zonisamide (Zonegran)

DRUGS THAT DELAY AN INFLUX OF CALCIUM

Succinimides	Miscellaneous
ethoxsuximide (Zarontin)	divalproex (Depakote)
methsuximide (Celontin)	valproic acid (Depakene)
phensuximide (Milontin)	zonisamide (Zonegran)

The benzodiazepines represent a major class of drugs used not only to control seizures but also anxiety (Chapter 7), skeletal muscle spasms (Chapter 30 ⬭), and alcohol withdrawal symptoms. For details on the actions and adverse effects of the benzodiazepines, refer to these chapters. Benzodiazepines used for seizures are summarized in Table 8.2.

Like benzodiazepines, barbiturates intensify the effect of GABA in the brain, thus suppressing abnormal neuronal discharges. Phenobarbital is one of the most commonly prescribed anti-seizure

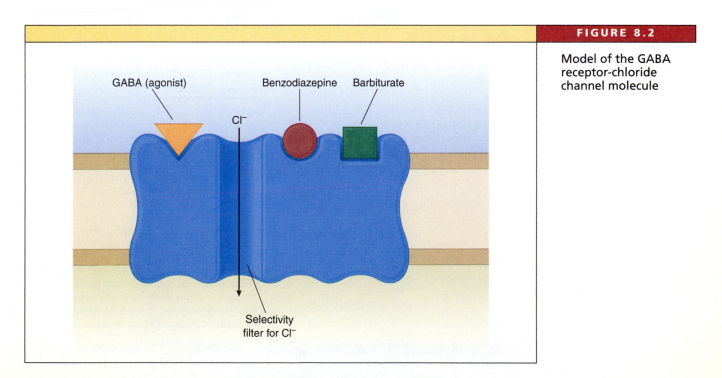

FIGURE 8.2

Model of the GABA receptor-chloride channel molecule

TABLE 8.2	Benzodiazepines Used for Seizures	
DRUG	**ROUTE AND ADULT DOSE**	**REMARKS**
diazepam (Valium)	IM/IV; 5–10 mg (repeat as needed at 10–15 min intervals up to 30 mg; repeat again as needed every 2–4 hrs). IV push; administer emulsion at 5 mg/min.	Drug of choice for status epilepticus; Also for anxiety and muscle spasms.
clonazepam (Klonopin)	PO; 1.5 mg/day in 3 divided doses, increased by 0.5–1 mg every 3 days until seizures are controlled.	For absence (petit mal) seizures and minor motor seizures; Also for panic disorder; Schedule IV drug.
clorazepate dipotassium (Tranxene)	PO; 7.5 mg tid.	For partial seizures; Also for anxiety; Schedule IV drug.
lorazepam (Ativan)	IV; 4 mg injected slowly at 2 mg/min. If inadequate response after 10 min, may repeat once.	Most potent of the available benzodiazepines; For management of status epilepticus; Also for nausea and vomiting, preoperative sedation, anxiety and insomnia; Schedule IV drug.

medications. It is also used for insomnia (see Chapter 7 ⬤▭). Barbiturates used for seizures are listed in Table 8.3.

Other drugs of importance that stimulate an influx of chloride ion are listed in Table 8.4. Many of these are newer medications approved by the FDA in the 1990s.

PHENYTOIN AND PHENYTOIN-LIKE DRUGS (HYDANTOINS)

Phenytoin-like drugs dampen neuronal activity by delaying an influx of sodium ions across neuronal membranes. Hydantoin is the chemical label sometimes used to describe drugs found within this group.

DRUG PROFILE:
Phenobarbital (Luminal)

Actions:

Phenobarbital is a longer-acting barbiturate used for the management of a variety of seizures and convulsions. It is also used for insomnia. Phenobarbital is not used for pain relief and may increase a client's sensitivity to pain.

Adverse Effects:

Barbiturates can cause physical and psychological dependence; therefore clients must be cautious with extended use of this drug (Chapter 6) ⬤▭ . Common side effects are drowsiness, vitamin deficiency (Vitamin D, folate—B_9 and B_{12}), and laryngospasms. With overdose, phenobarbital may cause respiratory depression, CNS depression, coma, and death. Phenobarbital should not be taken with alcohol, other sedatives, or CNS depressants. As with most barbiturates, phenobarbital increases the metabolism of many other drugs, thus reducing their effectiveness. If at all possible, pregnant clients should not take this drug because of its Category D status. Unlike other shorter-acting barbiturates that are given a Schedule II status, phenobarbital is a Schedule IV drug.

TABLE 8.3	Barbiturates Used for Seizures	
DRUG	**ROUTE AND ADULT DOSE**	**REMARKS**
Short Acting		
pentobarbital (Nembutal)	PO/IM; 150–200 mg in 2 divided doses. IV; 100 mg, may increase to 500 mg if necessary.	For emergency control of general seizure activity; Also for insomnia and preoperative sedation; Schedule II drug.
secobarbital (Seconal)	IM/IV; 5.5 mg/kg repeated 3–4 hrs if necessary (IV infusion at less than 50 mg/15 sec).	For emergency control of seizure activity caused by conditions such as tetanus or poisons; Also for insomnia and preoperative sedation; Schedule II drug.
Long acting		
Pr phenobarbital (Luminal)	For seizures: PO; 100–300 mg/day. IV/IM 200–600 mg up to 20 mg/kg. For status epilepticus: IV; 15–18 mg/kg in single or divided doses (max 20 mg/kg).	For the management of tonic-clonic seizures, partial seizures, status epilepticus, and eclampsia; Also for sedation; Schedule IV drug.
amobarbital (Amytal)	IV; 65–500 mg, not to exceed 1 g.	For control of status epilepticus or acute convulsive episodes; Also for insomnia and preoperative sedation; Schedule IV drug.

8.5 Phenytoin and phenytoin-like drugs delay sodium influx into neurons.

Understanding how neurons are stimulated by sodium is a challenging subject in physiology. Simply, sodium channels guide the movement of sodium into and out of cells. In the nervous system, sodium movement is important because it is a major factor that determines whether or not neurons will be able to support an *action potential*. If sodium channels are temporarily inactivated, neuronal activity will decrease. With this category of drugs, sodium channels are not blocked; they are just made to be less sensitive. If channels were completely blocked, neuronal activity would cease, as occurs with some pain-blocking drugs (Chapter 12 ⊂⊃).

TABLE 8.4	Other GABA-like Drugs Used for Seizures	
DRUG	**ROUTE AND ADULT DOSE**	**REMARKS**
gabapentin (Neurontin)	For additional therapy: PO; start with 300 mg on day 1; 300 mg bid on day 2; 300 mg tid on day 3; continue to increase over one week to a dose of 1200 mg/day (400 mg tid); may increase to 1800–2400 mg/day.	Chemical structure similar to GABA; speeds up the release of GABA from brain neurons; used for partial seizures or seizures that could become generalized.
primidone (Mysoline)	PO; 250 mg/day; increased by 250 mg/week up to max of 2 grams in 2–4 divided doses.	Produces an action similar to barbiturates; used in combination with other anticonvulsant agents; for complex partial and generalized tonic-clonic seizures.
tiagabine hydrochloride (Gabitril)	PO; start with 4 mg/day; may increase by 4–8 mg/day every wk up to 56 mg/day in 2–4 divided doses.	Inhibits uptake of GABA into pre-synaptic neurons, prolonging GABA action; for the treatment of partial seizures.
topiramate (Topamax)	PO; start with 50 mg/day; increase by 50 mg/week to effectiveness (max 1600 mg/day).	Sugar-like chemical molecule; enhances the action of GABA; for partial seizures.

DRUG PROFILE:

Phenytoin (Dilantin)

Actions:

Phenytoin's anti-seizure activity is probably related to its chemical structure, which is similar to phenobarbital. It is effective against most types of seizures except absence seizures. It reduces the spread of electrical discharges within the brain, controlling motor activity. It also has antidysrhythmic properties (Chapter 16 🔗).

Adverse Effects:

Phenytoin may cause an irregular heartbeat, similar to the effect caused by local anesthetics. It may also cause a rapid loss of blood pressure and is toxic to many types of blood cells. It should not be used for seizures resulting from lowered blood sugar. Common side effects are drowsiness and overgrowth of gum tissue around the teeth. Phenytoin either interacts or is incompatible with many drugs and dietary supplements, including alcohol, anticoagulants and oral contraceptives. Phenytoin has a Category D status.

Hydantoins are the major chemical group in this category. The most established hydantoin is phenytoin. Other drugs, that delay sodium influx across neuronal membranes are sometimes referred to as *phenytoin-like* medications. Common phenytoin-like drugs include carbamazepine (Tegretol), divalproex (Depakote), and valproic acid (Depakene). Carbamazepine is widely used for partial seizures because it produces less drowsiness. Because of the unique mechanism by which some drugs in this class work, valproic acid is listed as a separate profile drug. Zonisamide is a newer drug in this class, approved by the FDA in the year 2000. Drugs approved for use in the 1990s were Felbamate (Felbatol) and Lamotrigine (Lamictal). Phenytoin and phenytoin-like drugs are listed in Table 8.5.

SUCCINIMIDES

succin = chemical with two–CO-groups
imide = chemical with one =NH group

Succinimide is a chemical class from which anti-seizure drugs, such as ethosuximide, methsuximide, and phensuximide are derived. These medications delay calcium influx into neurons.

DRUG PROFILE:

Valproic acid (Depakene)

Actions:

Valproic acid has a chemical structure different than other antiseizure medications, and its mechanism of action is not clearly understood. It is useful for a wide range of seizure types, including absence seizures and mixed types of seizures. Other uses include prevention of migraine headaches and for treatment of manic-depressive (bipolar) disorders (Chapter 9 🔗).

Adverse Effects:

Side effects of valproic acid include CNS depression, drowsiness, upset stomach, and prolonged bleeding time. Alcohol, aspirin, and other anticoagulant medication should be avoided with this drug. Clonazepam (Klonopin) along with valproic acid may precipitate absence seizures. Simultaneous use of other anticonvulsants or antihistamines should be monitored to avoid toxicity.

8.6 Succinimides act by delaying calcium influx into neurons.

Several types of calcium channels guide the movement of calcium into and out of cells. Many factors determine calcium movement, including a change in voltage across cellular membranes, the binding of natural neurotransmitters, hormones, and drugs. Calcium influx is necessary for neuronal impulse transmission.

Succinimides delay the entry of calcium into neurons by blocking calcium channels. Simply, anti-seizure drugs of this group increase the electrical threshold and reduce the likelihood that neurons will reach a critical electrical level and transmit neuronal impulses if stimulated. A neuron's electrical threshold is an excitable level where there is no turning back: the neuron must fire. If the electrical threshold is increased, this reduces the possibility of abnormal firing. Examples of calcium blocking drugs are listed in Table 8.6.

Concept review 8.2

▪ Name three major pharmacological categories and at least four chemical categories of anti-seizure medication. Which drug examples do not conveniently fit into only one drug class, and why not?

TABLE 8.5	Phenytoin and Phenytoin-like Drugs Used for Seizures	
DRUG	**ROUTE AND ADULT DOSE**	**REMARKS**
Pr phenytoin (Dilantin)	PO; 15–18 mg/kg or 1 gram initial dose; then 300 mg/day in 1–3 divided doses; may be gradually increased 100 mg/week.	For tonic-clonic seizures, psychomotor seizures, and seizures after head trauma.
Pr valproic acid (Depakene)	PO/IV; 15 mg/kg/day in divided doses when total daily dose is greater than 250 mg; increase 5–10 mg every week until seizures are controlled (max 60 mg/kg/day).	Unrelated to most other anti-seizure drugs; for absence seizures and mixed generalized types of seizures.
carbamazepine (Tegretol)	PO; 200 mg bid, gradually increased to 800–1200 mg/day in 3–4 divided doses.	For grand mal and psychomotor seizures; useful in trigeminal neuralgia (condition characterized by intense pain along the angle of the jaw); also for manic-depressive disorder.
felbamate (Felbatol)	Lennox-Gastaut syndrome: PO; start at 15 mg/kg/day in 3 to 4 divided doses; may increase 15 mg/kg at weekly intervals to max of 45 mg/kg/day. Partial seizures: PO; start with 1200 mg/day in 3–4 divided doses; may increase by 600 mg/day every 2 weeks to max of 3600 mg/day.	For use in Lennox-Gastaut syndrome and partial seizures.
fosphenytoin sodium (Cerebyx)	IV; initial dose 15–20 mg PE/kg at 100–150 mg PE/min followed by 4–6 mg PE/kg/d. (PE = phenytoin equivalents).	Converted to phenytoin in the body; for control of status epilepticus; short-term substitute for oral phenytoin.
lamotrigine (Lamictal)	PO; 50 mg/day for 2 wks, then 50 mg bid for 2 wks; may increase gradually up to 300–500 mg/d in 2 divided doses (max 700 mg/d).	For partial seizures, generalized tonic-clonic seizures, and myoclonic seizures.
zonisamide (Zonegran)	PO; 100–400 mg/day.	Broad-spectrum medication; newer drug for partial seizures; it is a sulfonamide, which means that it may cause an allergic reaction in some clients.

DRUG PROFILE:
Ethosuximide (Zarontin)

Actions:

Ethosuximide depresses activity of the motor cortex by elevating the neuronal threshold. It is usually ineffective against psychomotor or tonic-clonic seizures. However, it may be given in combination with other medications that better treat these conditions. It is a drug of choice for absence seizures.

Adverse Effects:

Common side effects are abdominal distress and weight loss. Ethosuximide may impair mental and physical abilities. Behavioral changes are more prominent in clients with a history of psychiatric disturbances. Levels of anticonvulsants and other drugs may be altered with coadministration of this drug. Ethosuximide should be especially avoided if severe liver or kidney disease is present.

TABLE 8.6	Succinimide Drugs Used for Seizures	
DRUG	**ROUTE AND ADULT DOSE**	**REMARKS**
Pr ethoxsuximide (Zarontin)	PO; 250 mg, bid, increased every 4–7 days whenever necessary up to 1.5 grams/day.	For absence seizures, myoclonic seizures, and akinetic epilepsy.
methsuximide (Celontin)	PO; 300 mg/day; may increase every 4–7 days as needed (max 1.2 g/day in divided doses).	For absence seizures; may be used in combination with other anticonvulsants in mixed types of seizure activity.
phensuximide (Milontin)	PO; 0.5–1 g bid or tid.	For absence seizures; similar characteristics to methsuximide.

8.7 Some types of seizures are controlled by a preferred group of drugs.

The goal of anti-seizure therapy is to reduce the number of seizures to the lowest possible level without causing sedation or other major side effects. For some clients, it is unreasonable to expect complete eradication of seizures. Pharmacotherapy does not cure epilepsy; it just reduces the occurrence of seizures.

It would be ideal if one category of drugs was able to reduce all types of seizures on a regular basis. In reality, however, even seizures of the same class do not always respond to the same class of medication among different clients. That is why there are so many kinds of anti-seizure medications. Healthcare practitioners often have to try one type of anti-seizure medication first and then change to a second choice if the first does not work. The second medication choice is introduced while the first medication is reduced very slowly. In general, anti-seizure medication is withdrawn over a period of 6–12 weeks because abrupt withdrawal of these drugs can cause seizures. Sometimes a combination of drug therapies is necessary to provide the best level of treatment. Because drug-drug interactions are common with some of the anti-seizure medications, healthcare practitioners must make sure that all drugs are compatible.

Table 8.7 provides examples of drugs that many practitioners consider standard when determining the best course of treatment for their clients. To make the optimum choice, practitioners must rely on information such as the client's history, the type of seizure, and possible causes of the seizures.

NATURAL ALTERNATIVES

Scullcap for Epilepsy

Skullcap, also called *mad-dog weed, helmet flower* or *madweed,* is a wet ground herb of swampy origin found mainly in the eastern part of North America, from Florida to British Columbia to Ontario. Its scientific name is *Sculellaria laterifolia;* a closely related species called *Sculellaria glaericulata* may be found within temperate zones of Britain and most of Europe.

This herb has been used for centuries as a nervous system relaxant. It has many of the anti-anxiety effects of the benzodiazepines and the sedative properties of the barbiturates. Chemical constituents of this herb bind to the GABA receptor-chloride channel molecule. The main constituents of skullcap are flavonoid glycosides such as scutellarin and scutellarein in addition to volatile oils, which assist in absorption across gastrointestinal membranes. Scullcap is known for its treatment of epilepsy and for its ability to soothe nervous excitement or to induce sleep. Herbal components may also produce a calming effect in disorders such as depression, bipolar disorder, muscle pain, and inflammation. ▪

Concept review 8.3

▪ Give the names of six traditional drugs used for the management of specific seizure types. Match the drugs with the types of seizures they best control. Which one of these drugs is used for a broader range of seizures compared to the others?

8.8 Some anti-seizure drugs also control symptoms of alcohol withdrawal.

Symptoms of alcohol withdrawal include mild to moderate tremors, lack of sleep, confusion, anxiety, and depression. The same medications used to control seizures also treats these symptoms.

Muscle tension and increased brain activity are common symptoms treated with anti-seizure medication. The main difference between pharmacotherapy for seizures and other disorders is drug dosage and how frequently the drug is administered. With alcohol withdrawal, drugs are administered to control a broader range of symptoms from tremors, sleeplessness, confusion, anxiety, and depression. Symptoms usually last from five to seven days, with the most intense symptoms being observed from one to three days after a client has stopped drinking. Seizures are

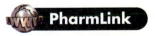

NATIONAL INSTITUTE ON ALCOHOL ABUSE AND ALCOHOLISM (NIAAA)

TABLE 8.7	Popular Drugs Used for the Management of Specific Types of Seizures			
	PARTIAL SEIZURES	**GENERALIZED SEIZURES**		
	(SIMPLE OR COMPLEX)	**(ABSENCE)**	**(ATONIC, MYOCLONIC)**	**(TONIC-CLONIC, STATUS EPILEPTICUS)**
Benzodiazepines				
diazepam (Valium)				✔
lorazepam (Ativan)				✔
Phenytoin-like				
phenytoin (Dilantin)	✔			✔
carbamazepine (Tegretol)	✔			✔
valproic acid (Depakene)	✔	✔	✔	✔
Succinimide				
ethoxsuximide (Zarontin)		✔	✔	

most likely to occur if withdrawal symptoms become intense. In severe cases, clients may hallucinate and develop a condition called DTs (short for delirium tremens). A serious condition such as this requires medical attention.

Because there is such an overlap of therapies with anti-seizure drugs, a list of similar drugs used for symptoms of alcohol withdrawal is provided in Table 8.8. A few other drugs used for the treatment of alcohol dependence have been added. A healthcare provider working in a detoxification unit might find this information helpful. Drugs for depression and hallucinations are covered in Chapter 9. Details regarding alcohol abuse were provided in Chapter 5 ⊂⊃.

TABLE 8.8	Drugs Used for Symptoms of Alcohol Withdrawal and Dependence	
DRUG	**ROUTE AND ADULT DOSE**	**REMARKS**
Alcohol Withdrawal Symptoms		
carbamazepine (Tegretol)	PO; 200 mg bid, gradually increased to 800–1200 mg/day in 3–4 divided doses.	Phenytoin-like drug used for alcohol withdrawal symptoms and rage outburst.
chlordiazepoxide hydrochloride (Librium)	PO; 50–100 mg prn (max 300 mg/day). IV/IM 50–100 mg every 3 hrs if needed.	Benzodiazepine used for symptoms of anxiety and tremors associated with alcohol withdrawal.
clonidine hydrochloride (Catapres)	PO; 0.1 mg bid or tid; may increase by 0.1–0.2 mg/day until desired response.	Antihypertensive agent; unlabeled use for alcohol withdrawal; reduces tremors and has a calming effect.
clorazepate dipotassium (Tranxene)	PO; 30–90 mg/day; reduce by 15 mg/day for 4 days to 7.5–15 mg/day.	Benzodiazepine used for short-term relief of anxiety associated with alcohol withdrawal and for the management of seizures.
diazepam (Valium)	PO; 2–10 mg bid to qid; IV/IM; 2–10 mg, repeat if needed in 3–4 hrs.	Benzodiazepine used for tremors, intense seizure activity, and muscle spasms.
hydroxyzine hydrochloride (Atarax; Vistaril)	PO; 25–100 mg/day tid or qid; IM; 25–100 mg every 4–6 hrs.	CNS depressant used for emotional stress or tension; useful in the treatment of chronic alcoholism where withdrawal symptoms are expressed.
lorazepam (Ativan)	PO; 2–6 mg/day in divided doses (max 10 mg/day).	Benzodiazepine used for anxiety, insomnia, and more serious types of seizures associated with alcohol withdrawal. Considered to be a drug of choice.
oxazepam (Serax)	PO; 15–30 mg tid or qid.	Benzodiazepine used to control anxiety and acute withdrawal symptoms such as restlessness and tremors.
Alcohol Dependence Symptoms		
disulfiram (Antabuse)	For alcoholism: PO; 500 mg/day for 1–2 weeks; then 125–500 mg/day (max 500 mg/day).	Inhibits alcohol dehydrogenase, which metabolizes alcohol in the body; acts as a classical conditioning deterrent to alcohol abuse; the client becomes extremely sick when exposed to alcohol; used after withdrawal.
naltrexone hydrochloride (Trexan, ReVia)	For alcohol dependence: PO; 50 mg/day.	A pure opiate antagonist; reduces the craving and euphoria associated with alcohol consumption; a deterrent to alcohol abuse; used after withdrawal.

ON THE JOB

Mental Health Worker in a Detoxification Unit

A mental health worker in a detoxification unit has much to do with respect to client care. One has to take vital signs and attend to symptoms that give verification that clients are recovering without incident. This is often a challenging situation. Clients are quite ill, and one of the last things on their mind is making the worker's shift an easy one. Sometimes clients have seizures, and in this situation, one must notify the unit nurse as soon as possible. One should give the client plenty of room and not try to restrain him or her. In addition, the healthcare provider should move any chairs or furniture so as to avoid injury to the client, and be prepared to assist with vital signs once the client regains his or her composure. One should reassure the client and provide whatever is needed to make him or her feel as comfortable as possible until the incident passes. For clients recovering from withdrawal, the mental health worker should also assist with any social adjustments necessary during their recovery period, preparing them for life outside the clinic environment. ■

CLIENT TEACHING

Clients taking anti-seizure medications need to know the following:

1. Never abruptly stop your medication; it can lead to seizures.
2. Avoid alcohol; it can increase sedation.
3. Until your response to the drug is determined, avoid driving and the use of machinery that could lead to injury. Anti-seizure drugs can make you drowsy.
4. It may require several dosage adjustments over many months to find the dosage that lets you perform usual daily activities while controlling seizures.
5. Report side effects to your healthcare practitioner:
   - excess fatigue or drowsiness with benzodiazepines
   - over sedation, agitation, or confusion with barbiturates
   - gum overgrowth (gingival hyperplasia) or skin rash with hydantoid derivatives such as phenytoin (Dilantin)
   - tremors, weight gain, diarrhea, or irregular menses with valproic acid (Depakene)
   - dizziness, nausea, or over-sedation with carbamazepine (Tegretol)
   - hiccups or epigastric pain with ethosuximide (Zarontin)
6. Hydantoins interact with many other drugs, so do not add any other prescription, OTC drugs, or herbal supplements until you consult your healthcare practitioner.
7. It is important to keep laboratory appointments because many anti-seizure medication requires blood testing to ensure that the drug is at a safe and effective level in your blood.
8. Consult your healthcare practitioner before trying to become pregnant; some anti-seizure medications are not safe to use during pregnancy. ■

CHAPTER REVIEW

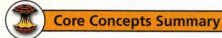 **Core Concepts Summary**

8.1 Seizures and convulsions are symptoms of epilepsy.

Seizures are often confused with convulsions. Seizures are abnormal or uncontrolled neuronal brain discharges. Convulsions are uncontrolled muscle contractions that may accompany major seizures.

8.2 Signs of seizures are easy to recognize.

Seizures fall into two major categories: partial seizures and generalized seizures. Within each major category, there are more specific types of seizures. Partial seizures may be simple or complex (called psychomotor or temporal lobe seizures). Generalized seizures may be classified as absence (petit mal), atonic (drop attacks), myoclonic, or tonic-clonic (grand mal) seizures. Status epilepticus is a medical emergency brought on by repeated seizures and convulsions.

8.3 Anti-seizure drugs may be grouped within three pharmacological categories.

Benzodiazepines, barbiturates, hydantoins, and succinimides represent the four major chemical categories of anti-seizure medication. They are grouped into three pharmacological categories: (1) drugs that stimulate an influx of chloride ion, an effect associated with the neurotransmitter GABA; (2) drugs that delay an influx of sodium; and (3) drugs that delay an influx of calcium.

8.4 By increasing the action of the inhibitory neurotransmitter GABA, abnormal neuronal activity can be suppressed.

Benzodiazepines, barbiturates, and other miscellaneous drugs reduce seizure activity by intensifying GABA action. GABA stimulates the influx of chloride ions into neurons, suppressing their ability to fire.

8.5 Phenytoin and phenytoin-like drugs delay sodium influx into neurons.

Drugs with an action like phenytoin (Dilantin) dampen neuronal activity by delaying an influx of sodium across neuronal membranes. Drugs with this kind of action are sometimes called hydantoins.

8.6 Succinimides act by delaying calcium influx into neurons.

Succinimides are drugs like ethosuximide, methsuximide, and phensuximide, with an ability to depress neuronal activity by delaying calcium influx into neurons. This causes the electrical threshold of individual neurons to be raised, making it more difficult for the neurons to fire.

8.7 Some types of seizures are controlled by a preferred group of drugs.

Many practitioners have a list of drugs that they rely on routinely to control certain types of seizures. When one medication doesn't work, they try another one. The goal of each practitioner is to determine the best course of treatment for the client.

8.8 Some anti-seizure drugs also control symptoms of alcohol withdrawal.

Most medications for seizures reduce brain activity and muscle tension. Because of this, anti-seizure medication is often very effective against symptoms of alcohol withdrawal, which include tremors, restlessness, anxiety, and inability to sleep. Some symptoms can be fatal, including severe convulsions and DTs.

EXPLORE PharMedia
www.prenhall.com/holland

Additional interactive resources and activities for this chapter can be found on the Companion Website. For animations, audio glossary, and review access the accompanying CD-ROM in this book.

Audio Glossary
Concept Review
NCLEX Review

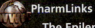

PharmLinks

The Epilepsy Foundation of America (EFA)

National Institute of Neurological Disorders and Stroke

Epilepsy Canada

National Institute on Alcohol Abuse and Alcoholism (NIAAA)

9 Drugs for Behavioral/Emotional Disorders, Mood Disorders, and Psychoses

CORE CONCEPTS

ADD/ADHD

9.1 Attention-deficit disorder (ADD) and attention-deficit/hyperactivity disorder (ADHD) are common in children.

CNS Stimulants

9.2 Methylphenidate (Ritalin) is the drug of choice for children with ADHD.

9.3 Common mood disorders are clinical depression and bipolar disorder (manic depression).

DEPRESSION

BIPOLAR DISORDER

Antidepressants

9.4 Antidepressants work by a variety of mechanisms.

Monoamine Oxidase (MAO) Inhibitors

Tricyclic Antidepressants (TCAs)

Selective Serotonin Reuptake Inhibitors (SSRIs)

Mood Stabilizers

9.5 Bipolar disorder may be effectively treated with lithium.

SCHIZOPHRENIA

9.6 Schizophrenia is the major psychosis.

9.7 Anti-psychotic medications attempt to stabilize clients with psychoses.

Conventional Anti-psychotics

Atypical Anti-psychotics

OBJECTIVES

After reading this chapter, the student should be able to:

1. Describe symptoms of attention deficit and hyperactivity in children and explain theories for why these disorders develop.

2. Know important drug treatments for attention-deficit/hyperactivity disorder, listing drug examples and giving details about their actions.

3. Identify two major types of mood disorders and explain their symptoms.

4. Describe the causes of clinical depression; explain the difference between clinical depression and major depression.

5. For each of the following mood enhancing drug classes, know representative drug examples, explain their mechanisms of action, primary actions, and important adverse effects.

   a. monoamine oxidase inhibitors
   b. tricyclic antidepressants
   c. selective serotonin reuptake inhibitors
   d. atypical antidepressant drugs

6. Know important mood-stabilizing drugs that treat bipolar disorder, explaining primary actions and adverse effects.

7. Identify the major type of psychosis and describe its symptoms; explain theories for why these symptoms develop.

8. Give examples of positive and negative symptoms of schizophrenia and explain why these are important for choice of drug therapy.

9. For each of the following anti-psychotic drug classes, know representative drug examples, explain their mechanisms of action, primary actions, and important adverse effects.

   a. phenothiazines and phenothiazine-like drugs
   b. atypical anti-psychotic medication

10. Categorize drugs used for behavioral disorders, mood disorders, and psychoses based on their classification and drug action.

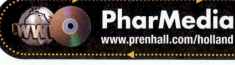

PharMedia
www.prenhall.com/holland

Additional interactive resources and activities for this chapter can be found on the Companion Website. For animations, audio glossary, and review access the accompanying CD-ROM in this book.

attention-deficit disorder (ADD): disorder often diagnosed in childhood and characterized by attention, organization, and behavior-control issues, that can extend into adulthood / *page 113*

attention-deficit/hyperactivity disorder (ADHD): disorder typically diagnosed in childhood and adolescence characterized by hyperactivity as well as attention, organization, and behavior-control issues / *page 113*

clinical depression: disorder characterized by depressed mood, lack of energy, abnormal eating patterns, and feelings of despair, guilt, and misery / *page 116*

major depression: disorder characterized by at least five symptoms of clinical depression / *page 117*

mania (MAY-nee-uh): disorder characterized by an expressive, impulsive, excitable, and over-reactive nature / *page 118*

manic (MAN-ik) **depression**: disorder characterized by extreme and opposite feelings, such as euphoria and depression or calmness and rage; also called bipolar disorder / *page 118*

mood disorders (affective disorders) (af-FEK-tiv): disorders involving a change in behavior such as clinical depression, emotional swings or manic-depression / *page 115*

mood enhancers (anti-depressants): drugs that combat depression by enhancing mood / *page 117*

mood stabilizers: drugs that level mood to treat bipolar disorder and mania / *page 118*

monoamine oxidase (mon-oh-AHM-een OK-see-daze) **inhibitors** (MAO inhibitors): drugs inhibiting monoamine oxidase, an enzyme that terminates the actions of neurotransmitters such as dopamine, norepinephrine, epinephrine, and serotonin; / *page 118*

narcolepsy (NAR-ko-lep-see): disorder characterized by uncontrolled attacks of sleep / *page 115*

negative symptoms: symptoms that subtract from normal behavior; signs that are used to assist with the diagnosis of schizophrenia / *page 127*

neuroleptic (noo-roh-LEP-tik) **malignant syndrome**: a potentially fatal condition caused by some anti-psychotic medications; symptoms include an extremely high body temperature, drowsiness, changing blood pressure, irregular heartbeat, and muscle rigidity / *page 128*

neuroleptics (noo-roh-LEP-ticks): drugs used to treat psychoses / *page 128*

positive symptoms: symptoms that add on to normal behavior; signs that are used to assist with the diagnosis of schizophrenia / *page 127*

schizoaffective (SKIT-soh-ah-FEK-tiv) **disorder**: disorder with symptoms similar to schizophrenia and mood disorders / *page 127*

schizophrenia (SKIT-soh-FREN-ee-uh): type of psychosis characterized by abnormal thoughts and thought processes, withdrawal from other people and the outside environment, and apparent preoccupation with one's own mental state / *page 126*

selective serotonin (sair-oh-TOE-nin) **reuptake inhibitors** (SSRIs): drugs that selectively inhibit the reuptake of serotonin into nerve terminals / *page 120*

serotonin syndrome: set of signs and symptoms associated with overmedication with antidepressants / *page 124*

tricyclic (treye-SICK-lick) **antidepressants** (TCAs): drugs with a three-ring chemical structure that inhibit the reuptake of norepinephrine and serotonin into nerve terminals / *page 119*

Disorders associated with emotional, unusual, or bizarre feelings are among the leading causes of mental health problems. Medical experts have become very adept at identifying symptoms that separate normal from abnormal behavior and more medications are available to treat these conditions than ever before. This chapter deals with three major disorders that fall within a broad range of ages from childhood to old age. These are behavioral/emotional disorders, mood disorders, and psychoses.

ADD/ADHD

Attention-deficit disorder (ADD) and **attention-deficit/hyperactivity disorder (ADHD)** are typically diagnosed in childhood and characterized by lack of attention, poor organization, and behavior-control issues and/or hyperactivity. These symptoms may extend into adulthood.

9.1 Attention-deficit disorder (ADD) and attention-deficit/hyperactivity disorder (ADHD) are common in children.

Attention-deficit disorder (ADD) and attention-deficit/hyperactivity disorder (ADHD) affect as many as 5% of all children. Many children diagnosed with ADD or ADHD are between the ages of three and seven years old, and these disorders are four to eight times more likely to occur in boys.

When one hears the words attention-deficit disorder, difficulty paying attention or focusing on tasks comes to mind. Small children are normally very active. However, when the child's activity level interferes with play, sleep, and learning, hyperactivity disorder may be diagnosed. Hyperactive children tend to interrupt, fidget, climb, and talk excessively for their developmental level, and so they are not able to interact successfully at school, on the playground, or at home. Symptoms of attention-deficit and hyperactivity are shown in the following list.

- distractibility
- difficulty following instructions
- failure to receive instructions properly
- inability to listen carefully
- inability to focus on one task at a time
- difficulty remembering
- frequent loss or misplacement of personal items

Most children who have ADD or ADHD have associated challenges. Many find it difficult to concentrate on tasks assigned in school. Even if they are gifted, their grades usually suffer because they have difficulty fitting into the conventional routine of a classroom. Discipline may also be a problem. Teachers are often the first to suggest that children be examined for ADD and receive medication for the disorder.

Fast Facts ADD/ADHD

- ADHD is the major reason why children are referred for mental health treatment.
- About one-half are also diagnosed with oppositional defiant or conduct disorder.
- About one-fourth are also diagnosed with anxiety disorder.
- About one-third are also diagnosed with depression.
- And about one-fifth also have a learning disability.

Source: National Mental Health Association

hyper = increased
kinetic = activity

The causes of ADD/ADHD are not clear; however, several theories have been proposed. For many years, scientists described these disorders as *minimal brain dysfunction (MBD)* and *hyperkinetic syndrome,* focusing on abnormal brain function and overactivity. More recent evidence suggests that hyperactivity may be related to dysfunction of a special group of neurotransmitters in the brain, including dopamine, norepinephrine, and serotonin. The specific location of neurotransmitter dysfunction is probably associated with the reticular activating system in the brain.

Within the past decade, experts have suggested that one-third to one-half of children diagnosed with ADD/ADHD will continue to experience symptoms of attention dysfunction in their adult years. Symptoms of ADD/ADHD in adults are similar to those of mood disorders and include anxiety, mania, restlessness, and depression. Some clients are perceived as lacking motivation and direction and have difficulty keeping a job or maintaining normal relationships with others. Frustration and problems with impulse control place the ADD/ADHD client at increased risk for alcohol and substance abuse.

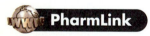

ADULTS WITH ADD

CNS STIMULANTS

Medications used to treat ADD/ADHD are central nervous system (CNS) stimulants. These drugs activate specific areas of the brain.

9.2 Methylphenidate (Ritalin) is the drug of choice for children with ADHD.

CNS stimulants are the main course of treatment for ADHD. Stimulant medication reverses many of the symptoms: it helps clients to focus on information given to them by teachers or parents and improves the likelihood of a child's finishing a task. The abuse potential of CNS stimulants was discussed in Chapter 5 ⊂⊃ .

DRUG PROFILE:
Methylphenidate (Ritalin)

Actions:

The exact mechanism by which methylphenidate produces its effects is not clear, but it stimulates the cerebral cortex in much the same way as amphetamine does. It activates the reticular activating system, causing heightened alertness in various regions of the brain. Activation is partially achieved by the release of neurotransmitters such as norepinephrine, dopamine, and serotonin. Because the child is better able to focus on tasks, impulsiveness, hyperactivity, and disruptive behavior are usually reduced within a few weeks. These changes support better focus on tasks and academic performance. Methylphenidate is also prescribed for narcolepsy a rare condition characterized by uncontrolled attacks of sleep.

Adverse Effects:

If given to a client not experiencing ADD/ADHD, methylphenidate causes nervousness and insomnia. All clients are at risk for irregular heatbeat, high blood pressure, and liver toxicity. Methylphenidate is a Schedule II drug, indicating its potential to cause dependence when used for extended periods. Periodic drug-free periods are recommended in order to reduce the risks of dependence and to assess the client's condition. Because methylphenidate reduces appetite, growth suppression is possible.

Mechanism in Action:

Methylphenidate (Ritalin) is a medication used for the treatment of attention-deficit disorder (ADD) in children, and narcolepsy in adults. Methylphenidate increases norepinephrine (NE) release in ascending pathways of the reticular activating system (RAS), which maintains arousal and alertness. Methylphenidate also directly stimulates dopamine release in areas of the brain responsible for concentration.

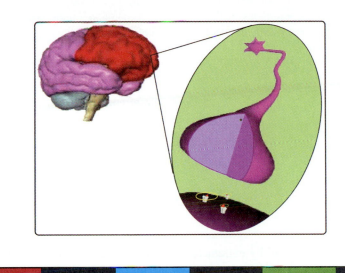

The most widely prescribed medication for ADD/ADHD is methylphenidate (Ritalin). In most cases, it is the only drug prescribed for ADHD disorder. (Dextro) amphetamine (Dexedrine, Adderall), methamphetamine (Dexoxyn), and pemoline (Cylert) may also occasionally be prescribed. Clonidine (Catapres) is useful when clients are aggressive, extremely active, and have difficulty with sleep. Antidepressants may also provide symptom relief. A list of these drugs is found in Table 9.1. Behavioral therapy may also be of value in reducing the symptoms of ADD/ADHD.

Concept review 9.1

▪ What are two major categories of symptoms observed with ADD/ADHD clients? Which drug is most often used in the treatment of these symptoms? What are the common symptoms of ADD/ADHD observed in adult clients?

9.3 Common mood disorders are clinical depression and bipolar disorder (manic depression).

One of the most common adult mental challenges is mood disorders, also called affective disorders. Although mood changes are a normal and expected part of life, when those changes become severe and/or rapid, the client may have a mood disorder.

TABLE 9.1	Drugs Used for Attention-Deficit/Hyperactivity Disorder	
DRUG	**ROUTE AND DOSE IN CHILDREN**	**REMARKS**
Pr methylphenidate hydrochloride (Ritalin)	Oral; 5–10 mg before breakfast and lunch, with gradual increase of 5–10 mg/week as needed (max 60 mg/day).	CNS stimulant; most widely used drug for ADHD clients; more dramatic effect on attention deficit than for hyperactivity.
clonidine hydrochloride (Catapres)	PO; 5 mg/kg/day in 4 divided doses, average dose is 0.15–0.2 mg/day.	Stimulates alpha-2 receptors in the brain; available in transdermal patch.
dextroamphetamine sulfate (Dexedrine)	3–5 years old—PO; 2.5 mg qd to bid; may increase by 2.5 mg at weekly intervals. ≥ 6 years old—PO; 5 mg qd to bid; increase by 5 mg at weekly intervals (max 40 mg/day).	CNS stimulant; potent appetite suppressant; should only be used for short-term treatment of ADHD; safety in children younger than three has not been established.
methamphetamine hydrochloride (Desoxyn)	≥ 6 years old—PO; 2.5–5 mg qd to bid; may increase by 5 mg at weekly intervals (max 20–25 mg/day).	CNS stimulant; abuse potential is high in adults.
pemoline (Cylert)	≥ 6 years old—PO; 37.5 mg/day; may increase by 18.75 mg at weekly intervals (max 112.5 mg/day).	Weak CNS stimulant; used in select cases as additional therapy; known hypersensitivity in children younger than six.
thioridazine hydrochloride (Mellaril)	> 2 years old—PO; 0.5–3 mg/kg/day in divided doses.	Anti-psychotic medication used for short-term treatment of ADD; for clients with symptoms of moderate depression; potent sedative.

Mood disorders are characterized by extremely elevated emotion, emotional swings, distorted thought processes, or depression. In some cases, clients may try to harm themselves or may cause themselves unintentional injury through impulsive behaviors. Two major types of mood disorders are depression and bipolar disorder (formerly called *manic depression*). More than 80% of clients who present symptoms of either disorder show improvement with drug therapy.

DEPRESSION

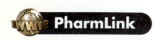

DIET AND DEPRESSION

Clinical depression is a disorder characterized by many symptoms, some of which are depressed mood, lack of energy, sleep disturbances, abnormal eating patterns, and feelings of despair, guilt, and misery. Clients become depressed for a variety of reasons. In some cases, depression may be *situational,* resulting from challenging circumstances such as severe physical illness, loss of a job, death of a loved one, divorce, or financial difficulties, coupled with inadequate psychosocial support. In other cases, the depression may be *biological,* associated with dysfunction of neurological processes leading to an imbalance in neurotransmitters. A family history of depression increases the risk for biological depression. Table 9.2 summarizes situational and biological causes of depression.

Women sometimes experience intense mood changes associated with hormonal changes during the menstrual cycle, pregnancy, childbirth, and menopause. If the mood is severely depressed and persists long enough to interfere with everyday functioning, the woman may benefit from medical treatment for premenstrual distress disorder (PMDD), postpartum depression, or menopausal distress. Some clients experience a type of depression during the winter months called *seasonal affective disorder (SAD)*. This type of depression is associated with the decreased release of the hormone melatonin in the brain in response to changes in the external environment.

TABLE 9.2	Situational and Biological Causes of Clinical Depression

SITUATIONAL CAUSES OF CLINICAL DEPRESSION

- Unpleasant life circumstances—grief over the loss of a loved one, divorce, loss of or dissatisfaction with a job, financial difficulty, excessive stress or responsibilities
- Negative thinking patterns—an environment that is likely to cause an individual to feel as if any attempts to escape or correct a situation are hopeless; poor self-image or lack of support from family or friends
- Substance abuse—substances that produce unpleasant side-effects or withdrawal symptoms, such as opiates, alcohol, or other CNS depressants
- Medication intended for therapeutic use—unfavorable side effects from medication intended to treat a medical disorder; for example, some anti-hypertensive drugs and oral contraceptives may cause depression

BIOLOGICAL (PHYSIOLOGICAL) CAUSES OF CLINICAL DEPRESSION

- Genetic—history of depression in one's family
- Hormonal changes in the body—fluctuations of reproductive or metabolic hormones
- Neurobiological dysfunction—chemical disturbances in the brain; usually related to abnormal functioning of the neurotransmitters or receptors for norepinephrine and/or serotonin
- Symptoms from a second disorder—almost any debilitating disorder, including head trauma, dementia, brain stroke or tumors, chronic pain, or thyroid dysfunction

Light therapy, exposing clients on a regular basis to specific wavelengths of light, can relieve SAD depression and can be used to prevent future episodes. This approach may allow the client to avoid the need for antidepressant drugs. Use of melatonin supplements for SAD treatment has not yet been thoroughly researched.

As with other mental health conditions, experts are aware of the many situations that can lead to depression, but they still do not completely understand the specific neurophysiological mechanisms underlying this disorder. In order to determine a course of treatment for the client, therapists often identify well-studied symptoms of depression, such as those in the following list. Clients diagnosed with **major depression** must show at least five of the symptoms listed.

- difficulty sleeping or sleeping too much
- extreme tiredness or listlessness
- abnormal eating patterns (eating too much or not enough)
- physical symptoms such as gastrointestinal pain, joint/muscle pain, or headaches
- inability to concentrate or make decisions
- feelings of despair, lack of self-worth, guilt, and misery
- obsession with death (expressing a wish to die or to commit suicide)
- avoidance of the company of other people
- lack of interest in personal appearance or sex
- hallucinations (experiencing things that are not real)
- delusions (false beliefs about one's situation)

Severe depression may respond to cognitive therapy or to a combination of psychotherapy with medication. Such counseling helps the client explore effective ways to deal with sources of stress. Medication does not completely restore chemical balance in the brain, but it does help to reduce depressive symptoms while the client develops effective means of coping. Drugs for depression are called **mood enhancers** or **antidepressants**.

Concept review 9.2

- What are the major causes of clinical depression? Identify symptoms of clinical depression. What is the name used to describe drugs that treat depression?

BIPOLAR DISORDER

bi *= two*
polar *= extremes*

Bipolar disorder (manic depression) is characterized by extreme and opposite moods, such as euphoria and depression. In addition to experiencing symptoms of clinical depression, clients display signs of mania. *Mania* refers to an expressive, impulsive, and hyper-excitable nature of an individual having a range of symptoms lasting for several months. Clients may shift quickly from emotions of extreme depression to extreme excitement, rage, and agitation. Symptoms of mania are, for the most part, exactly opposite those of depressive symptoms. Symptoms of mania include the following.

- lack of need for sleep
- extreme or prolonged activity or energy
- easy agitation, aggression, or other provoking behavior
- feelings of exaggerated confidence
- decision-making without regard for a long-term plan or consequences of action
- seeking the company or attention of others (intrusiveness)
- unusual interest in sex
- unwillingness or inability to see one's behavior as a problem (denial)
- possible abuse of drugs (alcohol, cocaine, or sleeping medication)

Like depression, symptoms of mania may be controlled by medication, although the choices of drugs are more limited. Drugs for bipolar disorder are called mood stabilizers because they have an ability to stabilize extreme shifts in emotions between mania and depression.

Concept review 9.3

- Identify the symptoms of mania. How do manic symptoms generally compare with depressive symptoms? Give the general name used to describe drugs used to treat bipolar disorder.

ANTIDEPRESSANTS

Antidepressants are medications that combat depression by enhancing mood.

9.4 Antidepressants work by a variety of mechanisms.

Clinical depression may be treated by a variety of drugs. The three primary classes of antidepressants are:

- monoamine oxidase (MAO) inhibitors
- tricyclic antidepressants (TCAs)
- selective serotonin reuptake inhibitors (SSRIs)

Antidepressants enhance the action of certain neurotransmitters in the brain, including norepinephrine and serotonin. For example, blocking the enzymatic breakdown of norepinephrine and slowing the reuptake of serotonin have been shown to alleviate signs of depression in many clients.

MONOAMINE OXIDASE (MAO) INHIBITORS

Monoamine oxidase (MAO) inhibitors are drugs that inhibit monoamine oxidase, an enzyme that terminates the actions of neurotransmitters such as dopamine, norepinephrine, epinephrine, and serotonin. When norepinephrine is released from the nerve terminal, one of the ways that the body naturally regulates how long this neurotransmitter acts is to break it down chemically by the enzyme *monoamine oxidase* (MAO). MAO is located within pre-synaptic nerve terminals as shown in Figure 9.1.

pre = *before*
synaptic = *the synapse*

Monoamine oxidase (MAO) inhibitors were once widely used in the drug treatment of depression. While MAO inhibitors increase the activity of norepinephrine within the brain, they also act everywhere else in the body. Thus, they accelerate heart rate, elevate blood pressure, cause hypotension with rapid changes in position, encourage weight gain, and interfere with sexual functioning. Eating foods containing tyramine while taking MAO inhibitors can cause a *hypertensive crisis.* Some foods containing tyramine are shown in Table 9.3.

MAO inhibitors also increase the effects of other substances in the bloodstream by blocking metabolic enzymes in the liver. Because of their adverse effects, MAO inhibitors are not the drugs of first choice for depression, but they are useful in cases where other drug therapies are ineffective. MAO inhibitors are listed in Table 9.4.

TRICYCLIC ANTIDEPRESSANTS (TCAS)

Tricyclic antidepressants are drugs with a three-ring chemical structure that inhibit the reuptake of norepinephrine and serotonin into nerve terminals. Tricyclic antidepressants were first used in the 1950s. These drugs produce their effect by inhibiting the reuptake of neurotransmitters into

tri = *three*
cyclic = *rings*

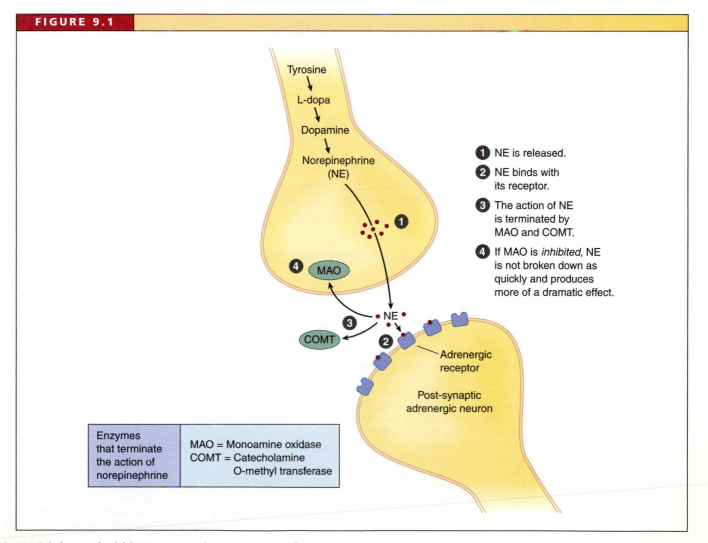

FIGURE 9.1

Tyrosine
↓
L-dopa
↓
Dopamine
↓
Norepinephrine
(NE)

1. NE is released.
2. NE binds with its receptor.
3. The action of NE is terminated by MAO and COMT.
4. If MAO is *inhibited*, NE is not broken down as quickly and produces more of a dramatic effect.

MAO

COMT

NE

Adrenergic receptor

Post-synaptic adrenergic neuron

| Enzymes that terminate the action of norepinephrine | MAO = Monoamine oxidase |
| | COMT = Catecholamine O-methyl transferase |

MAO is located within pre-synaptic nerve terminals

TABLE 9.3	Foods Containing Tyramine		
FRUITS	**DAIRY PRODUCTS**	**ALCOHOLIC BEVERAGES**	**MEATS**
avocados	cheese	beer	beef or chicken liver
bananas	sour cream	wines (especially red wines and Chianti)	pate
raisins	yogurt		meat extracts
papaya products, including meat tenderizers			pickled or kippered herring
canned figs			pepperoni
			salami
			sausage
			bologna/hot dogs
VEGETABLES	**SAUCES**	**YEAST**	**OTHER**
pods of broad beans (fava beans)	soy sauce	All yeast or yeast extracts	chocolate

pre-synaptic nerve terminals. The neurotransmitters particularly affected are norepinephrine and serotonin (see Figure 9.2). TCAs are used mainly for major depression and occasionally for milder situational depression. Clomipramine (Anafranil) is approved for treatment of obsessive-compulsive disorder, while other TCAs are unlabeled treatments for panic attacks. TCAs are occasionally used in the treatment of childhood eneuresis, or bedwetting. TCAs are listed in Table 9.5.

Tricyclic antidepressants produce fewer cardiovascular side effects and therefore are less dangerous than MAO inhibitors. However, TCAs produce a range of other adverse effects, including dry mouth, blurred vision, orthostatic hypotension, seizure activity, heart palpitations, and increased heart rate.

SELECTIVE SEROTONIN REUPTAKE INHIBITORS (SSRIS)

Ongoing efforts to find antidepressants with fewer side effects led to the development of a third category of antidepressants, the selective serotonin reuptake inhibitors (SSRIs). These drugs slow the reuptake of serotonin into nerve terminals. They are generally preferred over other drug classes because they treat depression effectively while avoiding sympathomimetic effects such as in-

DRUG PROFILE:
Phenelzine (Nardil)

Actions:

Phenelzine produces its effects by irreversible inhibition of monoamine oxidase (MAO), thus intensifying the effects of norepinephrine in the synapse. It may increase blood pressure, heart rate, and neural activity, leading to delirium, mania, anxiety, and convulsions. Its primary use is to manage symptoms of depression not responsive to more commonly used therapy and it is occasionally used for panic disorder. Drug effects may persist for two to three weeks after therapy is discontinued.

Adverse Effects:

Common side effects are constipation, dry mouth, orthostatic hypotension, insomnia, nausea, and loss of appetite. Severe high blood pressure is observed when ingesting foods containing tyramine. Many other drugs, especially those drugs that are altered by MAO, affect the action of phenelzine. Concurrent use of tricyclic antidepressants and selective serotonin reuptake inhibitors should be avoided, as the combination can cause temperature elevation and seizures. Opiate analgesics including meperidine (Demerol) should also be avoided because of the increased risk for respiratory collapse or hypertensive crisis.

TABLE 9.4	Monoamine Oxidase Inhibitors (MAOIs) Used for Clinical Depression	
DRUG	**ROUTE AND ADULT DOSE**	**REMARKS**
🅿 phenelzine sulfate (Nardil)	PO; 15 mg tid; may increase up to 90mg/day.	May cause a hypertensive crisis or respiratory depression; use cautiously in clients with epilepsy or diabetes, or who are likely to abuse drugs and alcohol.
isocarboxazid (Marplan)	PO; 10–30 mg/day (max dose 30 mg/day).	May cause peripheral edema and high blood pressure; used in cases where other approaches for treatment of depression are not successful.
tranylcypromine sulfate (Parnate)	PO; 30 mg/day; (give 20 mg in AM and 10 mg in PM), may increase by 10 mg/day at 3-week intervals up to max of 60 mg/day.	Used for severe depression in cases where clients have not responded to other medications.

creased heart rate and blood pressure or anticholinergic effects such as dry mouth, blurred vision, urinary retention, and constipation. However, they can cause other significant side effects including sexual dysfunction, nausea, headache, anxiety, weight gain, and insomnia.

It has become increasingly clear that serotonin has a more substantial role in depression than previously thought. Scientists already knew that antidepressants altered the sensitivity of serotonin to natural receptors in the brain, but they did not know how this was connected with depression. It

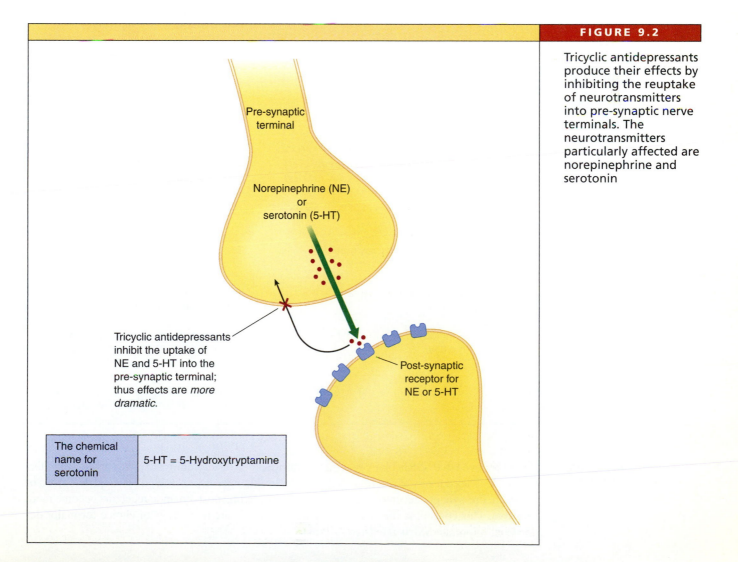

FIGURE 9.2

Tricyclic antidepressants produce their effects by inhibiting the reuptake of neurotransmitters into pre-synaptic nerve terminals. The neurotransmitters particularly affected are norepinephrine and serotonin

Pre-synaptic terminal

Norepinephrine (NE) or serotonin (5-HT)

Tricyclic antidepressants inhibit the uptake of NE and 5-HT into the pre-synaptic terminal; thus effects are *more dramatic.*

Post-synaptic receptor for NE or 5-HT

The chemical name for serotonin	5-HT = 5-Hydroxytryptamine

DRUG PROFILE:
Imipramine (Tofranil)

Actions:

Imipramine blocks the reuptake of serotonin and norepinephrine into presynaptic nerve terminals without affecting dopamine release. This stimulates nerves that normally respond to serotonin and norepinephrine. This explains the sensation of a full bladder experienced in some clients who take TCAs. Imipramine is mainly prescribed for clinical depression, although in some cases it is used for the treatment of chronic pain.

Adverse Effects:

Side effects of tofranil include sedation, drowsiness, blurred vision, dry mouth, and cardiovascular symptoms such as dysrhythmias, heart block, and higher blood pressure. Agents that mimic the action of norepinephrine or serotonin should be avoided. Alcohol enhances its sedative effects. Methylphenidate inhibits its metabolism and may produce toxicity. Some clients may experience photosensitivity.

TABLE 9.5	Tricyclic Antidepressants (TCAs) Used for Clinical Depression	
DRUG	**ROUTE AND ADULT DOSE**	**REMARKS**
Pr imipramine hydrochloride (Tofranil)	PO; 75–100 mg/day (up to 300 mg/day).	For biological depression or alcohol or cocaine dependence; may cause cardiac dysfunction and abnormal blood cell count; available IM; may control bedwetting in children.
amitriptyline hydrochloride (Elavil)	Adult: PO; 75–100 mg/day (may gradually increase to 150–300 mg/day). Geriatric: PO;10–25 mg at hs (may gradually increase to 25–150 mg/day).	For biological depression; inhibits gastric acid secretion by blocking histamine 2 receptors in the body.
amoxapine (Asendin)	Adult: PO; begin with 100 mg/day, may increase on 3rd day to 300 mg/day. Geriatric: PO; 25 mg at hs; may increase every 3–7 days to 50–150 mg/day (max 300 mg/day).	For situational and biological depression; not associated with cardiotoxicity; mild sedative.
desipramine hydrochloride (Norpramine)	PO; 75–100 day; may increase to 150–300 mg/day.	Active metabolite of imipramine.
doxepin hydrochloride (Sinequan)	PO; 30–150 mg/day at hs; may gradually increase to 300 mg/day.	For depression accompanying anxiety or alcohol dependence.
nortriptyline hydrochloride (Aventyl, Pamelor)	PO; 25 mg tid or qid; may increase 100–150 mg/day.	For biological depression; interactions similar to imipramine.
protriptyline hydrochloride (Vivactil)	PO; 15–40 mg/day in 3–4 divided doses (max 60 mg/day).	For symptoms of depression; very few sedative properties; causes increased heart rate.
trimipramine maleate (Surmontil)	PO; 75–100 mg/day (up to 300 mg/day).	For depression where there is a sleep disorder (has strong sedative effects).

post = *after*
synaptic = *the synapse*

is now believed that SSRIs block specifically the reuptake of serotonin into pre-synaptic nerve terminals. Increased levels of serotonin induce complex changes in pre- and post-synaptic neurons of the brain. Pre-synaptic receptors become less sensitive while post-synaptic receptors become more sensitive. This concept is illustrated in Figure 9.3. SSRIs are now drugs of choice for major depression. Important SSRIs are listed in Table 9.6.

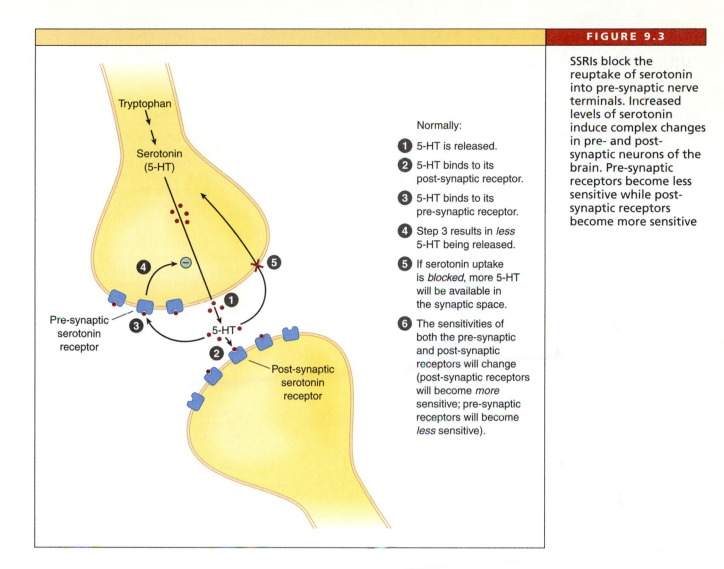

FIGURE 9.3

SSRIs block the reuptake of serotonin into pre-synaptic nerve terminals. Increased levels of serotonin induce complex changes in pre- and post-synaptic neurons of the brain. Pre-synaptic receptors become less sensitive while post-synaptic receptors become more sensitive

Normally:

1 5-HT is released.

2 5-HT binds to its post-synaptic receptor.

3 5-HT binds to its pre-synaptic receptor.

4 Step 3 results in *less* 5-HT being released.

5 If serotonin uptake is *blocked*, more 5-HT will be available in the synaptic space.

6 The sensitivities of both the pre-synaptic and post-synaptic receptors will change (post-synaptic receptors will become *more* sensitive; pre-synaptic receptors will become *less* sensitive).

A few drugs, known as atypical antidepressants, do not fall into the MAO inhibitor, TCA, or SSRI classes. Atypical antidepressants include tetracyclic agents. Some agents in this category, such as bupropion (Wellbutrin), not only inhibit the reuptake of serotonin, but also affect the activity of norepinephrine and dopamine. These miscellaneous antidepressants are listed in Table 9.7.

tetra = *four*
cyclic = *rings*

Concept review 9.4

■ What are the three major classes of antidepressants? Name representative drugs within each class and describe how each drug works pharmacologically.

MOOD STABILIZERS

Mood stabilizers are drugs that stabilize extreme shifts in mood. They prevent clients from becoming either depressed or manic.

9.5 Bipolar disorder may be effectively treated with lithium.

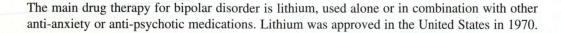

The main drug therapy for bipolar disorder is lithium, used alone or in combination with other anti-anxiety or anti-psychotic medications. Lithium was approved in the United States in 1970.

DRUG PROFILE:
Fluoxetine (Prozac)

Actions:

Actions of fluoxetine are attributed to its ability to selectively inhibit the reuptake of serotonin into pre-synaptic nerve terminals. It is mainly used for clinical depression, although it may also be used for obsessive-compulsive disorder and eating disorders. Actions include improved affect, mood enhancement, and reduced appetite, with maximum therapeutic effects taking several days to several weeks.

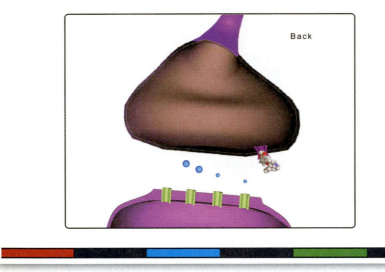

Back

Adverse Effects:

Fluoxetine may cause headaches, nervousness, insomnia, nausea, and diarrhea. Foods high in the amino acid, tryptophan should be avoided because tryptophan is the chemical precursor for serotonin synthesis. Coadministration with selegiline (Carbex, Eldepryl) may increase the risk of a hypertensive crisis. Tricyclic antidepressants administered simultaneously may produce serotonin syndrome. Serotonin syndrome is characterized by fever, confusion, shivering, sweating, and muscle spasms.

Mechanism in Action:

Fluoxetine (Prozac) is a selective serotonin reuptake inhibitor (SSRI). It acts by blocking the recycling of the brain neurotransmitter serotonin into pre-synaptic nerve terminals. At the synaptic cleft, serotonin continually binds with post-synaptic receptors and activates excitatory post-synaptic potentials (EPSPs). This is thought to restore the mental state of a depressed client to a normal level.

TABLE 9.6	Selective Serotonin Reuptake Inhibitors (SSRIs) Used for Clinical Depression	
DRUG	**ROUTE AND ADULT DOSE**	**REMARKS**
Pr fluoxetine hydrochloride (Prozac)	PO; 20 mg/day in the AM; may increase to max of 80 mg/day.	For obsessive-compulsive disorder and eating disorders.
citaprolam hydrochloride (Celexa)	PO; start at 20 mg/day; may increase to 40 mg/day if needed.	Does not mimic the sympathetic response; has no acetylcholine blocking properties; does not inhibit MAO.
fluvoxamine (Luvox)	PO; start with 50 mg/day; may increase up to 300 mg/day.	For obsessive-compulsive disorder; no severe cardiovascular side-effects; fewer acetylcholine blocking effects.
paroxetine (Paxil)	Depression: PO; 10–50 mg/day (max 80 mg/day). Obsessive-compulsive disorder: PO; 20–60 mg/day. Panic attacks: PO; 40 mg/day.	For obsessive-compulsive disorder and panic attacks.
sertraline hydrochloride (Zoloft)	Adult: PO; start with 50 mg/day; gradually increase every few weeks to a range of 50–200 mg. Geriatric: start with 25 mg/day.	Does not mimic sympathetic response; has no acetylcholine blocking properties; does not inhibit MAO.

TABLE 9.7	Atypical Drugs Used for Clinical Depression	
DRUG	**ROUTE AND ADULT DOSE**	**REMARKS**
bupropion hydrochloride (Wellbutrin)	PO; 75–100 mg tid (greater than 450 mg/day increases risk for adverse reactions).	For changing moods, schizoaffective disorders, and to quit smoking; increased risk for seizures; weaker blocker of serotonin and norepinephrine uptake.
maprotiline hydrochloride (Ludiomil)	Mild to moderate depression: PO; start at 75 mg/day; gradually increase every 2 weeks to 150 mg/day. Severe depression: PO; start at 100–150 mg/day; gradually increase to 300 mg/day.	Tetracyclic chemical structure; treats a broad range of depression from mild to severe.
mirtazapine (Remeron)	PO; 15 mg/day in a single dose at hs; may increase every 1–2 weeks (max 45 mg/day).	Tetracyclic chemical structure; potent blocker of serotonin type 2 and 3 receptors; use caution in cases where clients have kidney or liver dysfunction.
nefazodone (Serzone)	PO; 50–100 mg bid; may increase up to 300–600 mg/day.	Minimal cardiovascular effects; fewer effects in blocking acetylcholine; less sedation; less sexual dysfunction compared to other antidepressants.
trazadone hydrochloride (Desyrel)	PO; 150 mg/day; may increase by 50 mg/day every 3–4 days up to max of 400–600 mg/day.	Increases total sleep time; reduces night awakenings; has anxiolytic effects.
venlafaxine (Effexor)	PO; 25–125 mg tid.	Bicyclic chemical structure; does not cause sedative or cardiovascular effects; does not block acetylcholine effects.

Before this time, its benefit in manic-depressive illness had been known; however, its therapeutic safety had not been proven. Other drugs that stabilize mood have multiple uses. For example, carbamazepine (Tegretol) and valproic acid (Depakene) are also anti-seizure medications. Mood-stabilizing drugs including lithium are listed in Table 9.8.

Concept review 9.5

■ What is the main drug used to treat manic depression and how does it work pharmacologically? What other drugs treat manic depression?

NATURAL ALTERNATIVES

St. John's Wort for Depression

St. John's Wort (*Hypericum perforatum*) is an herb found throughout Britain, Asia, Europe, and North America that is commonly used as an antidepressant. It gets its name from a legend that red spots once appeared on its leaves on the anniversary of St. John's beheading. *Wort* is a British term for "plant." Researchers once claimed that it produced its effects the same way MAO inhibitors do: by increasing the levels of serotonin, adrenaline, and dopamine in the brain. More recent evidence suggests that it may selectively inhibit serotonin uptake. Some claim that it is more effective than fluoxetine (Prozac), paroxetine (Paxil), or sertraline (Zoloft) and produces fewer side effects. It has other purported uses including an anti-infective agent for conditions such as staph and strep, for nerve pains such as neuralgia and sciatica, and for mental burnout. It is extremely important to avoid combinations of St. John's Wort and antidepressant medications unless prescribed by a healthcare practitioner. ■

DRUG PROFILE:
Lithium (Eskalith)

Actions:

Although the exact mechanism of lithium's action is not clear, it is thought to alter the activity of neurons containing dopamine, norepinephrine, and serotonin. Simply, lithium reduces the activity of these neurotransmitters by influencing their release, synthesis, and reuptake. Therapeutic actions are stabilization of mood during periods of mania and antidepressant effects during periods of depression. Lithium has neither antimanic nor antidepressant effects in individuals without bipolar disorder. After taking lithium for two to three weeks, clients have an improved ability to concentrate and perform self care. To ensure therapeutic action, concentrations of lithium in the bloodstream must remain within a range of 0.6–1.5 mEq/L. Therefore, the monitoring of lithium serum levels is required on a regular basis. Close monitoring encourages compliance and helps to avoid toxicity.

Adverse Effects:

Lithium may cause dizziness, lack of energy, short-term memory loss, increased urination, nausea, vomiting, loss of appetite, abdominal aches, diarrhea, dry mouth, muscular weakness, and slight tremors. Some drugs increase the rate at which the kidneys remove lithium from the bloodstream, for example, diuretics, sodium bicarbonate, and potassium citrate. Other drugs, such as methyldopa and probenecid, inhibit the rate at which the kidneys excrete lithium. Clients should not have a salt-free diet with this therapy since this promotes lithium excretion.

TABLE 9.8	Drugs Used for Bipolar Disorder (Manic Depression)	
DRUG	**ROUTE AND ADULT DOSE**	**REMARKS**
Pr lithium carbonate (Eskalith)	PO; initial: 600 mg tid; maintenance 300 mg tid (max 2.4g/day).	For treatment of mania and depressive symptoms; must be used cautiously withclients having epilepsy or psychosis.
carbamazepine (Tegretol)	PO; 200 mg bid, gradually increased to 800–1200 mg/day in 3–4 divided doses.	For treatment of manic depressive and schizo-affective symptoms; used as anti-seizure medication.
valproic acid (Depakene)	PO; 250 mg tid (max 60 mg/kg/day).	For treatment of mania and prevention of migraine headache; used as anti-seizure medication.

SCHIZOPHRENIA

schizo = split
phrenia = mind

Schizophrenia is a type of psychosis characterized by abnormal thoughts and thought processes, disordered communication, withdrawal from other people and the outside environment, and a high risk for suicide.

9.6 Schizophrenia is the major psychosis.

Psychosis is a mental health condition characterized by delusions, hallucinations, disorganized behavior, and difficulty relating to others. Clients have a disorganized pattern of thinking and talking. Dementia, depression, chronic alcoholism, and childhood onset developmental disorder may be accompanied by psychosis, but schizophrenia is the major psychotic illness. Paranoia, extreme suspicion and delusions of persecution characterizes paranoid schizophrenia.

Clients with psychosis are usually unable to function normally in society without long-term medication. Schizophrenic clients see healthcare practitioners most often for medication adjustments. Family members and social organizations are important sources of help for clients who cannot function without continuous therapy.

Fast Facts Psychosis

- Psychotic symptoms are the most disruptive kinds of behaviors in a daily routine.
- Symptoms of psychosis are most often associated with other mental health problems including substance abuse, depression, and dementia.
- Psychotic disorders are among the most misunderstood mental health disorders in North America.
- Over 2,500,000 Americans have psychosis.
- Clients with psychosis often develop symptoms between the age of 13 and the early twenties.

Source: National Mental Health Association

Schizophrenia is the most common type of psychotic disorder. Clients experience many symptoms that may change over time; symptoms may appear quickly or take several months or years to develop. Symptoms of schizophrenia include those listed here.

- hallucinations (experiencing something that is not really there)
- delusions (false beliefs or ideas)
- paranoia (feeling that someone is "out to get" one)
- strange behavior, such as communicating in an unknown language
- being active for days without any sleep
- attitude of extreme indifference or detachment
- acting strangely or irrationally
- deterioration of appearance, hygiene, or academic performance

When observing clients with schizophrenia, practitioners look for two general types of symptoms: **positive symptoms** and **negative symptoms**. Positive symptoms are those that *add on* to normal behavior. These include hallucinations, delusions, and a disorganized thought or speech pattern. Negative symptoms are those that subtract from normal behavior. Symptoms include lack of interest, motivation, or responsiveness, and lack of pleasure in daily life. Negative symptoms are descriptive of the seemingly indifferent personality exhibited by many schizophrenics. Positive and negative symptoms are important because these often serve as a predictor of whether conventional or atypical anti-psychotic medication will best treat these behaviors.

The cause of schizophrenia has not been determined, although several theories have been proposed. One theory is the genetic theory. There is good evidence for this; many clients suffering from schizophrenia have family members who have been afflicted with the same disorder. Another theory is the neurotransmitter theory. This theory deals with the possibility of an overactive dopamine neurotransmitter pathway in the brain. Symptoms of schizophrenia seem to be associated with the dopamine type 2 (D_2) receptor because many drugs that control psychotic behavior also block this receptor. Computerized tomography (CT) and magnetic resonance (MR) scans often reveal a smaller hippocampus and larger ventricles in the brains of schizophrenics, especially males, but whether this is a cause or an effect of the disorder remains unclear.

Schizoaffective disorder is a condition in which the client exhibits symptoms of both schizophrenia and mood disorders. For example, an acute schizoaffective reaction may include distorted perceptions, hallucinations, and delusions, followed by extreme depression. Over a long time period, both positive and negative psychotic symptoms will appear. It is challenging to differentiate schizoaffective disorder from bipolar disorder or major depression with psychotic features, as individuals with affective disorders may also experience psychotic episodes.

schizo = *schizophrenia*
affective = *mood*

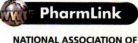

NATIONAL ASSOCIATION OF MENTAL ILLNESS

Concept review 9.6

- What are the major types of psychoses? Describe major symptoms associated with each type. What distinguishes a positive symptom from a negative symptom?

9.7 Anti-psychotic medications attempt to stabilize clients with psychoses.

neuro = nervous
leptic = state of mind

Anti-psychotic medications are sometimes called **neuroleptics**. There are two classes of neuroleptics: *conventional anti-psychotics* and *atypical anti-psychotics*. Conventional anti-psychotics are more effective in treating positive symptoms of schizophrenia. Atypical anti-psychotics treat both positive and negative symptoms. Atypical anti-psychotics are sometimes preferred because these address a broader range of symptoms and generally produce less dramatic side effects. Extrapyramidal side effects are distorted body movements and muscle spasms associated with conventional anti-psychotics. Extrapyramidal symptoms include severe spasms of the muscles of the face, tongue or back, lip-smacking movements, jerking motions, acute restlessness, and an induced Parkinson Syndrome (Chapter 10). If extrapyramidal effects are reported early after onset and the drug is withdrawn or the dosage is reduced, the side effects are reversible. With higher doses given for prolonged periods, the extrapyramidal symptoms may become permanent. With high dosages and during times of dosage increase, there is also risk for a rare but potentially fatal side effect: **neuroleptic malignant syndrome**. High fever, confusion, muscle rigidity, and high serum creatine kinase associated with this syndrome are treated with cooling, discontinuation of the anti-psychotic drug, and giving medications to increase brain dopamine levels. The biological basis for these side effects, also observed with Parkinson's disease, is explained more thoroughly in Chapter 10 ⬭. One of the most serious side effects with atypical anti-psychotics is severe reduction in white blood cells associated with clozapine (Clozaril).

CONVENTIONAL ANTI-PSYCHOTICS

Conventional anti-psychotic drugs (phenothiazines and phenothiazine-type drugs) treat positive symptoms of pychosis. The two major chemical groups of anti-psychotic medication are the phenothazines and phenothiazine-like drugs. Drug examples are listed in Table 9.9. Phenothiazines

DRUG PROFILE:
Chlorpromazine (Thorazine)

Actions:

Chlorpromazine provides symptomatic relief of positive symptoms in clients diagnosed with schizophrenia and controls manic symptoms in clients with schizoaffective disorder. Many clients must take chlorpromazine for seven or eight weeks before they experience improvement. Most clients do not realize the importance of drug therapy and, therefore, must be regularly encouraged to take this medication. With low to moderate doses, chlorpromazine can also control anxiety and vomiting. Many of the major effects of chlorpromazine can be attributed to blockade of dopamine receptors located throughout the brain.

Adverse Effects:

Strong blockade of alpha-adrenergic receptors and weak blockade of cholinergic receptors explain some of chlorpromazine's adverse effects. Common side effects are dizziness, drowsiness, and orthostatic hypotension. Concurrent use with sedative medications such as phenobarbital (Luminal) should be avoided. Taking chlorpromazine with tricyclic antidepressants might elevate blood pressure. Chlorpromazine is less effective when administered with anti-seizure medication or if the client smokes. Extrapyramidal side effects occur mostly in the elderly, women, and in pediatric clients who are dehydrated. Neuroleptic malignant syndrome, a potentially fatal condition caused by high doses of many anti-psychotic medications, may also be possible. Clients taking chlorpromazine and exposed to warmer temperatures should be monitored.

TABLE 9.9	Conventional Anti-psychotic Drugs	
DRUG	ROUTE AND ADULT DOSE	REMARKS
Phenothiazines		
(Pr) chlorpromazine hydrochloride (Thorazine)	PO; 25–100 mg tid or qid (clients may require up to 1000 mg/day). IM/IV; 25–50 mg (max 600 mg q 4–6 hours).	Strong sedative properties; controls nausea and vomiting, dementia and hiccups not treated by any other means; for agitated patients.
fluphenazine hydrochloride (Prolixin, Permitil)	PO; 0.5–10 mg/day up to a usual max of 20 mg/day.	Also for dementia; available in IM or SC forms.
mesoridazine besylate (Serentil)	PO; 10–50 mg bid or tid; may increase up to 400 mg/day.	Strong sedative properties; also for dementia, hyperactivity, alcohol dependence, and anxiety.
perphenazine (Phenazine, Trilafon)	PO; 4–16 mg bid to qid (max 64 mg/day).	Also for dementia and nausea; available in IM and IV forms.
prochlorperazine (Compazine)	PO; 5–10 mg tid or qid.	Also for severe nausea and vomiting; available as suppositories, IM or IV forms.
promazine hydrochloride (Prozine, Sparine)	PO/IM; 10–200 mg every 4–6 hours (max 1,000mg/day).	For agitated and paranoid clients; useful in clients withdrawing from alcohol; available in IM form.
thioridazine hydrochloride (Mellaril)	PO; 50–100 mg tid; (max 800 mg/day).	Strong sedative properties; for moderate to severe depression and dementia.
trifluoperazine hydrochloride (Stelazine)	PO; 1–2 mg bid; may increase up to 20 mg/day.	Used also for dementia; use cautiously in clients with seizure disorders; available in IM form.
Phenothiazine-like Drugs		
chlorprothixene (Taractan)	PO; 75–150 mg/day (max 600 mg/day).	Prominent sedative effects; less hypotensive than phenothiazines; available in IV form.
haloperidol (Haldol)	PO; 0.2–5 mg bid or tid.	For severe psychosis, dementia, and Tourette's disorder; available in IM form.
loxapine succinate (Loxitane)	PO; Start with 20 mg/day and rapidly increase to 60–100 mg/day in divided doses (max 250 mg/day).	Also for dementia.
molindone hydrochloride (Moban)	PO; 50–75 mg/day in 3–4 divided doses; may increase to 100 mg/day in 3–4 days (max 225 mg/day).	May produce insomnia and drowsiness.
pimozide (Orap)	PO; 1–2 mg/day in divided doses; gradually increase every other day to 7–16 mg/day (max 10mg/day).	For Tourette's disorder; use cautiously in clients with seizure disorders.
thiothixene hydrochloride (Navane)	PO; 2 mg tid; may increase up to 15 mg/day (max 60 mg/day).	Also for dementia; unlabeled use as an antidepressant.

have been used to treat psychoses for many years. Many phenothazines have a similar chemical structure to chlorpromazine (Thorazine). However, each medication varies slightly in potency, sedative properties, extrapyramidal side effects, and ability to block alpha adrenergic receptors. Drugs with a strong alpha-blocking component tend to raise blood pressure very quickly when the client suddenly changes position.

ATYPICAL ANTI-PSYCHOTICS

Because atypical anti-psychotics treat both the positive and negative symptoms of pychosis, a broader range of schizophrenic symptoms can be controlled with atypical anti-psychotics. Some drugs such as clozapine (Clozaril), for example, are especially useful in cases where conventional drug therapy is unsuccessful. Generally, there are fewer side effects with atypical anti-psychotics. However, side effects from the atypical antipsychotics are still significant and those clients must be carefully monitored in all cases. Examples of atypical anti-psychotics are shown in Table 9.10.

Concept review 9.6

■ What is a neuroleptic drug? What are the two major classes of drugs used to treat pychoses? How does each drug category generally affect positive and negative symptoms of schizophrenia?

TABLE 9.10	Atypical Antipsychotic Drugs	
DRUG	**ROUTE AND ADULT DOSE**	**REMARKS**
Pr clozapine (Clozaril)	PO; start at 25–50 mg/day and titrate to a target dose of 350–450 mg/day in 3 days; may increase further (max 900 mg/day).	For schizophrenia (adults older than 16 years).
olanzapine (Zyprexa)	Adult: PO; start with 5–10 mg/day; may increase by 2.5–5 mg every week (range 10–15 mg/day, max 20 mg/day).Geriatric: PO; start with 5 mg/day.	Blocks alpha-receptors and acetylcholine.
quetiapine fumarate (Seroquel)	PO; start with 25 mg bid; may increase to a target dose of 300–400 mg/day in divided doses.	Clients may experience hypotension when changing position; use cautiously in elderly clients.
risperidone (Risperdal)	PO; 1–6 mg bid; increase by 2 mg daily to an intial target dose of 6/mg/day.	Unlabeled use in behavioral disturbances (clients with mental retardation).

DRUG PROFILE:
Clozapine (Clozaril)

Actions:

Therapeutic effects of clozapine include remission of a range of psychotic symptoms including delusions, paranoia, and irrational behavior. Twenty-five percent of severely ill clients show improvement within six weeks of starting clozapine. Sixty percent of clients show improvement within six months. Clozapine seems to interfere with the binding of dopamine to its receptors located in the limbic system. Clozapine also binds to alpha-adrenergic, serotonergic, and cholinergic sites throughout the brain.

Adverse Effects:

Clozapine should not be used in clients with severe depression, in uncontrolled epilepsy, or with concurrent use of benzodiazepines. Common side effects are dizziness, drowsiness, headache, constipation, transient fever, salivation, flu-like symptoms, and fast or irregular heartbeat. Clozapine may also lower white blood count. This drug should not be taken with alcohol.

ON THE JOB

Teamwork in an Adult Psychiatric Facility

Working in an adult psychiatric facility is often an intimidating job because of a wide range of psychiatric disorders found within one confined area. Clients will have all kinds of disorders from depression to schizophrenia, and at any time, clients may become aggressive, agitated or suicidal. One has to be alert and familiar with the ways clients might behave while being confined in such a facility. Being familiar with behavioral symptoms and the types of medications clients are taking may be critical to the well-being and safety of everyone, including the staff. The healthcare practitioner might be tasked with a one-on-one observation of a client on suicide precautions for the entire duration of his or her shift. This kind of job is a situation where everyone—from the mental health worker to the charge nurse—must work together. ■

CLIENT TEACHING

Clients taking antidepressants need to know the following:

1. Tricyclics may increase appetite, cause dizziness with rapid change of position, and be sedating. Report dry mouth, constipation, urinary retention, or blurred vision if they occur.
2. MAO inhibitors may cause problems with sleep, agitation, dizziness when rapidly changing position, and dangerous interactions with other medications. Eating foods high in tyramine can cause a hypertensive crisis. Obtain a list of foods high in tyramine from your healthcare practitioner.
3. SSRIs may cause GI upset, dizziness, skin rash, and headache. Report these signs and symptoms to your healthcare practitioner.
4. Do not combine MAO inhibitors and SSRI antidepressants. Do not take St. John's Wort with any antidepressant. These combinations can cause serious side effects termed serotonin syndrome: confusion, mania, headache, respiratory problems, kidney failure, and possibly death.
5. Antidepressants may take one to four weeks to become fully effective.
6. Some antidepressants may decrease sexual interest or performance. If this occurs, discuss a change in medication with your healthcare practitioner.
7. If insomnia is a problem, take your medication in the morning.
8. If nausea is a problem, take your medication with food, unless ortherwise instructed.
9. Monitor your weight; an increase or a decrease may occur.
10. Avoid driving or operating machinery until you know your response to the medication. Its sedating effects can increase your risk for accidental injury.
11. Do not stop your medication without consulting your healthcare practitioner.

Clients taking anti-psychotics need to know the following:

1. It is imperative to report the development of tremors, involuntary repetitive movements, decreased muscle tone, or increased restlessness to your healthcare practitioner. These symptoms may indicate serious side effects that can be reversed if medication is changed soon after their onset.
2. If dry mouth, rapid heart rate, constipation, or urinary retention occur, consult your healthcare practitioner. An additional medication may be prescribed to relieve these signs and symptoms.
3. Avoid taking antacids with anti-psychotics: they delay or decrease anti-psychotic absorption.
4. Alcohol increases the depressant effects, so it should be avoided while taking anti-psychotics.
5. Extra protection from the sun is necessary: wear hats and sunscreen.
6. Avoid driving or operating machinery until you know your response to the medication. Its sedating effects can increase your risk for accidental injury.
7. If symptoms of your illness increase or are not relieved by the medication, contact your healthcare practitioner for guidance. Do not stop the medication unless directed to do so. ■

CHAPTER REVIEW

Core Concepts Summary

9.1 Attention-deficit disorder (ADD) and attention-deficit/hyperactivity disorder (ADHD) are common in children.

Difficulty paying attention is one of the main symptoms of ADD. Clients diagnosed with ADHD are also hyperactive. Unless helped or encouraged properly, clients with ADD may develop symptoms of maladjustment as they move into adulthood.

9.2 Methylphenidate (Ritalin) is the drug of choice for children with ADHD.

Symptoms of ADHD can be treated with CNS stimulants. Methylphinidate (Ritalin) is the drug choice for most clients.

9.3 Common mood disorders are clinical depression and bipolar disorder (manic depression).

Clients diagnosed with depression may have a range of symptoms. In cases of clinical depression, situational and biological causes have been identified. In the case of manic depression, the causes are less clear.

9.4 Antidepressants work by a variety of mechanisms.

Mood-enhancing drugs or antidepressants treat depression. There are three major classes of antidepressants: monoamine oxidase (MAO) inhibitors, tricyclic anti-depressants (TCAs), and selective serotonin reuptake inhibitors (SSRIs).

9.5 Bipolar disorder may be effectively treated with lithium.

Mood stabilizers treat manic depression or bipolar disorder mainly by lithium (Eskalith). Some anti-seizure medications may also be used. Each class of drug has a unique action and adverse effects.

9.6 Schizophrenia is the major psychosis.

The most common type of psychosis is schizophrenia. Schizoaffective disorder is characterized by psychosis and mood disorder. In addition, clients with mood disorders may experience psychotic episodes. Clients diagnosed with psychosis are treated based on the expression of positive and negative psychotic symptoms.

9.7 Anti-psychotic medications attempt to stabilize clients with psychoses.

Conventional anti-psychotic drugs (phenothiazines and phenothiazine-type medications) treat positive symptoms; atypical psychotic drugs treat both positive and negative symptoms. Healthcare providers must continually monitor the effectiveness of drug therapy and observe for extrapyramidal side effects.

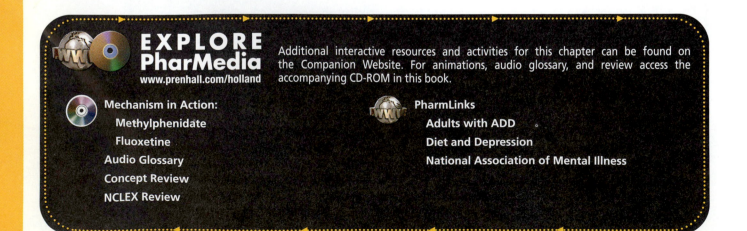

EXPLORE PharMedia
www.prenhall.com/holland

Additional interactive resources and activities for this chapter can be found on the Companion Website. For animations, audio glossary, and review access the accompanying CD-ROM in this book.

Mechanism in Action:
  Methylphenidate
  Fluoxetine
Audio Glossary
Concept Review
NCLEX Review

PharmLinks
  Adults with ADD
  Diet and Depression
  National Association of Mental Illness

10 Drugs for Parkinson's Disease and Dementia

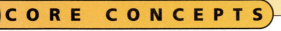

CORE CONCEPTS

PARKINSON'S DISEASE

10.1 Parkinson's disease is characterized by disturbances of muscle movement.

10.2 The symptoms of Parkinson's disease result from dysfunction of the dopamine neurotransmitter between various parts of the brain.

Anti-Parkinson's Drugs

10.3 Drug therapy for Parkinson's symptoms focuses mainly on dopamine and acetylcholine.

Dopaminergic Drugs

Cholinergic-Blockers

DEMENTIA

10.4 Dementia is a progressive and permanent loss of brain function.

Alzheimer's Drugs

10.5 Current medications for Alzheimer's disease result in only minor improvement of symptoms.

OBJECTIVES

After reading this chapter, the student should be able to:

1. Describe symptoms of Parkinson's disease and explain theories about why these symptoms develop.

2. Explain the neurochemical basis for Parkinson's disease, focusing on the roles of dopamine and acetylcholine in the corpus striatum.

3. Describe important pharmacological treatments for Parkinson's disease, listing drug examples and giving details about their actions.

4. Identify two main causes of dementia and explain the main goal of drug therapy in neurodegenerative disorders.

5. Describe symptoms of Alzheimer's disease and explain theories about why these symptoms develop.

6. Identify important pharmacological treatments for Alzheimer's disease.

7. Categorize drugs used for Parkinson's disease and dementia based on their classification and mechanism of action.

PharMedia
www.prenhall.com/holland

Additional interactive resources and activities for this chapter can be found on the Companion Website. For animations, audio glossary, and review access the accompanying CD-ROM in this book.

Degenerative neurobiologic disorders are often difficult to deal with pharmacologically. Parkinson's disease and Alzheimer's dementia, two common debilitating and progressive conditions, are the focus of this chapter. Vascular dementia, another common irreversible neurobiological disorder, results from stroke and is common among elderly clients. While symptoms and neurochemical mechanisms for these disorders continue to be intensively studied, cure is not presently possible. Despite this, drugs are available that provide some relief for the symptoms of these neurobiologic diseases.

Fast Facts Neurodegenerative Diseases

Parkinson's Disease

- 1,500,000 Americans have Parkinson's disease.
- Most clients with Parkinson's disease are above the age of 50.
- Greater than 50% of Parkinson's clients who have difficulty with voluntary movement are less than 60 years of age.
- More men than women develop this disorder.

Dementia

- 4,000,000 Americans have Alzheimer's disease.
- Alzheimer's disease mainly affects clients over the age of 65.
- 60–70% of all clients with dementia have Alzheimer's disease.

The National Parkinson's Foundation and the National Mental Health Association.

PARKINSON'S DISEASE

Parkinson's disease is a degenerative disorder of the CNS caused by death of neurons that produce the brain neurotransmitter dopamine.

10.1 Parkinson's disease is characterized by disturbances of muscle movement.

Parkinson's disease is a degenerative disorder affecting primarily clients older than 50 years of age and men slightly more than women; however, even teenagers can develop this disorder. After diagnosis, expression of full symptoms may take several years. The symptoms of Parkinson's disease are summarized in the following list.

- Tremors
  The hands and head develop a palsy-like motion or shakiness when at rest; pin rolling is a common behavior in progressive states where clients rub the thumb and forefinger together in a circular motion.

- Muscle rigidity
  Stiffness may resemble symptoms of arthritis; clients often have difficulty bending over or moving limbs. Some clients develop a rigid poker face. These symptoms may be less noticeable at first, but progress in later years.

brady = slow
kinesia = movement

- Bradykinesia
  This is the most noticeable of all symptoms. Clients may have difficulty chewing, swallowing, or speaking. Walking often becomes difficult. Clients shuffle their feet without taking large strides.

- Postural instability
  Clients may be humped over slightly and lose their balance. Stumbling commonly results in falling.

Although Parkinson's disease is a progressive disorder primarily affecting muscle movement, other health problems may develop. These include anxiety, depression, sleep disturbances, dementia, and disturbances of the autonomic nervous system such as difficulty urinating and performing sexually.

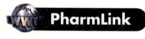

THE NATIONAL PARKINSON FOUNDATION

Several theories have been proposed to explain the development of Parkinson's disease. Because some clients with Parkinson's symptoms have a family history of this disorder, a genetic link is highly probable. Also, many different environmental toxins have been suggested as causes, but results have been inconclusive. Potentially harmful agents include carbon monoxide, cyanide, manganese, chlorine, and pesticides. Virus infections, head trauma, and stroke have also been proposed as causes of Parkinson's.

Concept review 10.1

- Parkinson's disease primarily affects which body functions? What are the four major symptoms of this disorder?

10.2 The symptoms of Parkinson's disease result from dysfunction of the dopamine neurotransmitter between various parts of the brain.

substantia = substance
nigra = substance

corpus = body
striatum = striped

Parkinson's symptoms develop due to the degeneration of dopamine-producing neurons found within an area of the brain known as the **substantia nigra**. When not enough dopamine is released, this neurotransmitter cannot make contact with other critical areas of the brain.

The most critical area for dopamine contact is the **corpus striatum**, an area responsible for controlling unconscious muscle movement. Clients with Parkinson's disease have a problem initiating movement and controlling movements. Balance, posture, muscle tone, and involuntary muscle movement depend on the proper balance of dopamine (inhibitory) and acetylcholine (stimulatory) in the corpus striatum. If dopamine is absent, acetylcholine has a more dramatic effect in this area. *For this reason, anti-Parkinson's drug therapy focuses not only on restoring* *striatal dopamine function, but also on blocking the effect of acetylcholine within the same area.* Thus, whenever the brain experiences a loss of dopamine within the substantia nigra or an overactive cholinergic influence in the corpus striatum, Parkinson's disease results.

Extrapyramidal symptoms (EPS) may develop for the same neurochemical reasons as Parkinson's disease. Anti-psychotic medications work through a mechanism involving blockade of dopamine receptors (pages 127–128). Extensive treatment with certain anti-psychotic drugs may induce artificial Parkinsonism or EPS by interfering with the same neural pathway and functions modified by the lack of dopamine.

With EPS, clients' muscles may spasm or become locked up. Fever and confusion are other signs and symptoms of this reaction. If EPS occurs in a healthcare facility, short-term medical treatment can be provided by administering diphenhydramine (Benadryl). If EPS is recognized outside the healthcare setting, the client should be taken to the emergency room, as untreated EPS can be fatal.

Tardive dyskinesia, a movement disorder often causing involuntary lip and tongue movements and less frequently causing involuntary movements of the trunk and extremities, is observed in clients who have been given anti-psychotic drugs for an extended length of time. Anticholinergic medications are sometimes prescribed concurrently with anti-psychotics to discourage development of tardive dyskinesia or to treat it once it develops.

tardive = late
dyskinesia = abnormal
movement

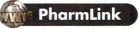

THE AMERICAN PARKINSON
DISEASE ASSOCIATION

PARKINSON SOCIETY CANADA

Concept review 10.2

- What is the major pathology of Parkinson's disease? What brain neurotransmitters are affected and how? What major drug category can produce Parkinson's-like symptoms with overmedication? What are Parkinson's-like symptoms called?

ANTI-PARKINSON'S DRUGS

Anti-Parkinson's drugs are agents given to restore the balance of dopamine and acetylcholine in specific regions of the brain.

10.3 Drug therapy for Parkinson's symptoms focuses mainly on dopamine and acetylcholine.

The goal of drug therapy for Parkinson's disease is to increase the ability of the client to perform normal daily activities such as eating, walking, dressing, and bathing. Drug therapy attempts to restore the balance of dopamine and acetylcholine in the brain, although this is an ongoing treatment and does not cure the disorder.

DOPAMINERGIC DRUGS

Dopaminergic drugs replace dopamine or increase its action in the brain. **Levodopa** is a dopaminergic drug that has been used more extensively than any other medication and is the main treatment for clients with Parkinson's disease. Its success has to do with its role in the biosynthesis of dopamine within nerve terminals. As shown in Figure 10.1, levodopa is a precursor of dopamine synthesis. Levodopa can cross the blood-brain barrier while dopamine cannot. Thus, dopamine cannot be used for therapy. Other approaches for therapy include increasing the action of dopamine by preventing its breakdown or by directly activating the dopamine receptor. Dopaminergic drugs of importance for Parkinson's disease are shown in Table 10.1.

CHOLINERGIC-BLOCKERS

A second approach to changing the balance between dopamine and acetylcholine in the brain is to give cholinergic-blocking drugs. Cholinergic drugs used for Parkinson's disease are centrally

DRUG PROFILE (Dopaminergic):
Levodopa (Larodopa)

Actions:

Levodopa restores the neurotransmitter dopamine in extrapyramidal centers of the brain, thus relieving some Parkinson's symptoms. To increase its effect, levopdopa is often combined with other drugs such as carbidopa (Lodosyn), which prevent its enzymatic breakdown. The trade name for the combination of levodopa-carbidopa is Sinemet.

Adverse Effects:

Side effects of levodopa include uncontrolled and purposeless movements such as extending the fingers and shrugging the shoulders, spasms of the eyelids, involuntary movements, loss of appetite, nausea, and vomiting. Blood pressure may be lowered when making sudden movements or rising too quickly from a seated position. Haloperidol (Haldol) may lower levodopa's effectiveness. Methyldopa (Aldomet) may increase toxicity.

Mechanism in Action:

Clients with Parkinson's disease have a reduction of dopamine and an elevation of acetylcholine in specific regions of the brain. This imbalance is responsible for symptoms such as slow movements, tremor, muscle rigidity, shuffling gait, flat facial expression, speech impairment, and lack of fine psychomotor skills. Levodopa, a precursor to dopamine, crosses the blood-brain barrier and restores the imbalance between dopamine and acetylcholine, thereby treating Parkinson's symptoms.

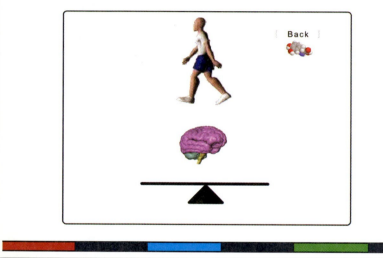

DRUG PROFILE (Cholinergic-Blocker):
Benztropine (Cogentin)

Actions:

Benztropine acts by blocking excess cholinergic stimulation of neurons not balanced by the presence of dopamine. This drug suppresses tremors but does not affect tardive dyskinesia. It is used for relief of Parkinson's symptoms and for the treatment of EPS brought on by antipsychotic drug therapy.

Adverse Effects:

Side effects of benztropine include sedation, dry mouth, constipation, and muscle weakness. Benztropine should not to be taken with alcohol because of combined sedative effects. OTC cold medicines should also be avoided. Other drugs that enhance dopamine release or activation of the dopamine receptor may produce additive effects. Similar sedative and muscle weakness effects are expected with tricyclic antidepressants, MAO inhibitors, phenothiazines, procainamide (Pronestyl), and quinidine (Quinedex). Therefore, these drugs should be avoided in combination with benztropine.

TABLE 10.1	Dopaminergic Drugs Used for Parkinson's Disease	
DRUG	**ROUTE AND ADULT DOSE**	**REMARKS**
Pr levodopa (L-Dopa, Larodopa)	PO; 500 mg to 1 gram/day; may be increased by 100–750 mg every 3–7 days.	Chemical precursor to dopamine; dosage can be reduced by 70%–80% if administered with carbidopa.
amantadine hydrochloride (Symmetrel)	PO; 100 mg qd or bid.	Also for infection with influenza A virus; for relief of drug-induced EPS; may cause release of dopamine from nerve terminals.
bromocriptine mesylate (Parlodel)	PO; 1.25–2.5 mg/day up to 100 mg/day in divided doses.	Also for suppression of lactation, for female infertility, and overproduction of growth hormone; activates the dopamine receptor directly.
carbidopa-levadopa	PO; 10 mg/100 mg levodopa; may increase this dose every day or every other day up to 6 times.	Prevents metabolism of levodopa, enhancing dopamine action(Sinemet).
pergolide (Permax)	PO; start with 0.05 mg daily for 2 days; increase by 0.1 or 0.15 mg/day every 3 days for 12 days; then increase by 0.25 mg every 3rd day until the desired effect.	Activates dopamine receptors.
pramipexole dihydrochloride (Mirapex)	PO; start with 0.125 mg tid for 1 week; double this dose for the next week; continue to increase by 0.25 mg/dose tid every week to a target dose of 1.5 mg tid.	Activates dopamine receptors.
ropinirole hydrochloride (Requip)	PO; start with 0.25 mg tid; may titrate up by 0.25 mg/dose tid every week to a target dose of 1 mg tid.	Activates dopamine receptors.
selegiline hydrochloride (L-Deprenyl,Eldepryl)	PO; 5 mg/dose bid (with breakfast and lunch); doses greater than 10 mg/day are potentially toxic.	Blocks MAO type B, the enzyme that degrades dopamine within the brain.
tolcapone (Tasmar)	PO; 100 mg tid (max 600 mg/day).	Blocks enzymes responsible for metabolizing dopamine.

TABLE 10.2	Cholinergic-Blockers Used for Parkinson's Disease	
DRUG	**ROUTE AND ADULT DOSE**	**REMARKS**
Pr benztropine mesylate (Cogentin)	PO; 0.5–1 mg/day; gradually increase as needed up to 6 mg/day.	Also used to relieve EPS from neuroleptic drugs; does not lighten tardive dyskinesia.
biperiden hydrochloride (Akineton)	PO; 2 mg qd to qid.	Blocks acetylcholine receptors; thus, actions associated with muscarinic blockade are observed, i.e., blurred vision and dry mouth; available in IM/IV forms.
diphenhydramine hydrochloride (Benadryl)	PO; 25–50 mg tid or qid (max 300/day).	Also for allergic reactions, motion sickness, sedation, and coughing; blocks cholinergic function even though it is an antihistamine; available in IM/IV forms.
procyclidine hydrochloride (Kemadrin)	PO; 2.5 mg tid pc; may be increased to 5 mg tid if tolerated with an additional 5 mg at hs (max 45–60 mg/day).	Blocks acetylcholine receptors in the brain.
trihexyphenidyl hydrochloride (Artane)	PO; 1 mg for day 1; double this for day 2; then increase by 2 mg every 3–5 days up to 6–10 mg/day (max 15 mg/day).	Also used to relieve EPS; unlabeled use for Huntington's chorea and spasmodic torticollis.

FIGURE 10.1

Levodopa's role in the biosynthesis of dopamine within nerve terminals. Levodopa is a precursor of dopamine synthesis. Levodopa can cross the blood-brain barrier while dopamine cannot

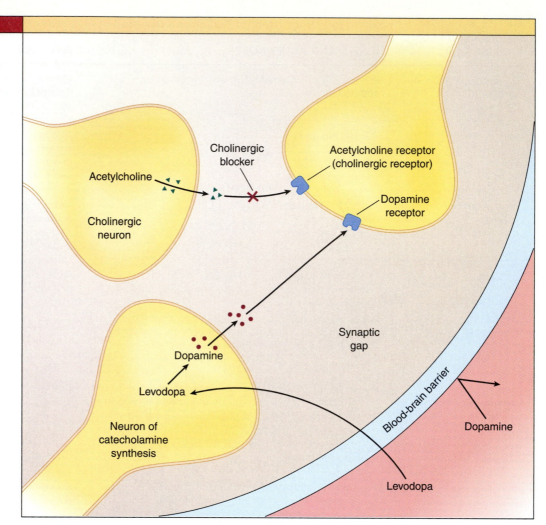

acting drugs that block the effect of acetylcholine. These agents prevent the overactivity of acetylcholine by blocking cholinergic receptors (Chapter 6 🔗). Only centrally acting anticholinergic drugs are effective for Parkinson's disease. The anticholinergics produce more side effects than the dopaminergic drugs and their primary use is for clients who cannot tolerate levodopa. Cholinergic-blocking drugs may also be used in combination with other anti-Parkinson's drugs. These drugs are shown in Table 10.2.

NATURAL ALTERNATIVES

Glutathione and Milk Thistle for the Treatment of Parkinson's Disease

The word is getting out about a natural alternative used for the treatment of Parkinson's disease: glutathione therapy. Glutathione is inexpensive and readily available; however, it is not available in oral form. IV therapy given by a qualified practitioner may dramatically reverse symptoms for up to four months. The primary role of glutathione is not to reverse neural damage after it has already begun, but to slow down the progression of damage by limiting the action of circulating free radicals. Free radicals are highly reactive molecules that are thought to produce molecular damage throughout the body, especially in vulnerable places including the brain. Glutathioine is an antioxidant, which means it is a molecular scavenger for molecules in the bloodstream that might cause serious cellular damage. Milk thistle (*Silybum marianum*) has been used to retain glutathione in the bloodstream during therapy. ■

Concept review 10.3

- Anti-Parkinson's drugs attempt to restore the balance of which two major central neurotransmitters? Describe the two approaches for restoring neurotransmitter balance in clients with Parkinson's disease.

DEMENTIA

Dementia is a degenerative disorder characterized by progressive memory loss, confusion, and inability to think or communicate effectively. Alzheimer's disease is the most common cause of dementia.

10.4 Dementia is a progressive and permanent loss of brain function.

The most common causes of dementia are **Alzheimer's disease** and multiple strokes. Dementia caused by stroke is sometimes called **multiple-infarct** or **vascular dementia**. An infarct is tissue damage resulting from a reduced blood supply. In the brain, the source of infarct is often blood clots in major vessels of the head and neck area. Medications to treat strokes are discussed in Chapter 17 ⬚ .

Currently, there is not an effective treatment for vascular dementia. Once degeneration of neuronal tissue has begun, little can be done to recover brain function. Prevention of additional strokes with more associated damage is a priority. Medications for anxiety, depression, or psychoses provide a level of comfort and safety to the client after the onset of dementia. These drugs were discussed in Chapters 7 and 9 ⬚ .

There is not a definitive diagnostic test for Alzheimer's disease. However, imaging techniques and documentation of multiple cognitive impairments not accounted for by other diseases lead to accurate diagnosis about 90% of the time. The only definitive diagnosis is based on the discovery of **amyloid plaques** and **neurofibrillary tangles** within the brain at autopsy.

Despite extensive research, the causes of Alzheimer's disease are still unknown. The early onset familial form of this disorder, accounting for about 10% of cases, is associated with gene defects on chromosome 1, 14, or 21. Chronic inflammation and excess free radicals may cause neuron damage in early and late onset dementia. Environmental, immunologic, and nutritional factors, as well as viruses are also considered as possible sources of brain damage.

Scientists do know that Alzheimer's clients experience a dramatic loss of cholinergic brain function. This means that clients eventually lose their ability to perform tasks that require acetylcholine as the neurotransmitter. Because acetylcholine is a major neurotransmitter within the **hippocampus**, an area of the brain responsible for learning and memory, and other parts of the cerebral cortex, neuronal function within these brain areas is especially affected. Thus, an inability to remember and to recall information is among the early symptoms of Alzheimer's disease. In more advanced stages, clients may become aggressive and agitated and require continuous care. Alzheimer's clients often are confused and wander off or get lost if left unattended. Some clients live for 20 years, but most die within 8 to 10 years of diagnosis. Symptoms of Alzheimer's disease are given in the following list.

- impaired memory
- confusion or disorientation
- inability to recognize family or friends
- impaired decision making
- need for constant care
- anxious, verbal, or combative behaviors

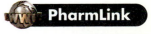

ALZHEIMER'S DISEASE INFORMATION PAGE

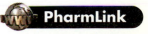

ALZHEIMER SOCIETY OF CANADA

ALZHEIMER'S DRUGS

Alzheimer's drugs attempt to slow memory loss or restore the client's ability to remember and provide relief for other symptoms. These are cholinergic drugs that enhance the action of acetylcholine in the brain.

10.5 Current medications for Alzheimer's disease result in only minor improvement of symptoms.

The FDA has approved only a few drugs for Alzheimer's symptoms. Most medications work by intensifying the effect of acetylcholine at the cholinergic receptor as shown in Figure 10.2. Acetylcholine is naturally degraded in the synapse by an enzyme called **acetylcholinesterase (AchE)**. When AchE is inhibited, acetylcholine levels become elevated and produce a more profound effect on the receptor.

Scientists believe that restoring cholinergic function in the brain will improve learning and memory. Thus, most research efforts have centered on restoring cholinergic function. However, some researchers are attempting to identify factors responsible for the appearance of amyloid plaques and neurofibrillary tangles. The hope is that if neuronal damage can be prevented, then the onset of dementia may also be prevented. Examples of medications approved for Alzheimer's disease are listed in Table 10.3.

FIGURE 10.2

Alzheimers medications work by intensifying the effect of acetylcholine at the receptor

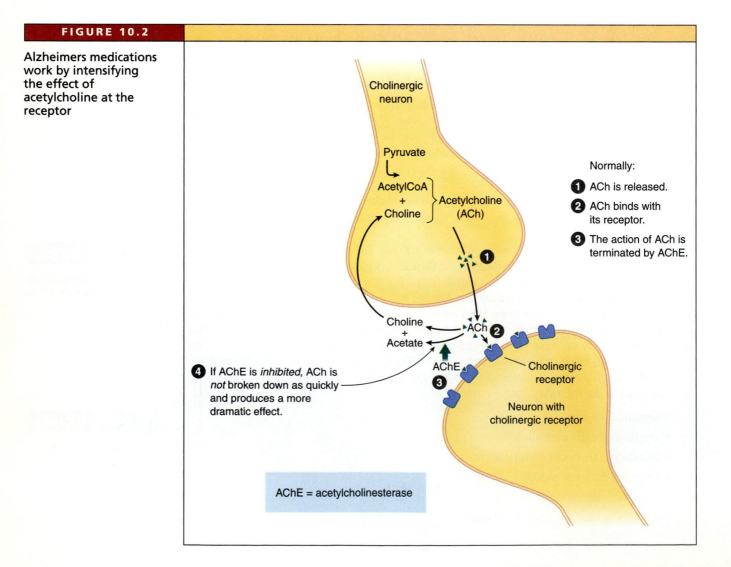

Normally:

1 ACh is released.

2 ACh binds with its receptor.

3 The action of ACh is terminated by AChE.

4 If AChE is *inhibited*, ACh is *not* broken down as quickly and produces a more dramatic effect.

AChE = acetylcholinesterase

DRUG PROFILE:

Tacrine (Cognex)

Actions:

Tacrine is an Ach inhibitor that improves memory in cases of mild to moderate Alzheimer's dementia. This is thought to occur by enhancing the effects of acetylcholine in neurons that have not yet been damaged. Clients should be monitored for improvement for at least six months prior to assessing maximum benefits of drug therapy. Improvement in memory may be observed as early as one to four weeks following medication. Unfortunately, the effects of Tacrine are short-lived and the degree of improvement is modest, at best.

Adverse Effects:

Common side effects of Tacrine are vomiting, diarrhea, obstruction of urinary flow, and darkened urine. The most serious side effect is hepatotoxicity, which often causes discontinuation of therapy. Tacrine increases the effects of neuromuscular blocking agents, theophylline, and cimetidine, and sensitizes the client to the effects of castor oil. This type of therapy should be used cautiously in clients who have glaucoma, diabetes, epilepsy, or cardiovascular disorders because of undesirable side effects such as hypotension, excessive urination, seizures, and bradycardia.

TABLE 10.3	Drugs of Importance for Alzheimer's Disease	
DRUG	**ROUTE AND ADULT DOSE**	**REMARKS**
donepezil hydrochloride (Aricept)	PO; 5–10 mg at hs.	For mild to moderate dementia; may cause nausea, diarrhea, muscle cramps, and weight loss.
ergaloid mesylate (Gerimal, Hydergine, Hydroloid-G, Niloric)	PO; 1 mg tid; doses up to 4.5–12 mg/day have been used.	Dilates blood vessels by a central action; increases cerebral blood flow; may reduce blood pressure and heart rate; also available in sublingual form.
Pr tacrine (Cognex)	PO; 10 mg qid; increase in 40 mg/day increments not sooner than every 6 weeks to a max of 160 mg/day.	For mild to moderate dementia; unlabeled use for severe dementia in clients with HIV infection; may cause nausea, vomiting, and liver toxicity.

Concept review 10.4

■ Alzheimer's disease is a dysfunction of which brain neurotransmitters? How do drugs for Alzheimer's disease restore neurotransmitter function and improve Alzheimer's symptoms?

ON THE JOB

Home Health Care Nursing of Clients with Dementia

Being a home health care nurse is a challenging but rewarding job. Dealing with dementia requires a tremendous amount of stamina and a positive outlook because clients often feel confused and abandoned. Also, family members are often anxious or concerned and rely on you to convey medical information about how their parent or loved one is doing. Daily tasks—taking a bath, going to the bathroom, or eating—will become more and more challenging as the condition worsens. Family members often feel burdened, guilty, or frustrated. An important role of the healthcare practitioner is to try to calm both the client and family members, informing them about any medications and adverse reactions that the client might experience. This covers a wide range of drugs from anxiolytics to anti-depressants and even anti-psychotic medication. Special diets will often be needed, and making the sure the family understands these limitations will be important. ■

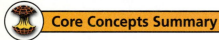

CLIENT TEACHING

Clients taking drugs for Parkinson's disease or dementia need to know the following:

1. Do not eat high protein foods or foods high in vitamin B$_6$ (such as wheat germ, liver, green leafy vegetables, bananas, and fish) if you are taking levodopa. These foods interfere with drug effectiveness.

2. Be extremely careful about getting up quickly from a seated position. Many dementia drugs cause dizziness, lightheadedness, blurred vision, and difficulty in concentrating.

3. Do not skip your medications or take OTC preparations (especially cold or cough medicines) without checking with your healthcare practitioner.

4. Do not worry if your urine becomes a little dark. This is a normal side effect of dopamine-like drugs.

5. Do not drink alcoholic beverages or take sedatives with dementia medications. Combined effects may be harmful.

6. Be familiar with adverse effects specific for the drugs you are taking.

7. Drugs may produce nausea, dry mouth, and diminished sweating in some cases. ■

CHAPTER REVIEW

Core Concepts Summary

10.1 Parkinson's disease is characterized by disturbances of muscle movement.

Four main disturbances are usually observed in Parkinson's clients: tremors, rigidity, bradykinesia, and postural instability. The cause of Parkinson's disease hasn't been found, but several theories have been proposed.

10.2 The symptoms of Parkinson's disease result from dysfunction of the dopamine neurotransmitter between various parts of the brain.

Parkinson's disease develops when dopamine is depleted from an area in the brain called the substantia nigra. Neurons from this area project to the corpus striatum where muscle movements are controlled. At the corpus striatum, the underlying chemical problem is lack of dopamine activity and a related overactivity of acetylcholine.

10.3 Drug therapy for Parkinson's symptoms focuses mainly on dopamine and acetylcholine.

Drug therapy for Parkinson's disease focuses on restoring dopamine function in the substantia nigra and dampening acetylcholine action at the corpus striatum. Two major drug therapies are levodopa (Larodopa) and benztropine (Cogentin).

10.4 Dementia is a progressive and permanent loss of brain function.

Two common types of dementia are Alzheimer's disease and vascular dementia. Restorative drug therapies for dementia mainly focus on Alzheimer's disease because this is the most common type of dementia.

10.5 Current medications for Alzheimer's disease result in only minor improvement in symptoms.

Some drugs for Alzheimer's disease block acetylcholinesterase, an enzyme responsible for inactivating acetylcholine. When acetylcholinesterase is inactivated, acetylcholine action is enhanced. Dementia from Alzheimer's disease and other disorders may also be treated by anxiolytics, mood enhancers, and anti-psychotic drugs.

EXPLORE PharMedia
www.prenhall.com/holland

Additional interactive resources and activities for this chapter can be found on the Companion Website. For animations, audio glossary, and review access the accompanying CD-ROM in this book.

Mechanism in Action:
  Levodopa
Audio Glossary
Concept Review
NCLEX Review

PharmLinks
  The National Parkinson Foundation
  The American Parkinson Disease Association
  Parkinson Society Canada
  Alzheimer's Disease Information Page
  Alzheimer Society of Canada

11 Drugs for the Control of Pain and Fever

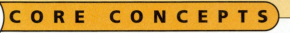

CORE CONCEPTS

ACUTE OR CHRONIC PAIN

11.1 Pain assessment is the first step to pain management.

11.2 Neural mechanisms of pain are well characterized.

11.3 Analgesics are classified as non-narcotics or narcotics.

Non-steroidal Anti-inflammatory Drugs (NSAIDS)

11.4 Non-steroidal anti-inflammatory drugs (NSAIDS) are effective in treating mild to moderate pain, inflammation, and fever.

Narcotic (Opioid) Analgesics

11.5 Opioids are substances extracted from the poppy plant that exert their effects through interaction with mu and kappa receptors.

11.6 Opioids are the drugs of choice for severe pain.

FEVER

Antipyretics

11.7 Fever is a defense mechanism of the body that can be effectively treated with antipyretic medications.

TENSION HEADACHE AND MIGRAINES

11.8 The goals of drug therapy for migraine headaches are to stop migraines in progress and to prevent them from occurring.

OBJECTIVES

After reading this chapter, the student should be able to:

1. Identify questions that a healthcare provider might ask a client in order to determine the type of pain he or she is experiencing.

2. Describe first and second pain and explain the neural mechanism for pain at the level of the spinal cord.

3. Explain two major ways that pain can be controlled involving the release of spinal neurotransmitters.

4. Explain the mechanism for pain at the nociceptor.

5. Identify the different classes of analgesics.

6. For each of the following drugs or drug classes, identify representative medications and explain the mechanism of drug action, primary actions, and important adverse effects.
   a. non-narcotic analgesics (NSAIDS): aspirin, ibuprofen, and ibuprofen-like drugs, and selective COX2 inhibitors
   b. narcotic analgesics and opioid blockers
   c. antipyretics
   d. triptans

7. Categorize drugs used in the treatment of pain and fever based on their classification and mechanism of action.

PharMedia
www.prenhall.com/holland

Additional interactive resources and activities for this chapter can be found on the Companion Website. For animations, audio glossary, and review access the accompanying CD-ROM in this book.

Aδ fibers: nerves that transmit sensations of sharp pain / *page 149*

acute pain: short-term sensation that is uncomfortable or hurtful; a sharp and intense pain / *page 148*

analgesic (an-ul-JEE-zik): drug used to reduce or eliminate pain / *page 149*

antipyretic (ANN-tee-pye-RETT-ik): drug that reduces fever / *page 158*

aura (AUR-uh): sensory cue such as bright lights, smells, or tastes that precede a migraine / *page 158*

bradykinin (bray-dee-KYE-nin): chemical mediator of pain released following tissue damage / *page 152*

C fibers: nerves that transmit dull, poorly localized pain / *page 149*

chronic pain: a long-term sensation that is uncomfortable or hurtful; a persistent, dull ache / *page 148*

cyclooxygenase (sye-klo-OK-sah-jen-ays): enzyme involved in the synthesis of prostaglandins / *page 151*

endogenous opioids (en-DAHJ-eh-nuss O-pee-oyds): chemicals produced naturally within the body that decrease or eliminate pain; they closely resemble the actions of morphine / *page 149*

kappa (CAP-uh): type of opioid receptor / *page 154*

migraine (MYE-grayne): severe headache preceded by auras that may include nausea and vomiting / *page 158*

mu (MYOO): type of opioid receptor / *page 154*

myelin (MYE-ul-in): fatty substance surrounding nerves that speeds up impulse transmission / *page 149*

narcotic (nar-KOT-ik): natural or synthetic drug related to morphine; may be used as a broader legal term referring to hallucinogens (LSD), CNS stimulants, marijuana, and other illegal drugs / *page 153*

nociceptors (no-si-SEPP-ters): receptors connected with nerves that receive and transmit pain signals to the spinal cord and brain / *page 149*

opiate (OH-pee-aht): morphine-like substance extracted from the poppy plant / *page 153*

opioid (OH-pee-oyd): natural or synthetic morphine-like substance / *page 153*

prostaglandins (pros-tah-GLAN-dins): chemicals released after tissue damage, leading to pain, inflammation, and other body reactions / *page 152*

substance P: a neurotransmitter within the spinal cord involved in the neural transmission of pain / *page 149*

tension headache: common type of head pain caused by stress and relieved by non-narcotic analgesics / *page 158*

Pain is an emotional experience characterized by unpleasant feelings, usually associated with trauma or disease. On a simple level, pain may be viewed as a defense mechanism that helps us to avoid potentially damaging situations and encourages us to seek medical help when necessary.

The perception of pain and the psychological reaction to pain are highly individualized. Although the neural and chemical mechanisms for pain are fairly straightforward, many psychological and emotional processes can modify this sensation. One of the goals of pharmacology is to alleviate pain and suffering by interrupting the process of pain transmission. This chapter deals with how pain can be controlled pharmacologically.

Fast Facts Pain

- Pain is a common symptom.

  16 million people experience chronic arthritic pain.

  31 million adults report low back pain, with 19 million people experiencing this on a chronic basis.

  50 million people are fully or partially disabled as a result of pain.

  Over 50% of adults experience muscle pain each year.

  Up to 40% of people with cancer report moderate to severe pain.

- About 28,000,000 Americans suffer from headaches and migraines.

  95% of migraines are controlled by drug therapy and other measures.

  After puberty, women have four to eight times more migraines than men.

  Before puberty, more boys have migraines than girls.

  Headaches and migraines appear mostly among people in their 20s and 30s.

  Persons with a family history of headache or migraine have a higher chance of developing these disorders.

TABLE 11.1	Factors Influencing a Client's Response to Pain
Age	Older clients may have a decreased perception of pain or simply ignore pain as a "natural" consequence of aging.
Emotional state	Anxiety, fatigue, and depression can increase the sensation of pain. Positive attitudes, support from caregivers, or intense focus or concentration may reduce the perception of pain.
Social/cultural influences	Some families, cultures, or social groups view expression of pain symptoms, such as crying as a sign of weakness. Other social units expect their members to freely express their feelings toward pain.
Past experiences with pain	If clients receive positive, supportive feedback from caregivers regarding their pain symptoms, they will more feely express these symptoms in the future. When clients are criticized for expressing their feelings or if their pain needs have been neglected, they will likely not express their emotions freely in the future.
Knowledge of pain	Clients are more likely to accept or tolerate their pain if they know the source of the sensation and the medical course of treatment designed to manage the pain. For example, if the client knows that the pain is temporary, such as during labor or after surgery, he or she is more likely to be accepting of the pain.

ACUTE OR CHRONIC PAIN

Acute pain is a short-term sensation that is uncomfortable or hurtful. When the sensation is longterm, it is called **chronic pain**. In some cases, pain may have a strong inflammatory component, or fever may be a major symptom. Factors influencing a client's response to pain are listed in Table 11.1.

11.1 Pain assessment is the first step to pain management.

An understanding of conditions that cause pain and an ability to recognize them is one of the most important aspects of medical therapy. Pain assessment has two main purposes. First, pain may only be a symptom of an underlying disorder. Assessment is necessary to help identify the cause of the pain so that the disorder can be effectively treated. In many cases, the pain will not diminish until the underlying problem is eliminated.

Secondly, selection of the correct pharmacological agent is dependent upon the nature and character of the pain. Sharp pain, referred to as *fast* or *first pain,* is usually treated differently than dull, throbbing pain, which is sometimes called *slow* or *second pain.* Acute pain, an intense pain occurring over a short time, is often treated differently than chronic pain, a lingering pain occurring over a longer time. Several numerical scales and survey instruments are available to help healthcare providers standardize the assessment of pain and predict the success of subsequent drug therapy. Successful pharmacotherapy depends upon an accurate and skillful assessment.

Pain can sometimes be managed using non-pharmacological techniques. This is important because drugs used to treat pain have the potential to cause serious adverse effects if taken in high doses for extended periods of time. Healthcare providers should encourage their clients to explore some of these methods to see if they help in eliminating the need for pain medication, or at least in lowering the necessary dose of pain-relieving drugs. Some techniques used for reducing pain are listed here.

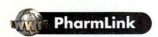

THE AMERICAN HOLISTIC NURSES ASSOCIATION

- acupuncture
- biofeedback therapy
- massage
- heat or cold packs
- meditation
- relaxation therapy
- art or music therapy
- imagery

- chiropractic manipulation
- hypnosis
- therapeutic touch
- healing touch
- transcutaneous electrical nerve stimulation (TENS)
- energy therapies such as Reiki and Qi gong

Concept review 11.1

- If you were a healthcare practitioner, what questions would you ask to identify a client's type of pain? How would you distinguish between acute pain and chronic pain? Which is the most difficult type of pain to treat?

11.2 Neural mechanisms of pain are well characterized.

The process of pain transmission begins when pain receptors are stimulated. These receptors, called **nociceptors**, are free nerve endings strategically-located throughout the body. The nerve impulse signaling the pain is sent to the spinal cord along two types of sensory neurons called Aδ and C fibers. **Aδ fibers** are wrapped in **myelin**, a lipid substance that speeds up nerve transmission. **C fibers** are unmyelinated. Thus, they carry information more slowly. The Aδ fibers signal sharp, well defined pain, whereas the C fibers conduct dull, poorly localized pain.

noci = pain or injury
ceptor = receiver

Once reaching the spinal cord, neurotransmitters are responsible for passing the pain message along to the next neuron. Here, a neurotransmitter called **substance P** is thought to be responsible for continuing the pain message, although other neurotransmitter candidates have been proposed. Scientific evidence suggests that in some locations throughout the nervous system, substance P may also be a pain modulator. Spinal substance P is critical because it controls whether or not pain signals will stop or continue to the brain. Substance P may be controlled by other neurotransmitters released from neurons in the CNS. One group of neurotransmitters called **endogenous opioids** include endorphins, dynorphins, and enkephalins. Figure 11.1 shows one point of contact where endogenous opioids modify sensory information at the level of the spinal cord.

endo = within
genous = coming from

The pain impulse may eventually reach the brain, which responds to the sensation. The possible responses to pain may vary extensively, ranging from signaling the skeletal muscles to jerk away from a sharp object to mental depression caused by thoughts of death or disability.

The fact that the pain signal begins at nociceptors located within peripheral tissues and organs allows several targets for the pharmacological modification of pain transmission. The two main classes of pain medications act at different locations: the non-steroidal anti-inflammatory drugs (NSAIDS) act at the peripheral level, whereas the opioids act centrally.

Concept review 11.2

- What is a nociceptor? Describe how pain can be regulated considering substance P and endogenous opioids.

11.3 Analgesics are classified as non-narcotics or narcotics.

Drugs used for pain relief are called **analgesics**. Analgesics may be classified as follows.

an = without
algesia = pain

- non-narcotic (non-opioid) analgesics
  - non-steroidal anti-inflammatory drugs (NSAIDS)
    - aspirin
    - ibuprofen and ibuprofen-like drugs
    - selective COX2 inhibitors

FIGURE 11.1

Neural pathways for
pain

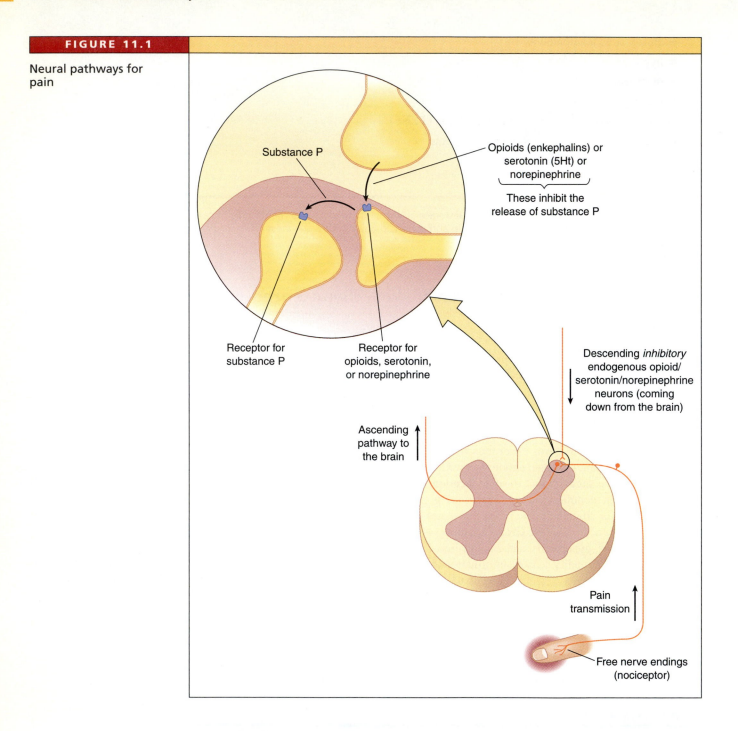

- narcotic (opioid) analgesics
- antipyretics (may have an anti-inflammatory action)
  - aspirin (NSAID)
  - acetaminophen
- drugs for migraine
  - triptans

Painful disorders having a strong inflammatory component, such as arthritis, are treated most effectively with the NSAIDS. Severe pain and pain that cannot be controlled with non-opioids are treated with narcotic analgesics. Minor headaches, body aches, fever, and other pain of less serious origin may be treated with the NSAIDS or acetaminophen. Triptans are used to control migraines.

NON-STEROIDAL ANTI-INFLAMMATORY DRUGS (NSAIDS)

NSAIDS are drugs that inhibit cyclooxygenase, an enzyme responsible for the formation of prostaglandins. Some prostaglandins activate peripheral nociceptors and thus produce pain. Other prostaglandins are associated with tissue damage and inflammation. When cyclooxygenase is inhibited, inflammation and pain are reduced.

11.4 Non-steroidal anti-inflammatory drugs (NSAIDS) are effective in treating mild to moderate pain, inflammation, and fever.

The drugs of choice for mild to moderate pain are the NSAIDS. These medications have many advantages. Aspirin and ibuprofen are available OTC and are inexpensive. They are available in many different formulations, including those designed for children. In most clients, they are very safe and produce adverse effects only at high doses. All the NSAIDS have antipyretic and anti-inflammatory activity, as well as analgesic properties. In fact, some of the NSAIDS, such as the selective COX2 inhibitors, are used primarily for their anti-inflammatory properties. The role of the NSAIDS in the treatment of inflammation is discussed in Chapter 20 ⊂⊃. Selected non-opioids used for analgesia are shown in Table 11.2.

TABLE 11.2	Selected Non-Opioid Analgesics	
DRUG	**RATE AND DOSE**	**REMARKS**
Pr acetaminophen (Tylenol)	PO; 325–650 mg every 4–6 hrs (max 4 grams/day).	Also for fever; available also in rectal form.
Pr aspirin (Acetylsalicylic acid, ASA)	PO; 350–650 mg every 4 hours (max 4 grams/day).	Also for fever, inflammation, and thromboembolic disorders; prevention of transient ischemic attacks and heart attacks; rectal form available.
ibuprofen (Advil, Motrin)	PO; 400 mg every 4–6 hours up to 1200 mg/day.	Also for fever and inflammation.
celecoxib (Celebrex)	PO; 100–200 mg bid or 200 mg/qd.	Also for inflammation; selective COX2 inhibitor.
diflunisal (Dolobid)	PO; 1000 mg followed by 500 mg bid to tid.	Also for inflammation; similar to ibuprofen.
etodolac (Lodine)	PO; 200–400 mg tid to qid.	Also for inflammation; similar to ibuprofen.
fenoprofen calcium (Nalfon)	PO; 200 mg every 4–6 hours.	Also for inflammation; similar to ibuprofen.
ketoprofen (Actron, Orudis)	PO; 12.5–50 mg tid to qid.	Also for inflammation; similar to ibuprofen.
ketorolac tromethamine (Toradol)	PO; 10 mg qid prn (max 40 mg/day).	Also for allergic conjunctivitis; available in IM/IV forms; similar to ibuprofen.
naproxen (Naprosyn; Anaprox)`	PO; 500 mg followed by 200–250 mg tid to qid (max 1250 mg/day).	Also for inflammation; similar to ibuprofen.
rofecoxib (Vioxx)	PO: 12.5–25 mg qd.	Also for inflammation; selective COX2 inhibitor.

FIGURE 11.2

Mechanisms of pain at the nociceptor level

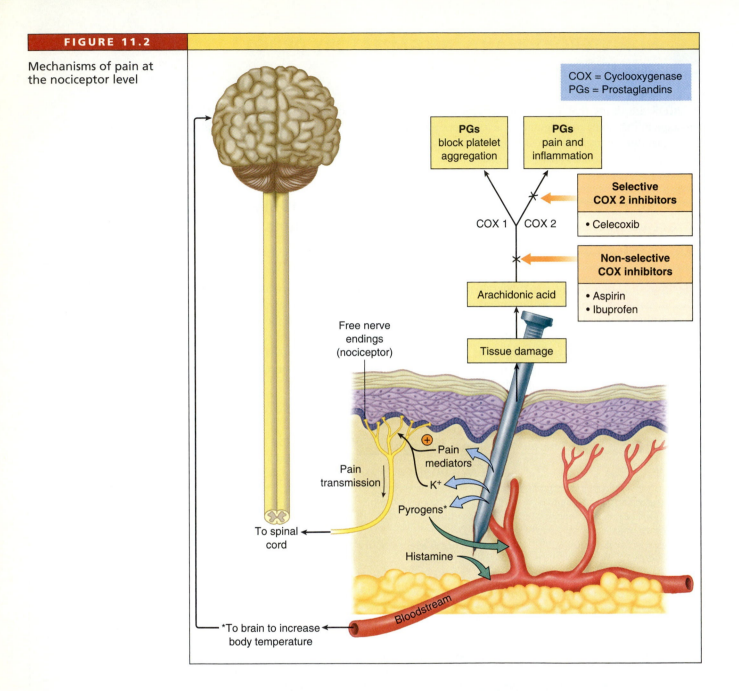

When tissue is damaged, chemical mediators are released including histamine, potassium, hydrogen ion, **bradykinin**, and **prostaglandins**. Bradykinin is connected with the sensory impulse of pain. The NSAIDS act by inhibiting pain mediators at the nociceptor level.

brady = slow
kinin = movement

Two types of prostaglandins are produced after injury, formed with the help of two enzymes called *cyclooxygenase type one* (COX1) and *cyclooxygenase type two* (COX2). Drugs that prevent prostaglandin formation are called cyclooxygenase inhibitors. The NSAIDS act by this mechanism. Aspirin inhibits both COX1 and COX2. Because the COX2 enzyme is more specific for the synthesis of prostaglandins that cause pain and inflammation, the selective COX2 inhibitors provide more specific pain relief and produce fewer side effects than aspirin. Figure 11.2 illustrates the mechanisms involved in pain at the nociceptor level.

Concept review 11.3

▪ Describe how pain might be regulated at the level of the nociceptor considering the following substances: cyclooxygenase inhibitors (NSAIDS) and prostaglandins. Explain how a client might develop fever from tissue damage.

DRUG PROFILE:
Aspirin (Acetylsalicylic acid, ASA)

Actions:

Aspirin inhibits prostaglandin synthesis involved in the production of pain and inflammation. It also produces mild to moderate relief of fever. Similar to acetaminophen, it has limited effects on peripheral blood vessels, causing vasodilation and sweating. Aspirin has significant anticoagulant activity and this property is responsible for aspirin's ability to reduce the risk of mortality following heart attacks and to reduce the incidence of strokes. Aspirin has also been found to reduce the risk of colorectal cancer, although the mechanism by which it affords this protective effect is unknown.

Adverse Effects:

At high doses, such as those used to treat inflammatory disorders, aspirin may cause gastric discomfort and bleeding because of its anti-platelet effects. Enteric-coated tablets and buffered preparations are available for clients who experience gastric distress. Aspirin should not be used during pregnancy, especially in the third trimester. Because of its association with Reye's syndrome, aspirin should not be used in children with fever, chicken pox, or influenza-like symptoms. Because aspirin increases bleeding time, it should not be given with anti-coagulants.

NARCOTIC (OPIOID) ANALGESICS

An opioid analgesic is a natural or synthetic morphine-like substance responsible for reducing pain. Opioids are **narcotic** substances, meaning that they can produce a numbness or stupor-like condition.

narc = *numbness or stupor*
otic = *like*

11.5 Opioids are substances extracted from the poppy plant that exert their effects through interaction with mu and kappa receptors.

Terminology associated with the narcotic analgesic medications is often confusing. These drugs are obtained from opium, an extract from the unripe seeds of the poppy plant, which contains over 20 different chemicals having pharmacologic activity. These natural substances, such as morphine and codeine, are called **opiates**. In a search for safer analgesics, chemists have created several dozen synthetic drugs with activity similar to that of the opiates. **Opioid** is a general term referring to any of these substances, natural or synthetic, and is often used interchangeably with the term opiate.

opi = *opium*
oid = *shape or form*

NATURAL ALTERNATIVES

Evening Primrose for Pain

Evening primrose (*Primula vulgaris*) was once considered a medicinal herb for rheumatism, gout, and paralysis. Among modern herbalists, it has several uses depending on which part of the flower is collected. Interestingly, one can find reports of many illnesses where primrose may be helpful, including arthritis, anxiety, high cholesterol levels, irritability, ADHD disorder, and fibromyalgia. Oil of primrose contains an essential fatty acid called *linoleic acid,* which is a natural precursor to gamma linolenic acid, a substance having a reputation for reducing breast tenderness and improving headaches resulting from premenstrual syndrome. Thus, evening primrose oil is sometimes suggested as a natural remedy for primary dysmenorrhea. Although some scientific reports are skeptical, other studies suggest that women with premenstrual syndrome are deficient in gamma linolenic acid. It may be that replacing this deficiency somehow blocks natural mechanisms for the transmission of pain. ■

FIGURE 11.3

Opiod receptors

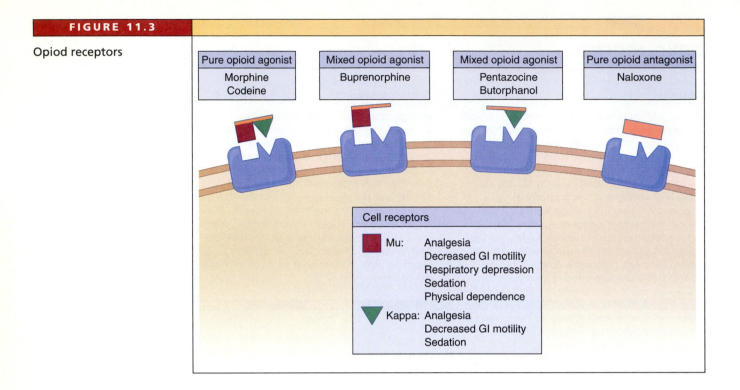

The term *opioid narcotic* is a more general term meant to describe morphine-like drugs that produce analgesia and CNS depression. These drugs may be natural, such as morphine, or synthetic such as meperidine (Demerol). In the context of drug enforcement, however, the term narcotic is often used to classify a broader range of abused illegal drugs such as hallucinogens, heroin, amphetamines, and marijuana. In medical environments, it is suggested that the health-care provider restrict use of the term narcotic to specifically refer to opioid medications.

Opioids exert their actions by activating at least six types of opioid receptors: mu (types one and two), kappa, sigma, delta, and epsilon. From the perspective of pain management, the **mu** and **kappa** receptors are the most important.

Some opioid agonists, such as morphine, activate both mu and kappa receptors. Other opioids such pentazocine (Talwin) exert mixed opioid agonist-antagonist effects by activating the kappa receptor but blocking the mu receptor. Opioid blockers such as naloxone (Narcan) inhibit both the mu and kappa receptors. Although it is often difficult to keep track of all the opioid receptors associated with the various narcotic analgesics and their actions, it is important because this is the body's natural way of providing the mechanism for a diverse set of body responses from one substance. Figure 11.3 illustrates opioid actions on the mu and kappa receptors.

11.6 Opioids are the drugs of choice for severe pain.

Opioids are the drugs of choice for severe pain that cannot be controlled with other analgesics. Over 20 different opioids are available, and these are classified by similarities in their chemical structures, by their mechanism of action, or by their efficacy. Perhaps the simplest method is by efficacy, which places opiates into categories of strong or moderate narcotic activity. Morphine is the prototype medication of choice for severe pain, and the drug to which all other opiates are compared. Opiate and opiate-blocking medications of importance for analgesia are listed in Table 11.3.

Opiates produce many important effects other than analgesia. They are effective at suppressing the cough reflex and at slowing down the motility of the GI tract for cases of severe diarrhea. As powerful CNS depressants, opioids can cause sedation, which may be either a therapeutic effect or a side effect, depending upon the client's disease state. Some clients experience euphoria, which is a reason why opiates are sometimes abused. Adverse effects include respiratory depression and nausea/vomiting.

eu = *true or good*
phoria = *feeling or bearing*

TABLE 11.3	Selected Opioids Used for Analgesia	
DRUG	**ROUTE AND ADULT DOSE**	**REMARKS**
Opioid Agonists with Moderate Efficacy		
codeine	PO; 15–60 mg qid.	Also for cough; available in IM and SC forms; combination drug with aspirin is called Empirin with codeine, or with acetaminophen is called Tylenol with codeine.
hydrocodone bitartrate (Hycodan)	PO; 5–10 mg every 4–6 hours prn (max 15 mg/dose).	Also for cough; combination drug with acetaminophen is called Amacodone C, Co-gesic, Vicodin, Dolacet, Norcet, and Norco.
oxycodone hydrochloride (OxyContin)	PO; 5–10 mg qid prn.	Combination drug with acetaminophen is called Percocet or Tylox, or with aspirin is called Percodan or Roxiprin.
propoxyphene hydrochloride (Darvon) propoxyphene napsylate (Darvon-N)	PO; 65 mg (HCl form) or 100 mg (napsylate form) every 4 hours prn (max 390 HCl/day; max 600 mg napsylate/day).	Combination drug with acetaminophen is called Darvocet or Propacet, or with aspirin and caffeine is called Darvon or Dolene.
Opiod Agonists with High Efficacy		
hydromorphone hydrochloride (Dilaudid)	PO; 1–4 mg every 4–6 hours prn.	Also for cough; available in IM, IV, SC, and rectal forms.
levorphanol tartrate (Levo-Dromoran)	PO; 2–3 mg tid to qid prn.	Also available in SC form.
meperidine hydrochloride (Demerol)	PO; 50–150 mg every 3–4 hours prn.	For preoperative medication or obstetric analgesia; available in IM, IV, and SC forms.
methadone hydrochloride (Dolophine)	PO; 2.5–10 mg every 3–4 hours prn.	For detoxification treatment of opioid dependency; available in IM and IV forms.
Pr morphine sulfate (Astramorph PF, Duramorph, and others)	PO; 10–30 mg every 4 hours prn.	Available in IM, IV, SC, intrathecal, epidural, and rectal forms.
oxymorphone hydrochloride (Numorphan)	SC/IM; 1–1.5 mg every 4–6 hours prn. PR; 5 mg every 4–6 hours prn.	Available in IM/IV, subcutaneous, and rectal forms.
Opioids with Mixed Agonist-Antagonist Effects		
buprenorphine hydrochloride (Buprenex)	IM/IV; 0.3 mg every 6 hours up to 0.6 mg every 4 hours.	For moderate to severe pain; available in SC, epidural, rectal, or IV forms.
butorphanol tartrate (Stadol)	IM; 1–4 mg every 3–4 hours prn (max 4 mg/dose).	For obstetrical analgesia during labor, cancer pain, renal colic, and burns; available in IV and intranasal forms.
dezocine (Dalgan)	IV; 2.5–10 mg (usually 5 mg) every 2–4 hours. IM; 5–10 mg (usually 10 mg) every 3–4 hours.	Causes less respiratory depression than morphine sulfate.
nalbuphine hydrochloride (Nubain)	SC/IM/IV; 10–20 mg every 3–6 hours prn (max 160 mg/day).	For moderate to severe pain.
pentazocine hydrochloride (Talwin)	PO; 50–100 mg every 3–4 hours (max 600 mg/day). SC/IM/IV; 30 mg every 3–4 hours (max 360 mg/day).	For moderate to severe pain (much lower dose for women in labor); available in IM, IV, and SC forms.

continues

TABLE 11.3	Selected Opioids Used for Analgesia—*continued*	
DRUG	**ROUTE AND ADULT DOSE**	**REMARKS**
Drugs with Opioid-Blocking Effects		
Pr naloxone hydrochloride (Narcan)	IV; 0.4–2 mg; may be repeated every 2–3 min up to 10 mg if necessary.	For opioid overdose and postoperative opioid depression.
nalmefene hydrochloride (Revex)	SC/IM/IV; Use 1 mg/ml concentration; non-opioid dependent: 0.5 mg/70 kg; opioid dependent; 0.1 mg/70 kg.	For opioid overdose and postoperative opioid depression; available in IV and SC forms.
naltrexone hyrdrochloride (Trexan, ReVia)	PO; 25 mg followed by another 25 mg in 1 hr if no withdrawal response; up to 800 mg/day.	For management of opiate or alcohol dependence; longer lasting effect than naloxone.

DRUG PROFILE (Opioid):
Morphine (Astramorph PF, Duramorph, and Others)

Actions:

In order to produce analgesia, morphine binds with both mu and kappa receptor sites. It causes euphoria, constriction of the pupils, and stimulation of cardiac muscle. It is used for symptomatic relief of severe pain and chronic pain after non-narcotic analgesics have failed, as pre-anesthetic medication, to relieve shortness of breath associated with heart failure and pulmonary edema, and for chest pain connected with a heart attack.

Adverse Effects:

Morphine may cause dysphoria (restlessness, depression, and anxiety), hallucinations, nausea, constipation, dizziness, and an itching sensation.

Overdose may result in severe respiratory depression or cardiac arrest. Morphine should not be mixed with alcohol or other CNS depressants. Tolerance develops to the analgesic, sedative, and euphoric effects of the drug. Cross-tolerance also develops between morphine and other narcotics such as heroin, methadone, and meperidine (Demerol). Physical and psychological dependence develops when high doses are taken for prolonged periods of time.

Mechanism in Action:

Morphine is an opioid that produces many actions throughout the central nervous system. One important action occurs at the level of the dorsal horn spinal cord. Here, morphine binds presynaptically to primary afferent neurons reducing the amount of released pain neurotransmitter. Simultaneously, morphine binds post-synaptically to second-order neurons responsible for transmitting ascending pain impulses to the brain.

DRUG PROFILE (Opioid-blocker):
Naloxone (Narcan)

Actions:

Naloxone is a pure opioid antagonist, blocking both the mu and kappa receptors. It is used for complete or partial reversal of opioid effects when acute opioid overdose is suspected. Given intravenously, it begins to reverse opioid symptoms such as CNS and respiratory depression within minutes. It will immediately cause opioid withdrawal symptoms in clients physically dependent on opioids. It is also used to treat post-operative opioid depression.

Adverse Effects:

Naloxone itself has minimal toxicity. However, in reversing the effects of opioids, the client may experience rapid loss of analgesia, increased blood pressure, tremors, hyperventilation, nausea/vomiting, and drowsiness. It should not be used for respiratory depression caused by non-opioid medications.

All of the narcotic analgesics cause physical and psychological dependence to some degree, as discussed in Chapter 5 ⬤. Many practitioners have been hesitant to administer the proper amount of opioid medication for fear of causing client addiction or of producing serious adverse effects such as sedation or respiratory depression. However, attitudes have changed mainly due to organized awareness groups, which feel that the medical community has not taken seriously clients who are in excruciating pain and have not medicated properly. It should now be understood that, when used according to accepted medical practice, clients can receive the pain relief they need without fear of addiction.

dys = abnormal
phoria = feeling or bearing

Some opioids are used primarily for conditions other than pain. For example, alfentanil (Alfenta), fentanyl (Sublimaze and others), remifentanil (Ultiva), and sufentanil (Sufenta) are used for general anesthesia; these are discussed in Chapter 12 ⬤.

Codeine is often prescribed as a cough suppressant and is covered in Chapter 24. Opiates of value in treating diarrhea are covered in Chapter 25 ⬤.

Concept review 11.4

- Distinguish between the following terms: *opioid, opiate,* and *narcotic.* Name six classes of opioid receptors and identify those that are connected with analgesia. Under what kinds of conditions should opioid medication should be used?

FEVER

Fever is a natural step in our body's defense system to remove foreign organisms. Persistent, high fever, however, can become quite dangerous. It is the job of the healthcare practitioner to determine whether the fever should be dealt with aggressively or if it should be allowed to run its course. Clients who take anti-fever medication might be doing more harm than good. In fact, many forms of bacteria are killed by an elevated fever.

anti = against
pyretic = fever

11.7 Fever is a defense mechanism of the body that can be effectively treated with antipyretic medications.

Prolonged, elevated fever can become a serious problem, especially in young children. For example, fever can stimulate febrile seizures in small children, as discussed in Chapter 8 ⬤. In adults, an elevated fever can be harmful in that it may break down body tissues, reduce mental

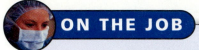

ON THE JOB

Hospice and Pain Medications

Being a hospice worker can be one of the most rewarding yet challenging jobs of any home care service. Being able to improve the quality of life for clients with a severe or terminal illness is an opportunity that requires a special gift. Certified nursing assistants, health workers, social workers, and nurses who travel to clients' homes or to a medical facility must be very in-tune with the emotions and thoughts of family members and people who have a need. Pain medications are often a part of that experience for clients and for the professionals administering care. Opioids are usually administered under conditions where clients must be allowed to experience the highest quality pain management while still being allowed to function as normally as possible. The right combination of medicine is required for proper support and respite. ■

acuity, and lead to delirium. It can even cause coma, particularly among elderly clients. In rare instances, an elevated fever may be fatal.

In most situations, however, fever is more of a discomfort than a life-threatening problem and can be controlled effectively by inexpensive, OTC medications. Examples of common brand-name medications taken for fever are Advil, Aleve, Bayer, Cope, Excedrin, Motrin, Orudis, and Tylenol. Many of these medications are marketed for different age groups, including special, flavored brands for infants and children. For fast delivery and effectiveness, drugs may come in various forms including gels, caplets (a combination capsule/tablet), enteric-coated tablets, or suspensions, and they may be provided in various strengths, including extra strength.

ANTIPYRETICS

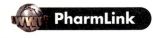

THE OXFORD PAIN INTERNET SITE

Antipyretics are drugs that reduce fever. Some antipyretics are also NSAIDS and, therefore, reduce pain and inflammation. Other antipyretics may reduce fever and pain without affecting the inflammatory component.

Concept review 11.5

■ Name three common types of disorders controlled by nonopioid analgesics. Which nonopioid analgesic controls fever only? Which control fever and inflammation?

TENSION HEADACHE AND MIGRAINES

Headaches represent a special type of pain that is common throughout the population and which requires a slightly different approach to pain management. There are different varieties of headaches, the most common type being the **tension headache**. This usually occurs when muscles of the head and neck area become very tight as a result of stress and tension, causing a steady and lingering pain. Most tension headaches last from minutes to hours, but they are generally considered an annoyance rather than a medical emergency. Tension headaches can usually be effectively treated with OTC analgesics such as aspirin, acetaminophen, or ibuprofen.

The most painful type of headache is the **migraine**. It is characterized by throbbing or pulsating pain, sometimes preceded by an aura. **Auras** are sensory cues that let the client know that a migraine attack is coming soon. Examples of sensory cues are jagged lines, flashing lights, special smells, tastes, or sounds. Most migraines are accompanied by nausea and vomiting. Triggers

DRUG PROFILE:
Acetaminophen (Tylenol)

Actions:

Acetaminophen reduces pain by an unknown pharmacological mechanism. It reduces fever by direct action at the level of the hypothalamus and causes dilation of peripheral blood vessels, enabling sweating and dissipation of heat. Acetaminophen and aspirin have equal efficacy in relieving pain and reducing fever. Acetaminophen has no anti-inflammatory action; therefore it is not effective in treating arthritis or pain caused by tissue swelling following injury. The primary therapeutic usefulness of acetaminophen is for the treatment of fever in children and for relief of mild to moderate pain when aspirin is contraindicated.

Adverse Effects:

Acetaminophen is quite safe and adverse effects are uncommon at therapeutic doses. Unlike aspirin, acetaminophen has no effect on blood coagulation and does not cause gastric irritation. Ingestion of this drug with alcohol is not recommended because of the possibility of hepatotoxicity. It is also not recommended in cases of malnutrition. In such cases, acute toxicity may result, leading to renal failure, which can be fatal. Other signs of acute toxicity include nausea, vomiting, chills, and abdominal discomfort.

for migraines include nitrates, monosodium glutamate (MSG) found in many oriental foods, food additives, caffeine, chocolate, and aspartame. By avoiding foods containing these substances, clients can often prevent the onset of a migraine attack.

11.8 The goals of drug therapy for migraine headaches are to stop migraines in progress and to prevent them from occurring.

There are two primary goals to the pharmacologic therapy of migraines. The first is to stop migraines in progress and the second is to prevent migraines from occurring. For the most part, the drugs used to abort migraines are different than those used to prevent migraines. Drug therapy is most effective if begun before a migraine has reached a severe level.

When OTC analgesics are unable to abort a migraine, the drugs of first choice are often the triptans. The oldest of the triptans, sumatriptan (Imetrex), was first marketed in the U.S. in 1993 and is available in oral, intranasal, and SC forms. Prefilled syringes of sumatriptan are available for clients who are able to self-administer the medication. For clients who are unresponsive to the triptans, ergotamine (Ergostat) or dihydroergotamine (Migranal) may be used. Ergotamine is an inexpensive, older medication that is available in oral, sublingual, and suppository forms. Dihydroergotamine is given parenterally and as a nasal spray. These two medications are pregnancy category X drugs. In unusual cases, where none of the above drugs is able to terminate migraine pain, opioids may be used.

Medications that prevent the onset of migraines include various classes of drugs that are discussed in other chapters of this text. These include beta-adrenergic blockers, calcium channel blockers, antidepressants, and anti-seizure drugs. Because all of these drugs have the potential to produce side effects, preventive therapy is only initiated if the incidence of migraines is high and the client is unresponsive to the drugs used to abort migraines in progress. Of the various drugs, propranolol (Inderal) is probably the most commonly prescribed. Amitriptyline is preferred for clients who may have a mood disorder or suffer from insomnia in addition to their migraines. Selected drugs used for migraines are shown in Table 11.4.

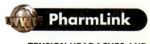

TENSION HEADACHES AND MIGRAINES

DRUG PROFILE:
Sumatriptan (Imetrex)

Actions:

Sumatriptan belongs to a relatively new group of antimigraine drugs known as the triptans. The triptans are serotonin agonists that act by causing vasoconstriction of cranial arteries. This vasoconstriction is moderately selective and does not usually affect overall blood pressure. The vasoconstriction terminates migraine attacks in 10 to 20 minutes after SC administration. If taken orally, sumatriptan should be administered as soon as possible after the migraine is suspected or begun.

Adverse Effects:

Some dizziness, drowsiness, or a warming sensation may be experienced after taking sumatriptan; however, these effects are not normally severe enough to warrant discontinuation of therapy. The drug should not be used in clients at risk for coronary artery disease or in clients taking ergotamine drugs.

TABLE 11.4	Selected Drugs used for Migraine Headaches	
DRUG	**ROUTE AND ADULT DOSE**	**REMARKS**
dihydroergotamine mesylate (D.H.E. 45, Migranal)	IM; 1 mg; may be repeated at 1 hr intervals to a total of 3 mg (max 6 mg/week).	Also available as nasal spray; pregnancy category X; for migraine termination. Also used in combination with low dose heparin to prevent post-op deep vein thrombosis.
ergotamine tartrate (Ergostat)	PO; 1–2 mg followed by 1–2 mg every 30 minutes until headache stops or a max of 6 mg/day or 10 mg/week is reached.	Also available in sublingual, inhalant, or rectal forms; may cause physical dependence; pregnancy category X; for migraine termination.
naratriptan (Amerge)	PO; 1–2.5 mg; may repeat in 4 hours if necessary (max 5 mg/day).	Serotonin agonist; for migraine termination.
Pr sumatriptan (Imitrex)	PO; 25 mg for 1 dose (max 100 mg).	Serotonin agonist; SC and intranasal forms available; for migraine termination.
zolmitriptan (Zomig)	PO; 2.5–5 mg; may repeat in 2 hours if necessary (max 10 mg/day).	Serotonin agonist; for migraine termination.
propranolol hydrochloride (Inderal)	PO; 80–240 mg/day in divided doses; may need 160–240 mg/day.	Beta-adrenergic blocker for migraine prevention.
amitryptyline hydrochloride (Elavil)	PO; 75–100 mg/ day.	Tricyclic antidepressant; unlabeled use for migraine prevention.
verapamil hydrochloride (Calan)	PO; 40–80 mg tid.	Calcium channel blocker; unlabeled use for migraine prevention.
methysergide (Sansert)	PO; 4–8 mg/day in divided doses.	Similar to ergotamine; for migraine prevention.
divalproex (Depakote)	PO; 250 mg bid; may increase to max of 1000 mg/day.	Anticonvulsant; for migraine prevention.

CLIENT TEACHING

Clients taking pain medication need to know the following:

1. Give careful consideration to the way you describe pain so that the analgesic medication given is suited to your complaint.

2. Any OTC medication taken for pain should be reported to your healthcare provider to minimize adverse effects and interactions.

3. Aspirin has many undesirable side effects, mainly related to gastric upset and bleeding. Carefully follow instructions and watch for drug interactions or contraindications.

4. Combining pain medications with alcohol and other CNS depressants (especially opioids) should be avoided.

5. Vital signs should be monitored with all opioid medication because of their CNS depressant effects.

6. Get up slowly from seated positions because some pain medications cause light-headedness.

7. If taking opiates, do not operate machinery or drive a car because of symptoms of dizziness, blurred vision, and drowsiness.

8. Abrupt discontinuation of opioids could result in withdrawal. Signs include chills, abdominal and muscle cramps, severe itching, sweating, restlessness, anxiety, yawning, and drug-seeking behavior. ▪

CHAPTER REVIEW

Core Concepts Summary

11.1 **Pain assessment is the first step to pain management.**

The healthcare practitioner's job is to try to find the source of pain by asking questions regarding the nature and extent of any particular discomfort. Whether a client feels acute or chronic pain is of importance to the selection of the correct pharmacological agent. Non-pharmacological techniques for reducing pain may be valuable supplements to pharmacologic therapy.

11.2 **Neural mechanisms of pain are well characterized.**

There are two types of pain: fast pain and slow pain. These may be explained by the way nerve impulses travel to the spinal cord. At the spinal level, substance P acts as a neurotransmitter for pain. Its release is influenced by other neurotransmitters, including endogenous opioids.

11.3 **Analgesics are classified as non-narcotics or narcotics.**

Minor to moderate pain is treated with non-narcotic analgesics like acetaminophen and NSAIDS such as aspirin, ibuprofen, and the selective COX2 inhibitors. Severe pain may require opioids.

11.4 **Non-steroidal anti-inflammatory drugs (NSAIDS) are effective in treating mild to moderate pain, inflammation, and fever.**

Following tissue injury, chemical mediators such as histamine, bradykinin, and prostaglandins are released and produce pain. Cyclooxygenase inhibitors or nonsteroidal anti-inflammatory drugs (NSAIDS) block the formation of prostaglandins, thus reducing pain. Aspirin inhibits both COX1 and COX2.

11.5 **Opioids are substances extracted from the poppy plant that exert their effects through interaction with mu and kappa receptors.**

Natural morphine-like substances called opiates are extracted from the poppy plant. These and other synthetic opioids cause their effects by interacting with receptors, the most important of which are the mu and kappa. Opioid blockers can reverse the effects of the narcotics in clients who have overdosed on the opiates.

11.6 **Opioids are the drugs of choice for severe pain.**

Morphine and related opioids are used to control severe pain. Opiates are also used for severe cough, diarrhea, and for induction of anesthesia. Opioids cause tolerance and have the potential to cause dependence if taken in high doses for prolonged periods.

11.7 **Fever is a defense mechanism of the body that can be effectively treated with antipyretic medications.**

When highly elevated for extended periods of time, fever can become dangerous and is treated with antipyretic medications. Acetaminophen is an anal-

gesic with antipyretic properties that is often used for this purpose.

11.8 **The goals of drug therapy for migraine headaches are to stop migraines in progress and to prevent them from occurring.**

Migraine headaches are treated with drugs that prevent the disorder and drugs that terminate the migraine in progress. Sumatriptan and ergotamine are drugs commonly used to abort migraines, while propranolol is one of the most common medications prescribed for migraine prevention.

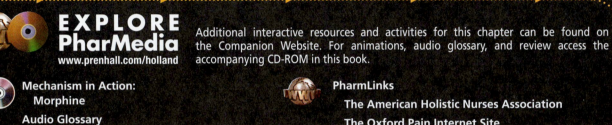

EXPLORE PharMedia
www.prenhall.com/holland

Additional interactive resources and activities for this chapter can be found on the Companion Website. For animations, audio glossary, and review access the accompanying CD-ROM in this book.

Mechanism in Action:
  Morphine
Audio Glossary
Concept Review
NCLEX Review

PharmLinks
  The American Holistic Nurses Association
  The Oxford Pain Internet Site
  Tension Headaches and Migraines

12 Drugs for Local and General Anesthesia

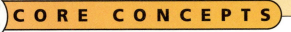

CORE CONCEPTS

LOCAL ANESTHESIA

12.1 Surface, local, or regional anesthesia is achieved by five major clinical techniques.

Local Anesthetics

12.2 Local anesthetics act by blocking the entry of sodium ions into neurons.

12.3 Local anesthetics are classified as amides or esters.

GENERAL ANESTHESIA

12.4 General anesthesia produces a complete loss of sensation accompanied by loss of consciousness.

General Anesthetics

12.5 Inhaled general anesthetics are used to maintain surgical anesthesia.

12.6 IV anesthetics are used either alone or to supplement inhalation anesthetics.

12.7 Non-anesthetic drugs are administered as adjuncts or supplements to surgery.

OBJECTIVES

After reading this chapter, the student should be able to:

1. Compare and contrast the five major clinical techniques involving local anesthetics.

2. Identify the two major classes of local anesthetics.

3. Explain why epinephrine and sodium hydroxide are sometimes included in local anesthetic cartridges.

4. Identify the actions of general anesthetics on the CNS.

5. Compare and contrast the two major ways that general anesthesia may be induced.

6. Identify the four stages of general anesthesia.

7. For each of the following classes, identify representative medications and explain the mechanism of drug action, primary actions, and important adverse effects.
   a. local anesthetics
   b. general anesthetics

8. Identify the classes of drugs used as adjuncts to anesthesia and explain their uses.

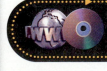

PharMedia
www.prenhall.com/holland

Additional interactive resources and activities for this chapter can be found on the Companion Website. For animations, audio glossary, and review access the accompanying CD-ROM in this book.

amide (AM-ide): type of chemical linkage found in some local anesthetics involving carbon, nitrogen, and oxygen (-NH-CO-) / *page 168*

anesthesia (ANN-ess-THEE-zee-uh): medical procedure involving drugs that block the transmission of nerve impulses and cause loss of sensation and/or consciousness / *page 165*

epidural anesthesia (ep-ee-DUR-ul): type of regional anesthesia where drugs are injected into the epidural space of the spinal cord / *page 167*

ester (ES-tur): type of chemical linkage found in some local anesthetics involving carbon and oxygen (-CO-O-) / *page 168*

general anesthesia: medical procedure that produces loss of sensation throughout the entire body and unconsciousness / *page 165*

infiltration anesthesia (in-fill-TRAY-shun): type of local anesthesia performed in preparation for a dental or medical procedure; local anesthetics are injected and infiltrate into the skin / *page 167*

local anesthesia: loss of sensation to a relatively small part of the body without loss of consciousness / *page 165*

nerve block anesthesia: technique for anesthetizing an area by injecting a blocking agent directly around a nerve / *page 167*

spinal anesthesia: regional anesthesia where drugs are injected into the spinal subarachnoid space / *page 167*

surface (topical) anesthesia (TOP-ik-ul): procedure where local anesthetics are applied to the surface of the body in order to numb the skin and mucous membranes / *page 167*

Anesthesia is a medical procedure performed by applying drugs that cause a loss of sensation. Local anesthesia occurs when clients lose sensation to a limited part of their body without losing consciousness. Because local anesthesia is not always applied to small, local body areas, some local anesthetic treatments are more accurately called surface anesthesia or regional anesthesia, depending on how the drugs are administered and their resulting effects.

an = without
thesia = sensation

General anesthesia requires a completely different class of drugs that cause loss of sensation to the entire body, usually resulting in a loss of consciousness. The purpose of this chapter is to examine drugs used for both local and general anesthesia. Some interesting facts about anesthesia are given in FastFacts.

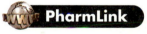

PharmLink

VIRTUAL ANESTHESIA TEXTBOOK

Fast Facts Anesthesia and Anesthetics

- Over 20 million people receive general anesthetics each year in the US.
- About half of the general anesthetics are administered by a nurse anesthetist.
- The first medical applications of anesthetics were in 1842 with ether and in 1846 with nitrous oxide.
- Herbal products may interact with anesthetics; St. John's Wort may intensify or prolong the effects of some opioids and anesthetics.

LOCAL ANESTHESIA

Local anesthesia is loss of sensation to a relatively small part of the body without loss of consciousness to the client. This type of technique may be necessary when a relatively brief dental or medical procedure is performed.

12.1 Surface, local, or regional anesthesia is achieved by five major clinical techniques.

The five major routes for applying local anesthetics are shown in Figure 12.1. The method to be employed is dependent upon the location and extent of the desired anesthesia. For example, some local anesthetics are applied topically prior to a needle-stick or minor skin surgery. Others are intended to block sensations to large areas such as an entire limb or the lower abdomen. The different methods of local and regional anesthesia are summarized in Table 12.1.

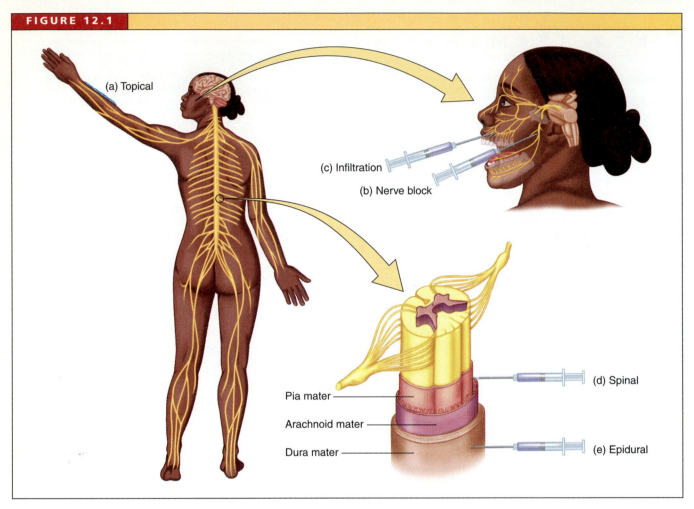

FIGURE 12.1

(a) Topical

(c) Infiltration

(b) Nerve block

(d) Spinal

(e) Epidural

Pia mater

Arachnoid mater

Dura mater

Techniques for applying local anesthesia: (a) topical; (b) nerve block; (c) infiltration; (d) spinal; (e) epidural

Concept review 12.1

■ What is local anesthesia? Name the five general methods of local and regional anesthesia.

LOCAL ANESTHETICS

Local anesthetics are drugs that produce loss of sensation to a limited part of the body. They produce this effect by blocking the entry of sodium ions into cells of the nervous system. Local anesthetics are sometimes called *sodium channel blockers*.

12.2 Local anesthetics act by blocking the entry of sodium ions into neurons.

The mechanism of action of local anesthetics is well known. Recall that the concentration of sodium ions is higher outside neurons compared to the inside. An influx of sodium into the cell is necessary for neurons to fire and conduct an electrical impulse. As depicted in Figures 12.2a and 12.2b, local anesthetics produce a numbing effect in a region by blocking sodium channels. Because the blocking of sodium channels is a non-selective process, both sensory and motor impulses are affected. Thus, both sensation and muscle activity will temporarily diminish in an area treated with a local anesthetic.

TABLE 12.1	Methods of Local and Regional Anesthesia	
ROUTE	**FORMULATION/METHOD**	**DESCRIPTION**
Surface (topical) anesthesia	Creams, sprays, suppositories, drops, and lozenges	Applied to mucous membranes including the eyes, lips, gums, nasal membranes, and throat. Very safe unless absorbed.
Infiltration (field-block) anesthesia	Direct injection into tissue immediate to the surgical site	Drug diffuses into tissue to block a specific group of nerves in a small area very close to the area to be operated upon.
Nerve block anesthesia	Direct injection into tissue that may be distant from the operation site	Drug affects the bundle of nerves serving the area to be operated upon. Used to block sensation in a limb or large area of the face.
Spinal anesthesia	Injection into the cerebral spinal fluid (CSF)	Drug affects large, regional area such as the lower abdomen and legs.
Epidural anesthesia	Injection into epidural space of spinal cord	Most commonly used in obstetrics during labor and delivery.

A primary concern during surgery is that the action of an anesthetic lasts long enough to complete the procedure. Adding small amounts of epinephrine to the anesthetic solution extends the duration of action of injectable local anesthetics. Epinephrine constricts blood vessels in the immediate area where the anesthetic is injected. This keeps the anesthetic in the area longer, thus extending the effect of the drug. The addition of epinephrine to lidocaine (Xylocaine), for example, increases its

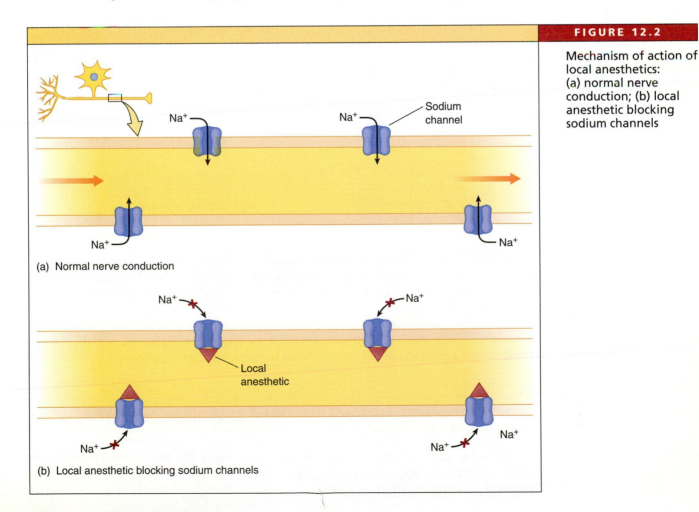

FIGURE 12.2

Mechanism of action of local anesthetics: (a) normal nerve conduction; (b) local anesthetic blocking sodium channels

(a) Normal nerve conduction

(b) Local anesthetic blocking sodium channels

TABLE 12.2	Selected Local Anesthetics	
DRUG	**USE**	**REMARKS**
Ester-type Drugs		
benzocaine (Americaine, Solarcaine, others)	topical anesthesia	for sunburn, sore throat, earache, hemorrhoids and other minor skin conditions
chloroprocaine (Nesacaine)	infiltration, nerve block, and epidural anesthesia	short duration
cocaine	topical anesthesia	for ear, nose, and throat procedures
procaine (Novocain)	infiltration, nerve block, epidural, and spinal anesthesia	short duration
tetracaine (Pontocaine)	topical and spinal anesthesia	long duration
Amide-type Drugs		
bupivicaine (Marcaine)	infiltration and epidural anesthesia	long duration
dibucaine (Nupercaine, Nupercainal)	topical or spinal anesthesia	long duration
etidocaine (Duranest)	infiltration, nerve block, and epidural anesthesia	long duration
Pr lidocaine (Xylocaine)	topical, infiltration, nerve block, epidural, and spinal anesthesia	may be combined as a mixture of lidocaine and prilocaine (EMLA cream) for topical application
mepivacaine (Carbocaine)	infiltration, nerve block, and epidural anesthesia	intermediate duration
prilocaine (Citanest)	infiltration, nerve block, and epidural anesthesia	intermediate duration
ropivacaine (Naropin)	infiltration, nerve block, and epidural anesthesia	long duration
Unrelated to Esters or Amides		
dyclonine (Dyclone)	topical anesthesia	for ear, nose, and throat procedures
pramoxine (Tronothane)	topical anesthesia	for minor medical procedures

numbing effect from 15–20 minutes to 45–60 minutes. This is important for dental or surgical procedures that take longer than 20 minutes; otherwise a second injection would be necessary.

Another chemical, sodium hydroxide, is sometimes added to the vial of anesthetic solution to increase the effectiveness of the anesthetic in regions that have extensive local infection or abscesses. Bacteria tend to acidify an infected site, and local anesthetics are less effective in an acidic environment. Adding an alkaline substance such as sodium hydroxide or sodium bicarbonate neutralizes the region and creates a more favorable basic environment for the anesthetic.

12.3 Local anesthetics are classified as amides or esters.

The two major classes of local anesthetics are esters and amides. The terms *ester* and *amide* refer to types of chemical linkages found within the anesthetic molecules. Esters have been used longer than amides for local anesthetic procedures.

DRUG PROFILE:
Lidocaine (Xylocaine)

Actions:

Lidocaine is the most frequently used injectable local anesthetic. It is available in solutions ranging from 0.5% to 2% for infiltration, nerve block, spinal, or epidural anesthesia. A topical form is also available. When given for anesthesia, its onset of action is 5–15 minutes. Several hours may be needed for complete sensation to reappear. Lidocaine is also given IV, IM, or SC to treat dysrhythmias, as discussed in Chapter 16 ⊂⊃ . Solutions of lidocaine containing preservatives or epinephrine are intended for local anesthesia and must never be given parenterally for dysrhythmias.

Adverse Effects:

When used for anesthesia, side effects are uncommon. An early symptom of toxicity is excitement, leading to irritability and confusion. Serious adverse effects include convulsions, respiratory depression, and cardiac arrest. Until the effect of the anesthetic diminishes, clients may injure themselves by biting or chewing areas of the mouth that have no sensation following a dental procedure.

Mechanism in Action:

Lidocaine acts as a local anesthetic to block neuronal pain impulses and as an antidysrhythmic to correct ventricular fibrillation and tachycardia. These actions are achieved by blocking sodium channels located within the membranes of neurons and cardiac tissue.

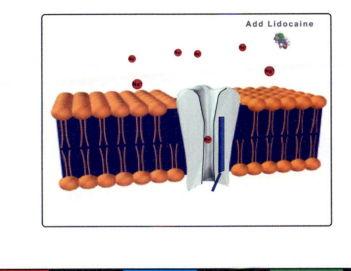

Add Lidocaine

The first local anesthetic to be discovered was cocaine. Cocaine is a natural ester, found in the leaves of the plant *Erythroxylon coca,* native to the Andes Mountains of Peru. As late as the 1880s, cocaine was routinely used for eye surgery, nerve blocks, and spinal anesthesia. Although still available for local anesthesia, cocaine is a Schedule II drug and rarely used therapeutically. The abuse potential of cocaine was discussed in Chapter 5 ⊂⊃ .

Another ester, procaine (Novocain) was once the drug of choice for dental procedures from the mid 1900s until the 1960s. The development of the amide-type drugs led to a significant reduction in procaine use. One ester, benzocaine (Solarcaine and others) is extensively used today as a topical OTC agent for treating a large number of conditions, including sunburn, insect bites, hemorrhoids, sore throat, and minor wounds.

Amides have largely replaced the esters because they generally have a longer duration of action and produce fewer side effects. Lidocaine (Xylocaine) is the most widely used amide for short surgical procedures requiring local anesthesia. Selected local anesthetics are summarized in Table 12.2.

Adverse effects to local anesthetics are uncommon. Allergy is rare. When it does occur, it is often due to sulfites, which are added as preservatives to prolong the shelf life of the anesthetic, or to methylparaben, which is sometimes added to retard bacterial growth in vials. Early adverse effects include symptoms of CNS stimulation such as restlessness or anxiety. Later effects, such as drowsiness and unresponsiveness, are due to CNS depression. Cardiovascular effects such as hypotension and dysrhythmias are possible. Clients with a history of cardiovascular disease are often given forms of local anesthetics that contain no epinephrine in order to reduce the potential

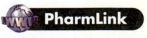

PATIENT'S GUIDE TO LOCAL AND REGIONAL ANESTHESIA

NATURAL ALTERNATIVES

Cloves and Anise as Natural Dental Remedies

You might not be aware that one natural remedy for tooth pain is oil of cloves. Extracted from the plant *Eugenia,* eugenol is the chemical extract found in cloves thought to produce its numbing effect. It works especially well for cavities. Soak a piece of cotton and pack it around the gums close to the painful area. Dentists sometimes recommend it for temporary relief of a toothache.

Another natural remedy is oil of anise, scientific name *Pimpinella,* for jaw pain caused by nerve pressure or gritting of teeth. Anise oil is an antispasmodic agent, which means it relaxes intense muscular pressure around the jaw angle, cheeks, and throat area. It has extra benefits in that it is also a natural expectorant, cough suppressant, and breath freshener. ▪

effects of this drug on the heart and blood pressure. CNS and cardiovascular side effects are not expected unless the local anesthetic is absorbed extremely rapidly or accidentally injected directly into a blood vessel rather than body tissues.

Concept review 12.2

- How does a local anesthetic work? How does the anesthetic action of lidocaine with epinephrine differ from that of lidocaine without epinephrine?

GENERAL ANESTHESIA

General anesthesia is a loss of sensation occurring throughout the entire body and unconsciousness resulting from the administration of an anesthetic. This medical procedure is often necessary when clients must remain still and without pain for a longer period of time than could be achieved with local anesthetics.

12.4 General anesthesia produces a complete loss of sensation accompanied by loss of consciousness.

The goal of general anesthesia is to provide a rapid and complete loss of sensation. Signs of general anesthesia include loss of pain, consciousness, memory, and body movement. Although all of these signs are similar to those of sleeping, general anesthesia and sleep are not exactly the same. General anesthetics depress all nervous activity in the brain, whereas sleeping depresses only very specific areas. In fact, some brain activity actually increases during sleep, as described in Chapter 7 ⊂⊃ .

General anesthesia is a progressive process that occurs in distinct stages. The most potent general anesthetics can quickly induce all four stages, whereas others are only able to induce Stage 1. Stage 3 is where most major surgery occurs; thus it is called *surgical anesthesia.* When seeking surgical anesthesia, it is desirable to progress through Stage 2 as rapidly as possible, as this stage produces uncomfortable symptoms. These stages are shown in Table 12.3.

GENERAL ANESTHETICS

General anesthetics are drugs that produce general anesthesia. These drugs are usually administered as IV medication or inhaled. When inhaled, two general types of medications may be used: gases and volatile agents. To supplement the effects of a general anesthetic, other non-anesthetic agents may be given before, during, and after surgery.

TABLE 12.3	Stages of General Anesthesia
Stage 1	Loss of pain; the client loses general sensation but may be awake. This stage proceeds until the client loses consciousness.
Stage 2	Excitement and hyperactivity; the client may be delirious and try to resist treatment. Heartbeat and breathing may become irregular and blood pressure can increase. This is the stage when some IV agents are administered to calm the client.
Stage 3	Surgical anesthesia; skeletal muscles become relaxed and delirium stabilizes; cardiovascular and breathing activities stabilize. Eye movements slow down and the patient becomes very still. This is the stage when surgery begins and remains until the procedure ends.
Stage 4	Paralysis of the medulla region in the brain responsible for controlling respiratory and cardiovascular activity. If breathing or the heart stops, death could result. This stage is usually avoided during general anesthesia.

12.5 Inhaled general anesthetics are used to maintain surgical anesthesia.

There are two primary methods of inducing general anesthesia. Intravenous agents are usually administered first to quickly induce anesthesia. After the client loses consciousness, inhaled agents are used to maintain the anesthesia. During short surgical procedures or those requiring lower levels of anesthesia, the IV agents may be used alone.

Inhaled general anesthetics may be gasses or volatile agents. Inhaled general anesthetics produce their affect by preventing the flow of sodium into neurons of the CNS. The exact mechanism for how this occurs is not exactly known, although recent evidence suggests that GABA receptors in the brain may be activated. It is not the same mechanism as is known for local anesthetics. There is some speculation that the mechanism may be related to how some anti-seizure medications work; however, this is still not conclusive. There is not a receptor that binds to general anesthetics, and they do not seem to affect neurotransmitter release. General anesthetics generally delay nerve impulses, producing a reduction in neural activity. Inhaled anesthetics are listed in Table 12.4.

The only gas used routinely for anesthesia is nitrous oxide, commonly called laughing gas. Nitrous oxide is used for dental procedures, obstetrics, and for brief surgical procedures. It may also be used along with other general anesthetics, making it possible to decrease their dosages with greater effectiveness.

Commonly administered volatile agents are halothane (Fluothane), enflurane (Ethrane), and isoflurane (Forane). The most potent of these is halothane. Some general anesthetics enhance the sensitivity of the heart to drugs such as epinephrine, norepinephrine, dopamine, and serotonin. Most volatile agents depress cardiovascular and respiratory function. Because it has less effect on the heart and does not damage the liver, isoflurane has become the most widely used inhalation anesthetic.

ON THE JOB

Surgical Technologists

Surgical technologists (ST) are an integral part of the operating room team that provide medical and surgical care to clients undergoing surgery. Prior to client arrival in the operating suite, the ST assembles necessary equipment and supplies specific to the particular operation. Upon the client's arrival, the ST may provide physical and emotional support, including taking vital signs, checking the client's chart, and positioning the client on the surgical table. During the procedure, the ST may don a sterile gown and pass the surgical team the necessary instruments. They may assist the surgeon in holding instruments or suctioning during surgery. Following the operation, the ST assists in counting the instruments, needles, and sponges. Surgical technology programs vary in length from 9–24 months. The training is most commonly available from community and technical colleges. ▪

DRUG PROFILE (Gas):
Nitrous Oxide

Actions:

The main action of nitrous oxide is analgesia caused by suppression of central pain mechanisms. This agent is much more useful as a supplemental anesthetic rather than as a primary anesthetic. It has a low potency and is unable to induce surgical anesthesia (Stage 3). Although it is unable to produce a complete loss of consciousness or muscle relaxation alone, it is sometimes combined with other surgical anesthetic agents. One advantage for dental procedures is that clients remain conscious and can follow instructions during the procedure. Nitrous oxide provides superior analgesia, thus making it an ideal dental drug.

Adverse Effects:

When used in low to moderate doses, adverse effects of nitrous oxide are uncommon. As the dose increases, clients may exhibit some signs of Stage 2 anesthesia such as anxiety, excitement, and combativeness. Lowering the inhaled dose will quickly reverse these adverse effects. As nitrous oxide is exhaled, the client may temporarily have some difficulty breathing at the end of a procedure. Nausea and vomiting following the procedure are more common with nitrous oxide than with other inhalation anesthetics. Nitrous oxide has the potential to be abused by users (sometimes medical personnel) who like the relaxed, sedated state that the drug produces.

TABLE 12.4	Selected Inhaled Anesthetics
DRUG	**USE**
(Pr) nitrous oxide	Used alone in dentistry, obstetrics, and short medical procedures; used in combination with more potent inhaled anesthetics.
desflurane (Suprane)	Induction and maintenance of general anesthesia.
enflurane (Ethrane)	Induction and maintenance of general anesthesia.
(Pr) halothane (Fluothane)	Induction and maintenance of general anesthesia; use has declined because safer agents are available.
isoflurane (Forane)	Induction and maintenance of general anesthesia; most widely used inhalation anesthetic.
methoxyflurane (Penthrane)	Used during labor because it does not suppress uterine contractionsas much as other agents.
servoflurane (Ultane)	Induction and maintenance of general anesthesia.

12.6 IV anesthetics are used either alone or to supplement inhalation anesthetics.

IV anesthetics are often used to supplement the effects of inhaled general anesthetics. Concurrent administration of IV and inhaled drugs allows the dose of inhaled anesthetic to be reduced,

DRUG PROFILE (Volatile Agent):
Halothane (Fluothane)

Actions:

Halothane, the prototype for the volatile anesthetics, produces a potent level of surgical anesthesia that is rapid in onset and in recovery. Although it is potent, it often does not produce as much muscle relaxation or analgesia as other volatile anesthetics. Therefore, halothane is often used with other anesthetic agents including muscle relaxants and analgesics. Nitrous oxide is sometimes combined with halothane.

Adverse Effects:

Halothane moderately sensitizes the heart muscle to epinephrine; therefore, cardiac dysrhythmias are a concern. This agent lowers both blood pressure and the respiratory rate. It also abolishes reflex mechanisms that normally keep the contents of the stomach from entering into the lungs. Because of its potential to cause liver damage, use of halothane has declined.

---

thus lowering the potential for serious side effects. They are also used to provide additional analgesia or muscle relaxation than could be provided by the inhaled anesthetic alone. Some are used alone in medical procedures that take less than 15 minutes. Drugs employed as IV anesthetics include barbiturates, opioids, and benzodiazepines. Selected IV anesthetics are shown in Table 12.5.

Concept review 12.3

■ What is the role of IV anesthetics in surgical anesthesia? Why are these drugs not used by themselves for general anesthesia?

12.7 Non-anesthetic drugs are administered as adjuncts or supplements to surgery.

Some non-anesthetic drugs are used either to complement the effects of the anesthetic or to treat expected side effects of the anesthetics. These agents are called *adjuncts* to anesthesia. They may be given prior to, during, or after surgery. Examples of surgical adjuncts are shown in Table 12.6.

Preoperative medications such as barbiturates or benzodiazepines are given to relieve anxiety and to provide mild sedation. Opioids such as morphine may be given to counteract pain that the client will experience after surgery. Anticholinergics such as atropine may be administered to dry secretions and to reverse the bradycardia caused by some anesthetics.

pre = before
operative = surgery

During surgery, the primary adjuncts are the neuromuscular blocking agents. So that surgical procedures can be carried out safely, it is necessary to administer medications that cause skeletal muscles to relax. Administration of these drugs allows the amount of anesthetic to be reduced. Neuromuscular blocking agents are classified as depolarizing blockers or non-depolarizing blockers. The major depolarizing blocker is succinylcholine (Anectine), which works by binding irreversibly to acetylcholine, the neurotransmitter responsible for skeletal muscle contraction. Mivacarium (Mivacron) is the shortest acting of the non-depolarizing blockers, while tubocurarine is a longer acting neuromuscular blocking agent.

Postoperative medications include analgesics for pain and antiemetics such as promethazine (Phenergan and others) for the nausea and vomiting that sometimes occur during recovery from the anesthetic. Occasionally a parasympathomimetic such as bethanechol (Urecholine) is administered to stimulate the smooth muscle of the bowel and the urinary tract to begin peristalsis following surgery.

post = after
operative = surgery
anti = against
emetic = vomiting

DRUG PROFILE:
Thiopental (Pentathol)

Actions

Thiopental is one of the oldest IV anesthetics. It is used for brief medical procedures or to induce anesthesia prior to administering inhaled anesthetics. It is classified as an ultra-short-acting barbiturate, having an onset time of less than one minute and duration of only 10–30 minutes. Unlike some agents, it has very low analgesic properties.

Adverse Effects

Like other barbiturates, thiopental can produce severe respiratory depression. It is used with caution in clients with cardiovascular disease because of its ability to depress the myocardium and cause dysrhythmias.

TABLE 12.5	Selected IV Anesthetics	
DRUG	CLASS	REMARKS
diazepam (Valium)	benzodiazepine	For induction of anesthesia; prototype drug for the benzodiazepines.
lorazepam (Ativan)	benzodiazepine	For induction of anesthesia and to produce conscious sedation; for short medical procedures or surgery.
midazolam hydrochloride (Versed)	benzodiazepine	For induction of anesthesia and to produce conscious sedation; for short diagnostic procedures.
ketamine (Ketalar)	dissociative agent	For sedation, amnesia, and analgesia; for short diagnostic, therapeutic, or surgical procedures; most often used in children.
etomidate (Amidate)	barbiturate-like	For induction of anesthesia; for short medical procedures.
propofol (Diprivan)	barbiturate-like	For induction and maintenance of general anesthesia; for short medical procedures.
methohexital sodium (Brevital)	barbiturate	Ultrashort-acting; for induction of anesthesia; used as a supplement to other anesthetic agents.
Pr thiopental sodium (Pentothal)	barbiturate	Ultrashort-acting; for induction of anesthesia; used as a supplement to other anesthetic agents.
alfentanil hydrochloride (Alfenta)	opiate	Rapid onset and short onset of action; for induction of anesthesia; used as a supplement to other anesthetic agents.
fentanyl citrate (Sublimaze and others)	opiate	Short acting analgesic used during the operative and perioperative period; used to supplement both general and regional anesthesia.
remifentanil hydrochloride (Ultiva)	opiate	Short acting analgesic; for induction and maintenance of general anesthesia.
sufentanil citrate (Sufenta)	opiate	Approximately seven times more potent than fentayl; onset and duration of action more rapid than fentanyl; for induction and maintenance of anesthesia.

TABLE 12.6	Selected Adjuncts to Anesthesia	
DRUG	**CLASS**	**REMARKS**
pentobarbital (Nembutal)	barbiturate	Short duration; for preoperative sedation; potent, causes respiratory depression.
secobarbital (Seconal)	barbiturate	Short duration; for preoperative sedation.
butabarbital sodium (Butisol)	barbiturate	Intermediate duration; for preoperative sedation.
amobarbital (Amytal)	barbiturate	Intermediate duration; for preoperative sedation.
alfentanil hydrochloride (Alfenta)	opioid	Short duration; for induction of anesthesia when endotracheal or mechanical ventilation is needed; provides analgesia.
fentanyl citrate (Duragesic, Actiq, others)	opioid	For analgesia during or after anesthesia; the combination of fentanyl and droperidol is called Innovar.
remifentanil hydrochloride (Ultiva)	opioid	For analgesia during or after anesthesia; shorter duration of action than fentanyl.
sufentanil citrate (Sufenta)	opioid	For primary anesthesia or to provide analgesia during or after anesthesia.
bethanecol chloride (Duvoid, Urebeth, Urecholine)	anti-cholinergic	For relief of constipation and urinary retention caused by opioids; stimulates GI motility.
droperidol (Inapsine)	dopamine blocker	For nausea and vomiting caused by opioids; reduces anxiety and relaxes muscles.
promethazine (Pentazine, Phenazine, Phenergan, others)	dopamine blocker	For nausea and vomiting associated with obstetric sedation and opioids.
succinylcholine choline	neuromuscular blocker	Short duration; depolarizing type (Anectine, Quelican, Sucostrin).
mivacurium (Mivacron)	neuromuscular blocker	Short duration; non-depolarizing type.
tubocurarine	neuromuscular blocker	Long duration; prototype for the non-depolarizing type.

CLIENT TEACHING

Clients treated with anesthetic medications need to know the following:

1. When using topical anesthetics for skin conditions, avoid touching your eyes:
2. Never apply topical medications to large patches of skin or to areas where there is an open lesion or cut.
3. If you have reacted adversely to a local anesthetic before, you should inform your dentist or healthcare practitioner before receiving additional anesthetic medications.
4. After receiving local anesthetic solutions for the mouth, food and drink should not be consumed until it is clear that the anesthetic has worn off.
5. Do not chew or pick at an area where a dental procedure has been performed while the area is still numbed.
6. Be careful not to inhale anesthetic sprays used for topical application.
7. Try to get immediate assistance if you feel drowsy, confused, or have blurred vision after receiving a local anesthetic. Other signs to look for include lightheadedness, an irregular heartbeat, or feeling like you are going to faint.
8. Clients who might be pregnant, prone to seizure activity, or who should not discontinue existing drug therapy, should communicate this with their practitioner before receiving anesthetics.
9. For outpatient dental or medical procedures involving anesthesia, it is best to plan for someone to assist you after the procedure. Follow your caregiver's instructions very carefully regarding what you should or should not do after anesthesia.
10. Make sure you have sufficient pain medication so that you can properly treat symptoms that might occur following the medical procedure. ▪

CHAPTER REVIEW

Core Concepts Summary

12.1 Surface, local, or regional anesthesia is achieved by five major clinical techniques.

The five common clinical techniques involving local anesthetics are topical (surface) anesthesia, infiltration (field block) anesthesia, nerve block anesthesia, spinal anesthesia, and epidural anesthesia.

12.2 Local anesthetics act by blocking the entry of sodium ions into neurons.

Blocking sodium entry into neurons prevents transmission of the electrical impulse along the nerve. Epinephrine is sometimes added to cartridges to increase the duration of action of the anesthetic. A base such as sodium hydroxide is added to make the tissue environment more alkaline.

12.3 Local anesthetics are classified as amides or esters.

The two major classes of local anesthetics are esters and amides. Esters are used less often because of allergic reactions among some clients. Benzocaine (Solarcaine, others) is the most commonly used ester, and lidocaine (Xylocaine) is the most widely prescribed amide.

12.4 General anesthesia produces a complete loss of sensation accompanied by loss of consciousness.

General anesthesia proceeds in stages from light sedation to total loss of consciousness and depression of neural conduction. The less potent anesthetics can only induce Stage 1, while more potent agents can induce all four stages.

12.5 Inhaled general anesthetics are used to maintain surgical anesthesia.

Inhaled anesthetics may be gasses, such as nitrous oxide, or volatile agents such as halothane. Nitrous oxide produces Stage 1, or conscious sedation. Halothane, and the more commonly used isoflurane, are capable of producing sustained surgical anesthesia.

12.6 IV anesthetics are used either alone or to supplement inhalation anesthetics.

Because of their short duration of action, IV anesthetics are used alone only for short medical procedures.

They are commonly used to rapidly induce general anesthesia, and are followed by inhaled agents.

12.7 Non-anesthetic drugs are administered as adjuncts or supplements to surgery.

Drugs are used to supplement general anesthetics. These may be used to provide pain relief, sedation, muscle relaxation, and reduction of nausea/vomiting or to stimulate smooth muscle following surgery.

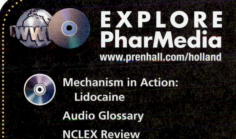

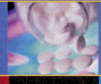

3 THE CARDIOVASCULAR SYSTEM

13 Drugs for Coagulation Disorders

CORE CONCEPTS

13.1 Hemostasis is a complex process involving multiple steps and a large number of enzymes and factors.

13.2 Removal of a blood clot is essential to restore normal circulation.

ABNORMAL COAGULATION

13.3 The normal coagulation process can be modified by a number of different mechanisms.

Anticoagulants

13.4 Anticoagulants prevent clot formation.

Antiplatelet Agents

13.5 Several drugs prolong bleeding time by interfering with platelet function.

Thrombolytics

13.6 Thrombolytics are used to dissolve existing clots.

Antifibrinolytics

13.7 Antifibrinolytics are used to promote the formation of clots.

OBJECTIVES

After reading this chapter, the student should be able to:

1. Explain the importance of hemostasis.
2. Construct a flow chart diagramming the important steps of hemostasis.
3. Identify the primary mechanisms by which coagulation-modifier drugs act.
4. For each of the following classes, identify representative medications and explain the mechanism of drug action, primary actions, and important adverse effects.
   a. anticoagulants
   b. antiplatelet agents
   c. thrombolytics
   d. antifibrinolytics
5. Categorize coagulation-modifying drugs based on their classification and mechanism of action.

PharMedia
www.prenhall.com/holland

Additional interactive resources and activities for this chapter can be found on the Companion Website. For animations, audio glossary, and review access the accompanying CD-ROM in this book.

activated partial thromboplastin time (APTT) (throm-bow-PLAS-tin): blood test used to determine how long it takes clots to form in order to regulate heparin dosage / *page 185*

anticoagulant (ANT-eye-co-AG-you-lent): an agent that inhibits the formation of blood clots / *page 184*

antifibrinolytics (ANT-eye-feye-brin-oh-LIT-iks): drugs used to prevent and treat excessive bleeding from surgical sites / *page 184*

antithrombin III (ANT-eye-THROM-bin): protein that prevents abnormal clotting by inhibiting thrombin / *page 187*

clotting factors: substances contributing to the process of blood clotting / *page 182*

coagulation (co-ag-you-LAY-shun): the process of blood clotting / *page 182*

coagulation cascade (koh-ag-you-LAY-shun cass-KADE): complex series of steps by which blood flow stops / *page 183*

embolus (EM-boh-luss): a blood clot carried in the bloodstream / *page 185*

fibrin (FEYE-brin): an insoluble protein formed from fibrinogen by the action of thrombin in the blood-clotting process / *page 183*

fibrinogen (feye-BRIN-oh-jen): blood protein converted to fibrin by the action of thrombin in the blood-clotting process / *page 183*

fibrinolysis (feye-brin-OL-oh-sis): removal of a blood clot / *page 183*

glycoprotein IIb/IIIa (GLEYE-koh-proh-teen): enzyme responsible for platelet aggregation / *page 189*

hemostasis (hee-moh-STAY-sis): the slowing or stopping of blood flow / *page 181*

low molecular weight heparins (LMWH): heparin-like drugs that inhibit blood-clotting / *page 187*

platelet (PLAY-tuh-let): cell involved in the blood-clotting process / *page 182*

plasmin (PLAZ-min): enzyme formed from plasminogen that dissolves blood clots / *page 183*

plasminogen (plaz-MIN-oh-jen): protein that prevents fibrin clot formation / *page 183*

prothrombin (PRO-throm-bin): blood protein converted to thrombin in the blood-clotting process / *page 183*

prothrombin activator: enzyme in the coagulation cascade that coverts prothrombin to thrombin; also called *prothrombinase* / *page 183*

prothrombin time (PRO-throm-bin): blood test used to determine the time needed for plasma to clot to regulate warfarin dosage / *page 184*

thrombin (THROM-bin): enzyme that causes clotting by forming thrombin / *page 183*

thromboembolic disease (THROM-bow-EM-bow-LIT-ik): disorders where clients have blood clots / *page 185*

thrombolytics (THROM-bow-LIT-iks): drugs used to dissolve existing blood clots / *page 184*

thrombus (THROM-bus): blood clot / *page 185*

tissue plasminogen activator (tPA): natural enzyme and a drug that dissolves blood clots / *page 183*

The process of hemostasis, or the stopping of blood flow, is an essential mechanism protecting the body from both external and internal injury. Without efficient hemostasis, bleeding from wounds would lead to shock and perhaps death. Too much clotting, however, can be just as dangerous as too little. Thus, hemostasis must maintain a delicate balance between fluidity and coagulation.

hemo = blood
stasis = stopping

A number of diseases and conditions can affect hemostasis. Some common disorders that may require pharmacologic therapy with coagulation-modifying drugs are described in Table 13.1.

TABLE 13.1	Disorders Commonly Treated with Coagulation-Modifying Drugs
DISORDER/CONDITION	**DESCRIPTION**
venous thrombus	clot within a vein
myocardial infarction	clot within a coronary artery
cerebrovascular accident/stroke	clot within an artery serving the brain
pulmonary embolus	clot within a pulmonary artery
valvular heart disease	disease of heart valves or replacement of a heart valve
angina	narrowing of the coronary vessels
indwelling devices	mechanical heart valves, stents
post-operative hemorrhage	bleeding following a surgical procedure

Fast Facts Clotting Disorders

- Von Willebrands is the most common hereditary platelet disorder, caused by a deficiency of a clotting protein.
- Hemophilia A is a hereditary lack of clotting factor VIII; it accounts for 80% of all hemophilia cases.
- Hemophilia B is a hereditary lack of clotting factor IX.
- More than 15,000 people in the U.S. have hemophilia A or B.
- Liver disease is one of the most common causes of coagulation disorders, as this organ supplies many of the clotting factors.

13.1 Hemostasis is a complex process involving multiple steps and a large number of enzymes and factors.

The process of hemostasis is complex and involves a number of substances called **clotting factors**. Hemostasis occurs in a series of sequential steps, sometimes referred to as a *cascade*. Drugs can be used to modify some of these steps.

When an injury occurs, cells lining the damaged blood vessel release chemicals that initiate the clotting process. The vessel immediately spasms or constricts in order to limit blood flow to the injured area. Small blood components called **platelets** become sticky, adhere to the injured area, and aggregate or clump to plug the damaged vessel. Blood flow is further slowed, thus allowing the process of **coagulation**, the formation of an insoluble clot, to occur. The three basic steps of hemostasis are shown in Figure 13.1.

FIGURE 13.1	
Basic steps in hemostasis	

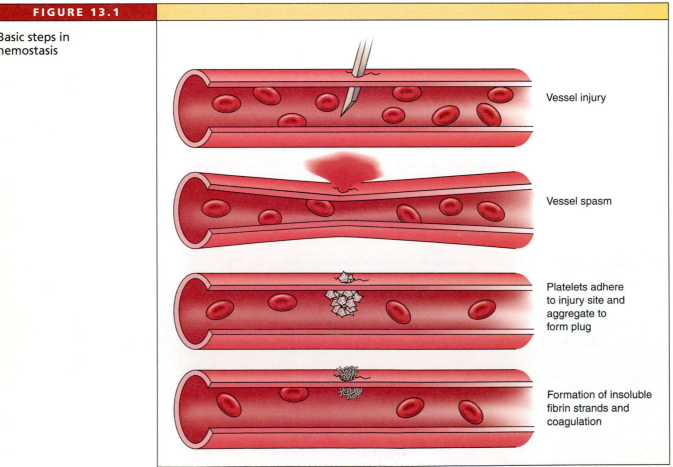

Vessel injury

Vessel spasm

Platelets adhere to injury site and aggregate to form plug

Formation of insoluble fibrin strands and coagulation

FIGURE 13.2

Major steps in the coagulation cascade

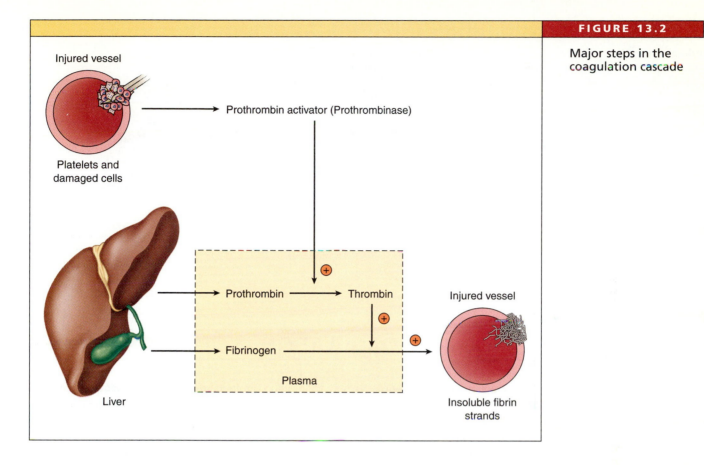

The **coagulation cascade** is a complex series of steps that begins when the injured cells release a chemical called **prothrombin activator** or *prothrombinase*. Prothrombin activator converts the clotting factor **prothrombin** to an enzyme called **thrombin**. Thrombin then converts **fibrinogen**, a plasma protein, to long strands of **fibrin**. Thus two of the factors essential to clotting, thrombin and fibrin, are only formed after injury to the vessels. The fibrin strands form an insoluble web over the injured area to stop blood loss. Normal blood clotting occurs in about six minutes. The primary steps in the coagulation cascade are shown in Figure 13.2.

thrombo = clot
plastin = to form
pro = before
thrombin = clot

It is important to note that several clotting factors, including thromboplastin and fibrinogen, are proteins made by the liver that are constantly circulating through the blood in an inactive form. Vitamin K is required for the liver to make four of the clotting factors. Because of the crucial importance of the liver in creating these clotting factors, clients with serious liver disorders often have abnormal coagulation.

13.2 Removal of a blood clot is essential to restore normal circulation.

The goal of hemostasis has been achieved once a blood clot is formed and the body is protected from excessive hemorrhage. The clot, however, stops most or all of the blood flow to the affected area; circulation must eventually be restored so that the tissue can resume normal activities. The process of clot removal is called **fibrinolysis**.

fibrin = fiber
lysis = break apart

Fibrinolysis also involves several cascading steps. When the fibrin clot is formed, nearby blood vessel cells secrete a chemical known as **tissue plasminogen activator (tPA)**. tPA converts the inactive protein **plasminogen**, which is present in the fibrin clot, to its active enzymatic form called **plasmin**. Plasmin then digests the fibrin strands to remove the clot. The body normally regulates fibrinolysis such that unwanted fibrin clots are removed, while fibrin present in wounds is left to maintain hemostasis. The steps of fibrinolysis are shown in Figure 13.3.

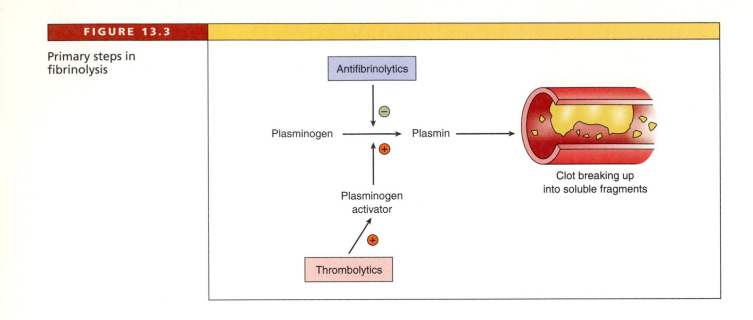

FIGURE 13.3

Primary steps in fibrinolysis

ABNORMAL COAGULATION

There are many types of disorders where abnormal coagulation might appear. Examples are when the blood becomes gelatinous or semi-solid, disrupting the normal flow of blood. Solid masses of blood or blood clots can place clients in extreme danger. Blood clots may become dislodged and move to another part of the body, for example the lungs or the brain. In some cases, the blood may not clot quickly enough, for example, following surgery. In this case, it is desirable to make the blood clot more quickly to prevent excessive bleeding.

13.3 The normal coagulation process can be modified by a number of different mechanisms.

anti = against
coagulation = clotting

Drugs can modify hemostasis in a number of ways. The four basic mechanisms of coagulation-modifying drugs are summarized in Table 13.2. The most commonly prescribed coagulation-modifiers, the class of drugs known as the anticoagulants, are used to prevent the formation of clots. To accomplish clot prevention, drugs can either inhibit specific clotting factors in the co-agulation cascade or diminish the clotting action of platelets. Regardless of the mechanism, all anticoagulant drugs will increase the normal time the body takes to form clots.

thrombo = clot
lytic = remove/destroy

Once an abnormal clot has formed, it may be critical to quickly remove it in order to restore normal function. This is particularly important for blood vessels serving the heart, lungs, and brain. A specific class of drugs, called thrombolytics, has been developed to dissolve such life-threatening clots.

anti = against
fibrin = fiber
lytic = remove/destroy

Occasionally, it is necessary to actually promote the formation of clots. These drugs, called antifibrinolytics, inhibit the normal removal of fibrin, thus keeping the clot in place for a longer period of time. These drugs are primarily used to speed clot formation in order to limit bleeding from a surgical site.

Because hemostasis involves a delicate balance of factors favoring clotting versus those inhibiting clotting, drug therapy with coagulation-modifiers is individualized to each client and must be carefully monitored. For example, prothrombin time (PT) is a laboratory test often used during therapy with the anticoagulant drug warfarin. While the normal range for PT is from 12–15 seconds, this value becomes prolonged with anticoagulant treatment. Daily PT tests may be conducted at the start of anticoagulant therapy to ensure optimum dose levels. The frequency of PT tests is increased to weekly or monthly as therapy progresses and the client's disease stabilizes. Because the method of performing PT tests varies from laboratory to laboratory, clotting time is

TABLE 13.2	Mechanisms by Which Coagulation Can Be Modified by Drugs	
TYPE OF MODIFICATION	**MECHANISM**	**DRUG CLASSIFICATION**
prevention of clot formation	inhibition of specific clotting factors	anticoagulant
prevention of clot formation	inhibition of platelet actions	anticoagulant/ antiplatelet
removal of an existing clot	clot is dissolved by the drug	thrombolytic
promotion of clot formation	inhibit the destruction of fibrin	antifibrinolytic

sometimes reported as an international normalized ratio (INR), which is the PT multiplied times a correction factor. Recommended post-treatment INR values range from 2 to 4.5. For the anticoagulant drug heparin, a different lab test called the **activated partial thromboplastin time** (APTT) is used. Normal values of this test range from 25–40 seconds.

Concept review 13.1

▪ Which of the clotting factors are always circulating in the blood? Which are only formed when coagulation is underway?

ANTICOAGULANTS

Anticoagulants are medications used to prolong bleeding time in order to prevent blood clots from forming. They are widely used for thromboembolic disease.

13.4 Anticoagulants prevent clot formation.

Once a stationary clot, called a thrombus, forms in a vessel, it often grows larger as more fibrin is added. Pieces of the thrombus may break off and travel in the bloodstream to affect other vessels. Traveling clots are called emboli. The term thromboembolic disease refers to these types of clotting disorders.

ON THE JOB

Dental Hygienists and Anticoagulants

The dental hygienist is trained to obtain accurate client medical histories because dental treatment may be contraindicated for clients taking certain medications. Perhaps the best example is that of clients taking warfarin. Because nearly all dental procedures result in some degree of bleeding, the decision to proceed with treatment will depend upon whether the procedure is elective or critical to the client's health. In most cases, the client will provide the dental office with recent INR or PT results. The client's physician may be consulted prior to initiating any treatment that could result in bleeding. The physician may ask the client to discontinue warfarin for a few days prior to the dental procedure so that clotting may return to a more normal state.

The dental hygienist is responsible for gathering drug data so that the dentist may make a rational decision on treatment. If treatment is rendered, the hygienist will take special care to limit the potential for bleeding. The hygienist is also responsible for educating the client about possible side effects of the treatment and the proper follow-up. For example, the hygienist will remind the client not to take aspirin, should pain be experienced following the procedure. ▪

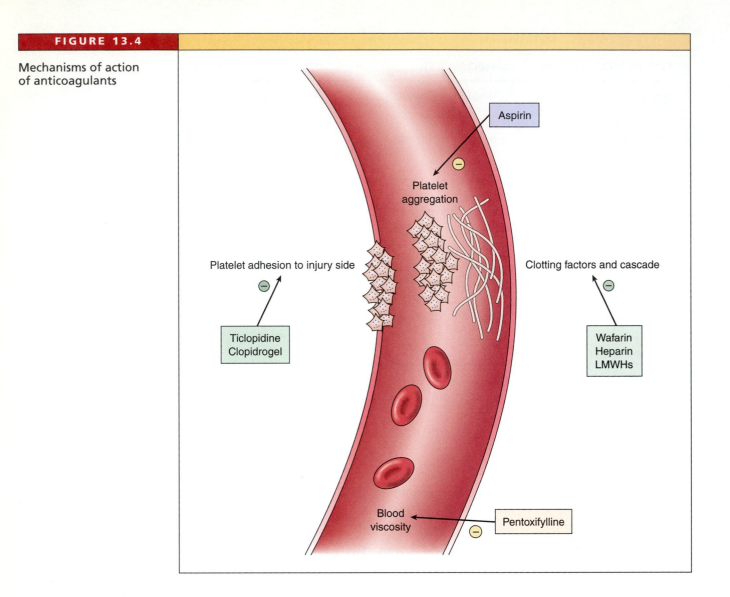

FIGURE 13.4

Mechanisms of action
of anticoagulants

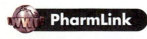

THE MIRACLES OF ASPIRIN

**IMMUNE
THROMBOCYTOPENIC
PURPURA (ITP)**

Anticoagulants are drugs that lengthen clotting time and prevent thrombi from forming or growing larger. Because thromboembolic disease can be life threatening, therapy is often begun by administering anticoagulants intravenously or subcutaneously. As the disease stabilizes, the client is switched to oral anticoagulants, with careful monitoring through the use of periodic PT tests. The most common anticoagulants are heparin and warfarin (Coumadin). Anticoagulants act by a number of different mechanisms, which are illustrated in Figure 13.4. Table 13.3 lists the primary anticoagulants.

ANTIPLATELET AGENTS

Antiplatelet medications exert an anticoagulant effect by interfering with various aspects of platelet function. Unlike the anticoagulants, which are used primarily to prevent thrombosis in veins, antiplatelet agents are used to prevent clot formation in arteries.

13.5 Several drugs prolong bleeding time by interfering with platelet function.

Platelets are a central component of the hemostasis process. Too few platelets or diminished platelet function can profoundly increase bleeding time. Three types of agents are called an-

DRUG PROFILE:
Heparin

Actions:

Heparin is a natural substance found in the lining of blood vessels. Its normal function is to prevent excessive clotting within blood vessels. When given as a drug, heparin provides immediate anticoagulant activity. The binding of heparin to a substance called antithrombin III results in an inactivation of some of the clotting factors and an inhibition of thrombin activity. Because heparin is not absorbed by the gastrointestinal mucosa, it must be given either subcutaneously (SC) or through intravenous (IV) infusion. The onset of action for IV heparin is immediate, whereas SC heparin may take up to an hour for maximum therapeutic effect.

In recent years, the heparin molecule has been shortened and modified to create a new class of drugs called low molecular weight heparins (LMWHs). LMWHs possess the same anticoagulant activity as heparin, but have several advantages. They produce a more stable response than heparin, thus fewer lab tests are needed, and family members or the client can be trained to give the necessary SC injections at home. LMWHs have become the drugs of choice for a number of clotting disorders, including the prevention of deep vein thrombosis following surgery.

Adverse Effects:

Abnormal bleeding is not uncommon during heparin therapy. Should APTT become prolonged or toxicity be observed, discontinuation of the drug will result in loss of anticoagulant activity within hours. If serious hemorrhage occurs, a specific antagonist, protamine sulfate, may be administered to neutralize the anticoagulant activity of heparin. Protamine sulfate has an onset of action of five minutes and is also an antagonist to the LMWHs.

TABLE 13.3	Anticoagulants	
DRUG	**ROUTE AND ADULT DOSE**	**REMARKS**
Pr heparin sodium (Heplock)	IV infusion: 5,000–40,000 units/day SC; 15,000–20,000 units bid.	For the prevention and treatment venous thrombosis and pulmonary embolus. Dose is adjusted according to PTT. Therapy begins with a higher dose, which is gradually reduced.
Pr warfarin sodium (Coumadin)	PO; 2–15 mg/day.	Same use as heparin sodium but effect is more prolonged. Dose is adjusted according to PT; IV form is available.
enoxaparin (Lovenox)	SC; 30 mg bid for 7–10 days.	Low molecular weight heparin (LMWH); used as deep vein thrombosis (DVT) prophylaxis prior to knee or hip replacement or abdominal surgery; unlabeled use is treatment of DVT or pulmonaryembolus; IM form available.
dalteparin sodium (Fragmin)	SC; 2,500–5,000 units/day for 5–10 days.	LMWH; see enoxaparin.
danaparoid sodium (Orgaran)	SC; 750 units bid for 7–10 days.	LMWH; see enoxaparin.
tinzaparin sodium (Innohep)	SC; 175 units/kg qd for at least 6 days.	LMWH; see enoxaparin.
pentoxifylline (Trental)	PO; 400 mg tid.	Reduces blood viscosity and increases the flexibility of red blood cells; for treatment of intermittent claudication.

DRUG PROFILE:

Warfarin (Coumadin)

Actions:

Unlike heparin, the anticoagulant activity of warfarin can take several days to reach its maximum effect. This explains why heparin and warfarin therapy are overlapped. Warfarin inhibits the action of vitamin K that is essential for the synthesis of several clotting factors. Because these clotting factors are normally circulating in the blood, it takes several days for them to clear the plasma and for the anticoagulant effect of warfarin to appear. Another reason for the slow onset is that 99% of the warfarin is bound to plasma proteins and is thus unavailable to produce its effect. This high protein binding is responsible for a significant number of drug-drug interactions that may occur during warfarin therapy.

Adverse Effects:

Like all anticoagulants, the most serious adverse effect of warfarin is abnormal bleeding. Upon discontinuation of therapy, the activity of warfarin can take up to 10 days to diminish. Should life-threatening bleeding occur during therapy, the anticoagulant effects of warfarin can be reduced in six hours through the IM or SC administration of its antagonist, vitamin K_1.

Mechanism in Action:

Many vitamin K-dependent clotting factors are essential for blood coagulation. The anticoagulant, warfarin, inhibits the amount of factors made available by the liver. Reducing vitamin K-dependent factors inhibits the formation of prothrombin, which is one of the final coagulation proteins in the clotting cascade. The result is slowed clot formation and increased bleeding time.

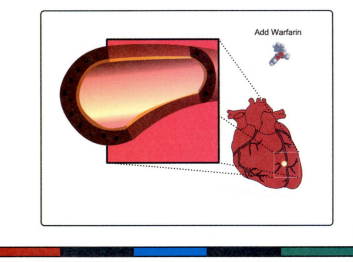

Add Warfarin

tiplatelet agents due to their inhibition of platelet function: (1) aspirin; (2) adenosine diphosphate (ADP) receptor blockers; and (3) glycoprotein IIb/IIIa receptor blockers.

Aspirin deserves special mention as an antiplatelet type of coagulation-modifier. Because it is available over-the-counter, clients may not consider aspirin a potent medication. However, its anticoagulant activity is well documented. Aspirin acts by inhibiting thromboxane$_2$, a powerful inducer of platelet aggregation. The anticoagulant effect of a single dose of aspirin may persist

NATURAL ALTERNATIVES

Garlic for Cardiovascular Disease

Garlic (*Allium sativum*) is one of the best-studied herbs. Purported indications for garlic include arteriosclerosis, common cold, cough/bronchitis, high cholesterol, hypertension, tendency to infection, and many other conditions. It has been proven to be of value in only a few of these disorders.

A number of different substances, known as *alliaceous oils,* have been isolated from garlic and shown to have pharmacologic activity. Dosage forms include eating prepared garlic oil or the fresh bulbs from the plant.

Garlic has been shown to decrease the aggregation or "stickiness" of platelets, thus producing an anticoagulant effect. Claims that garlic can reduce heart disease and the incidence of stroke may be related to this action. The healthcare provider may want to recommend that clients taking anticoagulant medications limit their intake of garlic to avoid bleeding complications. ■

DRUG PROFILE:
Abciximab (ReoPro)

Actions:

Abciximab is an antibody that interferes with the final step in platelet aggregation by binding to glycoprotein IIb/IIIa receptor sites on platelets. It is extremely effective, having the ability to reduce platelet function by as much as 90% in just two hours. Abciximab is only available by bolus injection and IV infusion.

Adverse Effects:

Like other drugs having an anticoagulant effect, contraindications for abciximab include active bleeding or recent trauma. The health-care provider must be observant for unusual bleeding. Abciximab is commonly used with aspirin and heparin, thus increasing the need for careful monitoring.

for as long as a week. Concurrent use of aspirin with other coagulation-modifiers should be avoided unless medically approved. The primary actions add adverse effects of aspirin are described in a Drug Profile in Chapter 11 ⊂⊃ .

The ADP receptor blockers comprise a small group of drugs that interfere with the plasma membrane of platelets, preventing them from aggregating. Both ticlopidine (Ticlid) and clopidogrel (Plavix) are given orally to prevent thrombi formation in clients who have experienced a recent thromboembolic event such as a stroke or MI.

Glycoprotein IIb/IIIa inhibitors are relatively new additions to the treatment of thromboembolic disease. Glycoprotein IIb/IIIa is an enzyme necessary for platelet aggregation. Inhibition of this enzyme has the effect of preventing thrombus formation in clients experiencing a recent myocardial infarction, stroke, or percutaneous transluminal coronary angioplasty (PTCA). Doses for the glycoprotein IIb/IIIa blockers and other antiplatelet agents are shown in Table 13.4.

TABLE 13.4	Antiplatelet Agents	
DRUG	**ROUTE AND ADULT DOSE**	**REMARKS**
aspirin (ASA, acetylsalicylic acid)	PO; 80 mg qd–650 mg bid.	Inhibits platelet aggregation; available without a prescription; higher doses are used to treat inflammation or pain.
dipyridamole (Persantine)	PO; 75–100 mg qid.	Platelet inhibitor to prevent embolism in clients with prosthetic heart valves; often used with warfarin; IV form available.
ADP Receptor Blockers		
ticlopidine (Ticlid)	PO; 250 mg bid.	Platelet aggregation inhibitor; prolongs bleeding time.
clopidrogrel Bisulfate (Plavix)	PO; 75 mg qd.	Prolongs bleeding time.
Glycoprotein IIb/IIIa Blockers		
(Pr) abciximab (ReoPro)	IV 0.25 mg/kg initial bolus over 5 min then 10 µg/min for 12 hr.	Used to prevent cardiac ischemia during coronary angioplasty; duration lasts up to 48 hr after infusion is stopped.
eptifibatide (Integrilin)	IV; 180µg/kg initial bolus over 1–2 min then 2µg/kg/min for 24–72 hr.	Also for unstable angina and other acute coronary syndromes; duration lasts up to 8 hr after infusion is stopped.
tirofiban hydrochloride (Aggrastat)	IV; 0.4 µg/kg/min for 30 min then 0.1µg/kg/min for 12–24 hr.	Similar to eptifibatide; duration lasts up to 8 hr after infusion is stopped.

THROMBOLYTICS

Unlike the anticoagulants, thrombolytics can dissolve existing fibrin clots. They are much more effective if given very soon after the clot forms.

13.6 Thrombolytics are used to dissolve existing clots.

It is often mistakenly believed that the purpose of anticoagulants such as heparin and warfarin is to dissolve preexisting clots. This is not the case: a totally different type of drug is needed for this purpose. These drugs, called *thrombolytics,* are administered quite differently than the anticoagulants and produce their effects by different mechanisms. Thrombolytics are prescribed for a number of different disorders, including the following.

- acute myocardial infarction (MI)
- pulmonary embolism
- acute ischemic cerebrovascular accident
- deep vein thrombosis (DVT)
- arterial thrombosis
- coronary thrombosis
- clear thrombi in arteriovenous cannulas and occluded IV catheters

Thrombolytics are non-specific: they will dissolve whatever clots they encounter. Because clotting is a natural and desirable process to prevent excessive bleeding, thrombolytics have a narrow margin of safety between dissolving "normal" and "abnormal" clots. Vital signs must be monitored continuously and any signs of bleeding may call for discontinuation of therapy. Because these medications are rapidly destroyed in the bloodstream, discontinuation normally

DRUG PROFILE:
Streptokinase (Streptase)

Actions:

The earliest drug in this class, streptokinase, was initially extracted from the bacterium *Streptococcus.* Later the drug was extracted from normal human blood. Like other thrombolytics, the primary action of streptokinase is to convert plasminogen to plasmin, which then degrades fibrin to dissolve preexisting clots. To achieve maximum effect, therapy should begin immediately after the onset of symptoms.

Adverse Effects:

Thrombolytics such as streptokinase are contraindicated in clients with active bleeding or with a history of recent trauma or stroke. The healthcare practitioner must check the client every 15–30 minutes during therapy for signs of bleeding. Because streptokinase is a foreign protein, allergic reactions may occur. Because the body will develop antibodies to streptokinase, repeat doses are often not recommended. The newer thrombolytics are not foreign proteins and some of these may be readministered if the initial dose is not effective.

TABLE 13.5	Thrombolytics	
DRUG	**ROUTE AND ADULT DOSE**	**REMARKS**
Pr streptokinase (Streptase, Kabikinase)	IV; 250,000–1.5 million units over a short period of time.	For acute deep vein thrombosis, pulmonary emboli, and MI.
alteplase recombinant (Activase)	IV; begin with 60 mg and then infuse 20 mg/hour over next 2 hours.	Naturally occurring tissue plasminogen activator; must be given within 6 hours of start of MI or 3 hours of thrombotic stroke.
anistreplase (Eminase)	IV; 30 units over 2–5 min.	Usually given at the onset of an acute MI.
reteplase recombinant (Retavase)	IV; 10 units over 2 min; repeat dose in 30 min.	Given during an acute MI to decrease chance of HF and death.
urokinase (Abbokinase)	IV; 4400–6000 units administered over several minutes to 12 hours.	For massive pulmonary emboli; restores patency in occluded IV catheters.

results in immediate termination of thrombolytic activity. After the clot is successfully dissolved with the thrombolytic, anticoagulant therapy is generally initiated to prevent the reformation of clots.

Since the discovery of streptokinase, the first thrombolytic, there have been a number of generations of thrombolytics. The newer drugs such as tenecteplase (TNK-tPA) are more fibrin-specific and may produce fewer side effects than streptokinase. Table 13.5 lists the major thrombolytics.

Concept review 13.2

■ Both warfarin and heparin are effective anticoagulants. Why would a physician choose heparin over warfarin?

ANTIFIBRINOLYTICS

Antifibrinolytics have an action opposite to that of anticoagulants: to shorten bleeding time. They are used to prevent excessive bleeding following surgery.

13.7 Antifibrinolytics are used to promote the formation of clots.

The final class of coagulation modifiers, the antifibrinolytics, is a small group of drugs used to prevent and treat excessive bleeding from surgical sites. All of the antifibrinolytics have very specific indications for use and none are commonly prescribed. Although their mechanisms differ, all drugs in this class prevent fibrin from dissolving, thus enhancing the stability of the clot. Because of their ability to slow blood flow, they are sometimes classified as hemostatic agents. Desmopressin differs from the others in being a hormone similar to vasopressin, a hormone naturally present in the body that promotes the renal conservation of water. Unlike the other antifibrinolytics it has uses beyond hemostasis that include the control of excessive or nocturnal urination (enuresis). The antifibrinolytics are listed in Table 13.6.

DRUG PROFILE:
Aminocaproic Acid (Amicar)

Actions:

Aminocaproic acid acts by inactivating plasminogen, the precursor of the enzyme plasmin that digests the fibrin clot. Aminocaproic acid is prescribed in situations where there is excessive bleeding as a result of clots being dissolved prematurely. During acute hemorrhages, it can be given IV to reduce bleeding in one to two hours. It is most commonly prescribed following surgery to reduce post-operative bleeding.

Adverse Effects:

Because aminocaproic acid tends to stabilize clots, it should be used cautiously in clients with a history of thromboembolic disease. Side effects are generally mild.

TABLE 13.6	Antifibrinolytics	
DRUG	**ROUTE AND ADULT DOSE**	**REMARKS**
Pr aminocaproic acid (Amicar)	IV; 4–5 g for 1 hour, then 1–1.25 g/hour until bleeding is controlled.	For control of excessive bleeding caused by pathologic condition known as *systemic hyperfibrinolysis;* oral form available.
aprotinin (Trasylol)	IV; 15,000 KIU as a test dose, then give 500,000 KIU during surgery.	Used prior to coronary bypass surgery to reduce perioperative blood loss.
desmopressin acetate (DDAVP)	IV; 0.3 µg/kg, repeated as needed.	To help control bleeding in patients with hemophelia A; infusion occurs over 15–30 minutes, usually immediately prior to surgery; PO, SC, and intranasal forms available. Also used for diabetes insipidus and nocturnal enuresis.
tranexamic acid (Cyklokapron)	PO; 25 mg/kg qid.	Used just prior to and following dental surgery; IV form available.

CLIENT TEACHING

Clients treated for coagulation disorders need to know the following:

1. Keep scheduled appointments for PT, APTT, and INR laboratory tests. Test results are used in making decisions about drug dose adjustments.
2. Report unusual bruising or bleeding such as nose bleeds, bleeding gums, black or red stool, heavy menstrual periods, or spitting up blood.
3. Inform your dental hygienist and dentist about use of anticoagulant medication.
4. Use caution when engaged in activities that can cause bleeding, such as shaving, brushing teeth, trimming nails, and using kitchen knives. A soft toothbrush and an electric razor are safe choices. Contact sports, with their high risk for injury, should be avoided.
5. Take medication on time and as directed. Do not skip a dose and do not double up on doses.
6. Speak with the practitioner before taking any other drugs, including OTC drugs or herbal supplements. Many drugs increase or decrease the action of anticoagulants. ■

CHAPTER REVIEW

 Core Concepts Summary

13.1 Hemostasis is a complex process involving multiple steps and a large number of enzymes and factors.

Hemostasis is an essential mechanism protecting the body from both external and internal injury that occurs in a number of steps that require a large number of clotting factors and enzymes. The final result of coagulation is the formation of the fibrin clot that protects the body from excessive bleeding.

13.2 Removal of a blood clot is essential to restore normal circulation.

During fibrinolysis, plasmin digests the fibrin strands thus restoring circulation to the injured area.

13.3 The normal coagulation process can be modified by a number of different mechanisms.

Anticoagulants prevent the formation of clots, thrombolytics dissolve existing clots, and antifibrinolytics promote the formation of clots. Coagulation is always carefully monitored through the use of PT or APTT laboratory tests.

13.4 Anticoagulants prevent clot formation.

Anticoagulants prolong coagulation time by inhibiting platelets or some specific clotting factor.

Heparin is given IV or SC to provide immediate activity and warfarin is given orally to offer more prolonged action. Protamine sulfate can reverse the anticoagulant activity of heparin and vitamin K_1 can reverse the effects of warfarin.

13.5 Several drugs prolong bleeding time by interfering with platelet function.

Aspirin, ADP receptor blockers, and glycoprotein IIb/IIIa receptor blockers prolong bleeding time by interfering with platelet function. They are used to prevent thrombus formation in arteries.

13.6 Thrombolytics are used to dissolve existing clots.

By dissolving existing clots, thrombolytics restore circulation to an injured area. For maximum effectiveness, they should be given as soon as possible after the thrombus is diagnosed.

13.7 Antifibrinolytics are used to promote the formation of clots.

Antifibrinolytics inhibit fibrin in a clot from dissolving and are used primarily to prevent excessive bleeding from surgical sites.

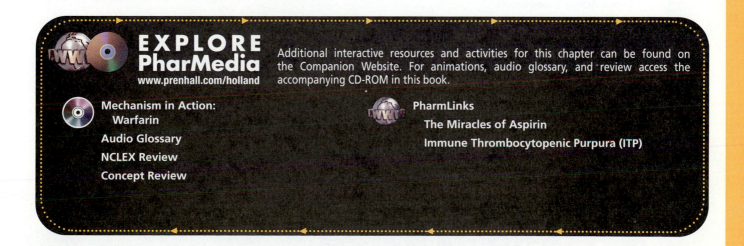

EXPLORE PharMedia
www.prenhall.com/holland

Additional interactive resources and activities for this chapter can be found on the Companion Website. For animations, audio glossary, and review access the accompanying CD-ROM in this book.

Mechanism in Action:
   Warfarin
Audio Glossary
NCLEX Review
Concept Review

PharmLinks
   The Miracles of Aspirin
   Immune Thrombocytopenic Purpura (ITP)

14 Drugs for Hypertension

CORE CONCEPTS

14.1 Hypertension is a major cause of death and disability.

14.2 Blood pressure is caused by the pumping action of the heart.

14.3 Three primary factors are responsible for blood pressure: cardiac output, the resistance of the small arteries, and blood volume.

14.4 Many factors help to regulate blood pressure.

14.5 Hypertension is well defined.

14.6 Non-pharmacologic therapy is often effective for minor hypertension.

Antihypertensives

14.7 Selection of specific antihypertension drugs depends upon the severity of the disease.

Diuretics

14.8 Diuretics are effective at reducing mild to moderate hypertension.

Calcium Channel Blockers

14.9 Calcium channel blockers have emerged as major drugs in the treatment of hypertension.

Angiotensin Converting Enzyme (ACE) Inhibitors

14.10 Blocking the renin-angiotensin pathway leads to a decrease in blood pressure.

Adrenergic Blockers

14.11 Organs innervated by the autonomic nervous system are a frequent target for antihypertensive drugs.

Direct Acting Vasodilators

14.12 Some drugs act directly on arteriolar smooth muscle to lower blood pressure.

OBJECTIVES

After reading this chapter, the student should be able to:

1. Identify the major risk factors associated with hypertension.

2. Summarize the long-term consequences of uncontrolled hypertension.

3. Describe how the pumping action of the heart creates blood pressure.

4. Explain the effects of cardiac output, peripheral resistance, and blood volume on blood pressure.

5. Discuss how the vasomotor center, baroreceptors, chemoreceptors, emotions, and hormones influence blood pressure.

6. Differentiate among mild, moderate, and severe hypertension.

7. Prescribe a method for controlling hypertension without drugs.

8. Apply "stepped care" principles as they pertain to antihypertension drugs.

9. For each of the following classes, identify representative medications and explain the mechanism of drug action, and primary actions, and important side effects.
   a. diuretics
   b. calcium channel blockers
   c. ACE inhibitors
   d. adrenergic-blockers
   e. direct-acting vasodilators

10. Categorize antihypertensive drugs based on their classification and mechanism of action.

PharMedia
www.prenhall.com/holland

Additional interactive resources and activities for this chapter can be found on the Companion Website. For animations, audio glossary, and review access the accompanying CD-ROM in this book.

aldosterone (al-DOH-stair-own): hormone released by the adrenal cortex that regulates sodium reabsorption / *page 205*

alpha$_1$-receptors (AL-fah): adrenergic receptors found in vascular smooth muscle / *page 209*

angiotensin II (AN-geo-TEN-sin): chemical released in response to falling blood pressure that causes vasoconstriction and release of aldosterone / *page 205*

angiotensin-converting enzyme (ACE) (angeo-TEN-sin): enzyme responsible for converting angiotensin I to angiotensin II / *page 205*

antidiuretic hormone (ADH) (ANT-eye-deye-your-ET-ik): hormone produced by the hypothalamus that stimulates the kidneys to conserve water / *page 199*

baroreceptors (BARE-oh-ree-sep-tours): nerves located in the walls of the atria, aortic arch, vena cava, and carotid sinus that sense changes in blood pressure / *page 199*

beta$_1$ receptors (BAY-tah): adrenergic receptors primarily found in the heart / *page 209*

beta$_2$ receptors: adrenergic receptors found in organs other than the heart / *page 209*

benign prostatic hyperplasia (BPH) (bee-NINE pross-TAT-ik heye-purr-PLAY-shah): non-malignant enlargement of the prostate gland / *page 210*

blood volume: amount of blood in the vascular system / *page 198*

bradycardia (bray-dee-KAR-DEE-ah): a condition of slow heartbeat / *page 209*

calcium channel blocker: drug that blocks the flow of calcium ions into myocardial cells / *page 204*

cardiac output: amount of blood pumped by each ventricle in one minute / *page 198*

chemoreceptors (KEE-moh-ree-sep-tors): nerves located in the aortic arch and carotid sinus that sense changes in oxygen content, pH, or carbon dioxide levels in the blood / *page 199*

diastolic pressure (DEYE-ah-stall-ik): blood pressure during the relaxation phase of heart activity / *page 197*

diuresis (deye-your-EE-sis): urine flow / *page 204*

diuretic (deye-your-ET-ik): substance that increases urine flow / *page 199*

electrolytes (ee-LEK-troh-lites): charged substances in the blood such as sodium, potassium, calcium, chloride, and phosphate / *page 203*

false neurotransmitter (NYUR-oh-TRANS-mitt-ur): chemical that simulates a natural neurotransmitter but does not produce the same physiologic effect / *page 209*

heart failure (HF): disease in which the heart muscle cannot contract with sufficient force to meet the body's metabolic needs / *page 196*

hyperkalemia (heye-purr-kah-LEE-mee-ah): high amounts of potassium in the blood / *page 203*

hypokalemia (heye-poh-kah-LEE-mee-ah): low amounts of potassium in the blood / *page 204*

hypertension (heye-purr-TEN-shun): high blood pressure / *page 195*

lumen (LOO-men): the inside diameter of a hollow tube such as a blood vessel / *page 198*

orthostatic hypotension (or-tho-STAT-ik): fall in blood pressure that occurs when someone changes position from recumbent to upright / *page 209*

peripheral resistance (per-IF-ur-ul): the amount of friction encountered by blood as it travels through the vessels / *page 198*

reflex tachycardia (ta-kee-CAR-dee-ah): temporary speeding up of heart rate that occurs when blood pressure falls / *page 206*

renin-angiotensin system (REN-in – an-geo-TEN-sin): series of enzymatic steps by which the body raises blood pressure / *page 199*

stepped care: a systematic approach to treatment of hypertension / *page 203*

stroke volume: volume of blood pumped out by a ventricle in a single beat / *page 198*

systolic pressure (SIS-tol-ik): blood pressure during the contraction phase of heart activity / *page 197*

vasomotor center (VAZO-mo-tor): area of the medulla that controls baseline blood pressure / *page 199*

Cardiovascular disease, which includes all conditions affecting the heart and blood vessels, is the most common cause of death in the United States. Hypertension or high blood pressure is the most common of the cardiovascular diseases. Because healthcare providers encounter numerous clients with this disease, a firm grasp of the underlying principles of antihypertensive therapy is critical.

hyper = high
tension = pressure

14.1 Hypertension is a major cause of death and disability.

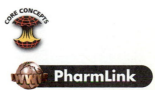

PharmLink

THE AMERICAN SOCIETY OF HYPERTENSION

The most common type of hypertension, accounting for 90% of all cases, is called *primary* or *essential*. Although the actual cause of primary hypertension is not known, many conditions or risk factors have been shown to be associated with the disease. Advancing age and weight gain, particularly around the hips and thighs, tends to be associated with hypertension. The disease is most prevalent in blacks and least prevalent in Mexican-Americans. Males in all ethnic groups experience more hypertension compared to females. The disease also has a heredity component, with family members of hypertensives having greater risk of acquiring the disease than non-family members. Other factors, such as tobacco use and high-fat diets, contribute to the disease.

Fast Facts Hypertension

- Hypertension increases with age. It affects approximately:
  30% of those over 50 years old; 64% of men over age 65; 75% of women over age 75
- Almost 13,000 people died of hypertension in the U.S. in 1996 (2 deaths per 100,000 population).
- Hypertension is responsible for over 10 million ambulatory care visits.
- Hypertension affects one in four Americans; 50–60 million people per year.
- Blacks have the highest rate of hypertension.
- Less than 25% of Americans diagnosed with hypertension keep their blood pressure within recommended parameters.
- Hypertension is the most common complication of pregnancy.

PharmLink

HERBAL THERAPIES FOR HYPERTENSION

DIETARY MODIFICATIONS FOR THE HYPERTENSIVE CLIENT

Because chronic hypertension may produce no identifiable symptoms for as long as 10 to 20 years, many people are not aware of their condition. Convincing clients to control their diets, spend money on medication, and take drugs on a regular basis when they are feeling healthy is a difficult task for the healthcare practitioner. Failure to control hypertension, however, can result in quite serious consequences. Prolonged high blood pressure can damage small blood vessels, leading to accelerated narrowing of the arteries resulting in strokes, kidney failure, and even cardiac arrest. One of the most serious consequences of chronic hypertension is that the heart must work harder to pump blood to the various organs and tissues. This excessive workload can cause the heart to fail and the lungs to fill with fluid, a condition known as **heart failure (HF)**. Drug therapy of HF is covered in Chapter 15 🔗 .

FIGURE 14.1	

Blood pressure changes throughout the circulation

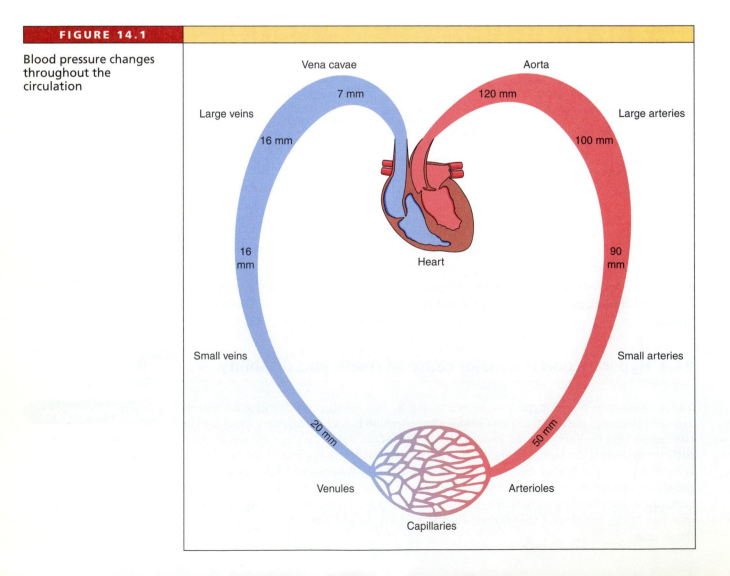

FIGURE 14.2

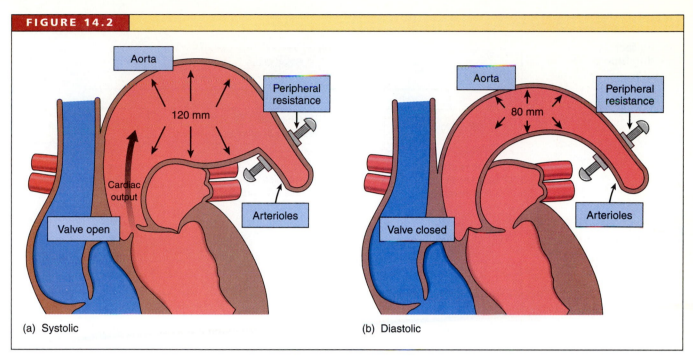

(a) Systolic   (b) Diastolic

Systolic and diastolic blood pressure

The death rate from cardiovascular-related diseases has dropped significantly over the past 20 years due, in large part, to the recognition and treatment of hypertension, as well as the acceptance of healthier lifestyle habits. Early treatment is essential; the long-term cardiovascular damage caused by hypertension may be irreversible if the disease is allowed to progress unchecked.

14.2 Blood pressure is caused by the pumping action of the heart.

Although pressure can be measured in nearly any vessel in the body, the term *blood pressure* commonly refers to pressure in the arteries. Because the pumping action of the heart is the source of blood pressure, those arteries closest to the heart, such as the aorta, have the highest pressure. Pressure decreases progressively as the blood travels further away from the heart, until it falls close to zero in the largest veins. This is illustrated in Figure 14.1.

When the ventricles of the heart contract and eject blood, the pressure created in the arteries is called **systolic pressure**. When the ventricles relax and the heart temporarily stops ejecting blood, pressure in the arteries will fall, and this is called **diastolic pressure**. Blood pressure is measured in units of millimeters mercury, abbreviated as mm Hg. (Hg is the chemical symbol for the element mercury.) The average systolic pressure in a healthy adult is considered to be 120 mm Hg, whereas the average diastolic pressure is 80 mm Hg. The systolic and diastolic pressures are usually measured and reported together, with the systolic given first. For example, average blood pressure is said to be 120/80 mm Hg. Figure 14.2 illustrates how the pumping action of the heart determines systolic and diastolic blood pressure.

14.3 Three primary factors are responsible for blood pressure: cardiac output, the resistance of the small arteries, and blood volume.

While many factors can influence blood pressure, three factors are truly responsible for creating the pressure. The three primary factors—cardiac output, peripheral resistance, and blood volume—are shown in Figure 14.3.

FIGURE 14.3

Primary factors affecting blood pressure

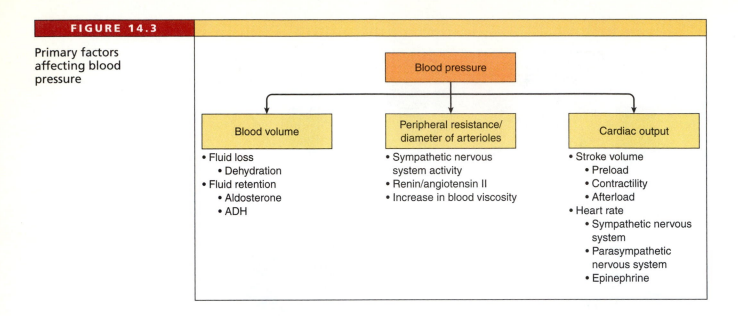

The volume of blood pumped per minute is called the **cardiac output**. While resting cardiac output is approximately five liters per minute (L/min), strenuous exercise can increase this output to as much as 35 L/min. The higher the cardiac output, the higher the blood pressure. Cardiac output is determined by heart rate and **stroke volume**, the amount of blood pumped by a ventricle in one contraction. This is important to pharmacology because drugs that change the cardiac output, stroke volume, or heart rate have the potential to influence a client's blood pressure.

As blood flows at high speeds through the vascular system, it bumps and drags across the walls of the vessels. Although the vessel walls, known as the endothelium, are extremely smooth, this friction reduces the velocity of the blood. This dragging or friction in the arteries is called **peripheral resistance**. Arteries have smooth muscle in their walls that, when constricted, will cause the inside diameter or **lumen** to become smaller, thus creating more resistance and higher pressure. This is how the body controls normal minute-by-minute changes in blood pressure. This is also important to pharmacology because a number of drugs affect this smooth muscle, causing vessels to constrict, thus raising blood pressure. Other drugs cause the smooth muscle to relax, thereby opening the lumen and lowering blood pressure. Some of these later drugs are among those used to treat hypertension. In Chapter 6, the role of the autonomic nervous system in controlling peripheral resistance was discussed ⊂⊃.

The third factor responsible for blood pressure is the total amount of blood in the vascular system, or **blood volume**. While the average person maintains a relatively constant blood volume of approximately five liters, this volume can change as a result of many regulatory factors and with

ON THE JOB

Paramedics and Maintaining Blood Pressure

At the scene of an automobile accident, paramedics are sometimes confronted by serious hemorrhaging in their clients. As blood pressure falls due to fluid loss, one of the treatments they may select is to start an IV of lactated Ringers solution. Lactated Ringers contains sodium chloride, potassium chloride, and calcium chloride in water. The concentration of electrolytes is similar to that in plasma and the solution is isotonic so that it does not cause fluid shifts between the intracellular and extracellular compartments.

Instead of lactated Ringers, paramedics may use other fluids to expand circulatory volume in order to restore fluid volume and blood pressure to normal. Normal saline is an isotonic solution of 0.9% sodium chloride and water that is sometimes preferred if the client is dehydrated. A third choice is 5% dextrose in water, known as D_5W. Unlike lactated Ringers or normal saline, D_5W is hypotonic and supplies calories for the client. Because the glucose moves rapidly into tissues with water quickly following, D_5W is less effective at expanding fluid volume. IV fluid therapy is discussed in Chapter 27. ■

certain disease states. More blood in the vascular system will exert additional pressure on the walls of the arteries and raise blood pressure. For example, high sodium diets cause water to be retained by the body, thus increasing blood volume and raising blood pressure. On the other hand, drugs called **diuretics** can cause fluid loss through urination, thus decreasing blood volume and lowering blood pressure. Diuretics are discussed later in this chapter and in Chapter 27 .

14.4 Many factors help to regulate blood pressure.

It is critical that the body maintains a normal range of blood pressure and that it has the ability to safely and rapidly change pressure as it proceeds through daily activities such as sleep and exercise. Too little blood pressure can cause dizziness and lack of urine formation, whereas too much pressure can cause vessels to rupture. A basic illustration of how the body maintains homeostasis during periods of blood pressure change is shown in Figure 14.4.

Blood pressure is regulated on a minute-to-minute basis by a cluster of neurons in the medulla oblongata called the **vasomotor center**. Nerves travel from the vasomotor center to the arteries, where the smooth muscle is directed to either constrict (raise blood pressure) or relax (lower blood pressure).

Clusters of neurons in the aorta and the internal carotid artery act as sensors to provide the vasomotor center with vital information on current conditions in the vascular system. Some of these neurons, called **baroreceptors**, have the ability to sense pressure within these large vessels. Others, called **chemoreceptors**, recognize levels of oxygen, carbon dioxide, and the acidity or pH in the blood. The vasomotor center reacts to information from baroreceptors and chemoreceptors by raising or lowering blood pressure accordingly.

baro = pressure
receptor = sensor

Emotions can also have a profound effect on blood pressure. Anger and stress can cause blood pressure to rise, whereas mental depression and lethargy may cause it to fall. Strong emotions, if present for a prolonged time period, may become important contributors to chronic hypertension.

A number of hormones and other agents affect blood pressure on a daily basis. When given as drugs, some of these agents may have a profound effect on blood pressure. For example, injection of epinephrine or norepinephrine will immediately raise blood pressure. **Antidiuretic hormone (ADH)** is a potent vasoconstrictor that can also increase blood pressure by raising blood volume. The **renin-angiotensin system** is particularly important in the drug therapy of hypertension

anti = against
diuretic = urination

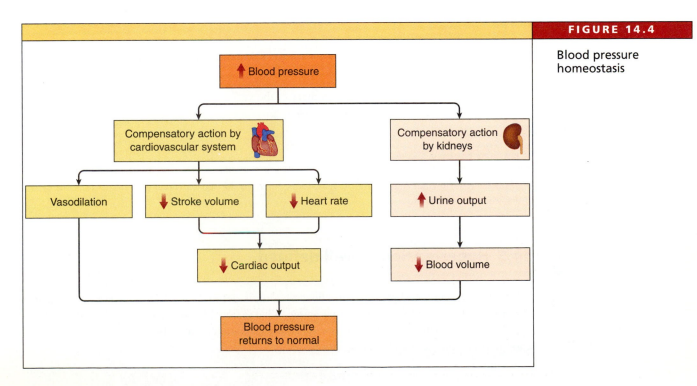

FIGURE 14.4

Blood pressure homeostasis

FIGURE 14.5

Hormonal and nervous factors influencing blood pressure

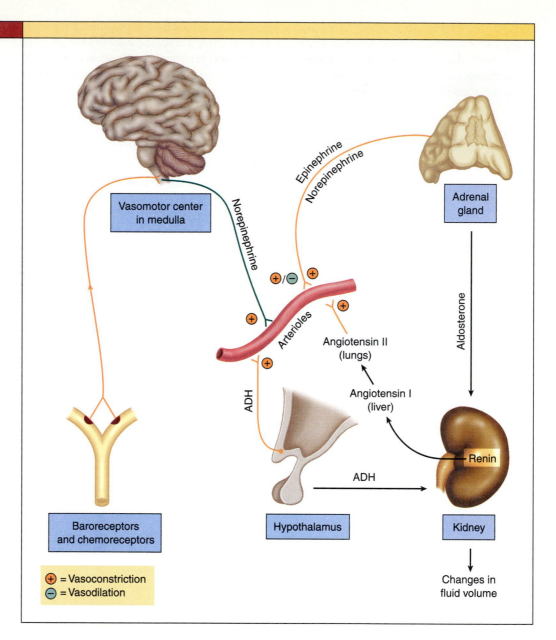

+ = Vasoconstriction
− = Vasodilation

and is discussed in Section 14.10. A summary of the various nervous and hormonal factors influencing blood pressure is shown in Figure 14.5.

Concept review 14.1

▪ Because hypertension may cause no symptoms, how would you convince a client to take his or her medication regularly?

14.5 Hypertension is well defined.

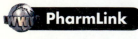

THE NATIONAL HEART, LUNG, AND BLOOD INSTITUTE

While the average blood pressure of a healthy adult is defined as 120/80 mm Hg, many factors affect blood pressure, including normal aging. What is considered normal blood pressure at one age may be considered abnormal in someone older or younger. Table 14.1 shows the normal variation in blood pressure that occurs throughout the life span.

TABLE 14.1	Variation in Blood Pressure Throughout the Lifespan	
AGE (YEARS)	**MALE**	**FEMALE**
1	96/66	95/65
5	92/62	92/62
10	103/69	103/70
20–24	123/76	116/72
30–34	126/79	120/75
40–44	129/81	127/80
50–54	135/83	137/84
60–64	142/85	144/85
70–74	145/82	159/85
80–84	145/82	157/83

The diagnosis of chronic hypertension is rarely made on a single blood pressure measurement. A client having a sustained blood pressure of 140/90 mm Hg after multiple measurements are made over several clinic visits is said to have hypertension. The disease is further subdivided according to the degree of pressure increase as shown in Table 14.2.

14.6 Non-pharmacologic therapy is often effective for minor hypertension.

When a client is first diagnosed with hypertension, the healthcare provider obtains a comprehensive medical history to determine if the disease can be controlled by non-pharmacologic means. Changing certain personal habits may eliminate the need for drug therapy altogether. Even if medications are needed to control the hypertension, it is important that the client continue these lifestyle changes so that dosages can be minimized, thus lowering the potential for drug side effects. Non-pharmacologic methods for controlling hypertension include the following.

- Clients 20% or more over normal body weight should implement a medically-supervised, safe weight-reduction plan.
- Stop using tobacco; smoking is a major contributor to hypertension.
- Watch mineral intake, limit salt (sodium) intake, and be sure to eat foods rich in potassium and magnesium.
- Limit alcohol consumption.
- Implement a medically-supervised aerobic exercise plan.
- Reduce sources of stress and learn to implement coping strategies.

TABLE 14.2	Definition of Hypertension
TYPE OF HYPERTENSION	**SYSTOLIC/DIASTOLIC BLOOD PRESSURE (MM HG)**
high normal	130–139/85–89
mild (Stage 1)	140–159/90–99
moderate (Stage 2)	160–179/100–109
severe (Stage 3)	180/110 or higher
crisis level (requires immediate intervention)	>210/>110

ANTIHYPERTENSIVES

14.7 Selection of specific antihypertension drugs depends upon the severity of the disease.

The goal of antihypertensive therapy is to reduce blood pressure to normal levels so that the long-term consequences of hypertension may be prevented. Keeping blood pressure within normal limits has been shown to reduce the risk of hypertension-related diseases such as stroke and heart failure. Several strategies are used to achieve this goal, and these are summarized in Figure 14.6.

Generally, pharmacologic therapy of hypertension begins with low doses of a single medication having few side effects, such as a diuretic. If this does not control blood pressure in two

---

FIGURE 14.6

Mechanism of action of antihypertensive drugs

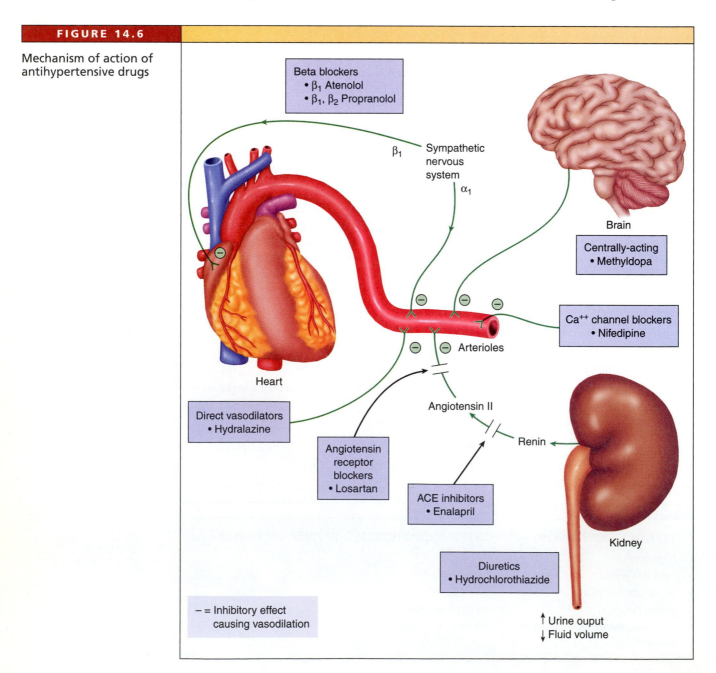

to four weeks, the healthcare practitioner may increase the dose of the initial drug or substitute another antihypertensive drug from a different drug class.

A common strategy used in controlling hypertension is **stepped care**. This involves using two drugs, from different classes, rather than one. The advantage of this approach is that it allows lower doses of each drug than would be needed if a single one were used. Lower doses usually produce fewer side effects and encourage better client compliance. Compliance decreases when clients need to take more than one drug or when they need to take them more often. In an effort to reduce non-compliance, drug manufacturers sometimes combine two drugs into a single pill or capsule. These combination drugs are quite common in the treatment of hypertension. One of the most widely used antihypertensive combinations is Dyazide, which contains two diuretics, hydrochlorothiazide (Hydrodiuril) and triamterene (Dyrenium). Another example is the drug Tarka that combines trandolapril (Mavik) and verapamil (Calan), two medications from different antihypertension classes.

The types of drugs used to treat chronic hypertension generally fall into five primary classes.

- diuretics
- calcium channel blockers
- angiotensin converting enzyme inhibitors
- autonomic nervous system agents
- direct-acting vasodilators

DIURETICS

Diuretics act by increasing the amount of urine production by the kidneys. They are widely used in the treatment of hypertension and heart failure.

14.8 Diuretics are effective at reducing mild to moderate hypertension.

Diuretics were the first class of drugs used to treat hypertension in the 1950s. Despite many advances in drug therapy since then, diuretics are still often considered first-line drugs for this disease because they produce few adverse effects and are very effective at controlling mild to moderate hypertension. For more advanced disease, they are frequently prescribed with other antihypertensive medications. Table 14.3 lists diuretics commonly used to treat hypertension. Diuretics are also used to treat heart failure (Chapter 15) and kidney disorders (Chapter 27 ⌕).

Many different diuretics are available for hypertension; however, all produce a similar result: the reduction of blood volume through the urinary excretion of water and electrolytes. **Electrolytes** are ions such as sodium (Na^+), calcium (Ca^{++}), chloride (Cl^-), and potassium (K^+). The mechanism by which diuretics reduce blood volume, specifically where and how the kidney is affected, differs among the various diuretics.

Whenever a drug changes urine composition or flow, electrolyte depletion is possible: the specific electrolyte lost is dependent upon the mechanism of action of the particular drug. Certain diuretics such as triamterene (Dyrenium) have less tendency to cause K^+ depletion, and for this reason are called *potassium-sparing diuretics*. Taking potassium supplements with potassium-sparing diuretics may lead to dangerously high potassium levels in the blood, or **hyperkalemia**, that can lead to cardiac conduction abnormalities.

hyper = high
hypo = low
ka = potassium
emia = blood

Concept review 14.2

- State the major reasons why a client should continue lifestyle changes even though their antihypertensive drug appears to be effective.

DRUG PROFILE:
Hydrochlorothiazide (Hydrodiuril)

Actions:

Hydrochlorothiazide is the most widely prescribed diuretic for hypertension, belonging to a class of about 12 drugs known as the thiazides. Like many diuretics, it produces few adverse effects and is quite effective at producing a 10–20 mm Hg reduction in blood pressure. Clients with severe hypertension, however, may require the addition of a second drug from a different class to control the disease. Hydrochlorothiazide acts on the kidney tubule to decrease the reabsorption of Na^+. Normally, over 99% of the sodium entering the kidney is reabsorbed by the body so that very little leaves via the urine. When hydrochlorothiazide blocks this reabsorption, more Na^+ is sent into the urine. Whenever sodium moves out, water flows with it, thus reducing blood volume and decreasing blood pressure. The volume of urine produced, or **diuresis,** is directly proportional to the amount of sodium reabsorption blocked by the diuretic.

Adverse Effects:

Hydrochlorothiazide has few serious adverse effects. The most common side effects involve potential electrolyte imbalances. In the case of hydrochlorothiazide, K^+ is lost along with the Na^+. Because potassium deficiency in the blood, or **hypokalemia,** may cause conduction abnormalities in the heart, clients are usually asked to increase their intake of dietary potassium as a precaution.

CALCIUM CHANNEL BLOCKERS

By blocking calcium ion channels, this class of drugs has a number of beneficial effects on the heart and blood vessels. They are widely used in the treatment of hypertension and other cardiovascular diseases.

14.9 Calcium channel blockers have emerged as major drugs in the treatment of hypertension.

Calcium channel blockers (CCBs) comprise a group of about 10 drugs that are used to treat a number of cardiovascular diseases, including angina pectoris, cardiac dysrhythmias, and hypertension. CCBs were first approved for the treatment of angina in the early 1980s, and it was quickly noted that a "side effect" of the drugs was the lowering of blood pressure in hypertensive clients. CCBs have since become one of the most widely prescribed classes of drugs for hypertension.

Contraction of muscle is regulated by the amount of calcium ion inside the muscle cell. When calcium enters the cell through channels in the plasma membrane, muscular contraction is initiated. CCBs block these channels and inhibit Ca^{++} from entering the cell, thus limiting muscular contraction. At low doses, CCBs cause the smooth muscle in arterioles to relax, thus lowering peripheral resistance and decreasing blood pressure. Some CCBs, such as nifedipine (Procardia), are selective for calcium channels in arterioles, while others, such as verapamil (Calan), affect channels in both arterioles and the myocardium. CCBs vary in their potency and by the frequency and types of side effects produced. The use of CCBs in the treatment of dysrhythmias and angina are discussed in Chapters 16 and 17, respectively ⊂▭⊃ . Table 14.4 lists CCBs commonly used to treat hypertension.

TABLE 14.3	Diuretics Used for Hypertension	
DRUG	**ROUTE AND ADULT DOSE**	**REMARKS**
furosemide (Lasix)	PO; 10–40 mg bid (max 480 mg/day).	Decreases blood potassium levels; acts by inhibiting sodium and chloride reabsorption in the loop of Henle; IV and IM forms available; loop diuretic.
Pr hydrochlorothiazide (Hydrodiuril, HCTZ)	PO; 12.5–100 mg in 1–2 divided doses (max 100 mg/day).	Acts by inhibiting sodium reabsorption in distal tubule; decreases blood potassium levels; thiazide-type.
spironolactone (Aldactone)	PO; 25–100 mg qd (max 200 mg/day).	Acts by inhibiting aldosterone in the distal tubule; postassium-sparing diuretic.
amiloride hydrochloride (Midamor)	PO; 5–20 mg in 1–2 divided doses (max 20 mg/day).	Potassium sparing; acts by directly inhibiting sodium-potassium exchange in the distal tubule.
chlorothiazide (Diuril)	PO/IV; 250 mg-1g in 1–2 divided doses (max 2 g/day).	Thiazide-type acts by inhibiting sodium reabsorption in distal tubule; decreases blood potassium levels.
chlorthalidone (Hygroton)	PO; 12.5–25 mg qd (max 100 mg/day).	Thiazide-type acts by inhibiting sodium reabsorption in distal tubule; decreases blood potassium levels.
indapamide (Lozol)	PO; 2.5 mg qd; may increase to 5mg qd if needed (max 5 mg/day).	Similar to thiazide-type, acts by inhibiting sodium reabsorption in distal tubule; decreases blood potassium levels.
torsemide (Demedex)	PO/IV; 5–10 mg qd (max 200 mg/day).	Sulfonamide loop diuretic; acts by inhibiting sodium and chloride reabsorption in the loop of Henle and distal tubule.
triamterene (Dyrenium)	PO; 100 mg bid (max 300 mg/day).	Potassium sparing; acts by directly inhibiting sodium-potassium exchange in the distal tubule.

ANGIOTENSION CONVERTING ENZYME (ACE) INHIBITORS

Drugs that affect the renin-angiotensin pathway decrease blood pressure and increase urine volume. They are widely used in the treatment of hypertension, heart failure, and myocardial infarction.

14.10 Blocking the renin-angiotensin pathway leads to a decrease in blood pressure.

The renin-angiotensin pathway is one of the primary homeostatic mechanisms controlling blood pressure and fluid balance in the body. Renin is an enzyme secreted by the kidneys when blood pressure falls or when there is a decrease in Na^+ flowing through the kidney tubules. In a series of enzymatic steps, angiotensin II, one of the most potent natural vasoconstrictors known, is formed. The enzyme responsible for the final step of this pathway is called angiotensin-converting enzyme (ACE). The intense vasoconstriction of arterioles caused by angiotensin II raises blood pressure by increasing peripheral resistance.

angio = vessels
tensin = pressure

A second, equally important effect of angiotensin II is its stimulation of the secretion of aldosterone, a hormone from the adrenal gland that increases sodium reabsorption in the kidney.

DRUG PROFILE:
Nifedipine (Procardia)

Actions:

Nifedipine is a CCB prescribed for angina as well as for hypertension. Nifedipine selectively blocks calcium channels in myocardial and vascular smooth muscle, including that in the coronary arteries. This results in less oxygen utilization by the heart, an increase in cardiac output, and a fall in blood pressure. Nifedipine is as effective as diuretics and beta-adrenergic blockers at reducing hypertension.

Adverse Effects:

Side effects of nifedipine are generally minor and related to vasodilation such as headache, dizziness, and flushing. Fast-acting forms of nifedipine can cause reflex tachycardia, a condition that occurs when the heart rate increases due to the rapid fall in blood pressure created by the drug. To avoid rebound hypotension, discontinuation of drug therapy should occur gradually.

Mechanism in Action:

Nifedipine is used to treat several cardiovascular disorders including angina pectoris, cardiac dysrythmias, and hypertension. Blocking calcium influx into smooth muscle cells results in arteriolar vasodilation. When arterioles are dilated, peripheral resistance and cardiac workload are reduced, and the blood pressure returns to normal.

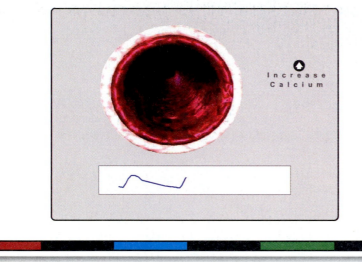

Increase Calcium

This increase in sodium reabsorption helps the body retain water, which raises blood volume and increases blood pressure. Drugs that inhibit ACE block the effects of angiotensin II, thus decreasing blood pressure through two mechanisms: lowering peripheral resistance and decreasing blood volume.

First detected in the venom of pit vipers in the 1960s, inhibitors of ACE have been approved as drugs for hypertension since the 1980s. Since then, the ACE inhibitors have become impor-

NATURAL ALTERNATIVES

Hawthorn for Hypertension

A number of botanicals have been claimed to have antihypertensive activity, including hawthorn, which is sometimes called *May bush.* Hawthorn (*Cretaegus*) is a thorny shrub or small tree that is widespread in North America, Europe, and Asia. Use of hawthorn dates back to ancient Greece. In some cultures, the shrub is used in magic and religious rites and is thought to ward off evil spirits. The ship *Mayflower* was named after this shrub.

Leaves, flowers, and berries of the plant are dried or extracted in liquid form. Active ingredients are flavonoids and procyanidins. Hawthorn has been purported to lower blood pressure after four weeks or longer of therapy, although the effect has been small. The mechanism of action may be inhibition of ACE or reduction of cardiac workload. Clients taking cardiac glycosides should avoid hawthorn, as it has the ability to decrease cardiac output. Clients should be advised not to rely upon any botanical for the treatment of hypertension without consulting with their healthcare practitioner, and frequent measurements of blood pressure must be taken to be certain that therapy is effective. ■

TABLE 14.4	Calcium Channel Blockers Used for Hypertension	
DRUG	**ROUTE AND ADULT DOSE**	**REMARKS**
Pr nifedipine (Procardia, Aldalat)	PO; 10–20 mg tid (max 180 mg/day).	Selective for calcium channels in blood vessels; decreases peripheral vascular resistance and increases cardiac output; also for angina; sustained release form available.
amlodipine (Norvasc)	PO; 5–10 mg qd (max 10 mg/day).	Works primarily on peripheral circulation; reduces systolic, diastolic, and mean blood pressure; also for angina.
diltiazem (Cardizem)	PO; 80–120 mg tid (max 360 mg/day).	Dilates coronary arteries; affects calcium channels in both heart and blood vessels; sustained release and IV forms available; also for angina and specific dysrhythmias.
felodipine (Plendil)	PO; 5–10 mg/day (max 20 mg/day).	Selective for calcium channels in blood vessels; also for angina and heart failure.
isradipine (DynaCirc)	PO; 1.25–10 mg bid (max 20 mg/day).	Affects calcium channels in both heart and blood vessels; also for angina.
nicardipine hydrochloride (Cardene)	PO; 20–40 mg tid (max 120 mg/day).	Selective for calcium channels in blood vessels; also for angina; sustained release and IV forms available.
nisoldipine (Nisocor, Solar)	PO; 10–20 mg bid (max 40 mg/day).	Structurally similar to nifedipine. Affects calcium channels in both the heart and blood vessels. Also for angina and heart failure.
verapamil hydrochloride (Calan, Isotopin, Verelan)	PO; 40–80 mg tid (max 360 mg/day).	Affects calcium channels in both heart and blood vessels; sustained release form available; IV form available for specific dysrhythmias.

tant drugs in the treatment of hypertension. Side effects are relatively minor and include persistent cough, and hypotension following the first dose of the drug. Some ACE inhibitors have also been approved for the treatment of heart failure and myocardial infarction, and these are discussed in Chapters 15 and 17, respectively ⊂▣⊃ . Table 14.5 lists ACE inhibitors commonly used to treat hypertension.

A second method of altering the renin-angiotensin pathway is by blocking the action of angiotensin II after it is formed. Several drugs, including irbesartan (Avapro), losartan (Cozaar), and valsartan (Diovan), block the receptors for angiotensin in arteriolar smooth muscle and in the adrenal gland, thus causing blood pressure to fall. Their actions of arteriolar dilation and increased renal sodium excretion are quite similar to those of the ACE inhibitors. Angiotensin receptor blockers have relatively few side effects, most of which are related to hypotension. Drugs in this class are often combined with drugs from other classes; for example, the drug Hyzaar combines losartan with the diuretic hydrochlorothiazide.

tachy = *rapid*
cardia = *heart*

ADRENERGIC-BLOCKERS

Blockade of adrenergic receptors results in a number of beneficial effects on the heart and vessels. These autonomic drugs are used for a wide variety of cardiovascular disorders.

DRUG PROFILE:
Enalapril (Vasotec)

Actions:

Enalapril is one of the most common ACE inhibitors prescribed for hypertension. Unlike captopril (Capoten), the first ACE inhibitor to be marketed, enalapril has a prolonged half-life, which permits administration once or twice daily. Enalapril acts by reducing angiotensin II and aldosterone levels to produce a significant reduction in blood pressure with few side effects. Enalapril has an efficacy comparable to the thiazide diuretics and the beta-adrenergic blockers and may be used by itself or in combination with other antihypertensives to minimize side effects.

Adverse Effects:

Unlike diuretics, ACE inhibitors such as enalapril have little effect on electrolyte balance, and unlike beta-adrenergic blockers, they cause few cardiac side effects. Like other antihypertensive drugs, enalapril may cause hypotension, especially when moving quickly from a supine to an upright position. This condition, known as postural or orthostatic hypotension, can cause light-headedness and even fainting. Care must be taken because a rapid fall in blood pressure may occur following the first dose. Other side effects include headache, dizziness, and postural hypotension.

TABLE 14.5 **ACE Inhibitors and Angiotensin Receptor Blockers Used for Hypertension**

DRUG	ROUTE AND ADULT DOSE	REMARKS
ACE Inhibitors		
captopril (Capoten)	PO; 6.25–25 mg tid (max 450 mg/day).	Also for heart failure and MI.
benazepril hydrochloride (Lotensin)	PO; 10–40 mg in 1–2 divided doses (max 40 mg/day).	May be used in combination with thiazide diuretics.
Pr enalapril maleate (Vasotec) enalaprilat (Vasotec IV)	PO; 5–40 mg in 1–2 divided doses (max 40 mg/day).	Also for heart failure; IV form available.
fosinopril (Monopril)	PO; 5–40 mg qd (max 80 mg/day).	Also for heart failure.
lisinopril (Prinivil, Zestril)	PO; 10 mg qd (max 80 mg/day).	Also for heart failure and MI.
moexipril hydrochloride (Univasc)	PO; 7.5–30 mg qd (max 30 mg/day).	Only approved for hypertension.
quinapril hydrochloride (Accupril)	PO; 10–20 mg qd (max 80 mg/day).	Also for heart failure.
ramipril (Altace)	PO; 2.5–5 mg qd (max 20 mg/day).	Also for heart failure.
trandolapril (Mavik)	PO; 1–4 mg qd (max 8 mg/day).	Only approved for hypertension; discontinue diuretics 2–3 days before starting therapy.
Angiotensin Receptor Blockers		
losartan potassium (Cozaar)	PO; 25–50 mg in 1–2 divided doses (max 100 mg/day).	Causes relaxation of smooth vascular muscle.
omesartan (Benicar)	PO; 20 mg qd (max 40 mg/day).	Approved in 2002.
irbesartan (Avapro)	PO; 150–300 mg qd (max 300 mg/day).	Maximum effect may take 6–12 weeks.
valsartan (Diovan)	PO; 80 mg qd (max 320 mg/day).	Evidence of effectiveness of therapy in 2–4 weeks.

14.11 Organs innervated by the autonomic nervous system are a frequent target for antihypertensive drugs.

As discussed in Chapter 6, the autonomic nervous system controls involuntary functions of the body such as heart rate, pupil size, and smooth muscle contraction, including that in the arterial walls ▭▭ . Stimulation of the sympathetic division causes fight-or-flight responses such as faster heart rate, an increase in blood pressure, and bronchodilation. Most organs also receive nerve signals from the parasympathetic division, which affects rest-and-digest actions that are generally the opposite of the sympathetic division. An important exception is the peripheral blood vessels that receive only sympathetic nerves.

Antihypertensive drugs have been developed that block the effects of the sympathetic division through a number of different mechanisms, although all have in common the effect of lowering blood pressure. These mechanisms include the following.

- blockade of alpha-receptors
- selective blockade of $beta_1$ receptors
- non-selective blockade of $beta_1$ and $beta_2$ receptors
- stimulation of $alpha_2$-receptors in the brainstem (centrally-acting)

Some drugs, such as epinephrine, affect all types of beta and alpha-adrenergic receptors and cause more side effects than those that are selective for only one type. Because of the reduced potential for side effects, drug developers have created medications specific to only one type of receptor. Prazosin (Minipress), for example, is specific to **alpha$_1$-receptors** and thus should have less effect on the heart, which contains **beta$_1$ receptors**. On the other hand, atenolol (Tenormin) and metoprolol (Toprol, Lopressor) are selective for $beta_1$ receptors and thus have little effect on the bronchi, which have **beta$_2$ receptors**.

The side effects of adrenergic-blockers are generally quite predictable, as they are extensions of the fight-or-flight response. The alpha$_1$-blockers tend to cause **orthostatic hypotension** when moving quickly from a supine to an upright position. Dizziness, nausea, **bradycardia**, and dry mouth are also common. Less common, though sometimes a major cause for non-compliance, is their adverse effect on male sexual function (impotence). Non-selective beta-blockers will slow the heart rate and cause bronchoconstriction: they should be used with caution in clients with asthma or heart failure.

ortho = straight
static = causing to stand
brady = slow
cardia = heart

Some adrenergic-blockers do not act directly on organs stimulated by peripheral autonomic nerves, but instead affect the production of neurotransmitters in the central nervous system. For example, methyldopa (Aldomet) is converted to a **false neurotransmitter** in the brainstem, thus causing a shortage of the "real" neurotransmitter and inhibition of the sympathetic nervous system. Clonidine (Catapres), an alpha$_2$-agonist, affects alpha-adrenergic receptors in the cardiovascular control centers in the brainstem. The centrally acting agents have a tendency to produce sedation. Adrenergic-blockers and centrally acting agents are listed in Table 14.6.

Concept review 14.3

- Why is it important for the client to weigh himself or herself on a regular basis when taking antihypertensive drugs?

hyper = high
plasia = growth

DIRECT-ACTING VASODILATORS

Drugs that direct affect arteriolar smooth muscle are very effective at lowering blood pressure but produce too many side effects to be drugs of first choice.

14.12 Some drugs act directly on arteriolar smooth muscle to lower blood pressure.

All the drugs discussed thus far lower blood pressure through indirect means: by affecting enzymes (ACE inhibitors), organs innervated by autonomic nerves (alpha and beta-blockers), or fluid volume (diuretics). It would seem that a more efficient way to reduce blood pressure would be to cause a

DRUG PROFILE (Adrenergic-Blocker):

Doxazosin (Cardura)

Actions:

Doxazosin is a selective alpha$_1$-adrenergic blocker available only in oral form. Because it is selective for blocking alpha$_1$-receptors in vascular smooth muscle, it has few adverse effects on other autonomic organs and thus is preferred over non-selective beta-blockers such as propranolol (Inderal). Doxazosin dilates both arteries and veins and is capable of causing a rapid, profound fall in blood pressure. Although prazosin (Minipress) was the first alpha-adrenergic blocker available for hypertension, other alpha-blockers such as doxazosin and terazosin (Hytrin) are more widely used because they have prolonged half-lives that allow them to be taken once daily.

Doxazosin and several other alpha-adrenergic blockers also relax smooth muscle around the prostate gland. Clients who have difficulty urinating due to an enlarged prostate, a condition known as benign prostatic hyperplasia (BPH) sometimes receive these drugs to relieve symptoms of this disease, as discussed in Chapter 29 ⊂▭⊃ .

Adverse Effects:

Upon starting doxazosin therapy, some clients experience orthostatic hypotension, although tolerance normally develops to this side effect after a few doses. Dizziness and headache are also common side effects, although they are rarely severe enough to cause discontinuation of therapy.

Mechanism in Action:

Doxazosin selectively blocks alpha$_1$-adrenergic receptors reversing any physiological effects brought on by increased smooth muscle tone. By dilating vascular smooth muscle alpha$_1$ antagonists reverse any frictional resistance to lower blood pressure. Alpha$_1$ blockers relax smooth muscle around the prostate gland allowing easier urination for clients with benign prostatic hypertrophy (BPH).

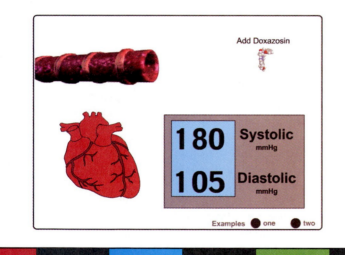

Add Doxazosin

180	Systolic
	mmHg
105	Diastolic
	mmHg

Examples ● one ● two

DRUG PROFILE (Direct-Acting Vasodilator):

Hydralazine (Apresoline)

Actions:

Hydralazine was one of the first oral antihypertensive drugs marketed in the United States. Although it produces an effective reduction in blood pressure, drugs in other antihypertensive classes have largely replaced hydralazine due to its many side effects.

Adverse Effects:

Hydralazine may produce many side effects, including severe reflex tachycardia. Clients taking hydralazine often receive a beta-adrenergic blocker that counteracts this effect on the heart. The drug may produce a lupus-like syndrome with extended use. Sodium and fluid retention is another potentially serious adverse effect. The use of hydralazine is mostly limited to clients whose hypertension cannot be controlled with other, safer medications.

TABLE 14.6	Adrenergic-Blockers and Central-Acting Agents Used for Hypertension	
DRUG	**ROUTE AND ADULT DOSE**	**REMARKS**
prazosin hydrochloride (Minipress)	PO; 1 mg hs; increase to 1 mg bid – tid (max 20 mg/day).	Used in combination with other antihypertensives; also for benign prostatic hypertrophy, Raynauds disease, and pheochromocytoma; alpha$_1$ blocker.
propranolol hydrochloride (Inderal)	PO; 40 mg bid but may be increased to 160–480 mg/day in divided doses (max 480/day).	Also for angina, MI, dysrhythmias, and migraine prophylaxis; IV form available; beta$_1$ and beta$_2$-blocker.
atenolol (Tenormin)	PO; 25–50 mg qd (max 100 mg/day).	Selective beta$_1$-blocker; IV form available for MI. Monitor apical pulse prior to administration.
bisoprolol fumarate (Zebeta)	PO; 2.5–5 mg qd (max 20 mg/day).	Selective beta$_1$-blocker; also for angina; discontinue drug gradually to avoid rebound hypertension.
clonidine hydrochloride (Catapres)	PO; 0.1 mg bid – tid (max 0.8 mg/day).	Central acting alpha$_2$-adrenergic agonist; transdermal patch available; epidural infusion form available for management of cancer pain.
(Pr) doxazosin mesylate (Cardura)	PO; 1 mg at hs; may increase to 16 mg/day in 1–2 divided doses (max 16 mg/day).	Alpha$_1$-blocker; also for benign prostatic hypertrophy.
methyldopa (Aldomet)	PO; 250 mg bid or tid (max 3 g/day).	Central acting alpha$_2$-adrenergic agonist; IV form available; lowers standing and supine blood pressure.
metoprolol tartrate (Toprol, Lopressor)	PO; 50–100 mg qd-bid. (max 450 mg/day)	Selective beta$_1$-blocker; sustained release and IV forms available; also for angina and MI.
terazosin (Hytrin)	PO; 1 mg at hs; increase 1–5 mg/day (max 20 mg/day).	Selective alpha$_1$-blocker; also for benign prostatic hypertrophy.

direct relaxation of arteriolar smooth muscle. Unfortunately, most drugs in this class of direct vasodilators produce reflex tachycardia that may be a serious concern for hypertensive clients.

One direct-acting vasodilator is specifically used for those clients who have an extremely high, life-threatening hypertension that must be quickly controlled. Nitroprusside (Nipride, Nitropress), with a half-life of only two minutes, has the capability of lowering blood pressure almost instantaneously upon IV administration. Careful monitoring is critical in order to avoid serious effects of over treatment, such as hypotension. The direct-acting vasodilators are listed in Table 14.7.

TABLE 14.7	Direct Acting Vasodilators Used for Hypertension	
DRUG	**ROUTE AND ADULT DOSE**	**REMARKS**
(Pr) hydralazine hydrochloride (Apresoline)	PO; 10–50 mg qid (max 300 mg/day).	Diastolic response usually greater than systolic; IV and IM forms available.
diazoxide (Hyperstat IV)	IV; 1–3 mg/kg by IV push (max 150 mg).	Dose may be repeated every 15 minutes until blood pressure falls; may be given as infusion or by push for malignant hypertension.
minoxidil (Loniten)	PO; 5–40 mg/day in a single or divided doses (max 100 mg/day).	Reserved for clients with severe hypertension; topical form used to promote hair growth.
nitroprusside sodium (Nipride, Nitropress)	IV; 0.5–10 μg/kg/min.	For hypertensive crisis; produces both arteriolar and venous dilation; infusion not to exceed 10 minutes.

CLIENT TEACHING

Clients treated for hypertension need to know the following:

1. Take your medication as prescribed, even if you feel well.
2. Never discontinue your medication without your healthcare provider's approval.
3. Try to incorporate lifestyle changes to control your hypertension, even if the medication brings your blood pressure to within normal limits.
4. Check your blood pressure on a regular basis and report any significant variations.
5. Get out of bed slowly to avoid dizziness.
6. Unless a potassium-sparing diuretic is prescribed, increase your intake of potassium-rich foods such as bananas, dried fruits, and orange juice.
7. Weigh yourself regularly and report abnormal weight gains or losses.
8. Do not take any OTC medications for colds, flu, or allergies without first checking with your healthcare provider. ■

CHAPTER REVIEW

 Core Concepts Summary

14.1   Hypertension is a major cause of death and disability.

High blood pressure is one of the most common diseases. Uncontrolled hypertension can cause chronic and debilitating disorders such as stroke, heart attack, and heart failure.

14.2   Blood pressure is caused by the pumping action of the heart.

As the heart pumps, it creates pressure that is greatest in the arteries closest to the heart. The pressure created by the heart's contraction is called systolic pressure, and that present during the heart's relaxation is called diastolic pressure.

14.3   Three primary factors are responsible for blood pressure: cardiac output, the resistance of the small arteries, and blood volume.

As blood leaves the heart, its pressure depends upon how much blood is present in the vessels (blood volume), how much is ejected per contraction (stroke volume), and how much resistance it encounters from the small arteries (peripheral resistance).

14.4   Many factors help to regulate blood pressure.

Clusters of neurons in the medulla known as the vasomotor center regulate blood pressure. Feedback is provided to the vasomotor center by baroreceptors and chemoreceptors in the aorta and internal carotid arteries. Agents such as epinephrine or ADH may have profound effects on blood pressure.

14.5   Hypertension is well defined.

A client having a sustained blood pressure of 140/90 mm Hg after multiple measurements made over several clinic visits is said to have hypertension.

14.6   Non-pharmacologic therapy is often effective for minor hypertension.

Because antihypertensive drugs may have uncomfortable side effects, lifestyle changes such as proper diet and exercise are often implemented prior to and during drug therapy to enable lower drug doses.

14.7 **Selection of specific antihypertension drugs depends upon the severity of the disease.**

Drug therapy of hypertension often begins with low doses of a single drug. If ineffective, a second drug from a different class may be added to the regimen. Multi-drug therapy is common.

14.8 **Diuretics are effective at reducing mild to moderate hypertension.**

Diuretics are often the first-line drugs for hypertension because they have few side effects and can control minor to moderate hypertension. Electrolytes should be carefully monitored in clients taking diuretics.

14.9 **Calcium channel blockers have emerged as major drugs in the treatment of hypertension.**

CCBs block calcium ions from entering cells and cause the smooth muscle in arterioles to relax, thus reducing blood pressure. Some CCBs may also be used to treat angina, heart failure, and dysrhythmias.

14.10 **Blocking the renin-angiotensin pathway leads to a decrease in blood pressure.**

Some antihypertensive agents block angiotensin-coverting enzyme (ACE), thus preventing the intense vasoconstriction caused by angiotensin. These drugs also decrease blood volume, which aids in producing their antihypertensive effect.

14.11 **Organs innervated by the autonomic nervous system are a frequent target for antihypertensive drugs.**

Antihypertensive autonomic drugs are available that block alpha$_1$-receptors, block beta$_1$ and/or beta$_2$ receptors, or stimulate alpha$_2$-receptors in the brainstem (centrally-acting). Although acting by different mechanisms, these drugs all lower blood pressure.

14.12 **Some drugs act directly on arteriolar smooth muscle to lower blood pressure.**

A few drugs lower blood pressure by acting directly to relax arteriolar smooth muscle, but these are not widely used because of their numerous side effects.

EXPLORE PharMedia
www.prenhall.com/holland

Additional interactive resources and activities for this chapter can be found on the Companion Website. For animations, audio glossary, and review access the accompanying CD-ROM in this book.

Mechanism in Action:
  Nifedipine
  Doxazofin
Audio Glossary
NCLEX Review
Concept Review

PharmLinks
  The American Society of Hypertension
  The National Heart, Lung, and Blood Institute
  Dietary Modifications for the Hypertensive Client
  Herbal Therapies for Hypertension

15 Drugs for Heart Failure

CORE CONCEPTS

15.1 Several disorders are associated with heart failure.

15.2 The central cause of heart failure is weakened heart muscle.

15.3 The three primary characteristics of heart function are force of contraction, heart rate, and speed of impulse conduction.

15.4 Non-pharmacologic therapy of early heart failure is sometimes effective.

Cardiac Glycosides

15.5 Cardiac glycosides increase the force of myocardial contraction and are the traditional drugs of choice for heart failure.

Angiotension Converting Enzyme Inhibitors

15.6 Angiotensin-converting enzyme (ACE) inhibitors are becoming first-line drugs for heart failure.

Vasodilators

15.7 Vasodilators can help reduce symptoms of heart failure by decreasing the oxygen demand on the heart.

Diuretics

15.8 Diuretics are effective at reducing fluid volume and relieving symptoms of heart failure.

Phosphodiesterase Inhibitors

15.9 Phosphodiesterase inhibitors increase the force of contraction and cause vasodilation.

Beta-Adrenergic Blockers

15.10 Beta-adrenergic blockers play a minor role in the treatment of heart failure.

OBJECTIVES

After reading this chapter, the student should be able to:

1. Identify the major risk factors associated with heart failure.

2. Relate how the classic symptoms associated with heart failure may be caused by weakened heart muscle.

3. Explain how preload and afterload affect cardiac function.

4. Define the terms inotropic, chronotropic, and dromotropic.

5. Explain several means by which clients may control their heart failure without drugs.

6. For each of the following classes, identify representative medications and explain the mechanism of drug action, primary actions, and important adverse effects.
   a. cardiac glycosides
   b. ACE inhibitors
   c. vasodilators
   d. diuretics
   e. phosphodiesterase inhibitors
   f. beta-adrenergic blockers

7. Categorize heart failure drugs based on their classification and mechanism of action.

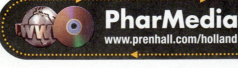

PharMedia
www.prenhall.com/holland

Additional interactive resources and activities for this chapter can be found on the Companion Website. For animations, audio glossary, and review access the accompanying CD-ROM in this book.

Heart failure (HF) is one of the most common and fatal of the cardiovascular diseases, and its incidence is expected to increase as the population ages. Despite the dramatic decline in death rates for most cardiovascular diseases that has occurred over the past two decades, the death rate for HF has only recently begun to decrease. Although improved treatment of myocardial infarction and hypertension has led to declines in mortality due to heart failure, approximately one in five clients still die within a year of diagnosis of HF and 50% die within five years. The incidence of sudden death is as much as nine times higher in HF clients than in the general population.

Fast Facts Heart Failure

- Heart failure increases with age. It affects:
  - 2% of those 40–50 years old
  - 5% of those 60–69 years old
  - 10% of those over age 70
- Over 40,000 people die of HF each year.
- Heart failure is responsible for over 2.9 million office care visits and 875,000 hospitalizations.
- Heart failure was the most common first-listed diagnosis in hospital clients aged 65 or older.
- Blacks have 1.5 to 2 times the incidence of HF as whites.
- Heart failure occurs slightly more frequently in men than women.
- Heart failure is twice as frequent in hypertensive clients and five times as frequent in persons who have experienced a heart attack.

15.1 Several disorders are associated with heart failure.

Heart failure is the inability of the ventricles to pump enough blood to meet the body's metabolic demands. It is not usually considered a distinct disease in itself, but is instead caused or worsened by certain underlying disorders. Indeed, while weakening of cardiac muscle is a natural consequence of aging, the process can be accelerated by a number of diseases associated with heart failure that are shown in Table 15.1. Because there is no cure for HF, the treatment goals are to prevent, treat, or remove the underlying causes, whenever possible, so that the client's quality of life can be improved and life expectancy extended. Effective drug therapy can relieve many of the distressing symptoms of heart failure and may prolong clients' lives.

TABLE 15.1	Types of Disorders Commonly Associated with Heart Failure
DISEASE	**DESCRIPTION**
mitral stenosis	inability of the mitral valve to open fully
myocardial infarction	clot within the coronary arteries
chronic hypertension	high systemic blood pressure
coronary artery disease	atherosclerosis of the coronary arteries
diabetes	lack of insulin or inability to tolerate carbohydrates

15.2 The central cause of heart failure is weakened heart muscle.

Although a number of diseases can lead to heart failure, the end result is the same: the heart is unable to pump out the volume of blood required to meet the body's metabolic needs. In order to understand how drugs act on the weakened heart muscle, it is essential to understand the underlying cardiac physiology.

The right side of the heart receives blood from the venous system and sends it to the lungs, where the blood receives oxygen and loses its carbon dioxide. The blood returns to the left side of the heart, which sends it out to the rest of the body through the aorta. The amount of blood received by the right side should exactly equal that sent out by the left side. If this does not happen, HF may occur. The amount of blood pumped by each ventricle per minute is the cardiac output. The relationship between cardiac output and blood pressure was explained in Chapter 14 ⬤⬤.

Although many variables affect cardiac output, the two most important factors are **preload** and **afterload**. Just before the chambers of the heart contract (systole), they are filled to their maximum capacity with blood. The degree to which the heart fibers are stretched just prior to contraction is preload. The more these fibers are stretched, the more forcefully they will contract—a principle called the **Frank-Starling law**. This is somewhat analogous to a rubber band: the more it is stretched, the more forcefully it will snap back. This strength of contraction of the heart is called **contractility**.

The second important factor affecting cardiac output is afterload. In order for the left ventricle to pump blood out of the heart, it must overcome a fairly substantial pressure in the aorta. The afterload is the pressure in the aorta that must be overcome for blood to be ejected from the left side of the heart.

In HF, the myocardium becomes weakened and the heart cannot eject all the blood it receives. This weakening may occur on the left side, the right side, or both sides of the heart. If it occurs on the left side, excess blood accumulates in the left ventricle. The wall of the left ventricle may become thicker (hypertrophy) in an attempt to compensate for the extra blood. Because the left ventricle has limits to its ability to compensate, blood "backs up" into the lungs, resulting in the classic symptoms of cough and shortness of breath, particularly when the client is lying down. Left heart failure is sometimes called *congestive heart failure*.

Although left heart failure is more common, the right side of the heart can also become weak, either simultaneously with the left side or independently from the left side. In right heart failure, the blood "backs up" into the peripheral veins. This results in swelling of the feet and ankles, a condition known as **peripheral edema**, and engorgement of organs such as the liver. Figure 15.1 illustrates the underlying pathophysiology of HF. Figure 15.2 illustrates the signs and symptoms of the client in HF.

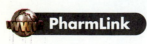

THE BEATING HEART

FIGURE 15.1

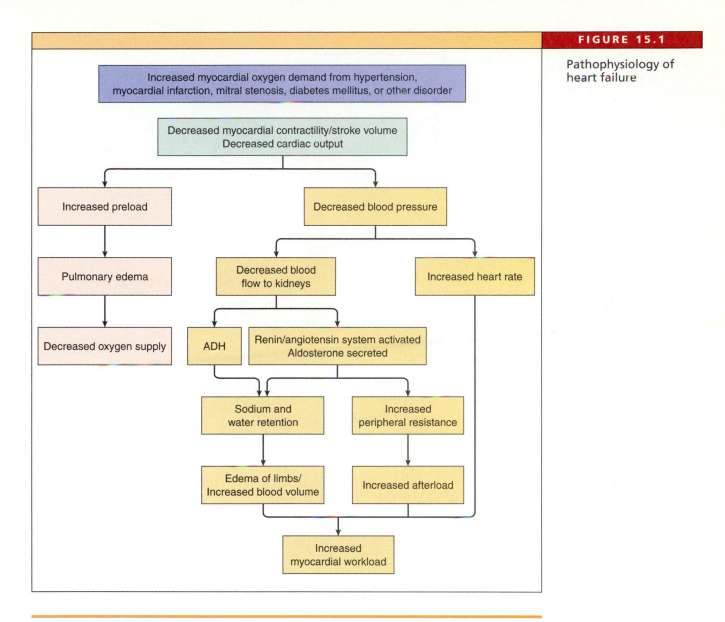

15.3 The three primary characteristics of heart function are force of contraction, heart rate, and speed of impulse conduction.

Cardiac physiology is quite complex, particularly when the heart is faced with a chronic disease such as heart failure. A simplified method for understanding cardiac function, and one that is quite useful for drug therapy, is to visualize the heart as having three fundamental characteristics.

- It contracts with a specific force or strength (contractility).
- It beats at a certain rate (beats per minute).
- It conducts electrical impulses at a particular speed.

The ability to affect the force of contraction is of particular interest to the pharmacotherapy of HF. Because the fundamental cause of heart failure is a weak myocardium, causing the muscle to

FIGURE 15.2

Signs and symptoms of the client with heart failure

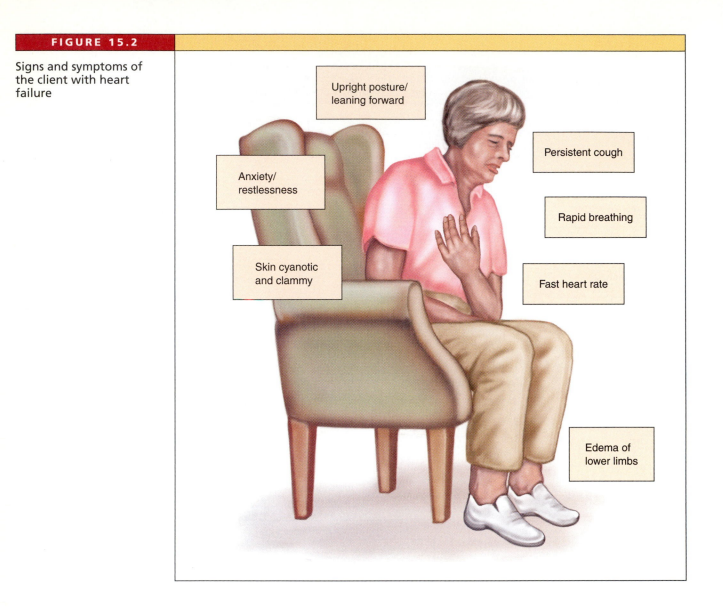

Upright posture/leaning forward

Persistent cough

Anxiety/restlessness

Rapid breathing

Skin cyanotic and clammy

Fast heart rate

Edema of lower limbs

beat more forcefully seems to be an ideal solution. The ability to increase the strength of contraction is called a positive **inotropic effect** and is a fundamental characteristic of the class of drugs known as the *cardiac glycosides*.

ino = fiber
tropic = to influence

The ability of the heart to speed up or slow down is a second characteristic important to pharmacology. A faster heart works harder, but not necessarily more efficiently. A slower heart has a longer time to rest between beats, known as the **refractory period**. The ability of a drug to change the heart rate is called a **chronotropic effect**.

chrono = time

A third fundamental characteristic of cardiac physiology is the electrical conduction through the heart. Some cardiovascular drugs influence the speed of this conduction, known as a **dromotropic effect**. These drugs are covered in Chapter 16 ▭.

dromo = running

These primary characteristics of cardiac function can be modified through pharmacothorapy to assist the heart in meeting the body's metabolic demands. The mechanisms by which heart failure medications accomplish this are shown in Figure 15.3.

15.4 Non-pharmacologic therapy of early heart failure is sometimes effective.

Although heart failure can be acute and require immediate treatment, it is often considered a progressive, chronic disorder. In its early stages, many of its symptoms can be alleviated through

FIGURE 15.3

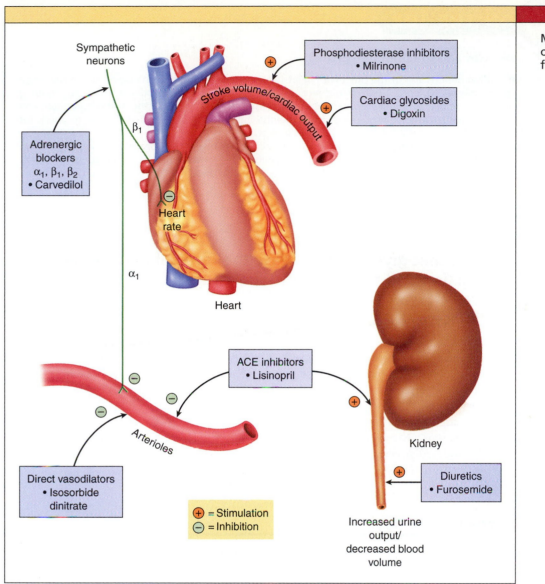

Mechanisms of action of drugs used for heart failure

Sympathetic neurons

Phosphodiesterase inhibitors
• Milrinone

Cardiac glycosides
• Digoxin

Stroke volume/cardiac output

β_1

Adrenergic blockers
$\alpha_1, \beta_1, \beta_2$
• Carvedilol

Heart rate

α_1

Heart

ACE inhibitors
• Lisinopril

Kidney

Arterioles

Direct vasodilators
• Isosorbide dinitrate

⊕ = Stimulation
⊖ = Inhibition

Diuretics
• Furosemide

Increased urine output/ decreased blood volume

non-pharmacological intervention. Through certain lifestyle changes, the client can experience a higher quality of life either without drug therapy, or with lower drug doses that have less risk for adverse effects. Signs and symptoms of HF are shown in Figure 15.3. Following are some non-pharmacological methods for controlling heart failure.

- stop using tobacco
- limit salt (sodium) intake and be sure to eat foods rich in potassium and magnesium
- limit alcohol consumption
- implement a medically-supervised exercise plan
- learn and use effective ways to deal with stress
- reduce weight to an optimum level
- limit caffeine consumption

CARDIAC GLYCOSIDES

The value of the cardiac glycosides in treating heart disorders has been known for over 2,000 years. They have been used as arrow poisons by African tribes and as medicines by the ancient Egyptians and Romans. The chemical classification draws its name from three sugars, or glycosides, which are attached to a steroid nucleus (Chapter 19 ⬭).

ON THE JOB

Digoxin and the Dental Hygienist

Providing dental care for the client with heart failure who is taking digoxin may present a challenge for the dental hygienist. The hygienist must be alert for common signs of digoxin toxicity, including digestive complaints, visual disturbances, and increased salivation. Prior to the start of treatment and periodically during long procedures, the hygienist should monitor the client's pulse to check for bradycardia.

Digoxin sensitizes the heart to rhythm abnormalities. Because of this, local anesthetics without epinephrine are normally used. Following the procedure, the dental hygienist should advise the client not to take tetracycline or erythromycin antibiotics because these may increase digoxin levels. ▪

15.5 Cardiac glycosides increase the force of myocardial contraction and are the traditional drugs of choice for heart failure.

Extracted from the common plants *Digitalis pupura* (purple foxglove) and *Digitalis lanata* (white foxglove), drugs from this class are sometimes called *digitalis glycosides.* Until the discovery of the ACE inhibitors, the cardiac glycosides were the mainstay of heart failure treatment. Indeed, they are still widely prescribed for this disorder. Digitalis helps the heart to beat more forcefully and more slowly.

The margin of safety between a beneficial dose and a toxic dose of cardiac glycosides is very small and severe adverse effects may result from unmonitored treatment. The two primary cardiac glycosides, digoxin and digitoxin, are quite similar in efficacy, the primary difference being that the latter has a more prolonged half-life. The route and doses of the cardiac glycosides are listed in Table 15.2.

Concept review 15.1

▪ How can the Frank-Starling law be used to explain the beneficial effects of the cardiac glycosides in treating heart failure?

ANGIOTENSIN CONVERTING ENZYME (ACE) INHIBITORS

Drugs affecting the renin-angiotensin system reduce the afterload on the heart and lower blood pressure. They are often drugs of choice in the treatment of heart failure.

15.6 Angiotensin-converting enzyme (ACE) inhibitors are becoming first-line drugs for heart failure.

The basic pharmacology of the ACE inhibitors and their effects on the renin-angiotensin pathway were discussed in Chapter 14 ▱ . Approved for the treatment of hypertension since the 1980s, ACE inhibitors have since been shown to slow the progression of heart failure and to reduce deaths from this disease. They have largely replaced digoxin as first-line drugs for the treatment of chronic HF. Table 15.3 lists the ACE inhibitors approved to treat HF.

The primary action of the ACE inhibitors is to lower peripheral resistance and to reduce blood volume by enhancing the excretion of sodium and water. The resultant reduction of arterial blood pressure diminishes the afterload required of the heart, thus increasing cardiac output. An additional effect of the ACE inhibitors is dilation of the veins returning blood to the heart. This action, which is probably not directly related to their inhibition of angiotensin, decreases preload and reduces peripheral edema. The combined reductions in preload, afterload, and blood volume

dys = difficult or bad
rhythmia = rhythm
hypo = below
kal = potassium
emia = blood

DRUG PROFILE (Cardiac Glycoside):
Digoxin (Lanoxin)

Actions:

The primary benefit of digoxin is its ability to increase the contractility or strength of cardiac contraction—a positive inotropic action. Digoxin accomplishes this by inhibiting Na^+-K^+ ATPase, the critical enzyme responsible for pumping Na^+ out of the myocardial cell in exchange for K^+. As Na^+ accumulates, calcium ions are released from their storage areas in the cell. The release of Ca^{++} produces a more forceful contraction of the muscle fibers.

By increasing myocardial contractility, digoxin directly increases cardiac output, thus alleviating symptoms of HF and improving exercise tolerance.

The increased cardiac output results in increased urine production and a desirable reduction in blood volume, thus relieving the distressing symptoms of lung congestion and peripheral edema.

In addition to its positive inotropic effect, digoxin also affects impulse conduction in the heart. It has the ability to suppress the SA node, the pacemaker of the heart, and slow down electrical conduction through the AV node. Because of these actions, digoxin is sometimes used to treat rhythm abnormalities known as **dysrhythmias**, as discussed in Chapter 16 ⊂⊃ .

Adverse Effects:

The most dangerous adverse effect of digoxin is its ability to create dysrhythmias, particularly in clients who have low potassium levels in the blood or hypokalemia. Because diuretics can cause hypokalemia and are also often used to treat HF, concurrent use of digoxin and diuretics must be carefully monitored. Other adverse effects of digoxin therapy include effects on the digestive system such as nausea, vomiting, anorexia, and abnormalities of the nervous system such as blurred vision. Periodic serum levels are obtained to determine if the digoxin level is within the therapeutic range, and the dosage may be adjusted based on the laboratory results. Digoxin also interacts with many other medications. Because small changes in digoxin levels can produce serious adverse effects, the healthcare provider must constantly be on the alert for drug-drug interactions.

Mechanism in Action:

Digoxin's primary action is to inhibit the $Na^+ - K^+$ ATPase enzyme. This enzyme is responsible for pumping sodium out of the myocardial cell in exchange for potassium. This increases the force of heart contraction, resulting in improved cardiac function and alleviation of heart failure symptoms.

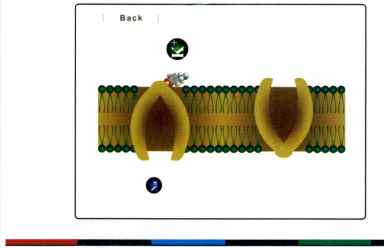

[Back]

TABLE 15.2	Cardiac Glycosides of Importance to Heart Failure	
DRUG	**ROUTE AND ADULT DOSE**	**REMARKS**
digitoxin (Crystodigin)	PO; 150 μg qd (max 0.3 mg/day).	Increases cardiac output; used to treat CHF and atrial dysrhythmias; larger dose is given to initiate therapy.
Pr digoxin (Lanoxin, Lanoxicaps)	PO; 0.1–0.375 mg qd (max 0.5 mg/day).	Increases the force and velocity of the myocardium; larger dose is given to initiate therapy; IV form available; also used for dysrhythmias.

DRUG PROFILE (ACE Inhibitor):
Lisinopril (Prinivil, Zestoric)

Actions:

Because of its value in the treatment of both heart failure and hypertension, lisinopril has become one of the most commonly prescribed drugs. Like other ACE inhibitors, doses of lisinopril may require two to three weeks of adjust-ment to reach maximum efficacy and several months of therapy may be needed for a client's functional status to return to normal. Because of their combined hypotensive action, concurrent therapy with lisinopril and diuretics should be carefully monitored.

Adverse Effects:

Although lisinopril causes few side effects, high potassium levels may occur during therapy. Thus, electrolyte levels are usually monitored periodically. Other side effects include cough, taste disturbances, and hypotension.

Mechanism in Action:

Angiotensin I is cleaved from the precursor molecule angiotensinogen. Following this reaction, angiotensin converting enzyme (ACE) catalyzes the conversion of angiotensin I to angiotensin II. Two major physiological actions result from this conversion: increased water/sodium retention and increased peripheral vascular resistance. Both physiological actions contribute to hypertension. Lisinopril lowers blood pressure by blocking ACE.

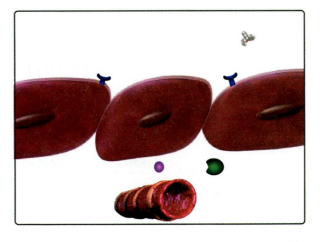

TABLE 15.3	ACE Inhibitors of Importance to Heart Failure	
DRUG	**ROUTE AND ADULT DOSE**	**REMARKS**
captopril (Capoten)	PO; 6.25–12.5 mg tid (max 450 mg/day).	Decreases central venous and pulmonary wedge pressure; also for hypertension and acute MI.
enalapril maleate (Vasotec) enalaprilat (Vasotec IV)	PO; 2.5 mg qd-bid (max 40 mg/day).	Increases cardiac output; IV form available; also for hypertension.
fosinopril (Monopril)	PO; 5–40 mg qd (max 40 mg/day).	Also for hypertension.
Pr lisinopril (Prinivil, Zestril)	PO; 10 mg qd (max 80 mg/day).	Therapy should not begin until two to three days after diuretics are stopped; also for hypertension and acute MI.
quinapril hydrochloride (Accupril)	PO; 10–20 mg qd (max 40 mg/day).	Observe for signs of hyperkalemia; also for hypertension.
ramipril (Altace)	PO; 2.5–5 mg bid (max 10 mg/day).	Also for hypertension.

substantially decrease the workload on the heart and allow it to work more efficiently. Several ACE inhibitors have been shown to reduce mortality following acute myocardial infarction when therapy is started soon after the onset of symptoms (Chapter 17 ⬤▭).

VASODILATORS

Vasodilators play a minor role in the drug therapy of heart failure. They are also used for hypertension and angina pectoris.

15.7 Vasodilators can help reduce symptoms of heart failure by decreasing the oxygen demand on the heart.

The two drugs in this class act directly on vascular smooth muscle to relax blood vessels and lower blood pressure. Hydralazine (Apresoline) acts on arterioles while isosorbide dinitrate (Isordil) acts on veins. Because the two drugs act synergistically, isosorbide dinitrate is usually combined with hydralazine in the treatment of HF. Because of the high incidence of side effects, they are generally reserved for clients who cannot tolerate ACE inhibitors. These two direct-acting vasodilators are listed in Table 15.4. The role of hydralazine in the treatment of hypertension is discussed in Chapter 14 ⬤▭ , and the use of isosorbide dinitrate for therapy of angina pectoris is presented in Chapter 17 ⬤▭ .

DIURETICS

Diuretics increase urine flow, thus reducing blood volume and cardiac workload. They are widely used in the treatment of cardiovascular disease.

DRUG PROFILE (Vasodilator):
Isosorbide dinitrate (Isordil)

Actions:

Isosorbide dinitrate acts directly on veins to cause venodilation, thus reducing venous return (preload), decreasing cardiac workload, and increasing cardiac output. Isosorbide dinitrate also dilates the coronary arteries to bring more oxygen to the myocardium. Isosorbide dinitrate belongs to a class of drugs called organic nitrates that are widely used in the treatment of angina, as discussed in Chapter 17 ⬤▭ .

Adverse Effects:

Side effects of isosorbide dinitrate include headache, hypotension, and reflex tachycardia. Use is contraindicated if the client is also taking sildenafil (Viagra) because serious hypotension may result.

TABLE 15.4	Direct Acting Vasodilators of Importance to Heart Failure	
DRUG	**ROUTE AND ADULT DOSE**	**REMARKS**
hydralazine hydrochloride (Apresoline)	PO; 10–50 mg qid (max 300 mg/day).	Increases heart rate, stroke volume, and cardiac output; also for hypertension; IV and IM forms available.
Pr isosorbide dinitrate (Isordil, Sorbitrate, Dilatrate)	PO; 2.5–30 mg qid administer ac and hs (max 160 mg/day).	Decreases myocardial oxygen consumption; sustained release form available; sublingual, chewable, and buccal forms available for angina.

NATURAL ALTERNATIVES

Carnitine and Heart Disease

Once thought to be a vitamin, carnitine is a natural substance structurally similar to amino acids. Its primary function in metabolism is to move fatty acids from the bloodstream into cells, where carnitine assists in the breakdown of lipids in the mitochondria. This breakdown produces energy and increases the availability of oxygen, particularly in muscle cells. A congenital deficiency of carnitine leads to severe brain, liver, and heart damage.

Although a normal diet supplies 300 mg. per day, certain clients may need additional amounts. Vegetarians are at risk to carnitine depletion, as plant protein supplies little or no carnitine. Endurance athletes and body-builders sometimes use carnitine supplements to build their muscle mass. Carnitine is available as a supplement in several forms, including L-carnitine, D L-carnitine, and acetyl L-carnitine. The best food sources of carnitine are organ meat, fish, muscle meats, and milk products.

L-carnitine supplementation has been shown to improve exercise tolerance in clients with angina. The use of L-carnitine may prevent the occurrence of dysrhythmias in the early stages of heart disease. L-carnitine has also been shown to decrease triglyceride levels while increasing HDL serum levels, thus helping to minimize one of the major risk factors associated with heart disease.

Carnitine has a number of additional purported effects including improvement of brain function in clients with Alzheimer's disease. Because of its role in fatty acid metabolism, some claim it assists in treating obesity, although this has not been medically demonstrated. ■

15.8 Diuretics are effective at reducing fluid volume and relieving symptoms of heart failure.

Diuretics are commonly used for the treatment of heart failure because they produce few adverse effects and are effective at reducing blood volume, edema, and congestion. As diuretics reduce fluid volume and lower blood pressure, the workload on the heart is reduced and cardiac output increases. Diuretics are rarely used alone, but instead are prescribed in combination with ACE inhibitors and other HF medications.

The mechanism by which diuretics reduce blood volume, specifically where and how the nephron of the kidney is affected, differs among the various drugs. Differences in mechanisms among the classes of diuretics are discussed in Chapter 27 ⬡ . The role of the thiazide diuretics in the treatment of hypertension is discussed in Chapter 14 ⬡ . Selected diuretics that are important to HF are listed in Table 15.5.

Concept Review 15.2

■ Why are the ACE inhibitors preferred over both the nitrates and the diuretics in the treatment of heart failure?

PHOSPHODIESTERASE INHIBITORS

Phosphodiesterase inhibitors have a brief half-life and are used for the short-term control of acute heart failure.

15.9 Phosphodiesterase inhibitors increase the force of contraction and cause vasodilation.

In the 1980s, two drugs became available that block the enzyme **phosphodiesterase** in cardiac and smooth muscle. Blocking phosphodiesterase has the effect of increasing the amount of calcium available for myocardial contraction. The inhibition results in two main actions that benefit

DRUG PROFILE (Diuretic):

Furosemide (Lasix)

Actions:

Furosemide is often used in the treatment of acute heart failure because it has the ability to remove large amounts of edema fluid from the client in a short period of time. Clients often receive quick relief from their distressing symptoms. Compared to other diuretics, furosemide is particularly beneficial when cardiac output and renal flow are severely diminished.

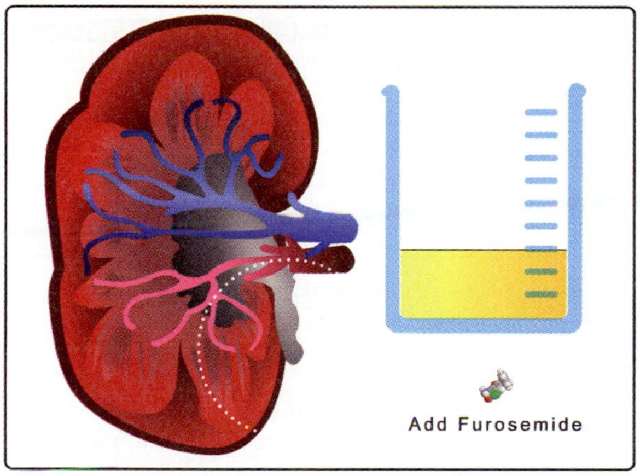

Adverse Effects:

Side effects of furosemide, like those of most diuretics, involve potential electrolyte imbalances, the most important of which is hypokalemia. Because hypokalemia may cause dysrhythmias in clients taking cardiac glycosides, combination therapy with furosemide and digoxin must be carefully monitored. Because furosemide is such a potent drug, fluid loss must be carefully monitored to avoid possible dehydration and hypotension.

Mechanism in Action:

Furosemide inhibits the combined transport of sodium, potassium, and chloride (called $Na^+-K^+-2Cl^-$ symport) across the ascending limb of the loop of Henle. By blocking active NaCl reabsorption, furosemide interferes with a concentrated medullary interstitium, which would normally attract water from the nephron. When water reabsorption is blocked, increased urination results.

TABLE 15.5 Selected Diuretics of Importance to Heart Failure

DRUG	ROUTE AND ADULT DOSE	REMARKS
Pr furosemide (Lasix)	PO; 20 – 80 mg in 1 or more divided doses (max 600 mg/day).	Monitor for signs and symptoms of hypokalemia; also for hypertension; IV and IM forms available; loop diuretic.
hydrochlorothiazide (Hydrodiuril, HCTZ)	PO; 25–200 mg in 1 to 3 divided doses (max 200 mg/day).	May precipitate diabetes in the prediabetic patient; also for hypertension; thiazide-type.
spironolactone (Aldactone)	PO; 25–200 mg in divided doses (max 200 mg/day).	For refractory edema with congestive heart failure; also for hypertension; potassium-sparing diuretic.
bumetanide (Bumex)	PO; 0.5–2 mg qd (max 10 mg/day).	Affects loop of Henle; diuretic activity is 40 times greater and duration of action is shorter than furosemide; IM and IV forms available.
chlorothiazide (Diuril)	PO; 250–1 g in 1–2 divided doses (max 2 g/day).	Initially reduces cardiac output; also for hypertension; thiazide type; IV form available.
triamterene (Dyrenium)	PO; 100 mg bid (max 300 mg/day).	Used as adjunct therapy to manage edema with congestive heart failure; also for hypertension; potassium sparing.
torsemide (Demadex)	PO; 10–20 mg qd (max 200 mg/day).	Affects Loop of Henle; also for hypertension; IV form available.

DRUG PROFILE (Phosphodiesterase Inhibitor):
Milrinone (Primacor)

Actions:

Of the two phosphodiesterase inhibitors available, milrinone is generally preferred because it has a shorter half-life and fewer side effects. It is only given intravenously and is primarily used for the short-term support of advanced HF. Peak effects occur in two minutes. Immediate effects of milrinone include an increased force of contraction and an increase in cardiac output.

Adverse Effects:

The most serious side effect of milrinone is ventricular dysrhythmia, which can occur in more than 1 out of every 10 clients taking the drug. The client's ECG is usually monitored continuously during the infusion of the drug.

TABLE 15.6	Phosphodiesterase Inhibitors	
DRUG	**ROUTE AND ADULT DOSE**	**REMARKS**
inamrinone lactate (Inocor)	IV; 0.75 mg/kg bolus given slowly over 2–3 min; then 5–10 µg/kg/min (max 10 mg/kg/day).	Larger dose is given to initiate therapy; peak effect is reached in 10 minutes.
Pr milrinone lactate (Primacor)	IV; 50 µg/kg over 10 min; then 0.375 – 0.75 µg/kg/min (no max dose given).	Larger dose is given to initiate therapy; peak effect reached in 2 minutes.

clients with HF: a positive inotropic response and vasodilation. Due to their toxicity, phosphodiesterase inhibitors are normally reserved for clients who have not responded to ACE inhibitors or cardiac glycosides, and they are generally used only for two to three days. The doses of phosphodiesterase inhibitors are given in Table 15.6.

BETA-ADRENERGIC BLOCKERS

A few beta-blockers are of value in the treatment of heart failure. They reduce the cardiac workload by decreasing afterload.

15.10 Beta-adrenergic blockers play a minor role in the treatment of heart failure.

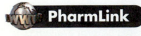

SUPPORT FOR HEART FAILURE CLIENTS AND HEALTH PROFESSIONALS

As has been seen with the cardiac glycosides, ACE inhibitors, and phosphodiesterase inhibitors, drugs that produce a positive inotropic effect play important roles in treating the diminished contractility that is the hallmark of HF. It may seem somewhat unusual, then, to find medications that exhibit a negative inotropic effect prescribed for this disease. Yet such is the case with the beta-adrenergic blockers. The basic pharmacology of the beta-blockers is presented in Chapter 6 ⊂⊃ . Other uses, routes, and dosages of the beta-adrenergic blockers are discussed elsewhere in this text: hypertension in Chapter 14, dysrhythmias in Chapter 16, and angina/myocardial infarction in Chapter 17 ⊂⊃ .

DRUG PROFILE (Beta-Adrenergic Blocker):
Carvedilol (Coreg)

Actions:

Carvedilol is the first beta-adrenergic blocker approved for the treatment of HF. It has been found to reduce symptoms, slow the progression of the disease, and increase exercise tolerance when combined with other heart failure drugs such as the ACE inhibitors. Unlike many drugs in this class, carvedilol blocks beta$_1$ and beta$_2$ as well as alpha$_1$-adrenergic receptors. The primary-therapeutic effects relevant to HF are a reduction in heart rate and a drop in blood pressure. The lower blood pressure decreases afterload and reduces the workload on the heart.

Adverse Effects:

Carvedilol's ability to decrease the heart rate combined with its ability to reduce contractility has the potential to worsen heart failure, and dosage must be carefully monitored. Because of the potential for adverse cardiac effects, beta-adrenergic blockers such as carvedilol are not considered first-line drugs in the treatment of HF.

CLIENT TEACHING

Clients treated for heart failure need to know the following:

1. It is important to check your pulse rate before taking digoxin. If the rate is <60 beats per minute, or the rate designated by your healthcare practitioner, the drug should not be taken.

2. Many drugs interact with digoxin to increase or decrease its effects on the heart. For this reason, it is important to consult with your healthcare provider before taking any other medication.

3. Visual disturbances (seeing halos or a yellow/green tinge, blurring), nausea, headaches, or irregular heartbeat should be reported without delay because they are signs and symptoms of digoxin toxicity.

4. Because many drugs for heart failure affect blood pressure, have this taken regularly and report any persistent changes.

5. Weigh yourself regularly and report abnormal weight gains or losses.

6. Your healthcare provider may advise eating foods high in potassium or prescribe a potassium supplement if you are taking certain diuretics. Taking potassium supplements with food reduces stomach irritation. ▪

CHAPTER REVIEW

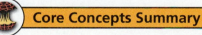 **Core Concepts Summary**

15.1 Several disorders are associated with heart failure.

Heart failure is not considered a distinct disease in itself. Instead, a number of diseases that affect the heart, such as chronic hypertension and diabetes, lead to this collection of symptoms known as HF.

15.2 The central cause of heart failure is weakened heart muscle.

Heart failure occurs when the heart cannot pump enough blood to meet the metabolic demands of the body. This usually occurs when the heart muscle cannot contract with sufficient force. Heart failure may occur on the right side, left side, or both sides of the heart, producing symptoms such as shortness of breath, coughing, and peripheral edema.

15.3 The three primary characteristics of heart function are force of contraction, heart rate, and speed of impulse conduction.

The ability of the heart to effectively pump blood is dependent upon the strength of contraction of the myocardial fibers. Heart rate and the speed of the impulse conduction across the myocardium also directly affect the ability of the heart to pump blood.

15.4 Non-pharmacologic therapy of early heart failure is sometimes effective.

Mild heart failure can be improved through lifestyle changes such as tobacco cessation and maintaining optimum weight. Clients receiving drug therapy for HF should also be encouraged to adopt these lifestyle changes.

15.5 Cardiac glycosides increase the force of myocardial contraction and are the traditional drugs of choice for heart failure.

Cardiac glycosides, long the mainstay for pharmacotherapy of HF, increase myocardial contractility and are very efficacious. The large number of drug-drug interactions and the potential for serious adverse effects such as dysrhythmias limit their use.

15.6 Angiotensin-converting enzyme (ACE) inhibitors are becoming first-line drugs for heart failure.

ACE inhibitors improve heart failure by reducing peripheral edema and increasing cardiac output.

Because of their effectiveness and their relatively low potential for serious adverse effects, they have become first-line drugs in the treatment of HF.

15.7 Vasodilators can help reduce symptoms of heart failure by decreasing the oxygen demand on the heart.

Direct vasodilators are effective at relaxing blood vessels, thus reducing myocardial oxygen demand on the heart. Their use is limited by their high incidence of side effects.

15.8 Diuretics are effective at reducing fluid volume and relieving symptoms of heart failure.

Diuretics produce few side effects and are often used in combination with other HF drugs to reduce client symptoms. Potent diuretics such as furosemide are particularly valuable in treating acute HF.

15.9 Phosphodiesterase inhibitors increase the force of contraction and cause vasodilation.

Phosphodiesterase inhibitors are a relatively new class of drugs used for the short-term treatment of HF. While effective, they are only given IV and can produce potentially serious adverse effects.

15.10 Beta-adrenergic blockers play a minor role in the treatment of heart failure.

Although beta-blockers decrease myocardial contractility, they also lower heart rate and blood pressure, which are beneficial to reducing the symptoms of HF. When treating clients with HF, they are nearly always used in combination with other drugs.

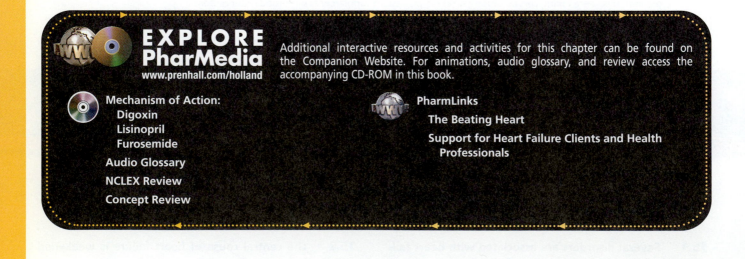

EXPLORE PharMedia
www.prenhall.com/holland

Additional interactive resources and activities for this chapter can be found on the Companion Website. For animations, audio glossary, and review access the accompanying CD-ROM in this book.

Mechanism of Action:
  Digoxin
  Lisinopril
  Furosemide
Audio Glossary
NCLEX Review
Concept Review

PharmLinks
  The Beating Heart
  Support for Heart Failure Clients and Health Professionals

16 Drugs for Dysrhythmias

CORE CONCEPTS

16.1 The frequency of dysrhythmias in the population is difficult to ascertain because many clients experience no symptoms.

16.2 Dysrhythmias are classified by their location and type of rhythm abnormality produced.

16.3 The electrical conduction pathway in the myocardium keeps the heart beating in a synchronized manner.

16.4 Changes in sodium and potassium levels generate the action potential in myocardial cells.

16.5 Non-pharmacologic therapy of certain dysrhythmias is often the treatment of choice.

Antidysrhythmics

16.6 Antidysrhythmic drugs are classified by their mechanism of action.

Sodium Channel Blockers

16.7 Sodium channel blockers slow the rate of impulse conduction through the heart.

Beta-adrenergic Blockers

16.8 Beta-adrenergic blockers reduce automaticity as well as slow conduction velocity in the heart.

Potassium Channel Blockers

16.9 Potassium channel blockers prolong the refractory period of the heart.

Calcium Channel Blockers

16.10 Two calcium channel blockers are available as antidysrhythmics.

Miscellaneous Drugs for Dysrhythmias

16.11 Digoxin and several other drugs are used for specific dysrhythmias, but do not act by blocking ion channels.

OBJECTIVES

After reading this chapter, the student should be able to:

1. Explain why the incidence of dysrhythmias in the population is difficult to ascertain.

2. Relate how rhythm abnormalities can affect cardiac function.

3. Illustrate the flow of electrical impulses through the normal heart.

4. Classify dysrhythmias based on their location and type of rhythm abnormality.

5. Explain how an action potential is controlled by the flow of sodium, potassium, and calcium ions across the myocardial membrane.

6. Specify the relationship between electrical conduction in the heart and cardiac output.

7. Identify the importance of non-pharmacologic therapies in the treatment of dysrhythmias.

8. Identify the primary mechanisms by which antidysrhythmic drugs act.

9. For each of the following classes, identify representative drugs, explain the mechanism of drug action, primary actions, and important adverse effects.
   a. sodium channel blockers
   b. beta-adrenergic blockers
   c. potassium channel blockers
   d. calcium channel blockers
   e. miscellaneous antidysrhythmic drugs

10. Categorize antidysrhythmic drugs based on their classification and mechanism of action.

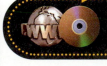

PharMedia
www.prenhall.com/holland

Additional interactive resources and activities for this chapter can be found on the Companion Website. For animations, audio glossary, and review access the accompanying CD-ROM in this book.

action potential: the change in electrical activity across the plasma membrane of a muscle or nerve cell due to changes in membrane permeability / *page 235*

atrioventricular bundle (ay-tree-oh-ven-TRIK-you-lur BUN-dul): specialized cardiac tissue that receives electrical impulses from the AV node and sends them to the bundle branches also known as the Bundle of His / *page 233*

atrioventricular (AV) node (ay-tree-oh-ven-TRIK-you-lur noad): mass of cardiac tissue that receives electrical impulses from the SA node and conveys them to the ventricles / *page 233*

automaticity (aw-toh-muh-TISS-uh-tee): ability of certain myocardial cells to spontaneously generate an action potential / *page 233*

bradycardia (bray-dee-KAR-DEE-uh): condition of slow heartbeat / *page 232*

bundle branches (BUN-dul BRAN-chez): electrical conduction pathway in the heart leading from the AV bundle and through the wall between the ventricles / *page 233*

calcium ion channel (KAL-see-um): pathway in a plasma membrane through which calcium ions enter and leave / *page 235*

cardioversion/defibrillation (kar-dee-oh-VER-shun/dee-fib-ree-LAY-shun): conversion of fibrillation to a normal heart rhythm / *page 236*

catheter ablation (kath-eh-tur uh-BLAY-shun): destruction of abnormal myocardial cells in order to restore normal cardiac rhythm / *page 236*

depolarization (dee-po-lur-eye-ZAY-shun): condition in which the plasma membrane charge is changed such that the inside is made less negative / *page 235*

dysrhythmia (diss-RITH-mee-uh): abnormality in cardiac rhythm / *page 231*

ectopic foci/pacemakers (ek-TOP-ik FO-si): cardiac tissue outside the normal cardiac conduction pathway that generates action potentials / *page 234*

electrocardiogram (ECG) (e-lek-tro-KAR-dee-oh-gram): device that records the electrical activity of the heart / *page 234*

fibrillation (fi-bruh-LAY-shun): type of dysrhythmia in which the chambers beat in a highly disorganized manner / *page 232*

flutter (FLUH-tur): type of dysrhythmia in which the contractions become extremely rapid / *page 232*

implantable cardioverter defibrillator (im-PLANT-uh-bul kar-dee-oh-VER-tur dee-FIB-ree-lay-tur): device placed in the patient to detect and correct dysrhythmias as they occur / *page 236*

polarized (POLE-uh-rized): condition in which the inside of a cell is more negatively charged than the outside of the cell / *page 235*

potassium ion channel (po-TASS-ee-um): pathway in a plasma membrane through which potassium ions enter and leave / *page 235*

Purkinje fibers (purr-KEN-gee FI-burrs): electrical conduction pathway leading from the bundle branches to all portions of the ventricles / *page 233*

refractory period (ree-FRAK-tor-ee): time during which the myocardial cells rest and are not able to contract / *page 235*

sinoatrial (SA) node (si-no-AYE-tree-ul noad): pacemaker of the heart located in the wall of the right atrium / *page 233*

sinus rhythm (SI-nuss): number of beats per minute normally generated by the SA node / *page 233*

sodium ion channel (SO-dee-um): pathway in a plasma membrane through which sodium ions enter and leave / *page 235*

supraventricular (sue-prah-ven-TRIK-you-lur): lying above the ventricles or in the atria / *page 232*

tachycardia (tack-ee-KAR-dee-uh): condition of fast heartbeat / *page 232*

Dysrhythmias *are abnormalities of electrical conduction or rhythm in the heart. Sometimes called arrhythmias, they encompass a number of different disorders that range from harmless to life threatening. Diagnosis is often difficult because clients usually must be connected to an electrocardiogram (ECG) and be experiencing symptoms in order to determine the exact type of rhythm disorder. Proper diagnosis and optimum pharmacologic treatment can significantly affect the frequency of dysrhythmias and their consequences.*

dys = difficult or bad
rhythmia = rhythm

Fast Facts Dysrhythmias

- Dysrhythmias are responsible for over 44,000 deaths each year.
- Atrial dysrhythmias occur more commonly in men than in women.
- The incidence of atrial dysrhythmias increases with age. They affect:
  less than 0.5% of those aged 25–3
  1.5% of those up to age 60
  9% of those over age 75
- About 15% of strokes occur in clients with atrial dysrhythmias.
- A large majority of sudden cardiac deaths are thought to be caused by ventricular dysrhythmias.
- Sudden cardiac death occurs three to four times more frequently in blacks.
- Atrial fibrillation affects 1.5 to 2.2 million people in the U.S.

16.1 The frequency of dysrhythmias in the population is difficult to ascertain because many clients experience no symptoms.

PharmLink

CHILDHOOD DYSRHYTHMIAS

a = no or not
symptomatic = symptoms

While some dysrhythmias produce no symptoms and have negligible effects on heart function, others are life threatening and require immediate treatment. Typical symptoms include dizziness, weakness, decreased exercise tolerance, shortness of breath, and fainting. Many clients report palpitations or a sensation that their heart has skipped a beat. Persistent dysrhythmias are associated with increased risk of stroke and heart failure. Severe dysrhythmias may result in sudden death. Because asymptomatic clients may not seek medical attention, it is difficult to estimate the frequency of the disease, although it is likely that dysrhythmias are quite common in the population.

16.2 Dysrhythmias are classified by the location and type of rhythm abnormality produced.

supra = above
ventricular = cardiac
ventricle

There are many types of dysrhythmias and they may be classified by a number of different means. The simplest method is to name dysrhythmias according to the type of rhythm abnormality produced and its location. A summary of the different types of dysrhythmias along with a brief description of each abnormality is given in Table 16.1. Dysrhythmias that originate in the atria are sometimes referred to as **supraventricular**. Those that originate in the ventricles are generally more serious because they more often interfere with the normal function of the heart. Although obtaining a correct diagnosis of the type of dysrhythmia is sometimes difficult, it is essential for effective treatment. Atrial **fibrillation**, a complete disorganization of rhythm, is thought to be the most common type of dysrhythmia.

While the actual cause of most dysrhythmias is elusive, dysrhythmias are associated with certain conditions, primarily heart disease and myocardial infarction. Following are some of the diseases commonly associated with dysrhythmias.

- hypertension
- cardiac valve disease, such as mitral stenosis
- coronary artery disease
- medications such as digitalis
- low potassium levels in the blood

TABLE 16.1	Types of Dysrhythmias
NAME OF DYSRHYTHMIA	**DESCRIPTION**
premature atrial or premature ventricular (PVC) contractions	an extra beat, often originating from a source other than the SA node; not normally serious unless it occurs in high frequency
atrial or ventricular **tachycardia**	rapid heart beat greater than 150 bpm; ventricular is more serious than atrial
atrial or ventricular **flutter** and/or fibrillation	very rapid, uncoordinated beats; atrial may require treatment but is not usually fatal; ventricular requires immediate treatment
sinus **bradycardia**	slow heartbeat, less than 50 beats per minute; may require a pacemaker
heart block	area of non-conduction in the myocardium; may be partial or complete; classified as first, second, or third degree

- myocardial infarction
- adverse effect from antidysrhythmic medication
- stroke
- diabetes mellitus
- congestive heart failure

16.3 The electrical conduction pathway in the myocardium keeps the heart beating in a synchronized manner.

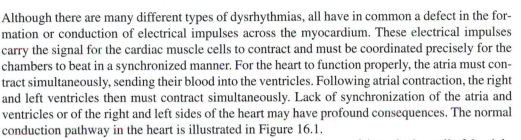

Although there are many different types of dysrhythmias, all have in common a defect in the formation or conduction of electrical impulses across the myocardium. These electrical impulses carry the signal for the cardiac muscle cells to contract and must be coordinated precisely for the chambers to beat in a synchronized manner. For the heart to function properly, the atria must contract simultaneously, sending their blood into the ventricles. Following atrial contraction, the right and left ventricles then must contract simultaneously. Lack of synchronization of the atria and ventricles or of the right and left sides of the heart may have profound consequences. The normal conduction pathway in the heart is illustrated in Figure 16.1.

Normal control of this synchronization begins in a small area of tissue in the wall of the right atrium known as the **sinoatrial (SA) node**. The SA node or pacemaker of the heart has a property called **automaticity**, the ability to spontaneously generate an electrical impulse known as an *action potential,* without instructions from the nervous system. The SA node generates a new action potential approximately 75 times every minute under resting conditions. This is referred to as the normal **sinus rhythm**.

Upon leaving the SA node, the action potential travels quickly across both atria to the **atrioventricular (AV) node**. The AV node also has the property of automaticity, although less so than the SA node. Should the SA node malfunction, the AV node has the ability to spontaneously generate action potentials and continue the heart's contraction.

As the action potential leaves the AV node, it travels rapidly to the **atrioventricular bundle** or bundle of His. The impulse is then conducted down the right and left **bundle branches** to the **Purkinje fibers**, which carry the impulse to all regions of the ventricles almost simultaneously.

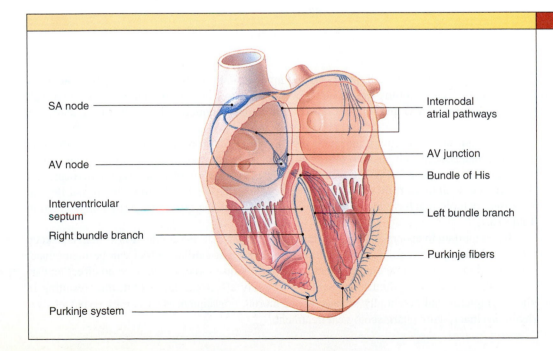

FIGURE 16.1

Normal conduction pathway in the heart
SOURCE: Pearson Education/PH College.

SA node

Internodal atrial pathways

AV node

AV junction

Bundle of His

Interventricular septum

Left bundle branch

Right bundle branch

Purkinje fibers

Purkinje system

FIGURE 16.2

Relationship of the electrocardiogram to electrical conduction in the heart   *SOURCE: Pearson Education/PH College*

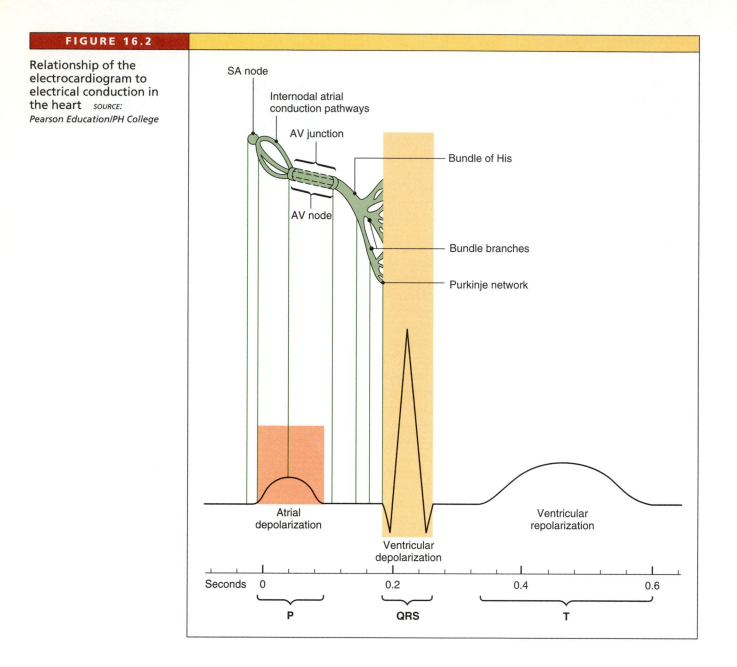

ec = outside
top = place
ic = pertaining to

The wave of electrical activity across the myocardium can be measured by the **electrocardiogram (ECG)**. The total time for the electrical impulse to travel across the heart is about 0.22 seconds. A normal ECG and its relationship to impulse conduction in the heart are shown in Figure 16.2.

Although action potentials normally begin at the SA node and spread across the myocardium in a coordinated manner, other regions of the heart may begin to initiate beats. These areas, known as **ectopic foci** or **ectopic pacemakers**, may send impulses across the myocardium that compete with those from the normal conduction system, thus affecting the normal flow of impulses. Ectopic foci have the potential to cause many of the types of dysrhythmias noted in Table 16.1.

It is important to understand that the underlying purpose of this conduction system is to keep the heart beating in a regular, synchronized manner so that cardiac output can be maintained. Some dysrhythmias occur sporadically, elicit no symptoms, and cause little or no effect on cardiac output. Some dysrhythmias, however, profoundly affect cardiac output, thus resulting in client symptoms and potentially serious, if not mortal, consequences. It is these types of dysrhythmias that require pharmacological treatment.

ON THE JOB

Paramedics and Antidysrhythmics

On a 911 call for a client complaining of chest pain, paramedics must quickly distinguish among the various possibilities. Is this client simply experiencing an acute anginal episode? Is the client suffering from an early myocardial infarction? Or is the pain something not even related to the heart, such as acid indigestion or heartburn?

One of the first pieces of data gathered by the paramedic is an ECG. But if an ECG suggests premature ventricular contractions (PVCs), is this a reason to begin aggressive treatment with a drug such as lidocaine? Many clients experience PVCs, but are asymptomatic. The paramedic must learn to interpret the ECG to determine if evidence exists for lidocaine treatment. More than six PVCs per minute, PVCs that may be coming from more than one area of the heart, or PVCs that occur in couplets are patterns that suggest the dysrhythmia may progress to a more life-threatening dysrhythmia. ■

Concept Review 16.1

■ Trace the flow of electrical conduction through the heart. What would happen if the impulse never reached the AV node?

16.4 Changes in sodium and potassium levels generate the action potential in myocardial cells.

Because most antidysrhythmic drugs act by interfering with the cardiac action potential, a firm grasp of this phenomenon is necessary for understanding drug mechanisms. **Action potentials** occur in both nervous and cardiac muscle cells because of changes in certain ions found inside and outside the cell. Under resting conditions, Na^+ and Ca^{++} are found in higher concentrations outside of myocardial cells, while K^+ is found in higher concentration within these cells. These imbalances are, in part, responsible for the inside of a myocardial cell membrane being slightly negatively charged, relative to the outside of the membrane. A cell having this negative membrane potential is said to be **polarized**.

An action potential begins when **sodium ion channels** located in the plasma membrane open and Na^+ rushes into the cell producing a rapid **depolarization**, or loss of membrane potential. During this period, Ca^{++} also enters the cell through **calcium ion channels**, although the influx is slower than that of sodium. It is this influx of Ca^{++} that is responsible for the contraction of cardiac muscle. During depolarization, the inside of the cell membrane temporarily reverses its polarity, becoming positive. The cell returns to its polarized state by the removal of K^+ through **potassium ion channels**. In cells located in the SA and AV nodes, it is the influx of Ca^{++}, rather than Na^+, that generates the rapid depolarization of the membrane. Blocking potassium, sodium, or calcium ion channels is a pharmacological strategy used to terminate or prevent dysrhythmias. Figure 16.3 illustrates the ion flows occurring during the action potential.

During depolarization and most of repolarization, the cell cannot initiate another action potential. This time, known as the **refractory period**, assures that the action potential finishes and the muscle cell contracts before a second action potential begins. The therapeutic effect of some antidysrhythmic agents is caused by their prolongation of the refractory period.

16.5 Non-pharmacologic therapy of certain dysrhythmias is often the treatment of choice.

The goals of antidysrhythmic pharmacotherapy are to terminate dysrhythmias and to reduce the frequency of abnormal rhythms in order to decrease the possibility of sudden death, stroke, or

FIGURE 16.3

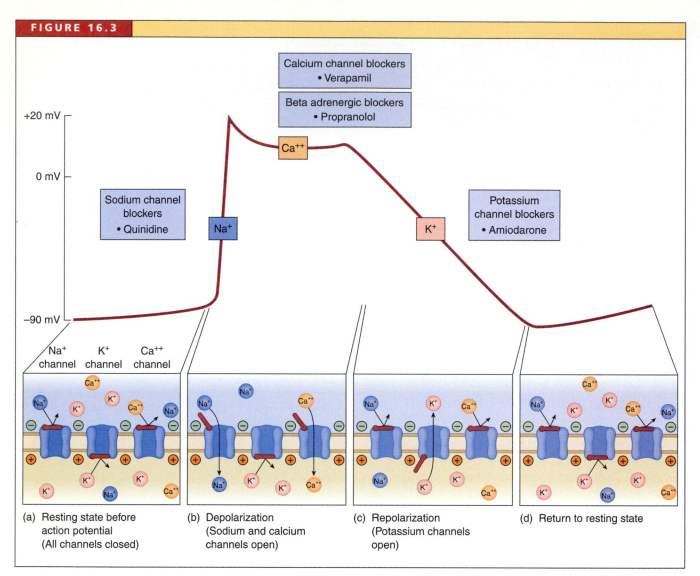

Ion channels in myocardial cells

other complications resulting from the disease. Because of their potential to cause serious side effects, antidysrhythmic drugs are normally reserved for those clients experiencing overt symptoms or for those whose condition cannot be controlled by other means. There is little or no benefit to the client in treating asymptomatic dysrhythmias with drugs. There are several non-pharmacologic strategies that physicians use to eliminate dysrhythmias.

The more serious types of dysrhythmias are corrected through electrical shock of the heart, a treatment called **cardioversion** or **defibrillation**. The electrical shock momentarily stops all electrical impulses in the heart, both normal and abnormal. Under ideal conditions, the temporary cessation of electrical activity will allow the SA node to automatically return conduction to a normal sinus rhythm.

Other types of non-pharmacologic treatment include identification and destruction of the myocardial cells responsible for the abnormal conduction through a surgical procedure called **catheter ablation**. Cardiac pacemakers are sometimes inserted to correct the types of dysrhythmias that cause the heart to beat too slowly. **Implantable Cardioverter Defibrillators** (ICDs) are placed in a client to restore normal rhythm by either pacing the heart or giving it an electric shock when dysrhythmias occur. In addition, the ICD is capable of storing information regarding the heart rhythm for the physician to evaluate.

NATURAL ALTERNATIVES

Coenzyme Q10 and Cardiovascular Disease

Coenzyme Q10 is a vitamin-like substance found in most animal cells. It is an essential component in the cell's mitochondria for producing energy, or ATP. Because the heart requires high levels of ATP, a sufficient level of coenzyme Q10 is particularly important to that organ.

A normal dietary intake of coenzyme Q10 is 2–5 mg/day. Foods richest in this substance are pork, sardines, beef heart, salmon, broccoli, spinach, and nuts. The elderly appear to have an increased need for coenzyme Q10. Although coenzyme Q10 can be synthesized by the body, many amino acids and other substances are required, thus clients having a number of different nutritional deficiencies may be in need of supplementation.

In 1978, a Nobel Prize was awarded for research proving the importance of coenzyme Q10 in energy transfer, but it was not until the 1990s that the substance became the top-selling supplement in health food stores. Coenzyme Q10 has been purported to aid a wide range of conditions, including heart failure, hypertension, dysrhythmias, angina, diabetes, neurological disorders, cancer, and aging. A considerable body of research has begun to accumulate, particularly regarding the role of coenzyme Q10 in heart disease. Some data have found below-normal levels of coenzyme Q10 in clients with heart failure. Studies suggest that the frequency of preventricular contractions may be reduced in some clients by supplementation with coenzyme Q10. Although most studies have demonstrated positive results, coenzyme Q10 has not been widely accepted by the conventional medical community. ▪

ANTIDYSRHYTHMICS

16.6 Antidysrhythmic drugs are classified by their mechanism of action.

Antidysrhythmic drugs are classified by the stage at which they affect the action potential. These drugs fall into four primary classes, referred to as Classes I, II, III and IV, and a miscellaneous group that does not act by one of the first four mechanisms. A typical action potential and the phases at which antidysrhythmic drugs act are shown in Figure 16.3. Categories of antidysrhythmics include the following.

- sodium channel blockers (Class I)
- beta-adrenergic blockers (Class II)
- potassium channel blockers (Class III)
- calcium channel blockers (Class IV)
- miscellaneous antidysrhythmic drugs

All antidysrhythmic drugs have the potential to profoundly affect the heart's conduction system. As such, they not only have the ability to correct dysrhythmias, they also have the ability to worsen or even create new dysrhythmias. The healthcare provider must carefully monitor clients taking antidysrhythmic drugs. Often, the patient is hospitalized during the initial stages of therapy so that doses can be accurately determined.

SODIUM CHANNEL BLOCKERS

The first medical uses of the sodium channel blockers were recorded in the 18th century. This is the largest class of antidysrhythmics and many are still widely prescribed.

DRUG PROFILE (Sodium Channel Blocker):
Quinidine sulfate (Quinidex)

Actions:

Quinidine, the oldest antidysrhythmic drug, was originally obtained as a natural substance from the bark of the South American *Cinchona* tree. Like other drugs in this class, quinidine blocks sodium ion channels in myocardial cells, thus reducing automaticity and slowing conduction of the electrical impulse through the myocardium. This slight delay in conduction velocity can suppress dysrhythmias. Quinidine is referred to as a broad-spectrum drug because it has the ability to correct many different types of atrial and ventricular dysrhythmias.

Adverse Effects:

The most common side effects of quinidine are gastrointestinal in nature and include nausea, vomiting, and diarrhea. A potentially serious interaction can occur when quinidine is given concurrently with digoxin. Because quinidine has the potential to double digoxin levels in the blood, the dose of digoxin must be reduced accordingly and carefully monitored. Like all antidysrhythmic drugs, quinidine has the ability to produce new dysrhythmias or worsen existing ones; thus clients should be frequently assessed for changes in cardiac status.

16.7 Sodium channel blockers slow the rate of impulse conduction through the heart.

Sodium channel blockers, the Class I drugs, are the largest group of antidysrhythmics. They are further divided into three subgroups, IA, IB, and IC, based on subtle differences in their mechanisms of action. Because progression of the action potential is dependent upon the opening of sodium ion channels, a blockade of these channels will slow the spread of impulse conduction across the myocardium. Sodium channel blockers used as antidysrhythmics are listed in Table 16.2.

Concept Review 16.2

■ Why does slowing the speed of the electrical impulse across the myocardium sometimes correct a dysrhythmia?

BETA-ADRENERGIC BLOCKERS

Beta-blockers are widely used for cardiovascular disorders. Their ability to slow the heart rate and conduction velocity can suppress several types of dysrhythmias.

16.8 Beta-adrenergic blockers reduce automaticity as well as slow conduction velocity in the heart.

The basic pharmacology of beta-adrenergic blockers was explained in Chapter 6 . Beta-blockers are used to treat a large number of cardiovascular diseases, including hypertension, MI, heart failure, and dysrhythmias. Because of potentially serious side effects, however, only a few beta-blockers are approved to treat dysrhythmias. Although the effects of beta-blockers on the heart are complex, their basic actions are to slow the heart rate and decrease conduction velocity through the AV node. Myocardial automaticity is reduced and many types of dysrhythmias are stabilized. The main value of beta-blockers as antidysrhythmic agents is to treat atrial dysrhythmias associated with heart failure. Beta-blockers of importance to dysrhythmias are listed in Table 16.3.

TABLE 16.2	Sodium Channel Blockers Used for Dysrhythmias (Class I)	
DRUG	**RATE AND ADULT DOSE**	**REMARKS**
Pr quinidine gluconate (Duraquin, Quinaglute) quinidine sulfate (Quinidex)	PO; 200–600 mg tid or qid (max 3–4 g/day).	Class 1A; gluconate salt is also available in IM and IV forms; sustained release forms available for the sulfate and gluconate salts.
disopyramide phosphate (Norpace, Nopamide)	PO; 100–200 mg qid (max 800 mg/day).	Class 1A; sustained release form available; usually reserved for serious ventricular dysrhythmias.
flecainide (Tambocor)	PO; 100 mg bid; increase by 500 mg bid every 4 days (max 400 mg/day).	Class 1C; usually reserved for serious ventricular dysrhythmias.
lidocaine hydrochloride (Xylocaine)	IV; 1–4 mg/min infusion; no more than 200–300 mg should be infused in a 1-hour period.	Class 1B; usually reserved for rapid control of ventricular dysrhythmias; IM, SC, and topical forms available; also widely used as a local anesthetic.
mexiletine (Mexitil)	PO; 200–300 mg tid (max 1200 mg/day).	Class 1B; usually reserved for serious ventricular dysrhythmias.
moricizine (Ethmozine)	PO; 200–300 mg tid (max 240 mg/day).	Class 1; usually reserved for serious ventricular dysrhythmias.
phenytoin (Dilantin)	IV; 50–100 mg every 10–15 min until dysrhythmia is terminated (max 1 g/day).	Class 1B; unlabeled use for dysrhythmias induced by cardiac glycosides; oral form is used to treat convulsions.
procainamide hydrochloride (Procan, Pronestyl, Procanbid)	PO; 1 g loading dose followed by 250–500 mg every 3 hours.	Class 1A; IM, IV, and sustained release forms available; for both supraventricular and ventricular dysrhythmias.
propafanone (Rythmol)	PO; 150–300 mg tid (max 900 mg/day).	Class 1C; usually reserved for serious ventricular dysrhythmias.
tocainide hydrochloride (Tonocard)	PO; 400–600 mg tid (max 2.4 g/day).	Class 1B; usually reserved for serious ventricular dysrhythmias.

Concept Review 16.3

■ Why are selective alpha-adrenergic blockers such as doxazosin (Cardura) of no value in treating dysrhythmias?

POTASSIUM CHANNEL BLOCKERS

Although it is a small class of drugs, the potassium channel blockers have very important applications to the treatment of dysrhythmias. These drugs prolong the resting stage of contraction, or the refractory period, which stabilizes certain types of dysrhythmias.

16.9 Potassium channel blockers prolong the refractory period of the heart.

The drugs in Class III exert their actions by blocking potassium ion channels in myocardial cells. After the action potential has passed and the myocardial cell is in a depolarized state, repolarization

DRUG PROFILE:
Propranolol (Inderal)

Actions:

Until 1978, propranolol was the only beta-blocker approved to treat dysrhythmias. Propranolol is a non-selective beta-adrenergic blocker, affecting both beta$_1$ receptors in the heart and beta$_2$ receptors in pulmonary and vascular smooth muscle. Propranolol reduces heart rate, slows conduction velocity, and lowers blood pressure. Propranolol is most effective against tachycardia and is often combined with other drugs such as digoxin (Lanoxin) or quinidine (Quinidex) in the treatment of cardiovascular disease. It is approved to treat a wide variety of disorders, including hypertension, angina, and migraine headaches. It is also used to help prevent myocardial infarction.

Adverse Effects:

Common side effects of propranolol include hypotension and bradycardia. Because of its ability to slow the heart rate, clients with other cardiac disorders such as heart failure must be carefully monitored. Side effects such as diminished sex drive and impotence may result in non-compliance.

Mechanism in Action:

Propranolol is a non-specific beta-blocker that reduces automaticity and conduction velocity in specialized conductive cells of the heart. These effects are achieved by interfering with the binding of natural adrenergic substances such as dopamine, epinephrine, and norepinephrine, all of which increase cardiac conduction, heart rate, force of contraction, and blood pressure.

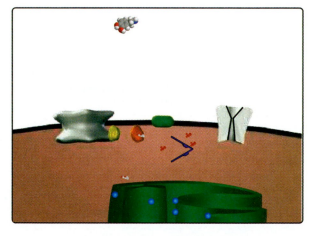

depends upon removal of potassium from the cell. The Class III drugs prolong the duration of the action potential by lengthening the refractory period, which tends to stabilize dysrhythmias. Drugs in this class generally have restricted uses because of potentially serious side effects. Drug manufacturers have been showing considerable interest in Class III drugs; in 1999, dofetilide was the first new antidysrhythmic drug approved in ten years and several others are in clinical trials. Potassium channel blockers used as antidysrhythmics are shown in Table 16.4.

TABLE 16.3	Beta-adrenergic Blockers Used for Dysrhythmias (Class II)	
DRUG	**ROUTE AND ADULT DOSE**	**REMARKS**
acebutolol hydrochloride (Sectral)	PO; 200–600 mg bid (max 1200 mg/day).	Cardioselective beta$_1$ blocker; usually reserved for ventricular dysrhythmias; also for hypertension and angina.
esmolol hydrochloride (Brevibloc)	IV; 50 μg/kg/min maintenance dose (max 200 μg/kg/min).	Very short half life of 9 min; cardioselective beta$_1$ blocker; usually reserved for immediate control of severe atrial dysrhythmias.
Pr propranolol (Inderal)	PO; 10–30 mg tid or qid (max 320 mg/day) IV; 0.5–3 mg every 4 hours prn.	Sustained release forms available; also for hypertension, prevention of MI, angina, and migraines.

DRUG PROFILE:
Amiodarone (Cardarone)

Actions:

Amiodarone is approved for the treatment of resistant ventricular tachycardia that may prove life threatening, and it has become a drug of choice for the treatment of atrial dysrhythmias in clients with heart failure. In addition to blocking potassium ion channels, some of amiodarone's actions on the heart relate to its blockade of sodium ion channels. Its onset of action may take several weeks when the drug is given orally. Its effects, however, can last four to eight weeks after the drug is discontinued because it has an extended half-life that may exceed 100 days.

Adverse Effects:

The most serious adverse effects from amiodarone occur in the lung, with the drug causing a pneumonia-like syndrome. The drug also causes blurred vision, rashes, photosensitivity, nausea, vomiting, anorexia, fatigue, dizziness, and hypotension. Amiodarone increases digoxin levels in the blood and enhances the actions of anticoagulants. As with other antidysrhythmics, clients must be closely monitored to avoid serious toxicity.

Mechanism in Action:

Amiodarone is effective in maintaining sinus rhythm in clients with atrial fibrillation, recurrent ventricular tachycardia, and fibrillation that are resistant to other types of drug therapy. Amiodarone blocks inactivated sodium channels, potassium channels, and interferes with myocardial cell-to-cell coupling.

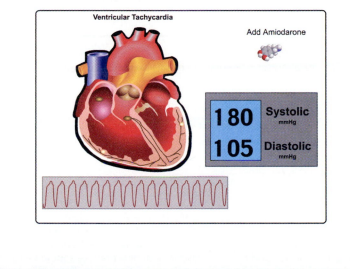

TABLE 16.4	Potassium Channel Blockers Used for Dysrhythmias (Class III)	
DRUG	**ROUTE AND ADULT DOSE**	**REMARKS**
Pr amiodarone hydrochloride (Cordarone, Pacerone)	PO; 400–600 mg/day in 1–2 divided doses; maintenance dose (max 1600 mg/day as loading dose).	IV form available; usually reserved for serious ventricular dysrhythmias.
bretylium tosylate (Bretylol)	IV; 1–2 mg/min continuous infusion (max 30 mg/kg/day).	Approved for hypotension in 1959 but no longer used for that purpose; usually reserved for serious ventricular dysrhythmias; IM form available.
dofetilide (Tikosyn)	PO; 125–500 µg bid based upon creatinine clearance (no max dose available).	Usually for atrial dysrhythmias.
sotalol (Betapace)	PO; 80 mg bid; (max 320 mg/day).	Usually reserved for serious ventricular dysrhythmias; also a non-selective beta-adrenergic blocker.

CALCIUM CHANNEL BLOCKERS

Like the beta-blockers, the calcium channel blockers are widely prescribed for various cardiovascular disorders. By slowing conduction velocity, they are able to stabilize certain dysrhythmias.

16.10 Two calcium channel blockers are available as antidysrhythmics.

Although about 10 calcium channel blockers (CCBs) are available to treat cardiovascular diseases, only a limited number have been approved for dysrhythmias. The basic pharmacology of this drug class was presented in Chapter 14 ⊂⊃ . Two important calcium channel blockers used for treating dysrhythmias are listed in Table 16.5.

Blockade of calcium ion channels has a number of effects on the heart, most of which are similar to those of beta-adrenergic blockers. Effects include reduced automaticity in the SA node and slowed impulse conduction through the AV node. This prolongs the refractory period and stabilizes many types of dysrhythmias. Calcium channel blockers are only effective against supraventricular dysrhythmias.

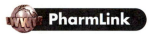

PharmLink

ALTERNATIVE ANTIDYSRHYTHMIC DRUGS

Concept review 16.4

▪ Remembering the effects of digitalis on the heart from Chapter 15, explain why most antidysrhythmic drugs have the potential to cause serious side effects in clients taking cardiac glycosides.

DRUG PROFILE:
Verapamil (Calan)

Actions:

Verapamil was the first CCB approved by the FDA. It acts by inhibiting the flow of Ca^{++} into myocardial cells and in vascular smooth muscle. In the heart, this action slows conduction velocity and stabilizes dysrhythmias. In the vessels, calcium ion channel inhibition lowers blood pressure. Verapamil also dilates the coronary arteries, an action that is important when the drug is used to treat angina (Chapter 17 ⊂⊃).

Adverse Effects:

Side effects are generally minor and may include headache, constipation, and hypotension. Because verapamil can cause bradycardia, clients with heart failure should be carefully monitored. Like many other antidysrhythmics, it has the ability to elevate blood levels of digoxin. Because both digoxin and verapamil have the effect of slowing conduction through the AV node, their concurrent use must be carefully monitored.

TABLE 16.5	Calcium Channel Blockers Used for Dysrhythmias (Class IV)	
DRUG	**ROUTE AND ADULT DOSE**	**REMARKS**
diltiazem (Cardizem, Dilacor, Tiamate, Tiazac)	IV; 5–15 mg/hr continuous infusion (max 15 mg/hour) for a maximum of 24 hr.	Oral and sustained release forms available for hypertension and angina.
Pr verapamil hydrochloride (Calan, Isoptin, Verelan)	PO; 80–160 mg tid (max 360 mg/day).	Sustained release and IV forms available; also for hypertension, angina, and migraines.

TABLE 16.6	Miscellaneous Drugs Used for Dysrhythmias	
DRUG	**ROUTE AND ADULT DOSE**	**REMARKS**
adenosine (Adenocard, Adenoscan)	IV; 6–12 mg given as a bolus injection.	Usually reserved for atrial dysrhythmias; half-life is only 10 seconds.
digoxin (Lanoxin)	PO; 0.125–0.5 mg qd; dose is individualized for each client.	Usually reserved for atrial dysrhythmias; IV and IM forms available; also for heart failure.
ibutilide fumarate (Corvert)	IV; 1 mg infused over 10 min.	Usually reserved for atrial dysrhythmias.

MISCELLANEOUS DRUGS FOR DYSRHYTHMIAS

Several other drugs are used to treat specific dysrhythmias, but do not act by the mechanisms described above. These drugs are summarized in Table 16.6.

16.11 Digoxin and several other drugs are used for specific dysrhythmias, but do not act by blocking ion channels.

Although digoxin (Lanoxin) is primarily used to treat heart failure, it is also prescribed for certain types of atrial dysrhythmias because it decreases automaticity of the SA node and slows conduction through the AV node. Excessive levels of digoxin can produce serious dysrhythmias, and interactions with other medications are common; therefore, clients must be carefully monitored during therapy. The mechanism of action and adverse effects of digoxin are described in Chapter 15 ⬜ .

Adenosine (Adenocard) and ibutilide (Corvert) are two additional drugs used for specific dysrhythmias. Adenosine is given as a one-to-two second bolus IV injection to terminate serious atrial tachycardia by slowing conduction through the AV node and decreasing automaticity of the SA node. Because of its 10-second half-life, side effects are generally self-limiting.

CLIENT TEACHING

Clients treated for dysrhythmias need to know the following:

1. Inform your healthcare practitioner if you experience very slow heart rate (<60 beats per minute), dizziness when standing up quickly, headache, or constipation while taking a CCB.
2. Inform your healthcare practitioner if systolic blood pressure is less than 90mm Hg., and do not take the next dose of CCB until you are instructed to do so.
3. Monitor your heart rate and blood pressure regularly during treatment with adenosine (Adenocard, Adenoscan) or ibutilide (Corvert).
4. Inform your dentist, surgeon, and eye doctor if you are taking propranolol (Inderal). This drug lowers intraocular pressure.
5. If you are diabetic, check your blood glucose regularly while taking beta-blockers. They can change how the body uses sugars and starches.
6. Check your pulse for decreased rate and changes in rhythm while taking antidysrhythmic drugs. Report changes to your healthcare provider. ▪

Ibutilide is also used as a short-acting IV intervention, infused over 10 minutes to quickly terminate atrial flutter and fibrillation. Ibutilide acts by prolonging the duration of the cardiac action potential. The infusion is stopped as soon as the dysrhythmia is terminated.

CHAPTER REVIEW

Core Concepts Summary

16.1 **The frequency of dysrhythmias in the population is difficult to ascertain because many clients experience no symptoms.**

Some dysrhythmias produce no symptoms and are harmless, while others are life threatening. The frequency of dysrhythmias is difficult to ascertain, although it is thought to be quite common, particularly in the geriatric population.

16.2 **Dysrhythmias are classified by the location and type of rhythm abnormality produced.**

Dysrhythmias are classified by their site of origin, either atrial or ventricular, and by the type of rhythm abnormality produced, such as tachycardia, flutter, or fibrillation. Dysrhythmias are associated with other diseases such as hypertension and heart failure.

16.3 **The electrical conduction pathway in the myocardium keeps the heart beating in a synchronized manner.**

The normal rhythm of the heart is established by the SA node, which ensures that the chambers beat in a synchronized manner. The central problem with dysrhythmias is their potential to affect the function of the heart, reduce cardiac output, and cause certain consequences such as stroke or heart failure.

16.4 **Changes in sodium and potassium levels generate the action potential in myocardial cells.**

Antidysrhythmic drugs affect the action potential in myocardial cells. They act by blocking sodium, potassium, or calcium channels in the cell membrane.

16.5 **Non-pharmacologic therapy of certain dysrhythmias is often the treatment of choice.**

All antidysrhythmic agents have the ability to cause rhythm abnormalities or worsen existing ones. Because of this, non-pharmacologic treatment is sometimes preferred over drug therapy. Dysrhythmias may be corrected using cardioversion or catheter ablation.

16.6 **Antidysrhythmic drugs are classified by their mechanism of action.**

Most antidysrhythmic medications are placed into one of five classes, based on their mechanism of action. Class I agents are further subdivided into IA, IB, and IC. Agents within the same class have similar actions and adverse effects.

16.7 **Sodium channel blockers slow the rate of impulse conduction through the heart.**

Sodium channel blockers stabilize dysrhythmias by slowing the spread of impulse conduction across the myocardium. Quinidine, a Class IA agent, is the oldest antidysrhythmic drug.

16.8 **Beta-adrenergic blockers reduce automaticity as well as slow conduction velocity in the heart.**

Beta-blockers such as propranolol stabilize dysrhythmias by slowing the heart rate and decreasing the conduction velocity through the AV node.

16.9 **Potassium channel blockers prolong the refractory period of the heart.**

Potassium channel blockers such as amiodarone stabilize dysrhythmias by prolonging the duration of the action potential and extending the refractory period.

16.10 Two calcium channel blockers are available as antidysrhythmics.

Calcium channel blockers such as verapamil have effects similar to those of beta-adrenergic blockers. These include reduced automaticity in the SA node, slowed impulse conduction through the AV node, and a prolonged refractory period.

16.11 Digoxin and several other drugs are used for specific dysrhythmias, but do not act by blocking ion channels.

Digoxin, adenosine, and ibutilide are used for specific dysrhythmias, but do not act by the mechanisms of Class I, II, III, or IV drugs. Adenosine and ibutilide are used for short-term, rapid termination of dysrhythmias.

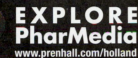 **EXPLORE PharMedia**
www.prenhall.com/holland

Additional interactive resources and activities for this chapter can be found on the Companion Website. For animations, audio glossary, and review access the accompanying CD-ROM in this book.

Mechanism in Action:
Propranolol
Amiodarone
Audio Glossary
Concept Review
NCLEX Review

 PharLinks
Childhood Dysrhythmias
Alternative Antidysrhythmic Drugs

17 Drugs for Chest Pain, Myocardial Infarction, and Stroke

CORE CONCEPTS

17.1 Chest pain is a common symptom that can have many different causes.

17.2 Heart muscle needs a continuous supply of oxygen from the coronary arteries to function properly.

ANGINA PECTORIS

17.3 Angina pectoris is characterized by severe chest pain caused by lack of sufficient oxygen to heart muscle.

17.4 Angina pain can often be controlled through lifestyle changes and surgical procedures.

17.5 The pharmacologic goals for the treatment of angina are usually achieved by reducing cardiac workload.

Organic Nitrates

17.6 The organic nitrates relieve angina by dilating veins and the coronary arteries.

Beta-adrenergic Blockers

17.7 Beta-adrenergic blockers relieve angina pain by decreasing the oxygen demands on the heart.

Calcium Channel Blockers

17.8 Calcium channel blockers relieve angina by dilating the coronary vessels and reducing the workload on the heart.

MYOCARDIAL INFARCTION

17.9 Early diagnosis of myocardial infarction increases chances of survival.

Thrombolytics

17.10 Thrombolytics are used to dissolve clots blocking the coronary arteries.

Beta-adrenergic Blockers

17.11 When given within 24 hours after the onset of myocardial infarction, beta-adrenergic blockers can improve chances of survival.

17.12 A number of additional drugs are used to treat the symptoms and complications of acute MI.

CEREBROVASCULAR ACCIDENT/STROKE

17.13 Stroke is a major cause of death and disability.

17.14 Aggressive treatment of thrombotic stroke with anticoagulants, antihypertensives, and thrombolytics can increase survival.

OBJECTIVES

After reading this chapter, the student should be able to:

1. Identify common diseases that may cause chest pain.

2. Describe how the myocardium receives its oxygen and nutrient supply.

3. Explain the pathophysiology of angina pectoris.

4. Prescribe lifestyle changes by which a client might control his/her angina.

5. For each of the following classes, identify representative drugs, explain the mechanism of drug action, primary actions, and important adverse effects as they relate to the treatment of angina.

   a. organic nitrates
   b. beta-adrenergic blockers
   c. calcium channel blockers

6. Explain the pathophysiology of myocardial infarction.

7. For each of the following classes, identify representative drugs, explain the mechanism of drug action, primary actions, and important adverse effects as they relate to the treatment of myocardial infarction.

   a. thrombolytics
   b. beta-adrenergic blockers
   c. anticoagulants and antiplatelet agents
   d. analgesics

8. Explain the pathophysiology of stroke.

9. Identify strategies used in the pharmacologic treatment of stroke.

10. Categorize drugs used to treat angina, myocardial infarction, and stroke based on their classification and mechanism of action.

PharMedia

www.prenhall.com/holland

Additional interactive resources and activities for this chapter can be found on the Companion Website. For animations, audio glossary, and review access the accompanying CD-ROM in this book.

angina pectoris (an-JEYE-nuh PEK-tore-us): acute pain in the chest upon physical or emotional exertion due to inadequate oxygen supply to the myocardium / *page 248*

atherosclerosis (ath-ur-oh-skler-OH-sis): a build-up of fatty substances and loss of elasticity of the arterial walls / *page 248*

cerebrovascular accident/stroke/brain attack (sir-ree-bro-VASK-u-lur): an acute condition of a blood clot or bleeding in a vessel in the brain / *page 259*

coronary arteries (KOR-un-air-ee AR-tur-ees): vessels that bring oxygen and nutrients to the myocardium / *page 248*

coronary arterial bypass graft (CABG): surgical procedure performed to restore blood flow to the myocardium by using a section of the saphenous vein or internal mammary artery to go around the obstructed coronary artery / *page 250*

hemorrhagic stroke (hee-moh-RAJ-ik): type of stroke caused by bleeding from a blood vessel in the brain / *page 260*

myocardial infarction (meye-oh-KAR-dee-ul in-FARK-shun): medical emergency of having a blood clot blocking a portion of a coronary artery / *page 254*

myocardial ischemia (meye-oh-KAR-dee-ul ik-SKEE-mee-uh): condition in which there is a lack of blood supply to the myocardium due to a constriction or obstruction of a blood vessel / *page 248*

percutaneous transluminal coronary angioplasty (PTCA) (per-cue-TAIN-ee-us trans-LOO-min-ul KOR-un-air-ee ANN-gee-oh-plas-tee): procedure by which a balloon-shaped catheter is used to compress fatty plaque against an arterial wall for the purpose of restoring normal blood flow / *page 250*

plaque (plak): fatty material that builds up in the lining of blood vessels and may lead to hypertension, stroke, myocardial infarction, or angina / *page 248*

reflex tachycardia (tak-ee-KAR-dee-ah): temporary speeding up of heart rate that occurs when blood pressure falls / *page 252*

stable angina: type of angina that occurs in a predictable pattern, usually relieved by rest / *page 248*

thrombotic stroke (throm-BOT-ik): type of stroke caused by a blood clot blocking an artery in the brain / *page 259*

unstable angina: type of angina that occurs frequently, with severe symptoms, and which is not relieved by rest / *page 248*

variant angina: chest pain that is caused by acute spasm of the coronary arteries rather than by physical or emotional exertion / *page 251*

All tissues in the body depend upon an adequate supply of oxygen and other nutrients that are delivered via an extensive arterial system. When these vessels become compromised—for example, clogged by fatty deposits or a clot—the tissues served by the affected arteries become starved for oxygen and their function will be affected. This chapter covers the pharmacotherapy of three such diseases: angina pectoris, myocardial infarction, and stroke.

17.1 Chest pain is a common symptom that can have many different causes.

Chest pain is a common complaint of clients seeking care in physician offices and emergency rooms. It is also one of the most frightening symptoms for clients, who often equate their pain to having a heart attack with a real risk of sudden death. The pain experienced by the client, however, is only a symptom of an underlying disorder; a large number of very diverse diseases can produce pain in the chest and some of these are unrelated to the heart. A major goal of the healthcare provider is to quickly determine the cause of the pain so that the proper treatment can be administered. Table 17.1 lists some of the common diseases that can produce chest pain as a symptom.

17.2 Heart muscle needs a continuous supply of oxygen from the coronary arteries to function properly.

The heart is the hardest-working organ in the body. While most organs' metabolism slows considerably during rest and sleep, the heart must continue pumping so that the tissues can receive the nutrients they need and dispose of the wastes they have accumulated. Being such a vital organ, the heart muscle or myocardium must receive a continuous supply of oxygen and nutrients; disturbing this flow for even brief periods can have serious and even fatal consequences.

TABLE 17.1	Examples of Disorders That May Produce Chest Pain
NAME OF DISEASE	**DESCRIPTION**
mitral stenosis	inability of the mitral valve to fully open
myocardial infarction	clot within the coronary arteries
hypertension	high systemic blood pressure
coronary artery disease	atherosclerosis of the coronary arteries
diabetes	lack of insulin or inability to tolerate carbohydrates
peptic ulcer disease	erosion of the mucosa of the stomach or small intestine
gastric reflux	backflow of stomach contents into the esophagus

myo = *muscle*
cardium = *heart*

Because the heart chambers fill with blood over 60 times per minute, one would think that the myocardium would have an ample supply of oxygen and nutrients. The myocardium, however, receives essentially no nutrients from the blood traveling through the heart's chambers. Instead, heart muscle receives its nutrients from the first two arteries branching off the aorta, the right and left coronary arteries. As these arteries branch, they circle the heart, bringing the myocardium its continuous supply of oxygen.

ANGINA PECTORIS

Angina pectoris is characterized by acute chest pain upon physical exertion or emotional stress. Although it produces many of the same symptoms as a heart attack, its pharmacological treatment is quite different.

17.3 Angina pectoris is characterized by severe chest pain caused by lack of sufficient oxygen to heart muscle.

athero = *fatty*
sclera = *hard*
osis = *condition of*

Angina occurs more frequently in women, in older clients, and in blacks. Its incidence peaks in the 65- to 74-year-old age group. The most common cause of angina is atherosclerosis: a buildup of fatty, fibrous material called plaque in the walls of arteries. Although plaque may take as long as 40 to 50 years to accumulate to a level that would cause symptoms, plaque deposition actually begins very early in life. If plaque accumulates in a coronary artery, the myocardium downstream from the affected artery begins to receive less oxygen than it needs to perform its metabolic functions. This condition of having a reduced blood supply to cardiac muscle cells is called myocardial ischemia. Figure 17.1 illustrates the progressive accumulation of plaque that is characteristic of atherosclerosis.

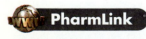

WOMEN AND HEART DISEASE

The classic presentation of angina pectoris is sharp pain in the heart region, often moving to the left side of the neck and lower jaw and down the left arm. Most often this pain is preceded by physical exertion or emotional excitement. These events increase the oxygen demand of the heart, and the clogged artery is unable to supply the nutrients needed by the stressed myocardium. With rest, anginal pain usually subsides in less than 15 minutes. Angina pectoris that is predictable in its frequency and duration is called stable angina. If angina episodes become more frequent or severe and occur during periods of rest, the condition is called unstable angina. Unstable angina requires more aggressive medical intervention. It is sometimes considered a medical emergency because it is associated with an increased risk of myocardial infarction (MI).

Angina pain may closely mimic that of an MI. It is necessary for the healthcare provider to quickly distinguish between the two diseases because the pharmacologic treatment of angina is much different from that of MI. While angina is rarely fatal, MI has a high mortality rate if treatment is delayed. Thus, drug therapy must begin immediately.

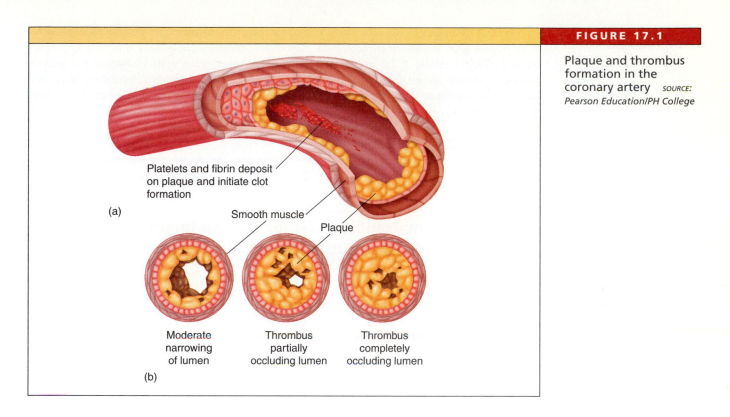

FIGURE 17.1

Plaque and thrombus formation in the coronary artery   *SOURCE: Pearson Education/PH College*

Platelets and fibrin deposit on plaque and initiate clot formation

(a)

Smooth muscle

Plaque

Moderate narrowing of lumen

Thrombus partially occluding lumen

Thrombus completely occluding lumen

(b)

Fast Facts Angina Pectoris

■ The incidence of angina peaks in the 75 to 84 age group:

4% of those 65 to 74 years old
6% of those 75 to 84 years old
4% of those over age 85

■ About 6,200,000 Americans have angina pectoris; 350,000 new cases occur each year.

■ Among ethnic groups, the incidence of angina is highest among blacks, intermediate in Mexican-Americans and lowest in non-Hispanic whites.

■ Angina occurs more frequently in women than men; black women have twice the risk of black men.

17.4 Angina can often be controlled through lifestyle changes and surgical procedures.

CORE CONCEPTS

A number of dietary and lifestyle factors have been found to be associated with an increased risk of angina. The healthcare provider should help the client control the frequency of anginal episodes by advising him/her to implement some or all of the following lifestyle changes.

■ stop using tobacco

■ limit salt (sodium) intake

■ eat foods rich in potassium and magnesium, such as bananas, beans, spinach, and tomatoes

■ limit alcohol consumption

■ implement a medically supervised exercise plan

■ reduce stress levels as much as possible

■ reduce dietary saturated fats and keep weight at an optimum level

■ if hyperlipidemia is present, have it treated

■ if hypertension is present, have it treated

angio = vessel
plasty = shaped or molded
by a surgical procedure

per = through
cutaneous = skin

When physicians discover that the coronary arteries are significantly occluded, **coronary arterial bypass graft (CABG)** or **percutaneous transluminal coronary angioplasty (PTCA)** may be performed. CABG involves the use of a surgically implanted vein graft to bypass the area of obstruction in the coronary artery. PCTA is a procedure whereby the area of narrowing is opened using either a balloon catheter or a laser. The procedure carries some risk and is not 100% effective; however, it is less invasive than CABG and many clients benefit from the procedure.

Concept review 17.1

■ How can a healthcare provider distinguish between stable angina and unstable angina?

17.5 The pharmacologic goals for the treatment of angina are usually achieved by reducing cardiac workload.

The treatment goals for a client with angina are twofold: to reduce the frequency of angina episodes and to terminate acute anginal pain in progress. The primary means by which antianginal drugs accomplish these goals is to reduce the myocardial demand for oxygen. This can be accomplished by at least four mechanisms.

- slowing the heart rate
- causing the heart to receive less blood (reduced preload) by dilating veins
- causing the heart to contract with less force (reduced contractility)
- lowering blood pressure, thus giving the heart less resistance in pushing the blood out of its chambers (reduced afterload)

Three classes of drugs—the organic nitrates, beta-adrenergic blockers, and calcium channel blockers—are used to treat angina. Drug therapy of stable angina is usually begun with the rapid-acting organic nitrates. If episodes become more frequent or severe, oral organic nitrates, beta-adrenergic blockers, or calcium channel blockers are added for prophylaxis. It is important to understand that antianginal medications only relieve symptoms and do not cure the underlying disorder. A summary of the means used to prevent and treat coronary artery disease is shown in Figure 17.2.

ORGANIC NITRATES

All drugs in this chemical class possess at least one nitrate (NO_2) group. The vasodilation effect of these agents is a result of the conversion of nitrate to its active form, nitric oxide (NO). Another nitrogen-containing drug, nitrous oxide (N_2O), is an inorganic agent used in anesthesia (Chapter 12 ⬤▬).

17.6 The organic nitrates relieve angina by dilating veins and the coronary arteries.

Since their medicinal properties were discovered in 1857, the organic nitrates have been the mainstay for the treatment of angina. The primary therapeutic action of the organic nitrates is the ability to relax both arterial and venous smooth muscle. When the organic nitrates cause venodilation, the amount of blood returning to the heart, or preload, is reduced and the chambers contain less blood. With less blood to eject, cardiac output (afterload) is reduced and the work required of the heart is decreased, thus lowering myocardial oxygen demand. This is the primary mechanism by which the organic nitrates reduce the frequency of anginal episodes and terminate chest pain in clients with stable angina.

FIGURE 17.2

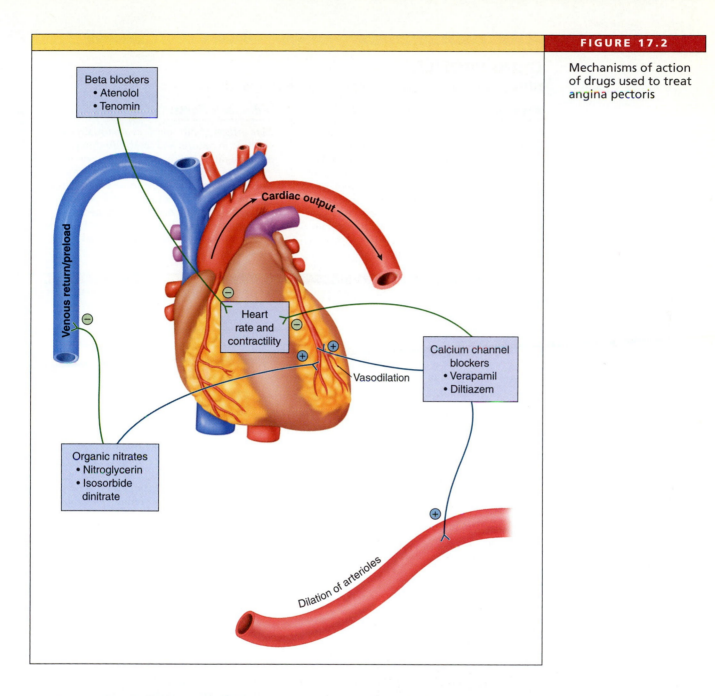

Mechanisms of action of drugs used to treat angina pectoris

Organic nitrates also have the ability to dilate coronary arteries, and this was once thought to be their primary mechanism of action. It seems logical that dilating a partially occluded coronary vessel would allow more oxygen to get to ischemic myocardial tissue. While this effect does indeed occur, is not believed to be the primary mechanism of nitrate action in stable angina. This action, however, is important in treating a less common form of angina known as variant angina, in which the chest pain is caused by spasm of a coronary artery. The organic nitrates can relax these spasms and terminate the pain.

Organic nitrates are of two types: short-acting and long-acting. The short-acting agents, such as nitroglycerin, are taken sublingually to quickly terminate an acute anginal attack in progress. Long-acting nitrates, such as isosorbide dinitrate, are taken orally or delivered through a transdermal patch to decrease the frequency and severity of anginal episodes.

trans = across or through
dermis = skin

Tolerance commonly occurs with the long-acting organic nitrates when they are taken for extended periods. The magnitude of the tolerance depends upon the dosage and the frequency of drug administration. Clients are often instructed to remove the transdermal patch for 6–12 hours each day or withhold the evening dose of the oral organic nitrate in order to delay the development of tolerance.

DRUG PROFILE:
Nitroglycerin (Nitrostat, Nitrobid, Nitro-Dur, and Others)

Actions:

Nitroglycerin, the oldest and most widely used of the organic nitrates, can be delivered by a number of different routes. It is normally taken while an acute anginal episode is in progress or just prior to physical activity. When given sublingually, it reaches peak plasma levels in only four minutes and thus can terminate anginal pain very rapidly. Chest pain that does not respond quickly to sublingual nitroglycerin may indicate myocardial infarction.

Adverse effects:

Side effects of nitroglycerin are usually cardio-vascular in nature, and rarely life threatening. Because nitroglycerin can dilate vessels in the head, headache is common and may be severe. Occasionally the venodilation created by nitro-glycerin causes reflex tachycardia. A beta-adrenergic blocker may be prescribed to diminish this undesirable increase in heart rate. The side effects of nitroglycerin often diminish after a few doses.

TABLE 17.2	Organic Nitrates Used for Angina	
DRUG	**ROUTE AND ADULT DOSE**	**REMARKS**
Pr nitroglycerin (Nitrostat, Nitrobid, Nitro-Dur, and others)	SL; 1 tablet (0.3–0.6 mg) or 1 spray (0.4–0.8 mg) q 3–5 min (max 3 doses in 15 min).	Dilates both arterial and venous blood vessels; sublingual, oral, translingual, IV, transmucosal, transdermal, and topical forms available; extended-release form available.
amyl nitrate (Vaporole)	Inhalation; 1 ampule (0.18–0.3 ml) prn.	Short-acting; onset is 10–30 seconds; may be repeated in 3–5 minutes; also used as treatment for cyanide poisoning.
erythrityl (Cardilate)	PO; 10–30 mg tid.	Sublingual form available.
isosorbide dinitrate (Isordil, Sorbitrate, Dilatrate SR)	PO; 2.5–30 mg qid.	Action similar to nitroglycerin; for both acute attacks and long term management; sublingual and chewable forms available; smaller dose is given to initiate therapy; extended-release form available.
isosorbide mononitrate (Monoket, Imdur, Ismo)	PO; 20 mg bid (max 240 mg/day with sustained release).	For the prevention of angina; a smaller dose is given to initiate therapy; extended-release form available.
pentaerythrityl (Peritrate, Duotrate, Pentylan)	PO; 10–20 mg tid or qid.	Extended-release form available.

tachy = rapid
cardia = heart

Long-acting nitrates are also useful in reducing the symptoms of heart failure. Their role in the treatment of this disease was discussed in Chapter 15 ⬭. Organic nitrates used to treat angina are listed in Table 17.2.

BETA-ADRENERGIC BLOCKERS

Beta-adrenergic blockers reduce the workload on the heart and are used for angina prophylaxis. Drugs for angina include cardioselective beta$_1$ blockers and mixed beta$_1$-beta$_2$ blockers.

17.7 Beta-adrenergic blockers relieve angina pain by decreasing the oxygen demands on the heart.

The pharmacology of the beta-adrenergic blockers was explained in Chapter 5 and in other chapters where the value of these drugs in the treatment of hypertension (Chapter 14), heart failure (Chapter 15), and dysrhythmias (Chapter 16) was presented ⚭ . Because of their ability to reduce the workload on the heart by slowing heart rate and reducing contractility, several beta-blockers are used to decrease the frequency and severity of anginal attacks caused by exertion. Clients should be advised against abruptly stopping beta-blocker therapy, as this may result in a sudden increase in workload on the heart. Selected beta-adrenergic blockers of importance to angina are listed in Table 17.3.

DRUG PROFILE:
Atenolol (Tenormin)

Actions:

Atenolol selectively blocks beta$_1$ receptors in the heart. Its effectiveness in angina is attributed to its ability to slow heart rate (negative chronotropic effect) and reduce contractility (negative inotropic effect), both of which lower myocardial oxygen demand. It is also used in the treatment of hypertension and in the prevention of MI. Because of its seven- to nine-hour half-life, it may be taken once a day.

Adverse effects:

Being a cardioselective beta$_1$ blocker, atenolol has few adverse effects on the lung and is useful for clients experiencing bronchospasm. Like other beta-blockers, therapy generally begins with low doses, which are gradually increased until the therapeutic effect is achieved. The most common side effects of atenolol include fatigue, weakness, and hypotension.

TABLE 17.3	Beta-adrenergic Blockers Used for Angina	
DRUG	**ROUTE AND ADULT DOSE**	**REMARKS**
propranolol hydrochloride (Inderal)	PO; 10–20 mg bid–tid (max 320 mg/day).	Non-selective beta$_1$ and beta$_2$ blocker; IV form available; also for hypertension, dysrhythmias, MI, and migraine prophylaxis.
🅿ʳ atenolol (Tenormin)	PO; 25–50 mg qd (max 100 mg/day).	Cardioselective beta$_1$ blocker; reduces rate and force of cardiac contractions; also for hypertension; IV form available for MI.
bisoprolol fumarate (Zebeta)	PO; 2.5–5 mg qd (max 20 mg/day).	Cardioselective beta$_1$ blocker; improves exercise tolerance in angina; may take 2–4 weeks for therapeutic effect; also for hypertension.
metoprolol tartrate (Toprol, Lopressor)	PO; 100 mg bid (max 400 mg/day).	Cardioselective beta$_1$ blocker; sustained-release form available; also for hypertension; IV form available for MI.
nadolol (Corgard)	PO; 40 mg qd (max 240 mg/day).	Non-selective beta$_1$ and beta$_2$ blocker; indicated for long-term prevention of angina; also for hypertension.
timolol maleate (Blocadren, Betimol, Timoptic)	PO; 15–45 mg tid (max 60 mg/day).	Non-selective beta$_1$ and beta$_2$ blocker; also for hypertension; topical form available for glaucoma.

CALCIUM CHANNEL BLOCKERS

Several calcium channel blockers reduce myocardial oxygen demand by both lowering blood pressure and slowing the heart rate. They are widely used in the treatment of cardiovascular disease.

17.8 Calcium channel blockers relieve angina by dilating the coronary vessels and reducing the workload on the heart.

Like beta-blockers, the calcium channel blockers (CCBs) have been discussed several times in this text for the treatment of hypertension (Chapter 14) and dysrhythmias (Chapter 16 ⬭). The first approved use of CCBs was for the treatment of angina. Blockade of calcium ion channels has a number of effects on the heart, most of which are similar to those of beta-adrenergic blockers.

CCBs cause arteriolar smooth muscle to relax, thus lowering peripheral resistance and reducing blood pressure. This reduction in afterload decreases the myocardial oxygen demand, thus reducing the frequency of anginal pain. Some CCBs are selective for arterioles. Others, such as verapamil and diltiazem, have an additional beneficial effect of slowing the heart rate (negative chronotropic effect). Because they relax arterial smooth muscle, the CCBs are useful in treating variant angina, where the coronary vessels are constricted by acute spasm. CCBs of importance to angina are listed in Table 17.4.

Concept review 17.2

■ How does decreasing the workload on the heart result in reduction in anginal pain?

MYOCARDIAL INFARCTION

A myocardial infarction (MI) is the result of a sudden occlusion of a coronary artery. Immediate pharmacologic treatment may reduce client mortality.

17.9 Early diagnosis of myocardial infarction increases chances of survival.

Heart attacks, or **myocardial infarctions**, are responsible for a substantial number of deaths each year. Some clients die before reaching a medical facility for treatment and many others die within

---

DRUG PROFILE (Calcium Channel Blocker):
Diltiazem (Cardizem)

Actions:

Diltiazem inhibits the transport of calcium ions into myocardial cells and has the ability to relax both coronary and peripheral blood vessels. It is useful in the treatment of atrial dysrhythmias and hypertension, as well as angina. When given as extended release capsules, it may be administered once daily.

Adverse Effects:

Side effects of diltiazem are generally not serious and are related to vasodilation: headache, dizziness, and edema of the ankles and feet. Although diltiazem produces few adverse effects on the heart or vessels, it should be used with caution in clients taking other cardiovascular medications, particularly digoxin or beta-adrenergic blockers; the combined effects of these drugs may cause heart failure or dysrhythmias.

TABLE 17.4	Calcium Channel Blockers of Importance to Angina	
DRUG	**ROUTE AND ADULT DOSE**	**REMARKS**
verapamil hydrochloride (Calan Isotopin, Verelan)	PO; 80 mg tid-qid (max 480 mg/day).	Dilates coronary arteries and inhibits coronary artery spasm; also for hypertension; sustained-release form available; IV form available for dysrhythmias.
amlodipine (Norvasc)	PO; 5–10 mg qd (max 10 mg/day).	Also for hypertension; combined with the ACE inhibitor benazopril to form the drug Lotrel.
bepridil hydrochloride (Vascor)	PO; 200 mg qd (max 400 mg/day).	Also blocks sodium channels; usually reserved for clients unresponsive to safer antianginals.
Pr diltiazem (Cardizem, Dilacor, Tiamate, Triazac)	PO; 30 mg qid (max 360 mg/day).	Dilates coronary arteries and decreases coronary artery spasm; sustained-release form available; also for hypertension; IV form available for dysrhythmias.
nicardipine hydrochloride (Cardene)	PO; 20–40 mg tid or 30–60 mg SR bid (max 120 mg/day).	Also for hypertension; sustained-release and IV forms available.
nifedipine (Procardia, Aldalat)	PO; 10–20 mg tid (max 180 mg/day).	Used in the treatment of vasospastic (Printzmetal's) angina; also for hypertension; sustained-release form available.

a day or two after the initial MI. Clearly, MI is a serious and frightening disease and one responsible for a large percentage of sudden deaths.

Fast Facts Myocardial Infarction

- About 1,100,000 Americans experience a new or recurrent MI each year.
- About one-third of clients experiencing an MI will die.
- About 250,000 Americans each year die of an acute MI within one hour of the onset of the symptoms.
- About 60% of clients who died suddenly of MI had no previous symptoms of the disease.
- Mortality from MI is slightly higher in males than females.
- Because women have heart attacks at older ages, they are more likely to die from them within a few weeks.
- More than 20% of men and 40% of women will die from heart attack within one year after being diagnosed.

ON THE JOB

The Nuclear Medicine Technologist and Heart Disease

The nuclear medicine technologist (NMT) is an essential healthcare provider who administers radioactive drugs, called *radioisotopes,* for the purpose of diagnosing disease. The NMT performs several tests that assist physicians in determining the degree of myocardial damage resulting from an MI.

Thallium-201 is a radioisotope that is taken up by myocardial cells in five to 15 minutes following IV administration. The patient is placed in front of a device called a *gamma camera* that measures the amount of thallium-201 in the heart muscle. Areas with diminished or absent blood flow will not contain thallium-201 and thus will appear blue or as "cold" spots. Generally, two scans are performed: one during treadmill exercise and one a few hours later under resting conditions.

Thallium itself is a toxic element. However, the amounts used in nuclear medicine scans are minute. The radioactivity is rapidly removed from the blood and excreted by the kidneys. Areas of decreased blood supply may retain thallium-201 for several hours. ▪

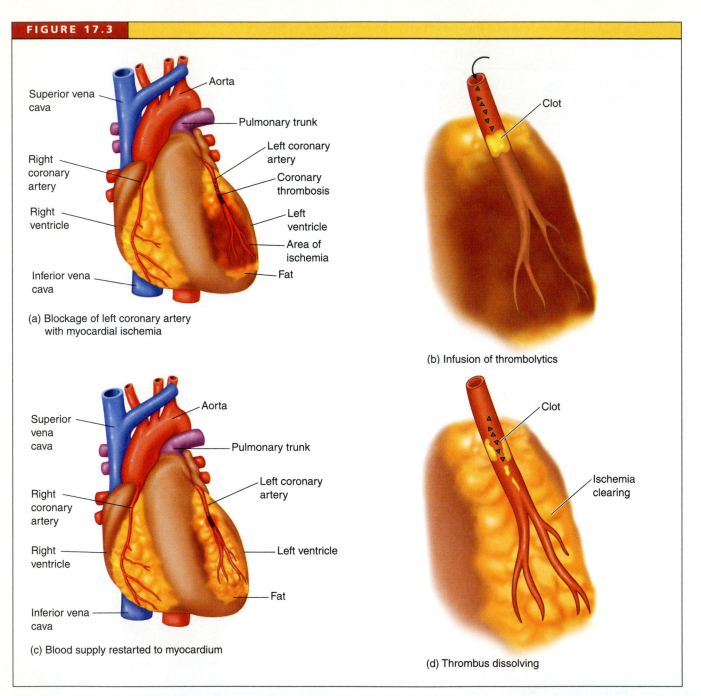

(a) Blockage of left coronary artery with myocardial ischemia

Superior vena cava — Aorta — Pulmonary trunk — Left coronary artery — Coronary thrombosis — Right coronary artery — Right ventricle — Left ventricle — Area of ischemia — Inferior vena cava — Fat

(b) Infusion of thrombolytics — Clot

(c) Blood supply restarted to myocardium

Superior vena cava — Aorta — Pulmonary trunk — Left coronary artery — Right coronary artery — Right ventricle — Left ventricle — Inferior vena cava — Fat

(d) Thrombus dissolving — Clot — Ischemia clearing

Blockage and reperfusion following myocardial infarction: (a) blockage of left coronary artery with myocardial ischemia; (b) infusion of thrombolytics; (c) blood supply returning to myocardium; (d) thrombus dissolving and ischemia clearing   SOURCE: (17.3A and 17.3C): Pearson Education/PH College

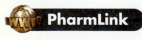 **PharmLink**

SEX AFTER HEART ATTACKS

The primary cause of myocardial infarction is advanced coronary artery disease. Plaque build-up can narrow the coronary arteries that supply the myocardium with its essential oxygen. Pieces of plaque may break off and lodge in a small vessel serving a portion of the myocardium. Deprived of its oxygen supply, this area becomes ischemic and cardiac cells can die unless their blood supply is quickly restored. Figure 17.3 illustrates this blockage and the resulting reperfusion process.

The goals of the pharmacologic treatment of acute MI include the following.

■ to restore blood supply (perfusion) to the damaged myocardium as quickly as possible through the use of thrombolytics

- to reduce myocardial oxygen demand with organic nitrates or beta-blockers in order to prevent subsequent MIs
- to control or prevent associated dysrhythmias with beta-blockers or other antidysrhythmics
- to reduce post-MI mortality with aspirin and ACE inhibitors
- to control MI pain and associated anxiety with analgesics

THROMBOLYTICS

Thrombolytics dissolve existing clots. Immediate treatment with these medications may restore circulation to the myocardium and reduce the high mortality associated with MI.

17.10 Thrombolytics are used to dissolve clots blocking the coronary arteries.

The basic pharmacology of the thrombolytics was presented in Chapter 13 ⬭ . In the treatment of MI, the goal of thrombolytic therapy is to dissolve clots that are obstructing the coronary arteries, thus restoring circulation to the myocardium. Quick restoration of cardiac circulation has been found to reduce mortality from the disease. After the clot is successfully dissolved, anticoagulant or antiplatelet therapy is initiated to prevent the formation of additional thrombi. Dosages and descriptions of the various thrombolytics are given in Chapter 13 ⬭ .

  Thrombolytics have a narrow margin of safety. The primary risk of thrombolytics is excessive bleeding from interference in the clotting process. Vital signs must be monitored continuously and any signs of bleeding generally call for discontinuation of therapy. Because these medications are rapidly destroyed in the blood, discontinuation of the drug normally results in the rapid termination of any adverse effects.

BETA-ADRENERGIC BLOCKERS

Like their use in angina, beta-blockers are used in MI clients to reduce the cardiac workload. Recent research suggests that their use may reduce mortality following an MI.

17.11 When given within 24 hours after the onset of myocardial infarction, beta-adrenergic blockers can improve chances of survival.

The basic pharmacology and usefulness of the beta-adrenergic blockers in the treatment of cardiovascular disease has been discussed in a number of chapters in this text. This section will focus on their use in the treatment of MI.

  Beta-blockers have the ability to slow the heart rate (negative chronotropic effect), decrease contractility (negative inotropic effect), and reduce blood pressure. These three actions reduce myocardial oxygen demand, which is beneficial for clients who experienced a recent MI. In addition, their ability to slow impulse conduction through the heart tends to suppress dysrhythmias, which can be serious and sometimes fatal complications following MI. When given within eight hours after the onset of acute MI, beta-blockers have been shown to reduce mortality in these clients. Beta-blockers of importance to MI are listed in Table 17.5.

17.12 A number of additional drugs are used to treat the symptoms and complications of acute MI.

A number of additional drugs have proven useful in treating the client presenting with an acute MI. Aspirin has been found to reduce mortality dramatically in the weeks following an acute MI.

DRUG PROFILE (Thrombolytic):
Reteplase (Retavase)

Actions:

Reteplase is one of the newer thrombolytics. Like other drugs in this class, reteplase is most effective if given within 30 minutes but not later than 12 hours after the onset of MI symptoms. It usually acts within 20 minutes and restoration of circulation to the ischemic site may be faster than with other thrombolytics. After the clot has been dissolved, heparin therapy is often started to prevent additional clots from forming.

Adverse Effects:

Reteplase is contraindicated in clients with active bleeding. Healthcare providers must be vigilant in recognizing and reporting any abnormal bleeding that may occur during thrombolytic therapy.

Mechanism in Action:

The thrombolytic, reteplase, dissolves blood clots by activating plasminogen, a protein found within many body tissues and the general circulation. Upon activation, plasminogen binds to fibrin, which is the mesh-like substance forming the insoluble clot. Thrombolytics remove clots and restore circulation to injured or occluded blood vessels.

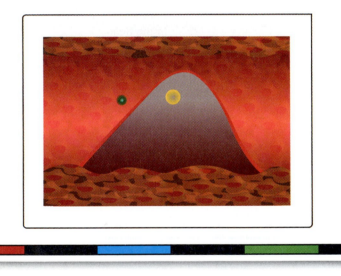

Unless contraindicated, 160–324 mg of aspirin is given as soon as possible following a suspected MI. The basic pharmacology of aspirin is covered in Chapters 11 and 20. Other coagulation modifiers, such as the glycoprotein IIb/IIIa blockers or the ADP receptor blockers, may be given to prevent further thrombi formation (Chapter 13 ⊂⊃).

DRUG PROFILE (Beta-adrenergic Blocker):
Metoprolol (Lopressor)

Actions:

Metoprolol is a selective beta$_1$ antagonist. When given intravenously, it quickly acts to reduce myocardial oxygen demand. Following an acute MI, metoprolol is infused slowly until a target heart rate is reached, usually 60 to 90 beats per minute. Upon hospital discharge, clients can be switched to oral forms of the drug. Metoprolol is also approved for angina, hypertension, and myocardial infarction.

Adverse Effects:

Because it is selective for blocking beta$_1$ receptors in the heart, metoprolol has few adverse effects on other autonomic organs and thus is preferred over non-selective agents such as propranolol for clients with lung disorders. Side effects are generally minor and relate to its autonomic activity, such as bradycardia and hypotension. Because of its multiple effects on the heart, clients with disorders such as heart failure should be carefully monitored.

TABLE 17.5	Beta-adrenergic Blockers Used for Myocardial Infarction	
DRUG	**ROUTE AND ADULT DOSE**	**REMARKS**
propranolol (Inderal)	PO; 60–80 mg tid (max 240 mg/day).	Non-selective beta$_1$ and beta$_2$ blocker; IV form available; also for hypertension, dysrhythmias, angina, and migraine prophylaxis.
acebutolol hydrochloride (Sectral)	PO; 400–800 mg qd (max 1200 mg/day).	Cardioselective beta$_1$ blocker; decreases cardiac output; also for hypertension, dysrhythmias, and angina.
atenolol (Tenormin)	IV; 5 mg q 5 min for 2 doses then begin PO 50 mg qd (give 1st dose 10 min after 2nd IV dose) (max 100 mg/day).	Cardioselective beta$_1$ blocker; also for hypertension.
Pr metoprolol (Toprol, Lopressor)	IV; 5 mg q 2 min for 3 doses followed by PO doses.	Cardioselective beta$_1$ blocker; also for hypertension and angina.
timolol maleate (Blocadren, Betimol)	PO; 10 mg bid (max 60 mg/day).	Non-selective beta$_1$ and beta$_2$ blocker; also for hypertension and angina; topical form available for glaucoma.

The ACE inhibitors, captopril (Capoten) and lisinopril (Prinivil, Zestoretic), have also been found to reduce mortality following MI. These drugs are most effective when therapy is started within a day or two after the onset of symptoms. Oral therapy with the ACE inhibitors normally begins after thrombolytic therapy has been completed and the patient's condition has stabilized. The pharmacology of the ACE inhibitors and the drug profile for lisinopril is presented in Chapter 15 ⊂⊃ .

Pain control is essential following acute MI in order to ensure client comfort and to reduce stress. Narcotic analgesics such as morphine sulfate are sometimes given to ease the pain associated with acute MI and to sedate the anxious client. Details on the pharmacology of the narcotic analgesics were presented in Chapter 11 ⊂⊃ .

Concept review 17.3

▪ Why is it important to treat an MI within the first 24 hours after symptoms have begun? What classes of drugs are used for this purpose?

CEREBROVASCULAR ACCIDENT (CVA)/STROKE

Stroke, a major cause of disability, is caused by a thrombus or bleeding within a vessel serving the brain. Although drug therapy is limited, immediate treatment may reduce the degree of permanent disability resulting from a stroke.

17.13 Stroke is a major cause of death and disability.

Cerebrovascular accident (CVA) or stroke is a major cause of permanent disability. The majority of strokes are caused by a thrombus in a vessel serving the brain (thrombotic stroke). Areas downstream from the clot lose their oxygen supply and neural tissue will begin to die unless circulation is quickly restored. A smaller percentage of strokes, about 20%, are caused by rupture of a

cerebro = head or brain
vascular = vessels

cerebral vessel and its associated bleeding into neural tissue (hemorrhagic stroke). Symptoms are the same for the two types of strokes. Specific symptoms will vary widely depending upon which area of the brain is affected and may include blindness, paralysis, speech problems, coma, and even dementia. Mortality from stroke is very high: as many as 40% of clients will die within the first year following the stroke.

Fast Facts Stroke (Brain Attack)

- Stroke is the third leading cause of death, behind heart disease and cancer.
- Between 1986 and 1996, the death rate due to stroke fell about 14%.
- Thirty percent of those who suffer stroke will die within one year of the attack.
- The incidence of brain attack increases with age (per 1000 population), although one-quarter of all strokes occur under age 65:

  14% of those 65–74 years old
  25% of those 75–84 years old
  28% of those over age 85
- About 4,400,000 stroke survivors are alive in the United States; 600,000 new cases occur each year.
- The highest incidence of stroke is in black men—more than double that of white women.
- Stroke occurs more frequently in men than women, although females account for about 60% of all deaths due to stroke.
- Over 160,000 Americans die of stroke each year.

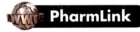
PharmLink

SUPPORT FOR STROKE VICTIMS

Many of the risk factors associated with stroke are the same as for other cardiovascular diseases such as hypertension and coronary artery disease. Lifestyle changes such as those in the following list may reduce the client's risk of experiencing a stroke.

- stop using tobacco
- limit salt (sodium) intake
- eat foods rich in potassium and magnesium, such as bananas, beans, spinach, and tomatoes
- limit alcohol consumption
- implement a medically supervised exercise plan
- reduce stress levels as much as possible
- reduce dietary saturated fats and keep weight at an optimum level
- if hyperlipidemia is present, have it treated
- if hypertension is present, have it treated

NATURAL ALTERNATIVES

Ginkgo Biloba for Cardiovascular Disease

Ginkgo biloba is a popular botanical that is often used for its effect on the brain. Ginkgo trees are native to China, Japan, and Korea and grow to be quite large. The trees are known for their extreme longevity, living to be over a hundred years old. They do not even flower for the first 20 years. The medicinal parts of the tree include the seeds and leaves. Ginkgo is available in liquid and solid forms and may be taken in drinks such as tea. The average daily dose is 120 mg of dried extract in two to three doses per day.

A considerable number of clinical studies have been conducted on ginkgo extracts. Active ingredients include flavenoids and terpenes. Effects include anticoagulant activity and an increase in blood flow to the brain and peripheral arteries. These effects are thought to be responsible for claims that ginkgo prevents strokes and improves cerebral blood flow following strokes. Controlled studies have not definitively proven these anti-stroke effects. ▪

17.14 Aggressive treatment of thrombotic stroke with anticoagulants, antihypertensives, and thrombolytics can increase survival.

Drug therapy of thrombotic stroke focuses on two main goals: prevention of strokes through the use of anticoagulants and antihypertensive agents, and restoration of blood supply to the affected portion of the brain as quickly as possible after an acute stroke through the use of thrombolytics.

As discussed in Chapter 14 ⬤▭ , sustained, chronic hypertension is closely associated with stroke. Antihypertensive therapy with beta-adrenergic blockers, calcium channel blockers, diuretics, and/or ACE inhibitors can help control blood pressure and reduce the probability of stroke.

Aspirin, through its anticoagulant properties, has been found to reduce the incidence of stroke. When given in very low doses, aspirin discourages the formation of thrombi by inhibiting platelet aggregation. Clients are sometimes placed on low-dose aspirin therapy on a continual basis following their first stroke. Ticlopidine (Ticlid) is an antiplatelet drug that may be used to provide anticoagulation in clients who cannot tolerate aspirin. Other anticoagulants such as warfarin may be given to prevent stroke in high-risk clients such as those with prosthetic heart valves. More detailed information on anticoagulant and antiplatelet agents is found in Chapter 13 ⬤▭ .

The single most important breakthrough in the treatment of stroke was development of the thrombolytic agents. Prior to the discovery of these drugs, the treatment of stroke was largely a passive, wait-and-see strategy. Now, stroke is aggressively treated with thrombolytics as soon as the client arrives at the hospital: these agents are most effective if administered within three hours of the attack. Use of aggressive thrombolytic therapy can completely restore brain function in a significant number of stroke clients. Because stroke is now viewed as a condition requiring immediate treatment, the disease has been renamed **brain attack**. Further information on the pharmacology of the thrombolytics can be found in Chapter 13.

CLIENT TEACHING

Clients treated for chest pain or stroke need to know the following:

1. As soon as you experience anginal pain, dissolve one nitroglycerin tablet under the tongue. If pain is not relieved in five minutes, use another. Many practitioners recommend a third nitroglycerin for pain not relieved five minutes after the second dose. If your chest pain/pressure is not relieved by three doses of nitroglycerin, call emergency medical services.

2. If you are using transdermal patches, rotate the application site and do not apply a new patch until after you have removed the old one.

3. Change positions slowly. Postural hypotension may cause dizziness and even fainting.

4. Monitor your blood pressure regularly and report any consistent changes to your healthcare provider.

5. Do not eat large or inconsistent amounts of foods high in vitamin K while taking warfarin, as this interferes with clotting time.

6. Do not take herbal supplements or OTC drugs before getting advice from your healthcare provider. Many drugs increase or decrease the effects of warfarin. ▪

CHAPTER REVIEW

 Core Concepts Summary

17.1 **Chest pain is a common symptom that can have many different causes.**

Chest pain is a common complaint and a frightening symptom for clients. The healthcare provider must quickly determine the cause of the pain so that appropriate treatment can be administered.

17.2 **Heart muscle needs a continuous supply of oxygen from the coronary arteries to function properly.**

The myocardium receives no oxygen or nutrients from the blood flowing through the atria or ventricles. The high metabolic rate of the heart requires that a continuous supply of oxygen be maintained in the coronary arteries.

17.3 **Angina pectoris is characterized by severe chest pain caused by lack of sufficient oxygen to heart muscle.**

The coronary arteries can become partially occluded with plaque, resulting in ischemia. Lack of sufficient oxygen to the myocardium causes sharp chest pain upon emotional or physical exertion, the characteristic symptom of angina.

17.4 **Angina pain can often be controlled through lifestyle changes and surgical procedures.**

A number of lifestyle changes can reduce the deposition of plaque in the coronary arteries and help prevent coronary artery disease.

17.5 **The pharmacologic goals for the treatment of angina are usually achieved by reducing cardiac workload.**

Reducing the workload on the heart can relieve anginal pain. This can be accomplished by slowing the heart rate, venodilation, reducing the force of myocardial contraction, or by reducing blood pressure.

17.6 **The organic nitrates relieve angina pain by dilating veins and the coronary arteries.**

Fast-acting organic nitrates can quickly terminate anginal pain by causing venodilation, which reduces the workload on the heart. They also dilate the coronary arteries, bringing more oxygen to the heart. Long-acting nitrates can prevent acute angina episodes, but the patient may become tolerant to their protective effect.

17.7 **Beta-adrenergic blockers relieve angina pain by decreasing the oxygen demands on the heart.**

Beta-blockers lower blood pressure, slow the heart, and reduce the force of contraction, thus reducing the workload on the myocardium. They are prescribed to reduce the frequency of acute anginal episodes.

17.8 **Calcium channel blockers relieve angina by dilating the coronary vessels and reducing the workload on the heart.**

CCBs are effective at lowering blood pressure, thus reducing the workload on the heart. They are prescribed to reduce the frequency of acute anginal attacks.

17.9 **Early diagnosis of myocardial infarction increases chances of survival.**

Myocardial infarction is caused by a thrombus in a coronary artery and is responsible for a substantial number of sudden deaths. Fast, effective diagnosis and treatment can reduce mortality.

17.10 **Thrombolytics are used to dissolve clots blocking the coronary arteries.**

When used within hours after the onset of MI, thrombolytics can dissolve the clot and restore circulation to the myocardium.

17.11 **When given within 24 hours after the onset of myocardial infarction, beta-adrenergic blockers can improve chances of survival.**

Beta-blockers can slow the heart and reduce blood pressure, which has been shown to reduce mortality when they are given soon after MI symptoms appear.

17.12 **A number of additional drugs are used to treat the symptoms and complications of acute MI.**

Aspirin and ACE inhibitors have been shown to reduce mortality when given soon after the onset of

MI. Narcotic analgesics are sometimes given to reduce the pain and anxiety associated with an MI.

17.13   Stroke is a major cause of death and disability.

Stroke, or brain attack, is caused by either a thrombus or bleeding in a cerebral vessel. It is a major cause of death and disability. Clients can lower their risk of stroke by adopting many of the same lifestyle changes as with coronary artery disease or hypertension.

17.14   Aggressive treatment of thrombotic stroke with anticoagulants, antihypertensives and thrombolytics can increase survival.

Stroke, or brain attack, is now viewed as an emergency condition requiring immediate treatment in order to improve client prognosis. Thrombolytics, when given quickly after the onset of stroke, can restore some or all brain function. Some degree of stroke prevention can be achieved by using anticoagulants and by controlling blood pressure.

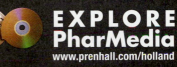 **EXPLORE PharMedia**
www.prenhall.com/holland

Additional interactive resources and activities for this chapter can be found on the Companion Website. For animations, audio glossary, and review access the accompanying CD-ROM in this book.

Mechanism in Action:
   Reteplase
Audio Glossary
Concept Review
NCLEX Review

 PharLinks
   Women and Heart Disease
   Sex After Heart Attacks
   Support for Stroke Victims

18 Drugs for Shock and Anaphylaxis

CORE CONCEPTS

18.1 Shock has many different causes.

18.2 Shock is a clinical syndrome characterized by collapse of the circulatory system.

18.3 The initial treatment of shock includes administration of basic life support and identification of the underlying cause.

Vasoconstrictor Agents

18.4 Vasoconstrictors are sometimes needed during shock to maintain blood pressure.

Cardiotonic Agents

18.5 Cardiotonic drugs are useful in reversing the decreased cardiac output resulting from shock.

18.6 Anaphylaxis is a special kind of shock involving a hyper-response of body defense mechanisms.

OBJECTIVES

After reading this chapter, the student should be able to:

1. Compare and contrast the different types of shock.

2. Relate the general symptoms of shock to their physiological causes.

3. Explain the initial treatment of a client with shock.

4. For each of the following classes, identify representative drug, explain the mechanism of drug action, primary actions, and important adverse effects.

   a. adrenergic-agonists and other vasoconstrictors
   b. cardiotonic agents
   c. antihistamines
   d. corticosteroids

5. Categorize drugs used in the treatment of shock based on their classification and mechanism of action.

PharMedia
www.prenhall.com/holland

Additional interactive resources and activities for this chapter can be found on the Companion Website. For animations, audio glossary, and review access the accompanying CD-ROM in this book.

Shock *is a condition in which vital tissues are not receiving enough blood to function properly. Without adequate oxygen and other nutrients, cells cannot carry on normal metabolism. Shock is considered a medical emergency; failure to reverse the causes and symptoms of shock may lead to irreversible organ damage and death. Most types of shock have a high mortality rate. This chapter will examine how drugs are used to aid in the treatment of different types of shock.*

Fast Facts Shock

- Cardiogenic shock occurs in 7–10% of the clients suffering acute MI.
- Cardiogenic shock is the leading cause of death in clients hospitalized with acute MI, with a mortality rate of 70–80%.
- The mortality rate for clients with sepsis who develop septic shock is 40–70%.
- Incidence of anaphylaxis may be twice as high in women as in men.

18.1 Shock has many different causes.

There are several types of shock, each having different causes. The most useful method for classifying the different types is by naming the underlying pathological process or organ system causing the disease. Table 18.1 lists the different types of shock and their primary causes. This chapter will examine the pharmacologic therapy of two common types of shock: cardiogenic and anaphylactic.

18.2 Shock is a clinical syndrome characterized by collapse of the circulatory system.

Shock is a collection of signs and symptoms, many of which are nonspecific. Although symptoms vary somewhat among the different kinds of shock, there are some similarities. For example, the client may appear pale and claim to feel sick or weak without reporting any specific symptoms. Behavioral changes are often some of the earliest symptoms and may include restlessness, anxiety, confusion, depression, and lack of interest. Thirst is a common complaint; the skin may feel cold or clammy.

Assessing the client's cardiovascular status may give some important signs for a diagnosis of shock. Blood pressure is often low with a diminished cardiac output. Heart rate may be rapid with a weak pulse. Breathing is usually rapid and shallow. Figure 18.1 shows some of the common symptoms of a client in shock.

TABLE 18.1	Classification of Shock	
TYPE OF SHOCK	**DEFINITION**	**UNDERLYING PATHOLOGY**
cardiogenic	Failure of the heart to pump sufficient blood to tissues	Left heart failure, myocardial ischemia, myocardial infarction, dysrhythmias, pulmonary embolism, myocardial, or pericardial infection
hypovolemic	Loss of blood volume	Hemorrhage, burns, profuse sweating, excessive urination, vomiting, or diarrhea
neurogenic	Vasodilation due to over-stimulation of the parasympathetic or under-stimulation of the sympathetic nervous systems	Trauma to spinal cord or medulla, severe emotional stress or pain, drugs that depress the central nervous system
septic	Multiple organ dysfunction as a result of pathogenic organisms in the blood	Widespread inflammatory response to bacterial, fungal, or parasitic infection
anaphylactic	Acute allergic reaction	Severe reaction to allergen such as penicillin, nuts, shellfish, or animal proteins

hypo = *below*
vol = *volume*
emic = *pertaining to the blood*

neuro = *nervous system*
genic = *origin*

cardio = *heart*
genic = *origin*

Diagnosis of shock is rarely made on the basis of such nonspecific symptoms. A careful medical history, however, will give the healthcare provider valuable clues as to what type of shock may be present. For example, obvious trauma or bleeding combined with the above symptoms would suggest hypovolemic shock. If trauma to the brain or spinal cord is evident, neurogenic shock may be suspected. A history of heart disease would suggest cardiogenic shock, while a recent infection may indicate septic shock. A history of allergy with a sudden onset of symptoms following food or drug intake may suggest anaphylactic shock.

A hallmark of most types of shock is the inability of the cardiovascular system to send sufficient blood to the vital organs, with the heart and brain being affected early in the progression of the disease. Lack of blood to the brain may result in fainting, whereas disruption of blood supply to the myocardium may cause permanent damage to these vital cells. Without immediate treatment, other organ systems will be affected and respiratory failure or renal failure may result.

18.3 The initial treatment of shock includes administration of basic life support and identification of the underlying cause.

Shock is treated as a medical emergency and the first goal is to provide basic life support. Rapid identification of the underlying cause is essential because the client's condition may deteriorate rapidly. Keeping the client quiet and warm until specific therapy can be initiated is important. Maintaining an open airway, adequate respiration, and normal blood pressure is critical. If the

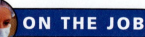

ON THE JOB

The Radiographer and Contrast Media

The radiographer is an integral member of the healthcare team who administers X-radiation for the purpose of obtaining images for the diagnosis of disease. In order to demonstrate the urinary tract, arteries, or veins, the radiographer must use drugs called radiopaque contrast media. This contrast media contains a relatively high percentage of iodine (14–48%) an element that is very dense and that will absorb X-rays.

Some clients are allergic to iodine, and administration of these iodine-based drugs may cause acute anaphylaxis. Radiographers must obtain a thorough drug history prior to administration of the contrast medium. This includes a history of food allergies, particularly to seafood and shellfish that contain high amounts of iodine. An accurate history will alert the X-ray physician, known as the *radiologist,* to potential adverse reactions and perhaps prevent serious effects from occurring. ■

FIGURE 18.1

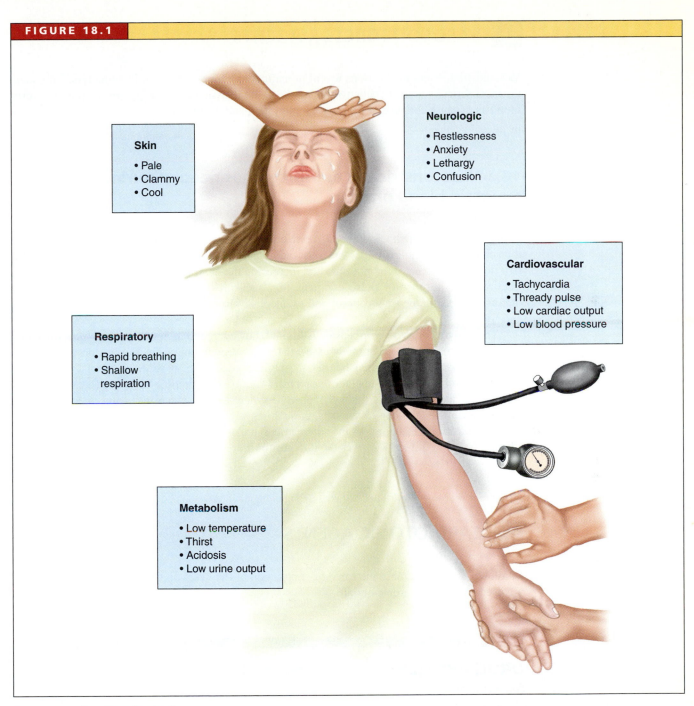

Skin
- Pale
- Clammy
- Cool

Neurologic
- Restlessness
- Anxiety
- Lethargy
- Confusion

Cardiovascular
- Tachycardia
- Thready pulse
- Low cardiac output
- Low blood pressure

Respiratory
- Rapid breathing
- Shallow respiration

Metabolism
- Low temperature
- Thirst
- Acidosis
- Low urine output

Symptoms of a client in shock

client has lost significant blood or other body fluids, immediate maintenance of blood volume through the administration of fluid and electrolytes or blood products is essential. Sodium bicarbonate may be administered to reverse the acidosis that may occur during shock. Details of fluid and electrolyte therapy are presented in Chapter 27 ⬭ . Once basic life support is established, the healthcare practitioner can begin more specific treatment of the underlying causes of the shock.

Concept review 18.1

■ How would a paramedic arriving on the scene of a motorcycle accident determine the cause of his/her client's shock?

VASOCONSTRICTOR AGENTS

Vasoconstrictors are medications useful in maintaining blood pressure. In some types of shock, the most serious medical challenge facing the client is hypotension, which may become so profound as to cause collapse of the circulatory system and death.

18.4 Vasoconstrictors are sometimes needed during shock to maintain blood pressure.

In the early stages of shock, the body compensates for the fall in blood pressure by increasing the activity of the sympathetic nervous system. This sympathetic activity results in vasoconstriction, thus raising blood pressure and increasing the heart rate and force of myocardial contraction. The purpose of these compensatory measures is to maintain blood flow to vital organs such as the heart and brain and to decrease flow to other organs such as the kidneys and liver.

The body's ability to compensate is limited, however, and as shock progresses, a profound hypotension may develop. In many cases, the developing hypotension requires drug therapy. A number of vasoconstrictors may be used to stabilize blood pressure in shock clients. Adrenergic-agonists used for shock include norepinephrine (Levarterenol, Levophed), metaraminol (Aramine), methoxamine (Vasoxyl), phenylephrine (Neo-Synephrine), and mephentermine (Wyamine). When given intravenously, these drugs have ability to immediately raise blood pressure. The basic pharmacology of the adrenergic-agonists, or sympathomimetics, was discussed in Chapter 6 ⬚⬚⬚ . Table 18.2 gives the dosages for these agents.

CARDIOTONIC AGENTS

Cardiotonic drugs increase the force of contraction of the heart. In the treatment of shock, they are used to increase cardiac output.

DRUG PROFILE (Vasoconstrictor):
Norepinephrine (Levarterenol, Levophed)

Actions:

Norepinephrine is a sympathomimetic that acts directly on alpha-adrenergic-receptors in the smooth muscle of blood vessels to rapidly raise blood pressure. Its stimulation of beta$_1$ receptors in the heart produces a positive inotropic response that increases cardiac output. The primary uses of this drug are for acute shock and cardiac arrest. Because it is only administered by the IV route, its onset of action is immediate.

Adverse Effects:

Norepinephrine is a very powerful vasoconstrictor; thus, continuous monitoring of the client's blood pressure is required in order to avoid hypertension. When first administered, a reflex bradycardia is sometimes experienced. It also has the ability to produce various types of dysrhythmias. Because of its potent effects on the cardiovascular system, it should be used with great caution on clients with heart disease.

TABLE 18.2	Vasoconstrictors of Importance to Shock	
DRUG	**ROUTE AND ADULT DOSE**	**REMARKS**
Pr norepinephrine bitartrate (Levarterenol, Levophed)	IV; 8–12 μg/min until pressure stabilizes, then 2–4 μg/min for maintenance.	Has both alpha and beta$_1$ adrenergic activity; also for cardiac arrest.
mephentermine sulfate (Wyamine)	IV; 20–60 mg as an infusion (1.2 mg/ml of D5W).	Has alpha and predominant beta-adrenergic activity; also for certain cardiac dysrhythmias.
metaraminol bitartrate (Aramine)	IV; 0.5–5 mg followed by infusion of 15–100 mg in 500 ml D5W.	Has both alpha and beta$_1$ adrenergic activity; effects similar to norepinephrine except slower onset and longer duration; SC and IM forms available.
methoxamine hydrochloride (Vasoxyl)	IV; 3–5 mg over 5–10 min.	Selective to alpha-receptors; used to maintain blood pressure during anesthesia; also for certain dysrhythmias; IM form available.
phenylephrine hydrochloride (Neo-synephrine and many others)	IV; 0.1–0.18 mg/min until pressure stabilizes, then 0.04–0.06 mg/min for maintenance.	Selective to alpha-receptors; used to maintain blood pressure during anesthesia; also for certain dysrhythmias, nasal congestion, glaucoma and to dilate the pupil during ophthalmic exams; SC, IM, ophthalmic, and nasal spray forms available.

18.5 Cardiotonic drugs are useful in reversing the decreased cardiac output resulting from shock.

As cardiogenic shock progresses, the heart begins to fail. Cardiac output decreases, lowering the amount of blood reaching vital tissues and deepening the degree of shock. Cardiotonic drugs, also known as **inotropic agents**, have the potential to reverse the cardiac symptoms of shock by increasing the force of myocardial contraction. In Chapter 15 ⬭ , the role of the cardiotonic drug digoxin (Lanoxin) in treating clients with heart failure was discussed. Digoxin increases myocardial contractility and cardiac output, thus rapidly bringing tissues their essential oxygen. Chapter 15 should be reviewed, as drugs prescribed for heart failure are sometimes used for the treatment of shock.

Dobutamine (Dobutrex) is a beta$_1$ adrenergic-agonist that has value in the short-term treatment of certain types of shock because of its ability to cause the heart to beat more forcefully without causing major effects on heart rate. The resulting increase in cardiac output assists in maintaining blood flow to vital organs. Dobutamine has a half-life of only two minutes.

18.6 Anaphylaxis is a special kind of shock involving a hyper-response of body defense mechanisms.

Anaphylactic shock involves an abnormality in a second body system—the immune system. Anaphylaxis is a condition in which the natural body defenses produce a hyper-response to an **antigen**. An antigen may be defined as anything that is recognized as foreign by the body. Certain foods, industrial chemicals, drugs, pollen, animal proteins, and even latex gloves can be antigens. A more detailed discussion of the immune system and the pharmacotherapy of immune disorders are included in Chapter 20 ⬭ .

Normally the body responds to an antigen by processes such as inflammation, antibody production, and activation of lymphocytes that rid the body of the foreign agent. During ana-

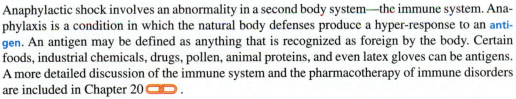

DRUG PROFILE:
Dopamine (Dopastat, Inotropin)

Actions:

Dopamine is the immediate metabolic precursor to norepinephrine. While classified as an adrenergic-agonist, the mechanism of dopamine's action is dependent upon the dose. At low doses, dopamine selectively stimulates dopaminergic receptors, especially in the kidneys, leading to vasodilation and an increased blood flow through the kidneys. This makes dopamine of particular value in hypovolemic and cardiogenic shock. At higher doses, dopamine stimulates beta$_1$ adrenergic-receptors, causing the heart to beat with more force and increasing cardiac output. Another beneficial effect of dopamine when given in higher doses is its ability to stimulate alpha-adrenergic-receptors, thus causing vasoconstriction and raising blood pressure.

Adverse Effects:

Because of its profound effects on the cardiovascular system, clients receiving dopamine are continuously monitored for signs of dysrhythmias and hypotension. Side effects are normally self-limiting because of the short half-life of the drug.

Mechanism in Action:

Dopamine is a naturally occurring neurotransmitter that relieves symptoms of heart failure or shock by increasing the force of cardiac contraction. This is accomplished through activation of beta$_1$ receptors and an influx of calcium into myocardial cells.

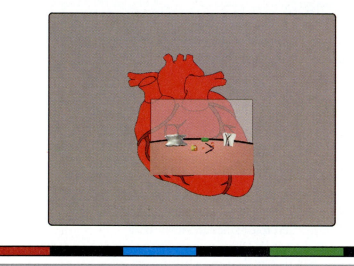

TABLE 18.3	Cardiotonic Drugs of Importance to Shock	
DRUG	**ROUTE AND ADULT DOSE**	**REMARKS**
digoxin (Lanoxin, Lanoxicaps)	IV; digitalizing dose-2.5 μg-5 μg q 6 hours × 24 hours; maintenance dose- 0.125–0.5 mg qd.	Doses are highly individualized for each client; oral forms available; also for dysrhythmias and heart failure.
dobutamine (Dobutrex)	IV; infused at a rate of 2.5–40 μg//kg/min for a max of 72 hours.	Selective beta$_1$ activity; for cardiac decompensation.
Pr dopamine hydrochloride (Dopastat, Intropin)	IV; 1.5 μg/kg/min initial dose; may be increased to 30 μg//kg/min.	May stimulate dopaminergic, beta$_1$ or alpha$_1$ receptors, depending on dose.

phylaxis, the body responds quickly—usually within 20 minutes after exposure to the antigen—by releasing massive amounts of histamine and other defense mediators. Shortly after exposure to the antigen, the client may experience itching, hives, and a tightness in the throat or chest. Swelling occurs around the larynx, causing the voice to become hoarse and a nonproductive cough. As anaphylaxis proceeds, the client presents acute symptoms such as a

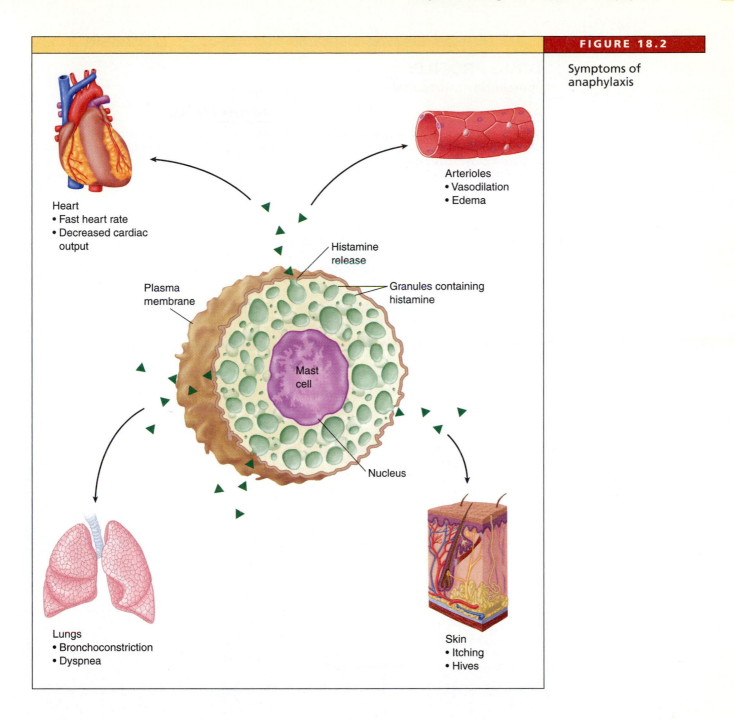

FIGURE 18.2

Symptoms of anaphylaxis

Heart
• Fast heart rate
• Decreased cardiac output

Arterioles
• Vasodilation
• Edema

Histamine release

Plasma membrane

Granules containing histamine

Mast cell

Nucleus

Lungs
• Bronchoconstriction
• Dyspnea

Skin
• Itching
• Hives

rapid fall in blood pressure and difficulty breathing due to bronchoconstriction. The fall in blood pressure causes a rebound speeding up of the heart known as *reflex tachycardia*. Untreated anaphylactic shock is often fatal. Figure 18.2 illustrates the symptoms of anaphylaxis.

Drug therapy of anaphylaxis is symptomatic and involves supporting the cardiovascular system and preventing further hyper-reaction of body defenses. Several drugs are used to treat the symptoms of anaphylactic shock, depending upon the severity of the condition. Oxygen is usually administered immediately. Antihistamines such as diphenhydramine (Benadryl) may be administered IM or IV to prevent additional release of histamine. A bronchodilator such as albuterol (Ventolin, Proventil) is sometimes administered by inhalation to relieve the acute shortness of breath caused by histamine. Corticosteroids such as hydrocortisone may be administered to dampen the inflammatory response. The effects of antihistamines, bronchodilators, and corticosteroids are discussed in detail in Chapters 20, 23, and 27, respectively ⟡ .

ana = *without*
phylaxis = *protection*

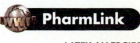

LATEX ALLERGIES

DRUG PROFILE:
Epinephrine (Adrenalin)

Actions:

Subcutaneous or intravenous epinephrine is a drug of choice for acute anaphylactic shock because it can reverse many of the distressing symptoms within minutes. Epinephrine is a non-selective adrenergic agonist, stimulating both alpha- and beta-adrenergic-receptors. Almost immediately after injection, blood pressure rises due to stimulation of alpha$_1$ receptors. Activation of beta$_2$ receptors in the bronchi opens the airway and relieves the client's shortness of breath. Cardiac output increases due to stimulation of beta$_1$ receptors in the heart.

Adverse Effects:

When administered parenterally, epinephrine may cause serious adverse effects. Hypertension and dysrhythmias may occur rapidly; therefore, the client is monitored continuously following IV or SC injections.

Concept review 18.2

■ How can cardiotonic drugs reduce the symptoms of shock without causing vasoconstriction?

CLIENT TEACHING

Clients treated for shock need to know the following:

1. If you suspect that you are experiencing signs or symptoms of shock, seek emergency medical assistance immediately.
2. While waiting for medical assistance, keep warm by using blankets.
3. If a healthcare provider is present, have him or her monitor your temperature, pulse, and blood pressure until emergency medical assistance arrives.
4. Do not move around. Lie down and elevate your feet.
5. Report any changes in your mental status, such as depression, confusion, or anxiety to your healthcare provider immediately.
6. If you know that you are allergic to bee or wasp stings, carry medication, such as an EpiPen, if you intend to go camping or hiking. Inform others of your allergy and be sure they know where you keep your medication and how to use it. ■

CHAPTER REVIEW

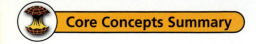

Core Concepts Summary

18.1 Shock has many different causes.

Shock is often classified by the underlying pathologic process or by the organ system that is primarily affected. Basic types include cardiogenic, hypovolemic, neurogenic, septic, and anaphylactic shock.

18.2 **Shock is a clinical syndrome characterized by collapse of the circulatory system.**

Non-specific symptoms of shock include hypotension, cold or clammy skin, reduced cardiac output, and behavioral changes such as confusion, apathy, or disorientation. A thorough medical history is essential for proper diagnosis.

18.3 **The initial treatment of shock involves administration of basic life support and identification of the underlying cause.**

Because shock may be life threatening if allowed to proceed without medical intervention, immediate therapy is targeted at restoring or maintaining vital processes such as respiratory function, blood pressure, and cardiac output.

18.4 **Vasoconstrictors are sometimes needed during shock to maintain blood pressure.**

An immediate concern for the client in shock is falling blood pressure. A variety of adrenergic-agonists, both selective and non-selective, are used to maintain blood pressure and cardiac function.

18.5 **Cardiotonic drugs are useful in reversing the decreased cardiac output resulting from shock.**

Circulatory failure can occur during shock if the cardiac output falls below a critical level. A number of cardiotonic drugs are used to strengthen myocardial function and improve cardiac output.

18.6 **Anaphylaxis is a special kind of shock involving a hyper-response of body defense mechanisms.**

When the body mounts a hyper-response to an antigen, anaphylactic shock may result. Epinephrine is a drug of choice for immediately reversing the cardiovascular symptoms. Other vasoconstrictors, antihistamines, and corticosteroids also serve roles in treating this form of shock.

EXPLORE PharMedia
www.prenhall.com/holland

Additional interactive resources and activities for this chapter can be found on the Companion Website. For animations, audio glossary, and review access the accompanying CD-ROM in this book.

Mechanism in Action:
  Dopamine
Audio Glossary
Concept Review
NCLEX Review

PharmLinks
  Latex Allergies

19 Drugs for Lipid Disorders

CORE CONCEPTS

19.1 High lipid levels can lead to cardiovascular disease and other serious disorders.

19.2 The three basic types of lipids are triglycerides, phospholipids, and sterols.

19.3 Lipids are carried through the blood as lipoproteins.

19.4 The ratio of LDL to HDL is an important factor in predicting cardiovascular disease.

19.5 Lipid levels can often be controlled through lifestyle changes.

HMG CoA Reductase Inhibitors (Statins)

19.6 Statins are drugs of first choice in reducing blood lipid levels.

Bile Acid Resins

19.7 Binding bile acids and accelerating their excretion can reduce cholesterol and LDL levels.

Nicotinic Acid

19.8 Nicotinic acid can reduce LDL levels, but side effects limit its usefulness.

Fibric Acid Agents

19.9 Fibric acid agents lower triglyceride levels, but have little effect on LDLs.

OBJECTIVES

After reading this chapter, the student should be able to:

1. Summarize the link between high blood cholesterol, LDL levels, and cardiovascular disease.

2. Compare and contrast the different types of lipids.

3. Illustrate how lipids are transported through the blood.

4. Compare and contrast the different types of lipoproteins.

5. Give examples of how cholesterol and LDL levels can be controlled through non-pharmacologic means.

6. For each of the following, identify representative drugs, explain the mechanism of drug action, primary actions, and important adverse effects.

   a. HMG CoA reductase inhibitors
   b. bile acid-binding agents
   c. nictotinic acid
   d. fibric acid agents

7. Categorize antilipidemic drugs based on their classification and mechanism of action.

PharMedia
www.prenhall.com/Holland

Additional interactive resources and activities for this chapter can be found on the Companion Website. For animations, audio glossary, and review access the accompanying CD-ROM in this book.

atherosclerosis (ath-ur-oh-sklur-OH-sis): condition characterized by a build-up of fatty plaque and loss of elasticity of the walls of the arteries / *page 276*

B-complex vitamin: group of water-soluble vitamins, including thiamine, riboflavin, pyridoxine, niacin, biotin, and cyanocobalamin that are essential for human nutrition / *page 283*

bile acid (BEYE-ul): chemicals secreted in bile that aid in the digestion of fats / *page 283*

bile acid resin: substance that binds bile acids to remove cholesterol from the body / *page 283*

cholesterol (koh-LESS-tur-ol): a natural lipid that is an integral part of cell membranes and that contributes to atherosclerotic plaque / *page 275*

enterohepatic recirculation (EN-tur-oh-hep-AT-ik): the recycling of bile acids, cholesterol, and other metabolites from the liver, to the bile, through the intestine, and back to the liver / *page 283*

high-density lipoprotein (HDL): lipid-carrying particle in the blood that contains high amounts of protein and lower amounts of cholesterol; considered to be "good" cholesterol / *page 276*

HMG CoA reductase (ree-DUCK-tase): primary enzyme in the biochemical pathway for the synthesis of cholesterol / *page 281*

hypercholesterolemia (HEYE-purr-koh-LESS-tur-ol-EEM-ee-uh): high levels of cholesterol in the blood / *page 275*

hyperlipidemia (HEYE-purr-LIP-id-EEM-ee-uh): excess amounts of lipids in the blood / *page 275*

lecithin (LESS-ih-thin): phospholipid that is an important part of cell membranes / *page 276*

lipoprotein (LIP-oh-PROH-teen): substance carrying lipids in the bloodstream / *page 276*

lipoprotein (a): a specific lipid-carrying protein that is associated with a high risk of atherosclerosis / *page 279*

low-density lipoprotein (LDL): lipid-carrying particle that contains lower amounts of protein and high amounts of cholesterol; considered to be "bad" cholesterol / *page 276*

omega-3 fatty acids (oh-MAY-gah): lipid found in high concentrations in certain fish that is associated with a lower risk of atherosclerosis / *page 280*

phospholipid (FOS-foh-LIP-id): type of lipid that contains two fatty acids, a phosphate group, and a chemical backbone of glycerol / *page 276*

plaque (PLAK): fatty material that builds up in the lining of blood vessels and may lead to hypertension, stroke, myocardial infarction, or angina / *page 275*

steroid (STAIR-oyd): type of lipid that consists of four rings that comprises certain hormones and drugs / *page 276*

sterol nucleus (STAIR-ol NUK-lee-us): ring structure common to all steroids / *page 276*

triglyceride (tri-GLISS-ur-ide): type of lipid that contains three fatty acids and a chemical backbone of glycerol / *page 276*

very low-density lipoprotein (VLDL): lipid-carrying particle that is converted to LDL in the liver / *page 278*

Research during the 1960s and 1970s brought about a nutritional revolution as new knowledge about lipids and their relationship to obesity and cardiovascular disease allowed people to make more intelligent lifestyle choices. Since then, advances in the diagnosis of lipid disorders have helped to identify clients at greatest risk for cardiovascular disease and those most likely to benefit from pharmacologic intervention. Research in pharmacology has led to safe, effective drugs for lowering lipid levels, thus decreasing the risk of cardiovascular-related diseases. As a result of this knowledge and the advancements in pharmacology, the incidence of death due to most cardiovascular diseases has been declining, although these disorders still remain the leading cause of death in the United States.

19.1 High lipid levels can lead to cardiovascular disease and other serious disorders.

Hyperlipidemia, the general term referring to high levels of lipids in the blood, is a major risk factor for cardiovascular disease. Elevated blood **cholesterol**, or **hypercholesterolemia**, is the type of hyperlipidemia that is most familiar to the general public. Cholesterol contributes to the fatty **plaque** that narrows arteries, thus contributing to angina, myocardial infarction (MI), and brain attack as discussed in Chapter 17 ⊂⊃ . Ingestion of saturated fats plays a role in raising cholesterol levels in the blood. It is important that the healthcare provider have a firm grasp of lipid physiology in order to understand the pharmacology of the antilipidemics and, indeed, cardiovascular disease itself.

hyper = above
lipid = fat
emia = blood

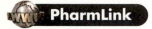

PharmLink

HOW CAN I LOWER MY
CHOLESTEROL BY CHANGING
MY DIET?

Fast Facts High Blood Cholesterol

- The incidence of high blood cholesterol increases until age 65.
- Moderate alcohol intake does not reduce LDL-cholesterol, but it does increase HDL-cholesterol.
- Prior to menopause, high blood cholesterol occurs more frequently in men, but after age 50, the disease is more common in women.
- In order to lower blood cholesterol, both dietary cholesterol and saturated fats must be reduced.
- Familial hypercholesterolemia affects 1 in 500 people and is a genetic disease that predisposes people to high cholesterol levels.

19.2 The three basic types of lipids are triglycerides, phospholipids, and sterols.

Three types of lipids are important to humans, and these are illustrated in Figure 19.1. The most common are the triglycerides. These are neutral fats that form a large family of different lipids, all having three fatty acids attached to a chemical backbone of glycerol. Triglycerides are the major storage form of fat in the body and the only type of lipid that serves as an important energy source. They account for 90% of total lipids.

A second class, called phospholipids, is formed when a phosphorous group replaces one of the fatty acids in a triglyceride. This class of lipids is essential to building plasma membranes. The best-known phospholipids are lecithins, which are found in high concentration in egg yolks and soybeans. Once promoted as a natural treatment for high cholesterol levels, controlled studies have not shown lecithin to be of any benefit for this disorder. Likewise, lecithin has been proposed as a remedy for nervous system diseases such as Alzheimer's disease and bipolar disorder, but there is no definite evidence to support these claims.

athero = fatty
sclera = hard
osis = condition of

The third class of lipids is the steroids, a diverse group of substances having a common chemical group called the sterol nucleus or ring. Cholesterol is the most widely known of the steroids. While its negative role in promoting atherosclerosis is well known, cholesterol also is a natural and vital component of plasma membranes. Unlike the triglycerides that provide fuel for the body during times of energy need, cholesterol serves as the building block for a number of essential biochemicals, including vitamin D, bile acids, cortisol, estrogen, and testosterone. While clearly essential for life, the body only needs minute amounts of cholesterol. Because the body is able to make cholesterol from other chemicals, it is not necessary to provide excess cholesterol in the diet. Dietary cholesterol is obtained solely from animal products; humans do not absorb the sterols produced by plants.

19.3 Lipids are carried through the blood as lipoproteins.

Because lipid molecules do not mix with water, they must be specially packaged for transport through the blood. To accomplish this, the body forms complexes called lipoproteins that consist of various amounts of cholesterol, triglycerides, and phospholipids, along with a protein carrier. The three most common lipoproteins are named based on their weight or density, which comes primarily from the amount of protein present in the complex. For example, high-density lipoprotein (HDL) contains the most protein, up to 50% by weight. The highest amount of cholesterol is carried by low-density lipoprotein (LDL). Figure 19.2 illustrates the three basic lipoproteins and their compositions.

To understand the pharmacologic treatment of hyperlipidemia, it is important to understand the functions of these lipoproteins and their roles in transporting cholesterol. LDL transports cholesterol from the liver to the tissues and organs, where it is used to build plasma membranes or to synthesize other steroids. Once in the tissues, it can also be stored for later use. However, storage of cholesterol in the lining of blood vessels is not desirable because it contributes to plaque build-up. LDL is often called "bad" cholesterol because this lipoprotein contributes significantly to

FIGURE 19.1

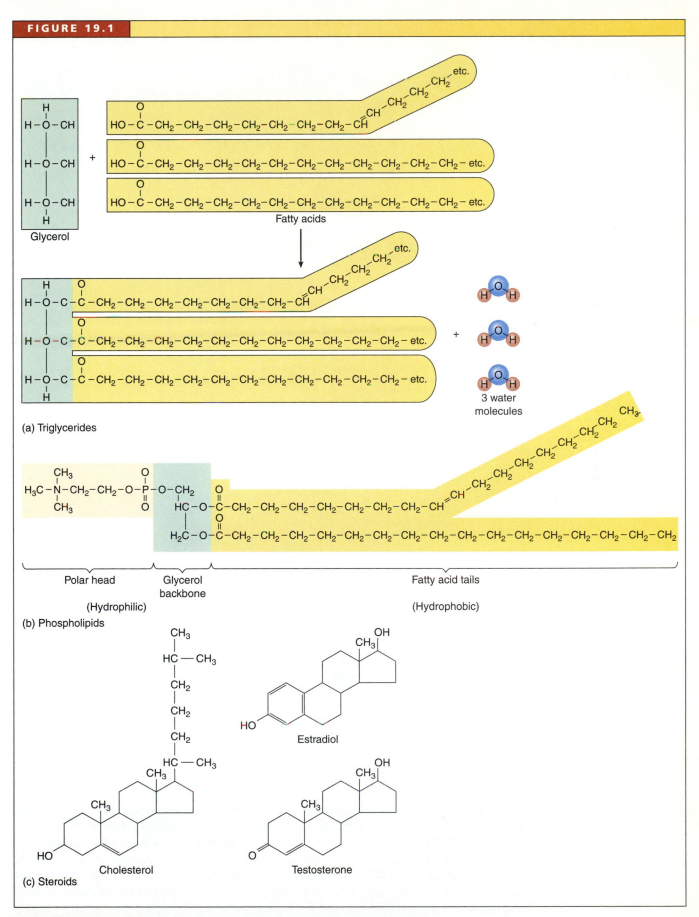

Chemical structure of lipids: (a) triglycerides; (b) phospholipids; (c) steroids

FIGURE 19.2

Composition of lipoproteins: (a) HDL; (b) LDL; (c) VLDL

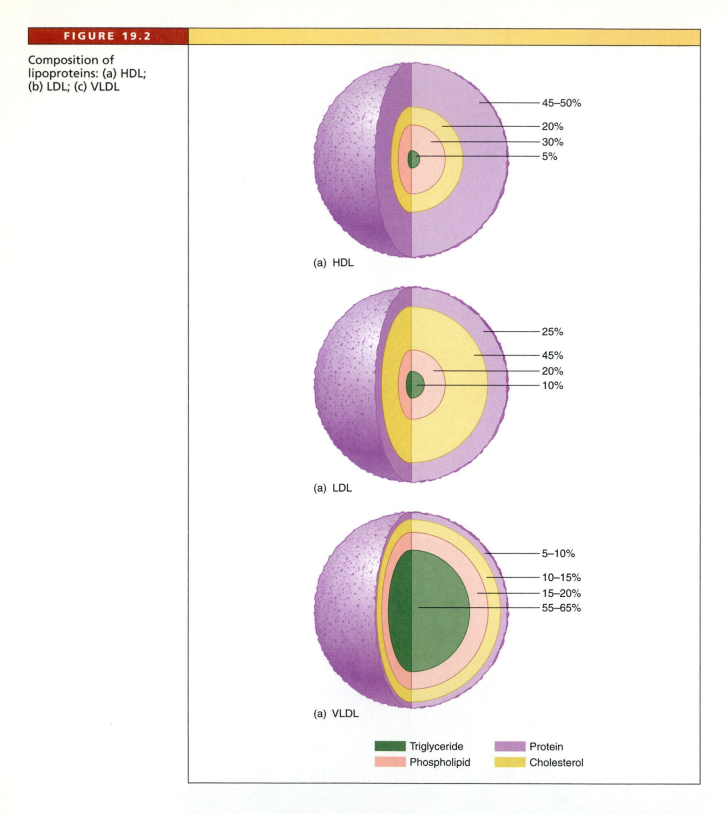

(a) HDL
- 45–50%
- 20%
- 30%
- 5%

(a) LDL
- 25%
- 45%
- 20%
- 10%

(a) VLDL
- 5–10%
- 10–15%
- 15–20%
- 55–65%

| Triglyceride | Protein |
| Phospholipid | Cholesterol |

plaque deposits and coronary artery disease. **Very low-density lipoprotein (VLDL)** is the primary carrier of triglycerides in the blood. VLDL is converted to LDL as it travels through the bloodstream. Lowering LDL levels has been shown to decrease the incidence of coronary artery disease.

Unlike LDL that is created in the liver, HDL is packaged in the tissues and other organs. The cholesterol component of the HDL is transported to the liver where it is broken down to become part of bile that is subsequently excreted in the feces. Excretion via bile is the only route the body uses to remove cholesterol. Because HDL transports cholesterol for destruction and removal from the body, it is considered "good" cholesterol.

TABLE 19.1	Standard Laboratory Lipid Profiles	
TYPE OF LIPID	**LABORATORY VALUE (mg/dL)**	**STANDARD**
total cholesterol	less than 200	desirable
	200–239	borderline high
	greater than 239	high
LDL-cholesterol	less than 130	desirable
	130–159	borderline high
	greater than 159	high
HDL-cholesterol	men: 37–70	desirable
	women: 40–85	desirable
	greater than 35 mg/dL	high
LDL-HDL ratio	men: 1.0	desirable
	women: 1.47	desirable
	men: greater than 5.0	high
	women: greater than 4.5	high
triglycerides	less than 200 mg/dL	desirable
	200–400	borderline high
	400–1000	high
	greater than 1000	very high

19.4 The ratio of LDL to HDL is an important factor in predicting cardiovascular disease.

Although high levels of cholesterol in the blood are associated with cardiovascular disease, it is not sufficient to simply measure total cholesterol in the blood. Because some cholesterol is being transported for destruction, a more accurate profile is obtained by measuring LDL and HDL. The goal in maintaining normal cholesterol levels is to maximize the HDL and minimize the LDL. This is sometimes stated as a ratio of LDL to HDL. If the ratio is greater than 5.0 (five times more LDL than HDL), the male client is considered at risk for cardiovascular disease. The normal ratio in women is slightly lower, at 4.5.

Scientists have further divided LDL into subclasses of lipoproteins. For example, one variety found in LDL, called lipoprotein (a), has been strongly associated with plaque formation and heart disease. It is likely that further research will find other varieties, with the expectation that drugs will be designed to be more selective toward the "bad" lipoproteins. Table 19.1 gives the desirable, borderline, and high laboratory values for each of the major lipids and lipoproteins.

19.5 Lipid levels can often be controlled through lifestyle changes.

Although the medications used to control lipid levels have few serious adverse effects, clients are usually urged to control their hyperlipidemia through non-pharmacologic means prior to initiating drug therapy. The following list provides a number of ways clients can reduce their blood cholesterol levels prior to and during drug therapy. It is important to note that most of these factors apply to cardiovascular disease in general. Because many clients taking lipid-lowering drugs also have underlying cardiovascular disease, these lifestyle changes are particularly important.

ON THE JOB

Home Health Aides and Client Teaching

Home health aides have a major advantage over most other healthcare providers: they get to observe the client in his or her natural home environment. This allows these professionals to make a real impact on the client's surroundings. The home health aide is able to educate the hyperlipidomic client about proper eating habits, using the kitchen, food, and utensils in the home. The aide can examine the foods purchased by the client and, using nutritional labels on the food containers, discuss how to limit cholesterol and saturated fats in the diet. For home-bound clients, the home health aide may assist with the grocery list by adding food lower in fat content. He/she may suggest cooking methods, such as using broiling and steaming rather than pan or deep-fat frying in order to add more vitamins and limit fats. Although hospital nurses and physicians may suggest such lifestyle changes, the home health aide is better able to help clients implement them. ■

Following are means by which clients can reduce cholesterol levels.

- obtain periodic blood cholesterol tests
- if high blood cholesterol is present, have it treated
- maintain weight at an optimum level
- implement a medically supervised exercise plan
- reduce sources of stress; learn and implement coping strategies
- reduce dietary saturated fats and cholesterol
- increase soluble fiber in the diet, as found in oat bran, apples, beans, grapefruit, and broccoli
- reduce or eliminate tobacco use

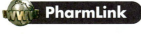 **PharmLink**

NATURAL METHODS FOR LOWERING BLOOD CHOLESTEROL

Nutritionists recommend that the intake of dietary fat be less than 30% of the total caloric intake. Cholesterol intake should be reduced as much as possible, but should not exceed 300 mg/day. It is interesting to note that restriction of dietary cholesterol alone will not result in a significant reduction in blood cholesterol levels. This is because the liver reacts to a low cholesterol diet by making more cholesterol and by inhibiting its excretion whenever saturated fats are present. Thus the client must reduce saturated fat in the diet, as well as cholesterol, in order to ultimately lower the level of blood cholesterol. Other factors can reduce blood cholesterol, including aerobic exercise, smoking cessation, general stress reduction, and the ingestion of **omega-3 fatty acids** found in certain cold-water fish.

Concept review 19.1

- Why is the cholesterol in high density lipoproteins considered to be "good" cholesterol?

HMG COA REDUCTASE INHIBITORS (STATINS)

The statin class of antihyperlipidemics interferes with a critical enzyme in the synthesis of cholesterol. They are first-line drugs in the treatment of lipid disorders.

19.6 Statins are drugs of first choice in reducing blood lipid levels.

In the late 1970s, compounds were isolated from various species of fungi that were found to inhibit cholesterol production in human cells in the laboratory. This class of drugs, known as the *statins*, has since revolutionized the treatment of lipid disorders. Statins can produce a dramatic

FIGURE 19.3

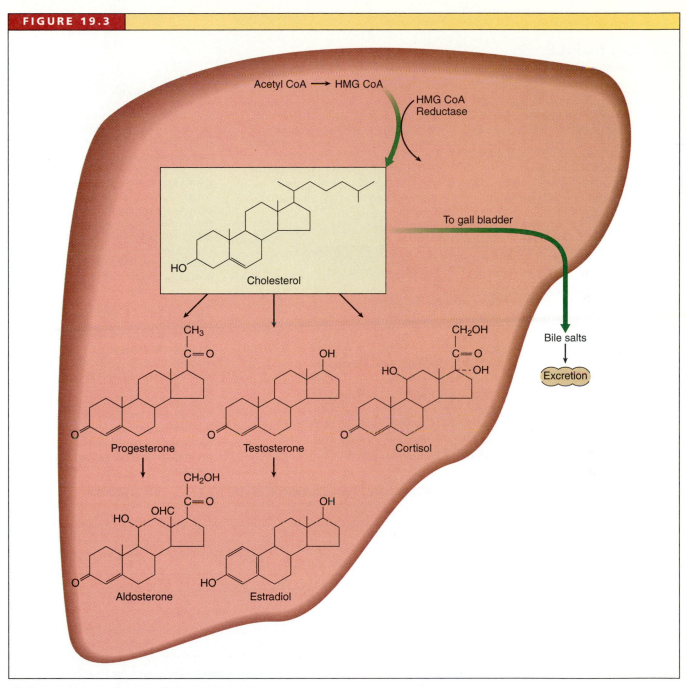

Cholesterol biosynthesis and excretion

20–40% reduction in LDL-cholesterol levels. In addition to dropping LDL-cholesterol levels in the blood, statins can also lower triglyceride levels, lower VLDL levels, and raise "good" HDL-cholesterol levels.

Cholesterol is made in the liver by a series of more than 25 metabolic steps, beginning with acetyl CoA, a two-carbon unit that is produced from the breakdown of fatty acids. Of the many enzymes involved in this complex pathway, HMG CoA reductase (hydroxymethlglutaryl-Coenzyme A reductase) serves as the primary regulatory site for cholesterol biosynthesis. Under normal conditions, this enzyme is controlled through negative feedback: high levels of LDL-cholesterol in the blood will shut down production of HMG Coenzyme A reductase, thus turning off the cholesterol pathway. Figure 19.3 illustrates some of the steps in cholesterol biosynthesis and the importance of HMG CoA reductase.

DRUG PROFILE:
Atorvastatin (Lipitor)

Actions:

Although lovastatin (Mevacor) was the first HMG CoA reductase inhibitor approved for use in the United States, newer statins have been developed that offer certain advantages. For example, atorvastatin has a longer half-life and may be administered without regard to food or time of day. Maximum effects from atorvastatin are seen in four to eight weeks, after which time a follow-up measurement of blood lipid levels is taken to determine whether the dosage is optimum.

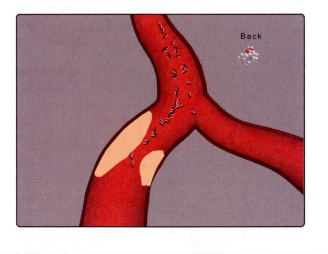

Adverse Effects:

Side effects of atorvastatin are rarely severe enough to cause discontinuation of therapy and include GI complaints such as intestinal cramping, diarrhea, and constipation. A small percentage of clients experience liver damage; thus, hepatic function is usually monitored periodically during therapy. Like other statins, atorvastatin is a pregnancy category X drug; birth defects have been noted in animal studies and the risks to the fetus outweigh any potential benefits to the client.

Mechanism in Action: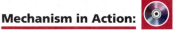

Atorvastatin slows the biosynthesis of cholesterol by blocking the rate-limiting enzyme, HMG CoA reductase. This enzyme is necessary for the availability of LDL (low-density lipoprotein) and VLDL (very-low-density lipoprotein) fragments to body cells including the liver. Atorvastatin also up-regulates LDL receptors in the liver. The net effect is reduced cholesterol and trigylceride blood levels.

TABLE 19.2	HMG CoA Reductase Inhibitors	
DRUG	**ROUTE AND ADULT DOSE**	**REMARKS**
Lovatstatin (Mevacor)	PO; 20–40 mg qd – bid.	Taken with meals in the evening.
(Pr) atorvastatin calcium (Lipitor)	PO; 10–80 mg qd.	May be taken with or without food any time of the day.
fluvastatin (Lescol)	PO; 20 mg qd (max 80 mg/day).	May be taken with or without food in the evening.
pravastatin (Pravachol)	PO; 10–40 mg qd.	May be taken with or without food in the evening.
simvastatin (Zocor)	PO; 5–40 mg qd.	May be taken with or without food in the evening.

The statins act by inhibiting HMG CoA reductase. As the liver makes less cholesterol, it responds by making more LDL receptors on the surface of liver cells. These, in turn, remove more LDL from the blood; thus, blood levels of both LDL and cholesterol are reduced. The drop in lipid levels is not permanent, however, so clients need to remain on these drugs during the remainder of their lives or until their hyperlipidemia can be controlled through dietary or lifestyle changes. Statins have been shown to slow the progression of coronary artery disease and to reduce mortality from cardiovascular disease. Doses of the HMG CoA reductase inhibitors are given in Table 19.2.

NATURAL ALTERNATIVES

Mukul Extracts for Lowering Blood Lipids

A number of herbal supplements are purported to lower blood cholesterol levels. One such botanical comes from the mukul tree (*Commiphora mukul*), a small, thorny shrub native to India. Extracts from the stems of this plant produce a thick resin called *guggul, guggul gum,* or *gugulipid.* The resin contains a number of active agents that are classified as steroids called *guggulsterones.*

The benefits of mukul extracts were reported in ancient Indian literature. Guggelsterones have been reported to lower both cholesterol and triglyceride levels while raising HDL levels. They are also reported to have some antiplatelet activity.

The powdered mukul resin is available in capsule form. Dosage depends upon the concentration of guggelsterones in the resin. However, a typical dosage is 25 mg three times daily. ■

All the statins are given orally and have few serious side effects. Many of them should be administered in the evening, as cholesterol biosynthesis in the body is higher at night.

BILE ACID RESINS

Bile acid resins bind bile acids, thus increasing the excretion of cholesterol. They are sometimes used in combination with the statins.

19.7 Binding bile acids and accelerating their excretion can reduce cholesterol and LDL levels.

Prior to the discovery of the statins, the primary means of lowering blood cholesterol was through use of **bile acid**-binding drugs. These drugs, sometimes called **bile acid resins**, bind bile acids, which contain a high concentration of cholesterol. Once bound in the intestine, the cholesterol cannot be reabsorbed through **enterohepatic recirculation** and thus is eliminated in the feces. Although effective at producing a 20% drop in LDL-cholesterol, the bile acid-binding drugs tend to cause more frequent side effects than the statins. Doses of the bile acid-binding agents are given in Table 19.3.

entero = intestine
heptic = liver

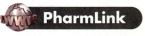
PharmLink

PSYLLIUM: A NATURAL BILE
ACID-BINDER

NICOTINIC ACID

Nicotinic acid is a vitamin that is occasionally used to lower lipid levels. It has a number of side effects that limit its use.

19.8 Nicotinic acid can reduce LDL levels, but side effects limit its usefulness.

Nicotinic acid, or niacin, is a water-soluble **B-complex vitamin**. Its ability to lower lipid levels, however, is unrelated to its role as a vitamin because much higher doses are needed to achieve an antilipidemic effect. For lowering cholesterol, the usual dose is 2 to 3 g per day. When taken as a vitamin, the dose is only 25 mg per day. The primary effect of nicotinic acid is to decrease VLDL levels. Because LDL is synthesized from VLDL, the patient experiences a reduction in

DRUG PROFILE:
Cholestyramine (Questran)

Actions:

Cholestyramine is a powder that is mixed with fluid before being taken once or twice daily. It is not absorbed or metabolized once it enters the intestine, thus it does not produce any systemic effects. It may take 30 days or longer to produce its maximum effect.

Adverse Effects:

Although cholestyramine rarely produces serious side effects, clients may experience constipation, bloating, gas, and nausea that sometimes limit its use. Because cholestyramine can bind to other drugs and interfere with their absorption, it should not be taken at the same time as other medications. Cholestyramine is sometimes combined with other cholesterol-lowering drugs such as the statins or nicotinic acid in order to produce additive effects.

TABLE 19.3	Bile Acid-binding Agents	
DRUG	**ROUTE AND ADULT DOSE**	**REMARKS**
Pr cholestyramine resin (Questran)	PO; 4–8 g bid-qid ac and hs.	Taken with large amounts of fluid; take other drugs 1 hour before or 4 hours after.
colestipol (Colestid)	PO; 5–15 g bid-qid ac and hs.	Taken with large amounts of fluid; take other drugs 1 hour before or 4 hours after.

LDL-cholesterol levels. It also has the desirable effects of reducing triglycerides and increasing HDL levels. As with other lipid-lowering drugs, its maximum effects may take a month or longer to achieve.

Although effective at reducing LDL-cholesterol by 20%, nicotinic acid produces more side effects than the statins. Flushing and hot flashes occur in almost every client. In addition, a variety of uncomfortable intestinal effects such as nausea, excess gas, and diarrhea are commonly reported. More serious side effects such as hepatotoxicity and gout are possible. Because of these adverse effects, nicotinic acid is most often used in lower doses in combination with a statin or bile acid-binding agent, as the beneficial effects of these drugs are additive.

Niacin is available without a prescription. However, clients should be instructed not to attempt self-medication with this drug. One form of niacin available over the counter as a vitamin supplement called *nicotinamide,* has no lipid-lowering effects. Clients should be informed that if nicotinic acid is used to lower cholesterol, it should be done under medical supervision.

Concept review 19.2

■ How does the mechanism of the statins differ from that of nicotinic acid?

FIBRIC ACID AGENTS

Once widely used to lower lipid levels, the fibric acid agents have been largely replaced by the statins. They are sometimes used in combination with the statins.

DRUG PROFILE:
Gemfibrozil (Lopid)

Actions:

Effects of gemfibrozil include up to a 50% reduction in VLDL with an increase in HDL. It is less effective than the statins at lowering LDL; thus, it is not a drug of first choice for reducing LDL-cholesterol levels. Gemfibrozil is taken orally at 600 to 1200 mg per day.

Adverse Effects:

Gemfibrozil produces few serious adverse effects, but it may increase the likelihood of gallstones and occasionally affect liver function. The most common side effects are GI related: diarrhea, nausea, and cramping. Figure 19.4 summarizes the mechanisms of the various drugs used to control lipid disorders.

FIGURE 19.4

Mechanisms of action of lipid-lowering drugs

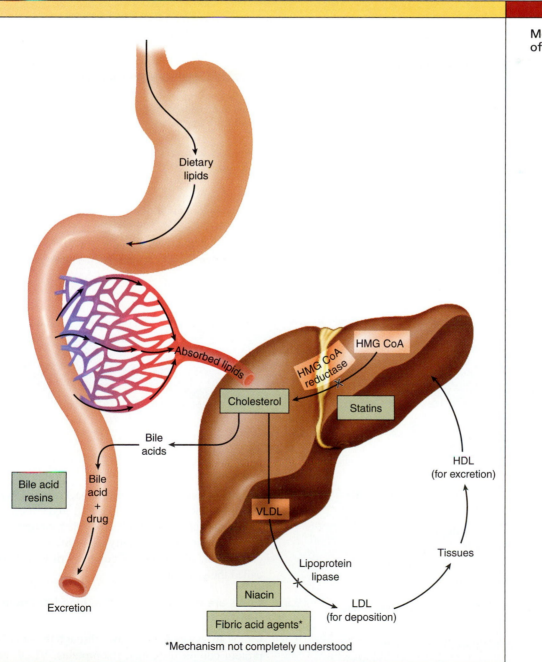

*Mechanism not completely understood

19.9 Fibric acid agents lower triglyceride levels, but have little effect on LDLs.

The first fibric acid agent, clofibrate (Atromid-S), was widely prescribed until studies demonstrated it did not reduce mortality from cardiovascular disease. Although clofibrate is now rarely prescribed, another fibric acid agent gemfibrozil is sometimes used for clients who have excessive triglyceride (VLDL) levels.

CLIENT TEACHING

Clients treated for lipid disorders need to know the following:

1. Because high cholesterol and triglyceride levels in the blood increase the risk for heart disease and stroke, you should follow your healthcare provider's instructions, even if you feel well.

2. Continuation of a low-fat, low-cholesterol diet while taking lipid-lowering drugs will provide the best results.

3. Atorvastatin (Lipitor) is the only statin drug that is effective regardless of the time of day it is taken. Taking other statin drugs in the evening makes them available to work on the higher amount of cholesterol that the body makes at night.

4. Self-medication with niacin can cause gout and liver damage from high doses, and failure to lower cholesterol from low doses. Supervision by a healthcare practitioner supports safe and effective use of this drug.

5. Your healthcare practitioner may prescribe a fibric acid agent to lower triglycerides and another drug to lower cholesterol. One drug should not be stopped when the second drug is ordered, except on practitioner advice.

6. Take prescribed bile acid-binding agents, such as psyllium (Metamucil), cholestyramine (Questran), and colestipol (Colestid) an hour after or four hours before other drugs to avoid counteracting drug effectiveness. Dissolving the bile acid-binding agent in water and keeping fluid intake high helps to avoid irritation of the mouth and constipation. ■

CHAPTER REVIEW

Core Concepts Summary

19.1 High lipid levels can lead to cardiovascular disease and other serious disorders.

Elevated levels of lipids in the blood can lead to plaque deposits on the walls of arteries. Narrowing of arteries may lead to angina pectoris, myocardial infarction, stroke, or hypertension.

19.2 The three basic types of lipids are triglycerides, phospholipids, and sterols.

Lipids can be classified into three types based on their chemical structures. Triglycerides contain three fatty acids connected to a backbone of glycerol. Phospholipids are similar to triglycerides, except a phosphate molecule and other components substitute for one of the fatty acids. Sterols, such as cholesterol, all contain a common ring structure called the sterol nucleus.

19.3 Lipids are carried through the blood as lipoproteins.

Lipids are packaged for travel through the blood in protein complexes called lipoproteins. VLDL and

LDL are associated with an increased incidence of cardiovascular disease, whereas HDL exerts a protective effect.

19.4 The ratio of LDL to HDL is an important factor in predicting cardiovascular disease.

A male client having an LDL to HDL ratio greater than 5.0 is at risk for cardiovascular disease. For females, a ratio greater than 4.5 indicates an increased cardiovascular risk.

19.5 Lipid levels can often be controlled through lifestyle changes.

Before starting pharmacotherapy for hyperlipidemia, clients should seek to control the condition through lifestyle changes such as restriction of dietary saturated fats and cholesterol, increased exercise, and smoking cessation.

19.6 Statins are drugs of first choice in reducing blood lipid levels.

Drugs in the statin class inhibit HMG CoA reductase, a critical enzyme in the biosynthesis of cholesterol. They are safe and effective at lowering LDL-cholesterol and are the most widely prescribed class of drugs for hyperlipidemias.

19.7 Binding bile acids and accelerating their excretion can reduce cholesterol and LDL levels.

The bile acid-binding drugs are effective at lowering LDL-cholesterol, although they produce more side effects than the statins. They should be taken separately from other medications because they can interfere with drug absorption.

19.8 Nicotinic acid can reduce LDL levels, but side effects limit its usefulness.

Nicotinic acid, or niacin, can be effective at lowering LDL-cholesterol when given in large amounts. It is not usually a first-line drug, but is sometimes combined in smaller doses with other lipid-lowering agents.

19.9 Fibric acid agents lower triglyceride levels, but have little effect on LDLs.

Fibric acids such as gemfibrozil are effective at lowering VLDLs, but less efficacious than the statins at lowering blood lipids. Their use is limited because of frequent side effects. However, they are sometimes combined with other agents to produce an additive effect.

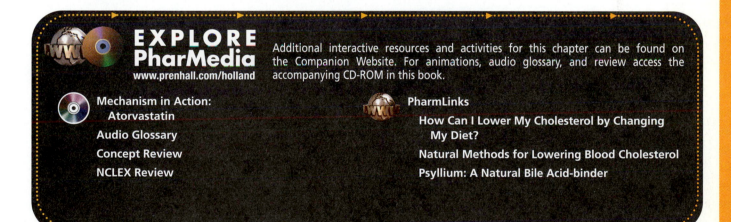

EXPLORE PharMedia
www.prenhall.com/holland

Additional interactive resources and activities for this chapter can be found on the Companion Website. For animations, audio glossary, and review access the accompanying CD-ROM in this book.

Mechanism in Action:
  Atorvastatin
Audio Glossary
Concept Review
NCLEX Review

PharmLinks
How Can I Lower My Cholesterol by Changing My Diet?
Natural Methods for Lowering Blood Cholesterol
Psyllium: A Natural Bile Acid-binder

4 THE IMMUNE SYSTEM

20 Drugs for Inflammation, Allergies, and Immune Disorders

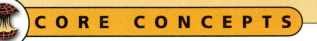

CORE CONCEPTS

INFLAMMATION

20.1 Inflammation is a natural response that limits the spread of invading microorganisms or injury.

20.2 Histamine is a key chemical mediator in inflammation.

20.3 Histamine can produce its effects by interacting with two different receptors.

20.4 Humoral immunity involves the production of antibodies.

20.5 Cell-mediated immunity involves the activation of specific T-cells.

ALLERGY

20.6 Allergic rhinitis is a disease characterized by sneezing, watery eyes, and nasal congestion.

H_1-Receptor Antagonists

20.7 Antihistamines, or H_1 receptor antagonists, are useful for treating allergic rhinitis and several other disorders.

Intranasal Glucocorticoids

20.8 Intranasal glucocorticoids have become drugs of choice in treating allergic rhinitis.

Sympathomimetics

20.9 Sympathomimetics are used to alleviate nasal congestion due to allergic rhinitis and the common cold.

Nonsteroidal Anti-inflammatory Drugs (NSAIDS)

20.10 Nonsteroidal anti-inflammatory drugs are the primary drugs for the treatment of simple inflammation.

Systemic Glucocorticoids

20.11 Systemic glucocorticoids are effective in treating acute or severe inflammation.

Immunosuppressants

20.12 Immunosuppressants are primarily used to avoid tissue rejection following organ transplant.

Vaccines

20.13 Vaccines are biological drugs used to prevent illness.

OBJECTIVES

After reading this chapter, the student should be able to:

1. Identify common signs and symptoms of inflammation.

2. Outline the basic steps in the acute inflammatory response.

3. Describe the central role of histamine in inflammation.

4. Compare and contrast the humoral and cell-mediated immune responses.

5. Differentiate between H_1 and H_2 histamine receptors.

6. Describe some common causes and symptoms of allergic rhinitis.

7. For each of the following classes, identify representative drugs, explain the mechanism of drug action, primary actions related to inflammation and/or the immune system, and important adverse effects:

   a. H_1-receptor antagonists,
   b. nonsteroidal anti-inflammatory drugs,
   c. intranasal and systemic glucocorticoids,
   d. intranasal and oral sympathomimetics,
   e. immunosuppressants,
   f. vaccines.

8. Categorize drugs used in the treatment of inflammation, allergies, and immune disorders based on their classification and mechanism of action.

9. For each of the major vaccines, give the recommended dosage schedule.

PharMedia
www.prenhall.com/holland

Additional interactive resources and activities for this chapter can be found on the Companion Website. For animations, audio glossary, and review access the accompanying CD-ROM in this book.

KEY TERMS

allergic rhinitis (rye-NYE-tis): syndrome of sneezing, itchy throat, watery eyes, and nasal congestion resulting from exposure to antigens; also known as hay fever / *page 297*

alternate-day therapy: taking a drug every other day in order to minimize side effects / *page 306*

anaphylaxis (ANN-ah-fah-LAX-iss): acute allergic response to an antigen that results in severe hypotension and may cause death if untreated / *page 293*

antibody (ANN-tee-BOD-ee): protein produced by the body in response to an antigen; used interchangeably with the term *immunoglobulin* / *page 294*

antigen (ANN-tih-jen): a foreign organism or substance that induces the formation of antibodies / *page 294*

B-cell: type of lymphocyte that is essential for the humoral immune response / *page 294*

booster: an additional dose of a vaccine given months or years after the initial dose to increase the effectiveness of the vaccine / *page 308*

bradykinin (BRAY-dee-KINE-in): a chemical released by cells during inflammation that produces pain and effects similar to those of histamine / *page 293*

complement (KOM-pluh-ment): a series of proteins that are involved in the non-specific defense of the body / *page 293*

Cushing's syndrome (KUSH-ings): a condition of having too much corticosteroids in the blood / *page 306*

cyclooxygenase (COX-1 and COX-2) (SEYE-kloh-OX-uh-jen-ase): key enzyme in the prostaglandin metabolic pathway that is blocked by aspirin and other NSAIDS / *page 305*

cytokines (SYE-toh-kines): chemicals produced by white blood cells, such as interleukins, leukotrienes, interferon, and tumor necrosis factor, that guide the immune response / *page 296*

cytotoxic T-cell: type of lymphocyte that directly attacks and destroys antigens / *page 295*

H_1-receptor: site located on smooth muscle cells in the bronchial tree that is stimulated by histamine / *page 294*

H_2-receptor: site located on cells of the digestive system that is stimulated by histamine / *page 294*

H_1-receptor antagonist: drug that blocks the effects of histamine in smooth muscle in the bronchial tree / *page 297*

helper T-cell: type of lymphocyte that coordinates both the humoral and cell-mediated immune responses and that is the target of the human immunodeficiency virus / *page 295*

histamine (HISS-tuh-meen): chemical released by mast cells in response to an antigen that causes dilation of blood vessels, smooth muscle constriction, tissue swelling, and itching / *page 293*

humoral immunity (HYOU-mor-ul eh-MEWN-uh-tee): a specific body defense mechanism involving the production and release of antibodies / *page 294*

hyperemia (HYE-purr-EEM-ee-uh): increase in blood supply to a part or tissue space causing swelling, redness, and pain / *page 293*

immunoglobulin (ih-MEW-noh-GLOB-you-lin): proteins produced by the body in response to an antigen; used interchangeably with the term *antibody* / *page 295*

immunosuppressant (ih-MEW-noh-suh-PRESS-ent): any drug, chemical, or physical agent that lowers the natural immune defense mechanisms of the body / *page 308*

inflammation (IN-flah-MAY-shun): non-specific body defense that occurs in response to an injury or antigen / *page 292*

leukotriene (LEW-koh-TRY-een): chemical released by cells during inflammation that produces effects similar to those of histamine / *page 293*

lymphocyte (LIM-foh-site): type of white blood cell formed in lymphoid tissue / *page 294*

mast cell: connective tissue cell located in tissue spaces that releases histamine following injury / *page 293*

memory B-cell: type of B-lymphocyte that remembers previous exposure to an antigen / *page 295*

memory T-cell: type of T-lymphocyte that remembers previous exposure to an antigen / *page 297*

plasma cell: type of cell derived from B-cells that produces antibodies / *page 294*

prostaglandins (PROSS-tuh-GLAN-dins): a class of chemicals that promotes inflammation and produces pain when released by cells in the body / *page 293*

rebound congestion: a condition of hypersecretion of mucous following use of intranasal sympathomimetics / *page 302*

salicylism (sal-IH-sill-izm): poisoning due to aspirin and aspirin-like drugs / *page 306*

T-cell: type of lymphocyte that is essential for the cell-mediated immune response / *page 295*

tinnitus (tin-EYE-tis): ringing in the ears / *page 306*

titer (TIE-ter): measurement of the amount of a substance in the blood / *page 308*

toxoid (TOX-oid): substance that has been chemically modified to remove its harmful nature but is still able to elicit an immune response in the body / *page 308*

transplant rejection: when the immune system recognizes a transplanted tissue as being foreign and attacks it / *page 308*

vaccine (vaks-EEN): preparation of microorganism particles that is injected into a client to stimulate the immune system, with the intention of preventing disease / *page 308*

vaccination/immunization (VAK-sin-AYE-shun/IH-mewn-ize-AYE-shun): receiving a vaccine or toxoid in order to prevent disease / *page 308*

The pain and redness of inflammation following minor abrasions and cuts is something everyone has experienced. Although there may be some discomfort from such scrapes, inflammation is a normal and expected part of our body's defense against injury. For some diseases, however, inflammation can be abnormal and rage out of control, producing severe pain, fever, and other distressing symptoms. It is these sorts of conditions for which drug therapy may be warranted.

Similarly, our bodies come under daily attack from a host of foreign agents that include viruses, bacteria, fungi, and even single-celled animals. In defending the body, our immune system may mount a rapid and effective response against these specific microbes. In some cases, vaccines *are given to stimulate the immune system so that disease can be prevented. On rare occasions, it is desirable to dampen the immune response to allow a transplanted organ to grow. The purpose of this chapter is to examine the pharmacotherapy of diseases and conditions affecting our body defenses.*

Fast Facts Anti-inflammatory and Immune Disorders

- Arthritis is the leading cause of disability.
- Costs of treating arthritis are nearly $65 billion annually.
- Arthritis is higher among women and older clients.
- Inflammatory bowel disease affects 300,000 to 500,000 Americans each year.
- Peptic ulcers affect 4.5 million Americans each year.
- Vaccines have eradicated smallpox from the world and the polio virus from the Western hemisphere.
- Vaccines have lowered the number of diphtheria cases in the U.S. from 175,000 in 1922 to 1 in 1998.
- Vaccines have lowered the number of measles cases in the U.S. from over 503,000 in 1962 to 89 in 1998.

INFLAMMATION

20.1 Inflammation is a natural response that limits the spread of invading microorganisms or injury.

The human body has developed many complex means to defend itself against injury and invading organisms. Inflammation is one of these defense mechanisms. Inflammation is a complex process that occurs in response to a large number of different stimuli, including physical injury, exposure to toxic chemicals, extreme heat, invading microorganisms, or death of cells. The central purpose of inflammation is to contain the injury or destroy the foreign agent. By removing cellular debris and dead cells, repair of the injured area can proceed at a faster pace. The physiological processes of inflammation proceed in the same manner, regardless of its cause. Signs of inflammation include swelling, pain, warmth, and redness of the affected area.

Inflammation may be classified as acute or chronic. During acute inflammation, such as that caused by minor physical injury, 8 to 10 days are normally needed for the symptoms to resolve and for repair to begin. If the body cannot contain or neutralize the damaging agent, inflammation may continue for prolonged periods and become chronic. In chronic diseases such as lupus and rheumatoid arthritis, inflammation may persist for years, with symptoms becoming progressively worse over time. Other disorders such as seasonal allergy arise at predictable times each year, and inflammation may produce only minor, annoying symptoms.

Treatment of inflammation may include drugs that dampen the natural inflammatory response. Most anti-inflammatory drugs are non-specific: it does not matter whether the inflammation is caused from injury or allergy, the drug will exhibit the same actions. A few anti-inflammatory drugs are specific to certain diseases, such as those used to treat gout. Following is a list of diseases that have an inflammatory component.

- allergic rhinitis
- anaphylaxis
- ankylosing spondylitis
- contact dermatitis

- Crohn's disease
- glomerulonephritis
- Hashimoto's thyroiditis
- multiple sclerosis
- peptic ulcers
- rheumatoid arthritis
- systemic lupus erythematosus
- type 1 diabetes
- ulcerative colitis

20.2 Histamine is a key chemical mediator in inflammation.

Whether the injury is due to microorganisms, chemicals, or physical trauma, the damaged tissue releases a number of chemical mediators that act as "alarms" to notify the surrounding area of the injury. Chemical mediators of inflammation include **histamine**, **leukotrienes**, **bradykinin**, **complement**, and **prostaglandins**. Table 20.1 lists the sources and actions of each of these mediators.

Histamine is a key chemical mediator of inflammation. It is primarily stored within **mast cells** that are located in tissue spaces under epithelial membranes such as the skin, the bronchial tree, the digestive tract, and along blood vessels. Mast cells detect foreign agents or injury and respond by releasing histamine, which initiates the inflammatory response within seconds. In addition, histamine directly stimulates pain receptors.

Histamine is a very potent vasodilator. When released at an injury site, it dilates nearby blood vessels, causing the capillaries to become more permeable or leaky. Plasma and components of the immune system such as complement and phagocytes can then enter the area to neutralize foreign agents. The affected area may become congested with blood because of the permeable capillaries, a condition called **hyperemia**, which can lead to significant swelling and pain. Figure 20.1 shows the basic steps in acute inflammation.

hyper = *above normal*
emia = *blood*

Rapid release of histamine on a larger scale throughout the body is responsible for the distressing symptoms of **anaphylaxis**, a life-threatening allergic response that may result in shock and death. A number of chemicals, insect stings, foods, and some therapeutic drugs can elicit this widespread release of histamine from mast cells. Drug therapy of anaphylactic shock was discussed in Chapter 18 ⬭ .

TABLE 20.1	Chemical Mediators of Inflammation
bradykinin	vasodilator that causes pain; effects are similar to those of histamine
complement	series of proteins that combine together in a cascade fashion to neutralize or destroy an antigen
histamine	stored and released by mast cells; causes dilation of blood vessels, smooth muscle constriction, tissue swelling, and itching
leukotrienes	stored and released by mast cells; effects are similar to those of histamine
prostaglandins	stored and released by mast cells; increase capillary permeability, attract white blood cells to site of inflammation, and cause pain

FIGURE 20.1

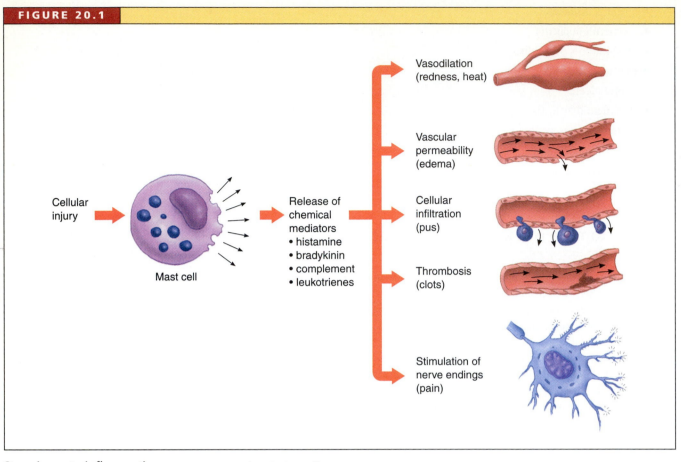

Steps in acute inflammation *SOURCE: Pearson Education/PH College.*

20.3 Histamine can produce its effects by interacting with two different receptors.

There are at least two different receptors by which histamine can elicit a response. **H₁-receptors** are present in the smooth muscle of the vascular system, the bronchial tree, and the digestive tract. Their stimulation results in itching, pain, edema, vasodilation, and bronchoconstriction. **H₂-receptors** are present in the stomach, and their stimulation results in the secretion of large amounts of hydrochloric acid.

Drugs that act as specific antagonists for H_1 and H_2 receptors are in widespread therapeutic use. H_1-receptor antagonists, used to treat allergies and inflammation, are discussed later in this chapter. H_2 receptor antagonists are used to treat peptic ulcers and are discussed in Chapter 25 ⬤▭ . A simplified mechanism of action for the antihistamines is illustrated in Figure 20.2.

20.4 Humoral immunity involves the production of antibodies.

anti = against
gen = formation

While inflammation is non-specific, the body has also developed elaborate mechanisms of protection that target specific foreign agents. Foreign substances that elicit a specific immune response are called **antigens**. Proteins, such as those present on the surfaces of pollen grains, bacteria, and viruses are the strongest antigens. The primary cell of the immune system that interacts with antigens is the **lymphocyte**.

Humoral immunity is initiated when an antigen encounters a type of lymphocyte known as a **B-cell**. The activated B-cell divides rapidly to form many copies, or clones, of itself. Most cells in this clone are called plasma cells. The primary function of the **plasma cells** is to secrete **antibodies**,

FIGURE 20.2

Mechanism of action of the antihistamines

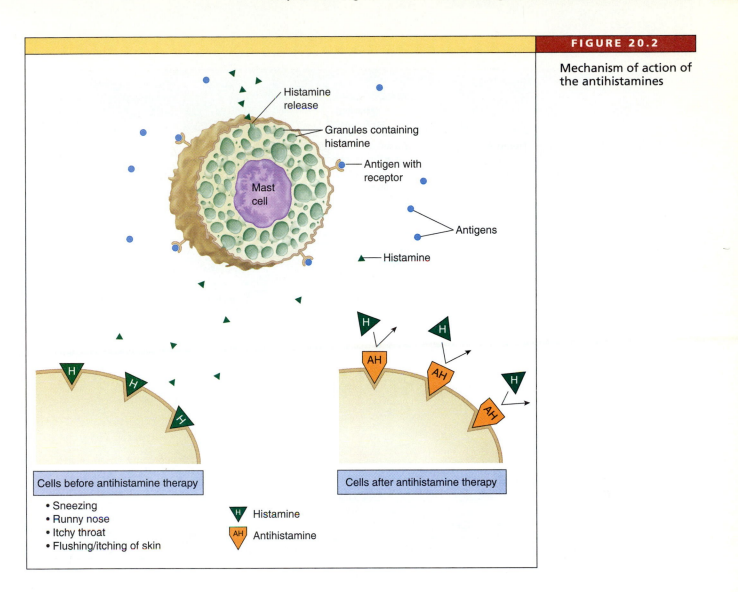

Histamine release

Granules containing histamine

Antigen with receptor

Mast cell

Antigens

▲— Histamine

Cells before antihistamine therapy

Cells after antihistamine therapy

• Sneezing
• Runny nose
• Itchy throat
• Flushing/itching of skin

H Histamine

AH Antihistamine

sometimes called **immunoglobulins**, which are specific to the antigen that initiated the challenge. As they circulate through the body, antibodies physically interact with the antigen to neutralize it or mark the foreign agent for destruction by other cells of the immune system. Peak production of antibodies occurs about 10 days after an antigen challenge. Figure 20.3 shows the basic steps in the humoral immune response.

Some B-cells, called **memory B-cells**, remember the initial antigen interaction. Should the body be exposed to the same antigen in the future, the body may secrete even higher levels of antibodies in a shorter time period, approximately two to three days. For some antigens, memory is retained for an entire lifetime. Vaccines, discussed later in this chapter, are sometimes administered to produce these memory cells in advance of exposure to the antigen, so that when the body is exposed to the real organism it can mount a fast, strong response.

20.5 Cell-mediated immunity involves the activation of specific T-cells.

The second branch of the immune system involves lymphocytes called **T-cells**. Two major types of T-cells are **helper T-cells** and **cytotoxic T-cells**. These cells are often named after a protein receptor on their plasma membrane; the helper T-cells have a CD4 receptor and the cytotoxic T-cells have a CD8 receptor. The helper T-cells are particularly important because they are responsible for activating most other immune cells, including B-cells.

FIGURE 20.3

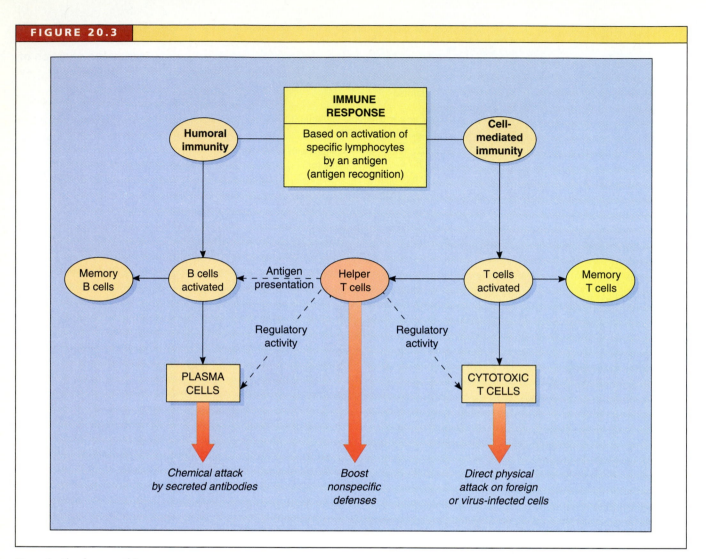

Steps in the humoral immune response   SOURCE: *Pearson Education/PH College.*

Like B-cells, activated or sensitized T-cells rapidly form clones after they encounter their specific antigen. Unlike B-cells, however, T-cells do not produce antibodies. Instead, T-cells produce huge amounts of chemicals called **cytokines**. Some cytokines kill foreign organisms directly, while others induce inflammation. Most cytokines act as messengers to the immune system, stimulating T-cells, B-cells, and other white blood cells to rid the body of the foreign agent. Specific

cyto = cell
kine(sis) = movement

NATURAL ALTERNATIVES

Echinacea for Boosting the Immune System

Echinacea purpurea, or purple coneflower, is one of the most popular medicinal botanicals. This plant is native to the midwestern U.S. and central Canada; its flowers, leaves, and stems are harvested and dried. Preparations include dried powder, tincture, fluid extracts, and teas. No single ingredient seems to be responsible for the herb's activity; a large number of active chemicals have been identified from the extracts.

Echinacea was used by Native Americans to treat various wounds and injuries. Echinacea is purported to boost the immune system by increasing phagocytosis and inhibiting the bacterial enzyme hyalouronidase. Some substances in echinacea appear to have antiviral activity; the herb is sometimes taken to prevent and treat the common cold and influenza, an indication for which it has received official approval in Germany. In general, it is used as a supportive treatment for any disease involving inflammation and to enhance the immune system. ■

cytokines released by activated T-cells include several interleukins, gamma interferon, and tumor necrosis factor (TNF). Several of these cytokines have been used to treat certain cancers. This new class of medications, called biologic response modifiers, is discussed in Chapter 23 ⊂⊃ .

Cytotoxic T-cells travel throughout the body searching for their specific antigen and can directly attack and kill certain bacteria, parasites, virus-infected cells, and cancer cells.

As with B-cells, some of the sensitized T-cells become memory cells. Should the body encounter the same antigen in the future, the memory T-cells will assist in mounting a more rapid immune response.

ALLERGY

Allergies are caused by a hyperresponse of body defenses. Many signs and symptoms are similar to those of inflammation, since histamine is released during an allergic response. Allergies may also involve mediators of the immune system.

20.6 Allergic rhinitis is a disease characterized by sneezing, watery eyes, and nasal congestion.

Allergic rhinitis, or hay fever, is a common disorder affecting millions of people annually. Symptoms resemble those of the common cold: tearing eyes, sneezing, nasal congestion, post-nasal drip, and itching of the throat. The exact cause of a client's allergic rhinitis is often difficult to pinpoint; however, common causes include pollen from weeds, grasses, and trees, molds, dust mites, certain foods, and animal dander. Non-allergenic factors such as chemical fumes, tobacco smoke, or air pollutants such as ozone may contribute to the symptoms. While some clients experience symptoms at specific times of the year, when pollen and mold are at high levels in the environment, other clients are afflicted throughout the year.

The fundamental problem of allergic rhinitis is inflammation of the mucous membranes in the nose, throat, and airways. Chemical mediators such as histamine are released that initiate the distressing symptoms. The mechanism of allergic rhinitis is illustrated in Figure 20.4.

Drugs used to treat allergic rhinitis may be grouped into two basic categories: preventers and relievers. Preventers are used for prophylaxis and include antihistamines, glucocorticoids, and mast cell stabilizers. Relievers are used to provide immediate, though temporary, relief for allergy symptoms once they have occurred. Relievers include the oral and intranasal sympathomimetics that are used as nasal decongestants.

rhin *= nose*
itis *= inflammation*

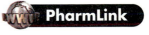

POLLEN AND ALLERGIC RHINITIS

H₁-RECEPTOR ANTAGONISTS

Antihistamines block the actions of histamine at the H₁-receptor. They are widely used OTC for relief of allergy symptoms, motion sickness, and insomnia.

20.7 Antihistamines, or H₁-receptor antagonists, are useful for treating allergic rhinitis and several other disorders.

H₁-receptor antagonists are commonly called *antihistamines*. Because the term antihistamine is non-specific and does not specify which of the two histamine receptors are affected, H₁-receptor antagonist is the more accurate term. Although a large number of H₁-receptor antagonists are available for use, their efficacies, therapeutic uses, and side effects are quite similar. A simple classification of these drugs is based on their ability to cause sedation. Older, first-generation H₁-receptor antagonists have the potential to cause significant drowsiness, whereas the newer, second-generation agents lack this effect in most clients. Care must be taken to avoid alcohol and other CNS depressants when taking antihistamines, as their sedating effects may be additive.

Allergic rhinitis

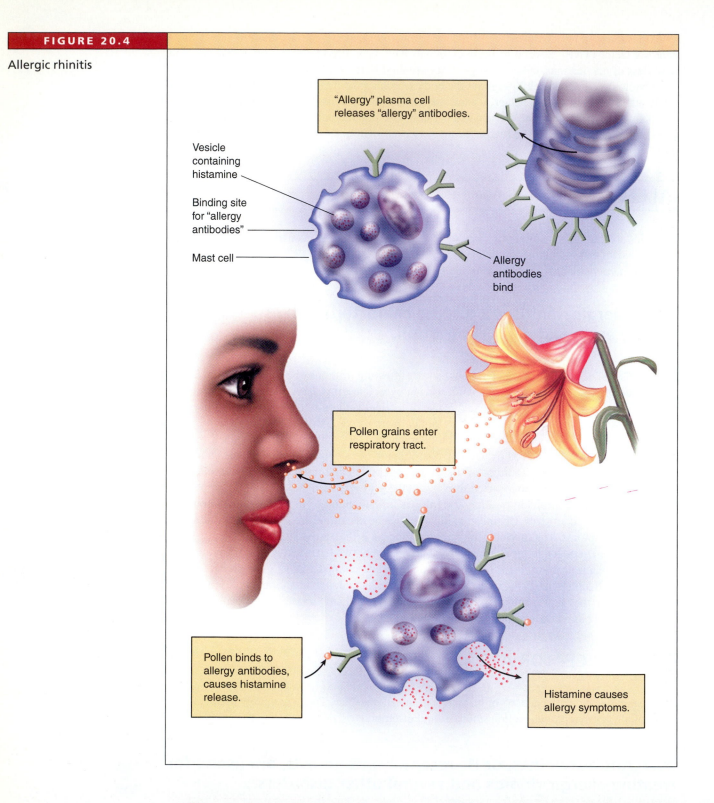

"Allergy" plasma cell releases "allergy" antibodies.

Vesicle containing histamine

Binding site for "allergy antibodies"

Mast cell

Allergy antibodies bind

Pollen grains enter respiratory tract.

Pollen binds to allergy antibodies, causes histamine release.

Histamine causes allergy symptoms.

The most common therapeutic use of H_1-receptor antagonists is for the treatment of allergies. These drugs provide relief from the sneezing, runny nose, and itching of the eyes, nose, and throat characteristic of allergic rhinitis. Many H_1-receptor antagonists are used in OTC cold and sinus medicines, often in combination with other drugs such as decongestants and antitussives. Some common OTC antihistamine combinations used to treat allergies are shown in Table 20.2.

Antihistamines are most effective when taken prophylactically to prevent allergic symptoms. Their effectiveness may diminish with long-term use. It should be noted that during severe allergic reactions such as anaphylaxis, histamine is just one of several chemical mediators released; thus, H_1-receptor antagonists are not very efficacious in treating this disorder.

TABLE 20.2	Selected Antihistamine Combinations Available OTC for Allergic Rhinitis		
BRAND NAME	**ANTIHISTAMINE**	**DECONGESTANT**	**ANALGESIC**
Actifed Cold and Allergy tablets	triprolidine	pseudoephedrine	
Actifed Cold and Sinus caplets	chlorpheniramine	pseudoephedrine	acetaminophen
Benadryl Allergy/Cold tablets	diphenhydramine	pseudoephedrine	acetaminophen
Chlor-trimeton Allergy-D tablets	chlorpheniramine	pseudoephedrine	
Dimetapp Cold and Fever liquid	brompheniramine	phenylpropanolamine	acetaminophen
Drixoral Cold and Allergy-12 hour	dexbrompheniramine	pseudoephedrine	acetaminophen
Sudafed Cold and Allergy tablets	chlorpheniramine	pseudoephedrine	
Tavist Allergy 12 hour tablets	clemastine		
Triaminic Cold/Allergy softchews	chlorpheniramine	pseudoephedrine	
Tylenol Allergy Sinus Nighttime caplets	diphenhydramine	pseudoephedrine	acetaminophen

While most antihistamines are given orally, azelastine (Astelin) was the first to be available by the intranasal route. Azelastine is considered to be as safe and effective as the oral antihistamines. Although a first-generation agent, it causes less drowsiness than others in its class because it is applied locally, with little systemic absorption.

H_1-receptor antagonists are also effective in treating a number of other disorders. Motion sickness responds well to these medications. It is also one of the few classes of drugs available to treat vertigo, a form of dizziness that causes significant nausea. Some of the older antihistamines are marketed as OTC sleep aids, taking advantage of their ability to cause drowsiness. Common H_1-receptor antagonists used to treat allergies and other disorders are shown in Table 20.3.

Concept review 20.1:

■ Why are the antihistamines most effective if given before inflammation occurs?

INTRANASAL GLUCOCORTICOIDS

Glucocorticoids may be applied directly to the nasal mucosa to prevent symptoms of allergic rhinitis. They have begun to replace antihistamines in the treatment of chronic allergic rhinitis.

20.8 Intranasal glucocorticoids have become drugs of choice in treating allergic rhinitis.

Glucocorticoids are hormones secreted by the cortex portion of the adrenal gland. They are used for a wide variety of disorders, including severe inflammation, adrenocortical deficiency (Chapter 28), neoplasia (Chapter 23), asthma (Chapter 24), and arthritis (Chapter 30). The basic pharmacology of the glucocorticoids is presented in Chapter 28 ⊂▭⊃ .

Intranasal glucocorticoids have joined antihistamines as first-line drugs in the treatment of allergic rhinitis. These medications are administered with a metered-spray device that delivers a consistent dose of drug per spray. Intranasal glucocorticoids produce none of the potentially serious adverse effects that are observed when these hormones are given orally. The most frequently reported side effects are an intense burning sensation in the nose immediately after spraying and drying of the nasal mucosa. The intranasal glucocorticoids and their doses are shown in Table 20.4.

DRUG PROFILE (First-generation Antihistamine):

Diphenhydramine (Benadryl and Others)

Actions:

Diphenhydramine is a first-generation H_1-receptor antagonist that is a component of some OTC medications. Its primary use is to treat symptoms of allergy and the common cold such as sneezing, runny nose, and tearing of the eyes. OTC preparations may combine diphenhydramine with an analgesic, decongestant, or expectorant. Diphenhydramine is also used as a topical agent to treat rashes and an IM form is available for severe allergic reactions. Other indications for diphenhydramine include Parkinson's disease, motion sickness, and insomnia.

Adverse Effects:

As with most older H_1-receptor antagonists, diphenhydramine causes significant drowsiness, although this usually diminishes with long-term use. Occasionally, a client will exhibit CNS stimulation and excitability rather than drowsiness. Anticholinergic effects such as dry mouth, tachycardia, and mild hypotension are seen in some clients.

Mechanism in Action:

Diphenhydramine is an antihistamine used to treat disorders such as allergic rhinitis, Parkinson's disease, and insomina. Diphenhydramine reduces inflammation by blocking H_1-receptors found within smooth muscle cells of the respiratory tract and the endothelial cells lining blood vessels located in the skin.

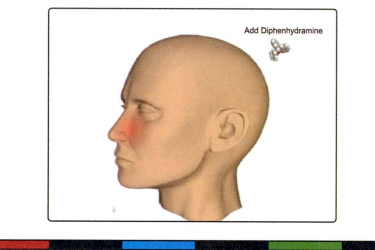

Add Diphenhydramine

DRUG PROFILE (Second-generation Antihistamine):

Fexofenadine (Allegra)

Actions:

Fexofenadine is a second-generation H_1-receptor antagonist with efficacy equivalent to that of diphenhydramine. Its primary action is to block the effects of histamine at H_1-receptors. When taken prophylactically, it reduces the severity of nasal congestion, sneezing, and tearing of the eyes. Its long half-life offers the advantage of being administered once or twice daily. Fexofenadine is only available in oral form. Allegra-D combines fexofenadine with pseudoephedrine, a decongestant.

Adverse Effects:

The major advantage of fexofenadine over first-generation antihistamines is that it causes less drowsiness. Although it is considered nonsedating, drowsiness can still occur in some clients. Other side effects are usually minor and include upset stomach.

TABLE 20.3	H₁-Receptor Antagonists	
DRUG	**ROUTE AND ADULT DOSE**	**REMARKS**
First-generation Agents		
Ⓟ diphenhydramine hydrochloride (Benadryl and others)	PO; 25–50 mg tid-qid (max 300 mg/day).	Topical, IV, IM, and SC forms available; also for motion sickness, Parkinson's disease, vertigo, and as an OTC sleep aid.
azatadine maleate (Optimine)	PO; 1–2 mg bid.	Trinalin is a combination of azatadine and pseudoephedrine.
azelastine hydrochloride (Astelin)	Intranasal; 2 sprays per nostril bid.	First-generation antihistamine.
brompheniramine maleate (Codimal A, Dimetapp)	PO; 4–8 mg tid-qid (max 40 mg/day).	Less sedative effects than diphenhydramine; IV, IM, and SC forms available; combined with other drugs for OTC use.
chlorpheniramine maleate (Chlor-Trimeton and others)	PO; 2–4 mg tid-qid (max 24 mg/day).	Also has antiemetic, antitussive, anticholinergic, and local anesthetic uses; IV, IM, SC, and extended release forms available; combined with other drugs for OTC use.
clemastine fumarate (Tavist)	PO; 1.34 mg bid (max 8.04 mg/day).	Central sedative effects are generally mild.
cyproheptadine hydrochloride (Periactin)	PO; 4 mg tid or qid (max 0.5 mg/kg/day).	Significant antipruritic, local anesthetic, and antiserotonin effects.
dexbrompheniramine (Drixoral)	PO; 6 mg bid.	Usually used in combination with pseudoephedrine and dextromethorphan as an over-the-counter drug for cold and allergy.
dexchlorpheniramine (Dexchlor, Poladex, Polargen, Polaramine)	PO; 2 mg q4–6h (max 12 mg/day).	Discontinue drug 72 hours before allergy skin tests.
promethazine (Phenergan, Phenazine)	PO; 12.5 mg qd (max 150 mg/day).	IV, IM, and rectal suppository forms available; also for preoperative sedation, motion sickness, nausea, and vertigo.
tripelennamine hydrochloride (PBZ-SR, Pelamine)	PO; 25–50 mg q4–6h (max 600 mg/day).	Also used to provide mucous membrane analgesia in young children with herpetic gingivo stomatitis; extended release form available.
triprolidine (Actifed, Actidil)	PO; 2.5 mg bid or tid.	Long-acting; combined with other drugs for OTC use.
Second-generation Agents		
cetirizine (Zyrtec)	PO; 5–10 mg qd.	Once-a-day dosing; non-sedating.
Ⓟ fexofenadine (Allegra)	PO; 60 mg qd – bid (max 120 mg/day).	Once-a-day dosing; non-sedating.
loratadine (Claritin)	PO; 10 mg qd.	Once-a-day dosing; non-sedating; take on an empty stomach.

DRUG PROFILE:
Fluticasone (Flonase)

Actions:

Fluticasone is typical of the intranasal glucocorticoids used to treat allergic rhinitis. Therapy usually begins with two sprays in each nostril twice daily, and decreases to one dose per day. Fluticasone acts to decrease local inflammation in the nasal passages, thus decreasing nasal stuffiness.

Adverse Effects:

Side effects to fluticasone are rare. Small amounts of the intranasal glucocorticoids are sometimes swallowed, thus increasing the potential for systemic side effects. Nasal irritation and bleeding occur in a small number of clients.

TABLE 20.4	Intranasal Glucocorticoids	
DRUG	**ROUTE AND ADULT DOSE**	**REMARKS**
beclomethasone (Beconase, Vancenase)	Intranasal; 1 spray bid-qid.	Oral inhaler available (Beclovent) for asthma.
budesonide (Rhinocort)	Intranasal; 2 sprays bid.	Oral inhaler available (Pulmicort) for asthma.
flunisolide (Nasalide, Nasarel)	Intranasal; 2 sprays bid may; increase to tid if needed.	Oral inhaler available (AeroBid) for asthma.
Pr fluticasone (Flonase)	Intranasal; 1 spray qd-bid (max qid).	Oral inhaler available (Flovent) for asthma; Topical form available (Cutivate) for dermatologic use.
mometasone (Nasonex)	Intranasal; 2 sprays qd.	Topical form available (Elocon) for dermatologic use.
triamcinolone (Nasacort AQ)	Intranasal; 2–4 sprays qid.	Oral inhaler available (Nasacort) for asthma. Also available in IM, SC, intradermal, and intraarticular forms.

SYMPATHOMIMETICS

Sympathomimetics stimulate the sympathetic nervous system. They may be administered orally or intranasally to dry the nasal mucosa.

20.9 Sympathomimetics are used to alleviate nasal congestion due to allergic rhinitis and the common cold.

Sympathomimetics are effective at relieving the nasal congestion associated with allergic rhinitis. Both oral and intranasal preparations are available. The intranasal drugs such as oxymetazoline (Afrin and others) are available OTC as sprays or drops and produce an effective response within minutes. Because of their local action, intranasal sympathomimetics produce few systemic effects. The most serious, limiting side effect of the intranasal preparations is rebound congestion; prolonged use causes hypersecretion of mucous and nasal congestion to worsen once the drug effects wear off. This sometimes leads to a cycle of increased drug use as the condition worsens.

Because of this rebound congestion, intranasal sympathomimetics should be used for no longer than three to five days.

When administered orally, sympathomimetics do not produce rebound congestion. Their onset of action by this route, however, is much slower than the intranasal preparations and they are less effective at relieving severe congestion. The possibility of systemic side effects is also greater with the oral drugs. Potential side effects include hypertension and CNS stimulation that may lead to insomnia or anxiety. Pseudoephedrine is the most common sympathomimetic found in OTC cold and allergy medicines. Because sympathomimetics only relieve nasal congestion, they are often combined with antihistamines in order to control the sneezing and tearing of allergic rhinitis. It is interesting to note that some OTC drugs having the same basic name (Neo-Synephrine, Afrin, Vicks) may contain different sympathomimetics. For example, Neo-Synephrine preparations with a 12-hour duration contain the drug oxymetazoline; preparations with the same name that last four to six hours contain phenylephrine. Some common combination drugs are shown in Table 20.2. Sympathomimetics used to treat allergic rhinitis are given in Table 20.5.

DRUG PROFILE:
Oxymetazoline (Afrin and Others)

Actions:

Oxymetazoline stimulates the alpha-adrenergic receptors of the sympathetic nervous system. This causes small arterioles in the nasal passages to constrict, producing a drying of the mucous membranes. Relief from the symptoms of nasal congestion occurs within minutes and lasts for 10–12 hours. The drug is administered with a metered spray device or by nose drops.

Adverse Effects:

Rebound congestion is common when oxymetazoline is used for longer than three to five days. Minor stinging and dryness in the nasal mucosa may be experienced. Systemic side effects are unlikely, unless the client swallows a considerable amount of the medicine. Clients with thyroid disorders, hypertension, diabetes, or heart disease should only use sympathomimetics upon the direction of their healthcare practitioner.

TABLE 20.5	Sympathomimetics of Value in Treating Allergic Rhinitis	
DRUG	**ROUTE AND ADULT DOSE**	**REMARKS**
ephedrine hydrochloride (Eledron)	Intranasal (0.5%); 2–4 drops no more than qid for 3–4 consecutive days.	Oral, IV, IM, and SC forms available. Also for acute asthma, hypotension, myasthenia gravis, and urinary incontinence.
epinephrine (Primatene)	Intranasal (0.1%); 1–2 drops bid.	SC, IV, and topical forms available. Also for anaphylaxis, cardiac arrest, asthma, and glaucoma.
naphazoline hydrochloride (Privine)	Intranasal; 2 drops q3–6 hours.	Also available as spray.
Pr oxymetazoline hydrochloride (Afrin/12 hr, Neo-Synephrine/12 hr and others)	Intranasal (0.05%); 2–3 sprays bid for up to 3–5 days.	Also available as drops.
phenylephrine hydrochloride (Neo-synephrine)	Intranasal (0.25–0.5%); 1–2 sprays q3–4h.	Also available as drops, chewable tablets, and hemorrhoidal cream. Also for hypotension and shock.
pseudoephedrine hydrochloride (Sudafed)	PO; 60 mg q4–6h (max 120 mg/day).	Produces little congestive rebound or irritation; also available as drops and in extended-release form.
xylometazoline hydrochloride (Otrivin)	Intranasal (0.1%); 1–2 sprays bid (max 3 doses/day).	Also available as drops.

■ The sympathomimetics are the most effective drugs for relieving nasal congestion, but physicians often prefer to prescribe antihistamines or intranasal glucocorticoids. Why?

NONSTEROIDAL ANTI-INFLAMMATORY DRUGS (NSAIDs)

NSAIDS such as aspirin and ibuprofen have analgesic, antipyretic, and anti-inflammatory effects. They are drugs of choice in the treatment of mild to moderate inflammation.

20.10 Nonsteroidal anti-inflammatory drugs are the primary drugs for the treatment of simple inflammation.

The analgesic effect of the nonsteroidal anti-inflammatory drugs (NSAIDS) was discussed in Chapter 11 ⬤▭. This class includes some of the most widely used drugs, such as aspirin, ibuprofen, and the newer COX-2 inhibitors. Although acetaminophen shares the analgesic and antipyretic properties of these other drugs, it has no anti-inflammatory action and is thus not considered an NSAID. Some of the NSAIDs used for inflammation are listed in Table 20.6.

DRUG PROFILE:
Naproxen (Naprosyn) and Naproxen Sodium (Aleve, Anaprox)

Actions:

Naproxen is an NSAID that inhibits prostaglandin synthesis through the non-selective inhibition of COX-1 and COX-2. Its efficacy at relieving pain and inflammation is similar to that of aspirin. Common indications include both rheumatoid arthritis and osteoarthritis, gout, and bursitis. In treating rheumatoid arthritis, the therapeutic effects may take three to four weeks to appear.

Adverse Effects:

Side effects of naproxen are generally not serious and include GI upset, dizziness, and drowsiness. Administration with food will decrease the incidence of stomach upset, which is the most common side effect. Because naproxen may prolong bleeding time, the drug should be administered with caution to those with bleeding disorders. Clients taking naproxen should notify their dental hygienist before dental procedures are performed.

Mechanism in Action:

Naproxen is a nonsteroidal antiinflammatory drug (NSAID) that inhibits prostaglandin synthesis through the non-selective inhibition of cyclooxygenase type-1 (COX-1) and cyclooxygenase type-2 (COX-2) enzymes. It is effective is treating arthritis and primary dysmenorrhea where symptoms of inflammation and/or pain are expressed. It also inhibits platelet aggregation and prolongs bleeding time without affecting whole blood clotting, prothrombin time, or platelet count.

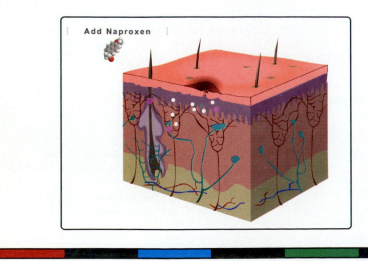

[Add Naproxen]

TABLE 20.6	Selected Nonsteroidal Anti-inflammatory Drugs	
DRUG	**ROUTE AND ADULT DOSE**	**REMARKS**
aspirin (ASA and others)	PO; 350–650 mg q 4 hours (max 4 g/day).	Inhibits the formation of prostaglandins; also for fever, pain, prevention of stroke, and MI.
celecoxib (Celebrex)	PO; 100–200 mg bid (max 400 mg/day).	Selective COX-2 inhibitor.
diclofenac sodium (Voltaren, Cataflam)	PO; 50 mg bid-qid (max 200 mg/day).	Extended-release form available.
diflunisal (Dolobid)	PO; 250–500 mg bid (max 1500 mg/day).	Similar to ibuprofen.
etodolac (Lodine)	PO; 200–400 mg tid-qid (max 1200 mg/day).	Extended-release form available.
fenoprofen calcium (Nalfon)	PO; 300–600 mg tid-qid (max 3200 mg/day).	Similar to ibuprofen.
flurbiprofen sodium (Ansaid)	PO; 50–100 tid-qid (max 300 mg/day).	Similar to ibuprofen.
ibuprofen (Motrin, Advil, and many others)	PO; 400–800 mg tid-qid (max 3200 mg/day).	Blocks prostaglandin synthesis as well as modulates T-cell function; also for dysmenorrhea.
ketoprofen (Actron, Orudis, Oruvail)	PO; 75 mg tid or 50 mg qid (max 300 mg/day).	Extended-release form available; similar to ibuprofen; also for dysmenorrhea.
nabumetone (Relafen)	PO; 1000 mg qd (max 2000 mg/day).	Inhibits COX-2 more than COX-1.
(Pr) naproxen (Naprosyn)	PO; 250–500 mg bid (max 1000 mg/day).	Also for dysmenorrhea.
naproxen sodium (Aleve, Anaprox)	PO; 275 mg bid (max 1100 mg/day).	Also for dysmenorrhea.
oxaprozin (Daypro)	PO; 600–1200 mg qd (max 1800 mg/day).	Similar to naproxen; once-a-day dosage.
piroxicam (Feldene)	PO; 10–20 mg qd-bid (max 20 mg/day).	Has prolonged half-life.
rofecoxib (Vioxx)	PO; 12.5–25 mg qd (max 50 mg/day).	Selective COX-2 inhibitor.
tolmetin sodium (Tolectin)	PO; 400 mg tid (max 2 g/day).	Exact mode of antiinflammatory action unknown.

The basic pharmacology and a drug profile of aspirin were presented in Chapter 11 ⬭ . Aspirin is useful in treating inflammation because it inhibits **cyclooxygenase (COX)**, a key enzyme in the pathway of prostaglandin synthesis that is found in every tissue. Aspirin causes irreversible inhibition of both forms of cyclooxygenase, COX-1 and COX-2. Because it is readily available, inexpensive, and efficacious, aspirin is usually a drug of first choice for treating mild inflammation.

Unfortunately, large doses of aspirin are necessary to suppress severe inflammation, and this results in a greater incidence of side effects than when the drug is used for pain or fever. The most common adverse effects observed during high-dose aspirin therapy relate to the digestive system. By increasing gastric acid secretion and irritating the stomach lining, high doses of aspirin may produce pain, heartburn, and even bleeding due to ulceration. Some aspirin formulations are buffered or given an enteric coating to minimize GI side effects. Because aspirin also has an anticoagulant effect (Chapter 13 ⬡), the potential for bleeding must be carefully monitored by the healthcare provider. High doses may produce salicylism, a syndrome that includes symptoms such as tinnitus, or ringing in the ears, dizziness, headache, and sweating. Clients with pre-existing kidney disease should be monitored carefully because aspirin and other NSAIDS may affect kidney function.

A large number of NSAIDS, such as ibuprofen, have been developed as alternatives to aspirin. Like aspirin, they exhibit their effects through inhibition of COX-1 and COX-2. Because of their similar mechanisms, they all have quite similar pharmacologic properties and a low incidence of adverse effects. The most common side effects of these drugs are nausea and vomiting, although the incidence of gastric ulceration and bleeding is less than that of aspirin. Most have no significant effect on blood coagulation and thus are safe to use for clients who may be at risk to bleeding.

The newest class of NSAIDS is that which selectively inhibits COX-2, and includes celcoxib (Celebrex) and rofecoxib (Vioxx). Inhibition of COX-2 produces the analgesic, anti-inflammatory, and antipyretic effects seen with the NSAIDS. Because they do not inhibit COX-1, celecoxib and rofecoxib do not produce the adverse effects on the digestive system seen with aspirin. Because they have no GI side effects and do not affect blood coagulation, these drugs are becoming drugs of choice for the treatment of moderate to severe inflammation.

SYSTEMIC GLUCOCORTICOIDS

Glucocorticoids have wide therapeutic application when given orally or parenterally. They have a potent anti-inflammatory action that can suppress severe cases of inflammation.

20.11 Systemic glucocorticoids are effective in treating acute or severe inflammation.

Glucocorticoids are natural hormones released by the cortex of the adrenal gland that have powerful effects on nearly every cell in the body. When used to treat inflammatory disorders, the drug doses are many times higher than those naturally present in the blood. The uses of glucocorticoids in treating hormonal imbalances are presented in detail in Chapter 28 ⬡ .

Glucocorticoids have the ability to suppress histamine and prostaglandins. In addition, they can inhibit the immune system by suppressing a certain functions of phagocytes and lymphocytes. These multiple effects have the ability to markedly reduce inflammation; thus, glucocorticoids are quite effective at treating severe inflammatory disorders.

Unfortunately the glucocorticoids have a number of serious adverse effects that limit their use in treating inflammation. These include suppression of the normal functions of the adrenal gland (adrenal insufficiency), elevated blood glucose, mood changes, cataracts, peptic ulcers, electrolyte imbalances, and osteoporosis. Because of their effectiveness at reducing the signs and symptoms of inflammation, glucocorticoids can mask infections that may be present in the client. This combination of masking inflammation and suppressing the immune system creates a potential for existing infections to grow rapidly and undetected. An active infection is usually a contraindication for glucocorticoid therapy.

Because the appearance of these adverse effects is a function of the dose and duration of therapy, treatment is often limited to the short-term control of acute disease. When longer therapy is indicated, doses are kept as low as possible and alternate-day therapy is sometimes used; the medication is taken every other day to encourage the client's adrenal gland to function on the days when no drug is given. During long-term therapy, the healthcare provider must be alert for signs of over-treatment, a condition referred to as Cushing's syndrome. In addition, the body becomes accustomed to the high doses of glucocorticoids and clients must discontinue the drug gradually, as abrupt withdrawal can result in lack of adrenal function. Selected glucocorticoids used to treat severe inflammatory disease are listed in Table 20.7.

IMMUNOSUPPRESSANTS

Drugs used to inhibit the immune response are called immunosuppressants. They are used for clients receiving transplanted tissues or organs.

DRUG PROFILE:
Prednisone (Meticorten and Others)

Actions:

Prednisone is a synthetic glucocorticoid. Its actions are the result of being metabolized to an active form, which is also available as a drug called *prednisolone* (Deltacortef and others). When used for inflammation, a 4–10 day duration for therapy is common. Alternate-day dosing is used for longer-term therapy. Prednisone is occasionally used to terminate acute bronchospasm in clients with asthma (Chapter 24) and for clients with certain cancers such as Hodgkin's disease, acute leukemia, and lymphomas (Chapter 23 ⊂⊃).

Adverse Effects:

When used for short-term therapy, prednisone has few adverse effects. Long-term therapy may result in Cushing's syndrome, a condition that includes elevated blood glucose, fat redistribution to the shoulders and face, muscle weakness, bruising, and bones that easily fracture. Diabetic clients must be aware that glucocorticoids can raise blood glucose levels. Gastric ulcers may occur with long-term therapy, and the client must report any potential infections immediately.

TABLE 20.7	Selected Glucocorticoids Used to Treat Severe Inflammation	
DRUG	**ROUTE AND ADULT DOSE**	**REMARKS**
hydrocortisone (Cetacort, Cortaid)	Topical; 0.5% cream applied qd-qidPO; 10–320 mg tid-qid.	Used widely for skin inflammation; IM, PO, rectal, and IV forms available; may be injected intraarticular.
betamethasone (Celestone, Betacort, and many others)	PO; 0.6–7.2 mg/day.	Topical, IM, and IV forms available.
cortisone acetate (Cortistan, Cortone)	PO; 20–300 mg/day in divided doses.	IM form available; also for adrenal insufficiency.
dexamethasone (Decadron and others)	PO; 0.25–4 mg bid-qid.	IM and IV forms available; also for adrenal insufficiency and immunosuppression.
methylprednisolone (Medrol)	PO; 4–48 mg/day in divided doses.	Available in IM, IV, and rectal, forms; also for neoplasia and adrenal insufficiency.
Pr prednisolone (Delta-Cortef, Keypred, Prelone, and others)	PO; 5–60 mg qd-qid.	Available in IM and IV forms; also for neoplasia, and adrenal insufficiency.
prednisone (Deltatsone)	PO; 5–60 mg qd-qid.	Only available in oral form; also for neoplasia.
triamcinolone (Kenalog, Azmacort, and many others)	PO; 4–48 mg qd-qid.	Available in IM, SC, intradermal, intraarticular and aerosol forms.

20.12 Immunosuppressants are primarily used to avoid tissue rejection following organ transplant.

The immune system is normally viewed as a life-saver, protecting clients from a host of foreign organisms in the environment. For those receiving organ or tissue transplants, however, the immune system is the enemy. Transplanted organs always contain some antigens that trigger the client's immune response. This response, called transplant rejection, is sometimes acute, with antibodies rushing to destroy the transplanted tissue within a few days. The cell-mediated immune system reacts more slowly to the transplant, attacking it about two weeks following surgery. Even if the organ survives these attacks, chronic rejection of the transplant may occur months or even years after surgery.

Immunosuppressants are medications given to dampen the immune response. Transplantation would be impossible without the use of effective immunosuppressant drugs. In addition, these agents may be prescribed for severe cases of rheumatoid arthritis or other inflammatory diseases. The immunosuppressants are quite toxic. Due to the suppressed immune system, infections are common and the client must be protected from situations where exposure to infection is likely. Certain tumors such as lymphomas occur more frequently in transplant clients than in the general population. The mechanism of action of each of the immunosuppressant drugs differs, although most are toxic to bone marrow. Drugs used to produce immunosuppression are listed in Table 20.8.

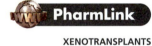

XENOTRANSPLANTS

Concept review 20.3:

■ Why are oral glucocorticoids usually used concurrently with the immunosuppressant drugs following a transplant operation?

VACCINES

20.13 Vaccines are biological drugs used to prevent illness.

The immune system reacts to an antigen by recognizing or attacking certain proteins on the surface of the invader. Sometimes it recognizes a toxin or secretion produced by a foreign organism. Pharmacologists have used this knowledge to create biological products that prevent disease called vaccines. Vaccines consist of suspensions of one of the following: (a) microbes that have been killed; (b) microbes that are alive but weakened (attenuated) so they are unable to produce disease; or (c) bacterial toxins, called *toxoids,* that have been modified to remove their hazardous properties.

Vaccination or immunization is performed in order to expose the client to the modified, harmless microorganism or its toxoid so that an immune response occurs in the following weeks or months. Memory B-cells remember the exposure and react quickly by producing large amounts of antibodies when later exposed to the real infectious organism. While some immunizations are only needed once, most require follow-up vaccinations, called boosters, in order to provide continuous protection. The effectiveness of a vaccine can be assessed by measuring the amount of antibody produced by the body after the vaccine has administered, a quantity called titer.

Most vaccines are administered with the goal of preventing illness. In the case of HIV infection, however, experimental vaccines are given after infection has occurred for the purpose of enhancing the immune system, rather than preventing the disease. While vaccines for some viral diseases are extremely effective, experimental vaccines for HIV have thus far been unable to prevent the disease. Drug therapy of HIV is discussed in Chapter 22 Chapter 22.

DRUG PROFILE:
Cyclosporine (Neoral, Sandimmune)

Actions:

Cyclosporine is a complex chemical obtained from a soil fungus. Its primary mechanism of action is to inhibit helper T-cells. Unlike some of the more cytotoxic immunosuppressants, it has little effect on bone marrow cells. When prescribed for transplant recipients, it is usually used in combination with high doses of a gluco-corticoid such as prednisone.

Adverse effects:

The primary adverse effect of cyclosporine occurs in the kidney, with up to 75% of clients experiencing reduction in urine flow. Frequent laboratory tests of kidney function are necessary. Other common side effects are tremor, hypertension, and elevated hepatic enzyme values. Although infections are common during cyclosporine therapy, they are fewer than with some of the other immunosuppressants. Periodic blood counts are necessary to be certain that WBCs do not fall below 4,000 or platelets below 75,000.

TABLE 20.8	Immunosuppressants	
DRUG	**ROUTE AND ADULT DOSE**	**REMARKS**
Pr cyclosporine (Sandimmune, Neoral)	PO; initial dose 14–18 mg/kg just prior to surgery; continue this dose for 1–2 weeks; then 5–10 mg/kg/day.	IV form available; inhibits T-cells; also for rheumatoid arthritis and severe psoriasis.
azathioprine (Imuran)	PO; 3–5 mg/kg qd.	IV form available; inhibits DNA, RNA, and protein synthesis; also for severe rheumatoid arthritis.
lymphocyte immune globulin (Antithymocyte Globulin)	IV; 10–30 mg/kg qd by slow infusion.	Alters the formation of T-cells and reduces their numbers.
methotrexate (Amethopterin, Folex, Rheumatrex)	PO; 2.5–5 mg bid 3 x week.	IV, IM, and intrathecal forms available; blocks metabolism of folic acid; also for neoplasia, severe psoriasis, and severe rheumatoid arthritis.
muromonab-CD3 (Orthoclone OKT3)	IV; 5 mg/day administered in less than 1 minute for 10–14 days.	Antibodies specific for the CD3 receptor on T-cells; for treatment of renal transplant rejection.
mycophenolate mofetil (CellCept)	PO; 1 g bid; begin within 24 hours of transplant.	IV form available; inhibits B- and T-cells and antibody formation.
tacrolimus (FK-506) (Prograf)	PO; 75–150 μg/kg bid; begin 6 hours after transplant.	IV form available; inhibits T-cells; also for severe psoriasis.

Vaccines are not without adverse effects. Common side effects include redness and discomfort at the site of injection and fever. Although severe reactions are uncommon, anaphylaxis is possible. Vaccinations may be contraindicated for clients who have a weak immune system or who are currently experiencing symptoms such as diarrhea, vomiting, or fever.

Effective vaccines have been produced for a number of debilitating diseases. The widespread use of vaccines has prevented serious illness in millions of clients, particularly children. One disease—smallpox—has been virtually eliminated from the planet through immunization, and others such as polio have diminished to extremely low levels. Table 20.9 gives some common vaccines and their recommended schedules.

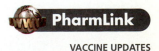

PharmLink

VACCINE UPDATES

TABLE 20.9	Common Childhood Vaccines and Their Schedules
VACCINE NAME	**SCHEDULE AND AGE**
diphtheria, tetanus, and pertussis (Tri-Immunol, Tripedia, Acel-Imune, Infanrix, Certiva)	First: 2 months Second: 4 months Third: 6 months Fourth: 15–18 months Fifth: 4–6 years
haemophilus influenza (HibTITER, OmniHIB, PedvaxHIB, ComVax))	First: 2 months Second: 4 months Third: 6 months Fourth: 12–15 months
hepatitis B (Recombivax HB, Energix-B)	First: birth to 2 months Second: 1 to 4 months Third: 6–18 months
measles, mumps and rubella (MMR II)	First: 12–15 months Second: 4–6 years
poliovirus, oral (Orimune)	First: 2 months Second: 4 months Third: 6–18 months Fourth: 4–6 years
varicella zoster/chicken pox (Varivax)	One dose: 12–18 months

ON THE JOB

Nursing in Family Practice

The nurse involved in family practice is in the unique position of seeing the same clients over an extended period of time. Watching children grow and knowing that one is playing a pivotal role in maintaining their health is a satisfying part of the job. Vaccinations are a critical part of that role.

Teaching parents the importance of maintaining up-to-date vaccinations for themselves and for their children is a dynamic responsibility of the nurse. It is important that the nurse stress the importance of preventing illness, rather than treating illness. Staying current on the latest recommendations regarding vaccination schedules is vital because these may change frequently. Also important is the role that the nurse plays in helping parents to organize their children's vaccination records so that they are complete and readily accessible when children enter school or change grades. ■

CLIENT TEACHING

Clients treated for inflammatory or immune disorders need to know the following:

1. If you are taking antihistamines for the first time, avoid operating machinery or performing other tasks requiring alertness, as drowsiness may occur.

2. Hard candies, chewing gum, or ice chips may be used to reduce the dry mouth caused by antihistamines.

3. Stop taking antihistamines and notify your healthcare provider if excessive sedation, wheezing, chest tightness, or bleeding/bruising occur.

4. Do not take OTC cold or allergy medicines containing antihistamines at the same time as prescription antihistamines.

5. Take NSAIDS with food in order to decrease stomach irritation.

6. Avoid drinking alcohol when taking high doses of NSAIDS or aspirin because it increases stomach irritation.

7. If signs of bleeding or bruising occur, discontinue aspirin use immediately and report the incident to your physician.

8. Take glucocorticoids exactly as prescribed, as improper use may lead to serious adverse effects.

9. Keep an accurate, written record of your child's vaccinations, including the date of the vaccination, route and site of vaccination, type of vaccine (including manufacturer and lot number) and the address of the physician's office where the vaccination occurred.

10. Keep immunizations up to date to prevent illness. Because recommendations can change, seek current information from a healthcare provider periodically.

11. Vaccines may contain a number of additives, including antibiotics, formaldehyde, thimersol, and monosodium glutamate. If you know or suspect you are allergic to any of these, notify your healthcare provider before getting a vaccination.

12. Cyclosporine should never be taken with grapefruit juice; blood levels of the drug are increased by this combination. ■

CHAPTER REVIEW

 Core Concepts Summary

20.1 Inflammation is a natural response that limits the spread of invading microorganisms or injury.

Inflammation is a non-specific response designed to rid the body of invading organisms or to contain the spread of injury. Acute inflammation occurs over a period of several days, whereas chronic inflammation may continue for months or years.

20.2 Histamine is a key chemical mediator in inflammation.

Inflammation is initiated by chemical mediators, one of the most important of which is histamine.

Release of histamine causes vasodilation, allowing capillaries to become leaky, thus causing tissue swelling. Extremely rapid release of histamine throughout the body can cause anaphylaxis.

20.3 Histamine can produce its effects by interacting with two different receptors.

The classic antihistamines used for allergies block H_1 histamine receptors in vascular smooth muscle, the bronchi, and on sensory nerves. The H_2 receptor inhibitors are used to treat peptic ulcers.

20.4   Humoral immunity involves the production of antibodies.

When B-cells encounter their specific antigen, they become plasma cells and secrete large quantities of antibodies. The antibodies are specific to the antigen and neutralize the foreign agent or destroy it. Some B-cells remember the antigen for many years.

20.5   Cell-mediated immunity involves the activation of specific T-cells.

T-cells also recognize specific antigens, but instead of producing antibodies, they produce cytokines, which rid the body of the foreign agent. Memory T-cells will remember the antigen for many years and mount a faster immune response upon subsequent exposures.

20.6   Allergic rhinitis is a disease characterized by sneezing, watery eyes, and nasal congestion.

Allergic rhinitis, also known as hay fever, is a chronic allergy triggered by a wide variety of antigens. The release of chemicals mediating the immune response can result in seasonal symptoms for some clients and chronic, continuous symptoms for others.

20.7   Antihistamines, or H₁-receptor antagonists, are useful for treating allergic rhinitis and several other disorders.

The H_1-receptor antagonists, commonly known as antihistamines, are used to treat allergies and inflammation. Newer drugs in this class are non-sedating and offer the advantage of once-a-day dosage.

20.8   Intranasal glucocorticoids have become drugs of choice in treating allergic rhinitis.

Intranasal glucocorticoids have become a treatment of choice for allergic rhinitis because of their high efficacy and wide margin of safety. When used by this route, they do not produce the serious adverse effects observed when they are given orally.

20.9   Sympathomimetics are used to alleviate nasal congestion due to allergic rhinitis and the common cold.

Oral and intranasal sympathomimetics are effective at relieving nasal congestion. Use of the intranasal preparations, however, is usually limited to three to five days because of the potential for rebound congestion.

20.10   Nonsteroidal anti-inflammatory drugs are the primary drugs for the treatment of simple inflammation.

NSAIDS are drugs that inhibit the enzyme cyclooxygenase. Nonselective cycloxygenase inhibitors, including aspirin, are very effective at reducing inflammation and pain, but cause significant GI side effects in some clients. The newer selective COX2 inhibitors cause less GI disturbance.

20.11   Systemic Glucocorticoids are effective in treating acute or severe inflammation.

Glucocorticoids are hormones that are extremely effective at reducing inflammation. Because overtreatment with these drugs can cause a serious syndrome called Cushing's syndrome, therapy for inflammation is generally short-term.

20.12   Immunosuppressants are primarily used to avoid tissue rejection following organ transplant.

In order for an organ or tissue transplant to be successful, the client's immune system must be suppressed for a period of time following surgery. Immunosuppressants are very effective at dampening the client's immune system, but must be monitored very carefully because loss of immune function can lead to infections and cancer.

20.13   Vaccines are biological drugs used to prevent illness.

Vaccines are biological products usually given to prevent a serious illness. Vaccines are of several types: live, attenuated, or toxoid. They are very effective when taken according to schedule and rarely produce serious adverse effects.

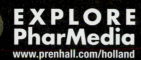

EXPLORE PharMedia
www.prenhall.com/holland

Additional interactive resources and activities for this chapter can be found on the Companion Website. For animations, audio glossary, and review access the accompanying CD-ROM in this book.

Mechanism in Action:
  Diphenhydramine
  Naproxen
Audio Glossary
Concept Review
NCLEX Review

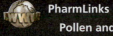

PharmLinks
  Pollen and Allergic Rhinitis
  Xenotransplants
  Vaccine Updates

21 Drugs for Bacterial Infections

CORE CONCEPTS

21.1 Pathogens are described by their virulence, pathogenicity, and mechanism of action.

21.2 Bacteria are described by their shape, their ability to utilize oxygen, and by their staining characteristics.

21.3 Antiinfective drugs are classified by their chemical structure or by their mechanism of action.

21.4 Antiinfective drugs act by affecting the target organism's metabolism or life cycle.

21.5 Acquired resistance is a major problem with antiinfective drugs.

21.6 Careful selection of the correct antibiotic is essential for effective pharmacotherapy and to limit adverse effects.

Penicillins

21.7 The penicillins are one of the oldest and safest groups of antiinfectives.

Cephalosporins

21.8 The cephalosporins are similar in structure and function to the penicillins and are one of the most widely prescribed antiinfective classes.

Tetracyclines

21.9 The tetracycline class has one of the broadest spectrums, but they are drugs of choice for relatively few diseases.

Macrolides

21.10 The macrolides are safe alternatives to penicillin for many diseases.

Aminoglycosides

21.11 The aminoglycosides are narrow-spectrum drugs that have the potential to cause serious toxicity.

21.12 A number of additional antiinfectives have specific indications.

TUBERCULOSIS

Antitubercular Agents

21.13 Pharmacotherapy of tuberculosis requires a unique set of specific drugs because of the slow-growing, complex microbes.

OBJECTIVES

After reading this chapter, the student should be able to:

1. Compare and contrast the terms pathogenicity and virulence.

2. Describe how bacteria are classified.

3. Compare and contrast the terms bacteriostatic and bacteriocidal.

4. Using a specific example, explain how resistance can develop to an antiinfective drug.

5. Explain the importance of culture and sensitivity testing to antiinfective chemotherapy.

6. Identify the mechanism of development and symptoms of superinfections caused by antiinfective therapy.

7. For each of the following, identify representative drugs, explain the mechanism of drug action, primary actions, and important adverse effects:
   a. penicillins
   b. cephalosporins
   c. tetracyclines
   d. macrolides
   e. aminoglycosides
   f. miscellaneous antibiotics

8. Categorize antibacterial drugs based on their classification and mechanism of action.

9. Explain how the pharmacotherapy of tuberculosis differs from that of other infections.

PharMedia
www.prenhall.com/holland

Additional interactive resources and activities for this chapter can be found on the Companion Website. For animations, audio glossary, and review access the accompanying CD-ROM in this book.

acquired resistance: when a microbe is no longer affected by a drug following treatment with antiinfectives / *page 320*

aerobic (air-OH-bik): pertaining to an oxygen environment / *page 316*

anaerobic (AN-air-oh-bik): pertaining to an environment without oxygen / *page 316*

antagonism: type of drug interaction where one drug inhibits the effectiveness of another / *page 321*

antibiotic (ann-tie-bye-OT-ik): substance produced by a microorganism that inhibits or kills other microorganisms / *page 317*

antiinfective (ann-tie-in-FEK-tive): general term for any medication effective against pathogens / *page 317*

bacilli (bah-SILL-eye): bacteria that are oblong in shape; also called *rods* / *page 316*

bacteriocidal (bak-teer-ee-oh-SY-dall): substance that kills bacteria / *page 319*

bacteriostatic (bak-teer-ee-oh-STAT-ik): substance that inhibits the growth of bacteria / *page 319*

beta-lactam ring (bay-tuh LAK-tam): chemical structure found in most penicillins and some cephalosporins / *page 322*

beta-lactamase/penicillinase (bay-tuh-LAK-tam-ace/pen-uh-SILL-in-ace): enzyme present in certain bacteria that is able to inactivate many penicillins and some cephalosporins / *page 322*

broad-spectrum antibiotic: antiinfective that is effective against many different gram positive and gram negative organisms / *page 321*

chemoprophylaxis: (kee-moh-pro-fill-AX-is): use of a drug to prevent an infection / *page 321*

cocci (KOK-si): bacteria that are spherical in shape / *page 316*

culture and sensitivity test: laboratory test used to identify bacteria and to determine which antibiotic is most effective / *page 321*

gram-negative: bacteria that do not retain a purple stain because they have an outer envelope / *page 316*

gram-positive: bacteria that stain purple because they have no outer envelope / *page 316*

host flora (host FLOR-uh): normal microorganisms found in or on a client / *page 321*

mutations (myou-TAY-shuns): permanent, inheritable changes to DNA / *page 319*

narrow-spectrum antibiotic: antiinfective that is effective against only one or a small number of organisms / *page 321*

nephrotoxicity (NEF-row-toks-ISS-ih-tee): an adverse effect on the kidneys / *page 329*

nosocomial infections (noh-soh-KOH-mee-ul): infection acquired in a healthcare setting such as a hospital, physician's office, or nursing home / *page 321*

ototoxicity (OH-toh-toks-ISS-ih-tee): an adverse effect on hearing / *page 329*

pathogen (PATH-oh-jen): organism that is capable of causing disease / *page 316*

pathogenicity (path-oh-jen-ISS-ih-tee): ability of an organism to cause disease in humans / *page 316*

photosensitivity: condition that occurs when the skin is very sensitive to sunlight / *page 324*

plasmid (PLAZ-mid): small piece of circular DNA found in some bacteria that is able to transfer resistance from one bacterium to another / *page 320*

red-man syndrome: rash on the upper body caused by certain antiinfectives / *page 330*

spirilla (speer-ILL-ah): bacteria that have a spiral shape / *page 316*

superinfection: condition caused when a microorganism grows rapidly as a result of having less competition in its environment / *page 321*

toxin (TOX-in): chemical produced by a microorganism that is able to cause injury to its host / *page 316*

tubercles (TOO-burr-kyouls): cavity-like lesions in the lung characteristic of infection by *Mycobacterium tuberculosis* / *page 332*

virulence (VEER-you-lens): the severity of disease that an organism in able to cause / *page 316*

The human body has adapted quite well to living in a world teeming with microorganisms. In the air, water, food, and soil, microbes are an essential component to life on the planet. In some cases, microorganisms such as those in the colon play a beneficial role in human health. When in an unnatural environment or when present in unusually high numbers, however, microorganisms can cause a wide variety of ailments ranging from mildly annoying to fatal. The development of the first antiinfective drugs in the mid 1900s was a milestone in the field of medicine. In the last 50 years, pharmacologists have attempted to keep pace with microbes that rapidly become resistant to therapeutic agents. This chapter examines two groups of antiinfectives: the antibacterial agents and the specialized drugs used to treat tuberculosis.

Fast Facts Bacterial Infections

- Infectious diseases are the third most common cause of death in the U.S. and the most common cause of death worldwide.
- Foodborne illness is responsible for 76 million illnesses, 300,000 hospitalizations, and 5,000 deaths each year. About 500 people die of Salmonella each year in the U.S.
- Urinary tract infections (UTI) are the most common infection acquired in hospitals. Nearly all are associated with the insertion of a urinary catheter. Hospital-acquired urinary infections add an average of 3.8 days to a hospital stay and can cost $3,803 per infection.

- Over 2 million nosocomial infections are acquired each year. These infections adds one day for UTI, seven to eight days for surgical site infections, and six to thirty days for pneumonia.
- Two hundred thousand nosocomial infections of the bloodstream occur annually.
- Pneumococcal infections are the most common invasive bacterial infections in children, accounting for 1400 meningitis infections, 17,000 bloodstream infections, and 71,000 pneumonia infections in clients under the age of 5.
- Up to 30% of all *S. pneumoniae* found in some areas of the U.S. are resistant to penicillin.
- Nearly all strains of *S. aureus* in the U.S. are resistant to penicillin.
- About 73,000 cases of *E. coli* poisoning are reported annually in the U.S. with the most common source being ground beef.

21.1 Pathogens are described by their virulence, pathogenicity, and mechanism of action.

path = *disease*
gen = *producing*

A microbe that can cause disease in humans is called a **pathogen**. Human pathogens include viruses, bacteria, fungi, unicellular organisms, and multicellular animals. Examples of these pathogens are illustrated in Figure 21.1. In order to infect humans, pathogens must bypass a number of elaborate body defenses, such as those described in Chapter 20 ⊂▭⊃ . Pathogens may enter through broken skin, or by ingestion, inhalation, or contact with a mucous membrane such as the nasal, urinary, or vaginal mucosas.

The ability of an organism to cause infection is called its **pathogenicity**. Pathogenicity depends upon an organism's ability to bypass or overcome the body's immune system. Another common word used to describe a pathogen is **virulence**. A highly virulent organism is one that can produce disease when present in very small numbers.

After gaining entry, pathogens generally cause disease by one of two basic mechanisms. Some pathogens grow extremely rapidly and cause disease by their sheer numbers. This rapid growth can overcome the immune system and negatively impact cellular function. A second mechanism is the production of **toxins**, or chemicals that disrupt human cells. Even very small amounts of some bacterial toxins may disrupt normal cellular activity and, in extreme cases, result in death.

21.2 Bacteria are described by their shape, their ability to utilize oxygen, and by their staining characteristics.

Because of the huge number of different bacterial species, several descriptive systems have been developed to simplify their study. It is important for healthcare providers to learn these basic organizational schemes because antiinfective drugs that are effective against one organism in a class are likely to be effective against other pathogens in the same class. A list of common bacterial pathogens and the types of diseases that they cause is shown in Table 21.1.

Some bacteria contain a thick cell wall and retain a purple color after a violet stain is applied to them. These are called **gram-positive** bacteria. Bacteria that have thinner cell walls will lose the violet stain and are called **gram-negative**. The distinction between gram-positive and gram-negative bacteria is a profound one that reflects important biochemical, physiological, and genetic differences between the two groups.

Bacteria assume several basic shapes. Those with rod shapes are called **bacilli**, those that are spherical are **cocci**, and those that are spiral are called **spirilla**.

A third factor used to classify bacteria is their ability to use oxygen. Those that thrive in an oxygen environment are called **aerobic** and those that grow best without oxygen are called **anaerobic**. Some organisms have the ability to change their metabolism and survive in either aerobic or anaerobic conditions, depending upon their external environment.

FIGURE 21.1

Types of pathogenic organisms:
(a) bacterium; (b) virus;
(c) protozoan pathogens;
(d) multicellular parasites; (e) fungi
SOURCE: (21.1 A-D): Pearson Education/PH College.

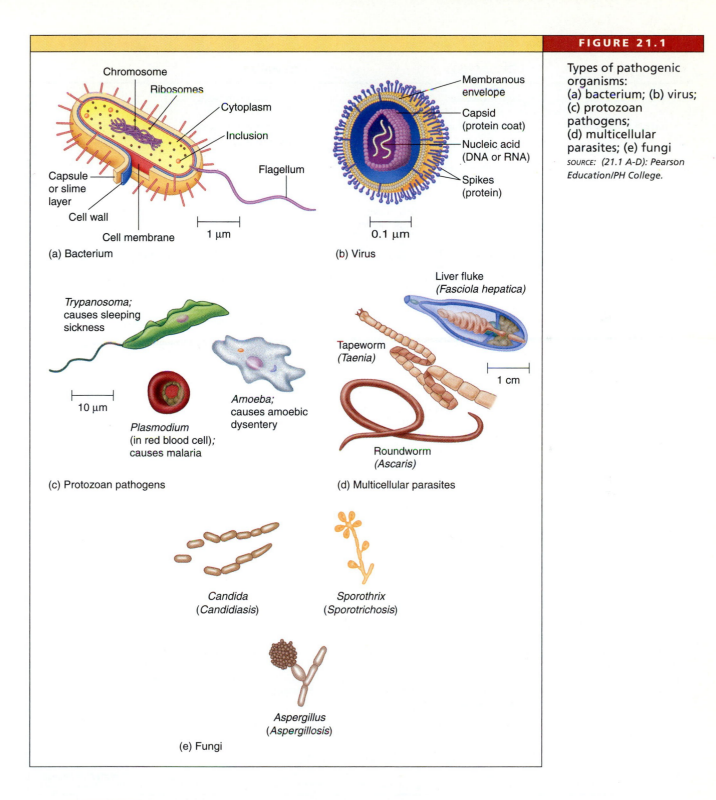

(a) Bacterium

Chromosome
Ribosomes
Cytoplasm
Inclusion
Capsule or slime layer
Cell wall
Cell membrane
Flagellum
1 μm

(b) Virus

Membranous envelope
Capsid (protein coat)
Nucleic acid (DNA or RNA)
Spikes (protein)
0.1 μm

(c) Protozoan pathogens

Trypanosoma; causes sleeping sickness
10 μm
Plasmodium (in red blood cell); causes malaria
Amoeba; causes amoebic dysentery

(d) Multicellular parasites

Liver fluke (*Fasciola hepatica*)
Tapeworm (*Taenia*)
1 cm
Roundworm (*Ascaris*)

(e) Fungi

Candida (*Candidiasis*)
Sporothrix (*Sporotrichosis*)
Aspergillus (*Aspergillosis*)

21.3 Antiinfective drugs are classified by their chemical structure or by their mechanism of action.

Antiinfective is a general term that applies to any drug that is effective against pathogens. Although **antibiotic** is a more frequently used word, this term technically refers only to natural substances produced by a microorganism that can kill other microorganisms. In current practice, the terms *antiinfective, antimicrobial,* and *antibiotic* are often used interchangeably, as they are in this text.

anti = against
bio = life
ic = pertaining to

TABLE 21.1	Common Bacterial Pathogens	
NAME OF ORGANISM	**DISEASE(S)**	**REMARKS**
Borrelia burgdorferi	Lyme disease	Acquired from ticks.
Chlamydia trachomatus	venereal disease, endometriosis	Most common cause of sexually transmitted diseases in the U.S.
Escherichia coli	traveler's diarrhea, UTI, bacteremia, endometriosis	Part of normal flora of GI tract.
Haemophilus	pneumonia, meningitis in children, bacteremia, otitis media, sinusitis	Some *Haemophilus* species are normal flora in the upper respiratory tract.
Klebsiella	pneumonia, UTI	Usually infects immunosuppressed clients.
Mycobacterium leprae	leprosy	Most cases in the U.S. occur in immigrants from Africa or Asia.
Mycobacterium tuberculosis	tuberculosis	Incidence very high in HIV-infected clients.
Mycoplasma pneumoniae	pneumonia	Most common cause of pneumonia in clients age 5 to 35.
Neisseria gonorrhoeae	gonorrhea and other sexually transmitted diseases, endometriosis, neonatal eye infection	Some *Neisseria* species are normal host flora.
Neisseria meningitides	meningitis in children	Some *Neisseria* species are normal host flora.
Pneumococci	pneumonia, otitis media, meningitis, bacteremia, endocarditis	Part of normal flora in upper respiratory tract.
Proteus mirabilis	UTI, skin infections	Part of normal flora in GI tract.
Pseudomonas aeroginosa	UTI, skin infections, septicemia	Usually infects immunosuppressed clients.
Rickettsia rickettsii	Rocky Mountain spotted fever	Acquired from tick bites.
Salmonella entertidis	food poisoning	From infected animal products, raw eggs, or undercooked meat or chicken.
Salmonella typhii	typhoid fever	From inadequately treated food or water supplies.
Staphylococci aureus	pneumonia, food poisoning, impetigo, abscesses, bacteremia, endocarditis, toxic shock syndrome	Some *Staphyloccoccus* species are normal host flora.
Streptococci	pharyngitis, pneumonia, skin infections, septicemia, endocarditis	Some *Streptococci* species are normal host flora.
Vibrio cholerae	cholera	From inadequately treated food or water supplies.

With well over 300 antiinfective drugs available, it is helpful to group these drugs into classes that have similar chemical or therapeutic properties. Chemical classes are widely used and the student will see names such as *aminoglycoside, fluoroquinolone,* and *sulfonamide* that refer to the fundamental chemical structure of a group of antiinfectives. Antiinfectives belonging to the same chemical class share similar mechanisms of action and side effects.

Another method of classifying antiinfectives is by mechanism of action. Examples include cell wall inhibitors, protein synthesis inhibitors, folic acid inhibitors, and reverse transcriptase inhibitors. These are used in this text, where appropriate.

21.4 Antiinfective drugs act by affecting the target organism's metabolism or life cycle.

The primary goal of antimicrobial therapy is to rid the body of the infectious organism. Drugs that accomplish this goal by killing bacteria are called bacteriocidal. Some medications do not kill the bacteria, but instead slow their growth so that the body's immune system can dispose of the microorganisms. These growth-slowing drugs are called bacteriostatic.

bacterio = bacteria
cidal = killing

static = staying the same

Bacterial cells are quite different from human cells. Bacteria have cell walls and contain certain enzymes and cellular structures that human cells lack. Antibiotics exert selective toxicity on bacterial cells by targeting these unique differences. In that way, bacteria can be killed or their growth severely hampered without major effects on human cells. Of course, there are limits to this selective toxicity, depending upon the specific antibiotic and the dose employed, and side effects can be expected from all the antiinfectives. The basic mechanisms of action of antimicrobial drugs are shown in Figure 21.2.

21.5 Acquired resistance is a major problem with antiinfective drugs.

Microorganisms have the ability to replicate extremely rapidly. During cell division, bacteria make frequent errors duplicating their genetic code. These errors, called mutations, occur spontaneously

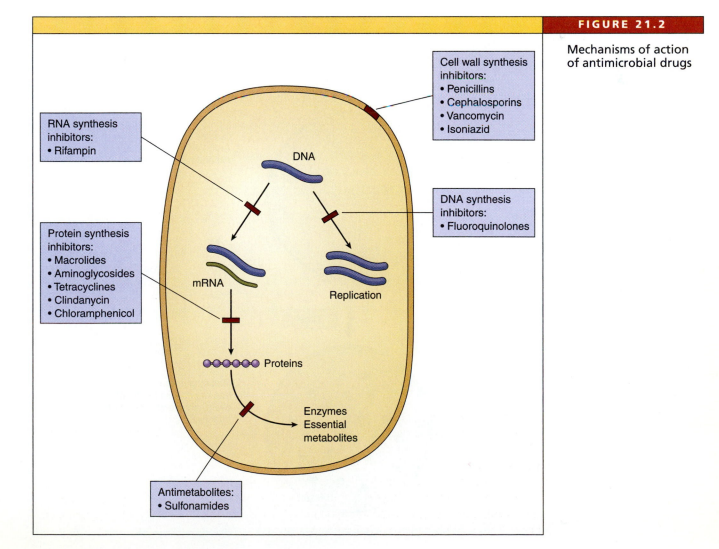

FIGURE 21.2

Mechanisms of action of antimicrobial drugs

Cell wall synthesis inhibitors:
• Penicillins
• Cephalosporins
• Vancomycin
• Isoniazid

RNA synthesis inhibitors:
• Rifampin

DNA

DNA synthesis inhibitors:
• Fluoroquinolones

Protein synthesis inhibitors:
• Macrolides
• Aminoglycosides
• Tetracyclines
• Clindanycin
• Chloramphenicol

mRNA

Replication

Proteins

Enzymes
Essential
metabolites

Antimetabolites:
• Sulfonamides

and randomly in the bacterial cell. Although most mutations are harmful to an organism, mutations occasionally result in a bacterial cell that has reproductive advantages over its neighbors. The mutated bacterium may be able to survive in harsher conditions or perhaps grow faster than other cells. One such mutation that is of particular importance to medicine is that which confers drug resistance upon a microorganism.

Antibiotics promote the development of drug-resistant bacterial strains by killing the masses of bacteria that are sensitive to the drug. The only bacteria remaining may be the microbes that underwent mutations to make them insensitive to the effects of the antibiotic. These drug-resistant bacteria are then free to grow, unrestrained by their neighbors that were killed by the antibiotic. Soon the client develops an infection that is resistant to conventional drug therapy. This phenomenon, called **acquired resistance**, is illustrated in Figure 21.3. Bacteria may pass the resistance gene to other bacteria by transferring small pieces of circular DNA called **plasmids**.

FIGURE 21.3

Acquired resistance

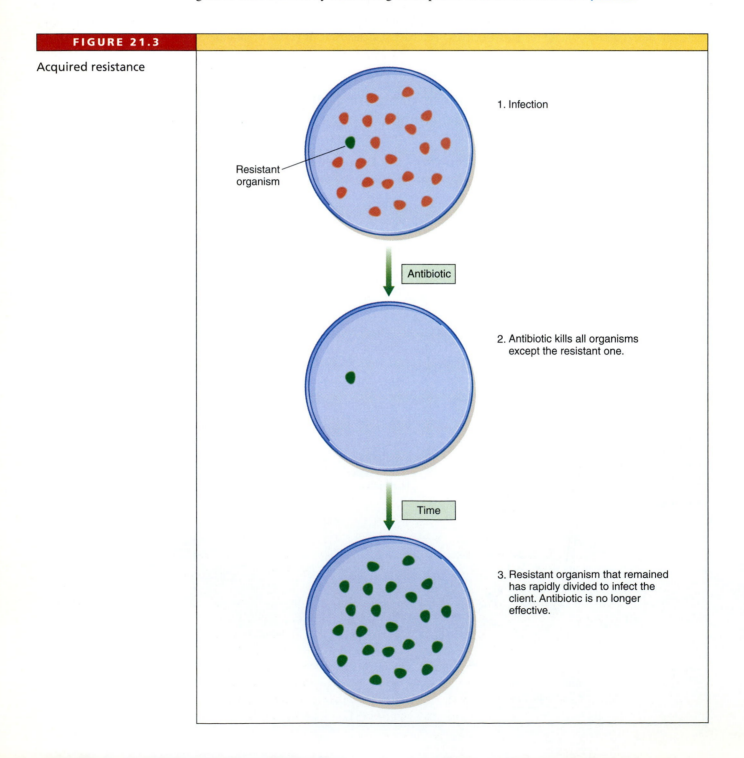

It is important to understand that the antibiotic did not create the mutation that conferred resistance. The mutation occurred randomly. The role of the antibiotic was to kill the surrounding cells that were susceptible to the drug, leaving the mutated one plenty of room to divide and infect.

The widespread and sometimes unwarranted use of antibiotics has led to a large number of resistant strains. For example, 60% of all *Staphylococcus* bacteria are now resistant to penicillin. The longer an antibiotic is used in the population and the more often it is prescribed, the larger will be the percentage of resistant strains. Infections acquired in a hospital or other healthcare setting, called nosocomial infections, are often resistant to common antibiotics. In an effort to delay the development of resistance, healthcare practitioners should restrict the use of antibiotics to those conditions deemed medically necessary.

In most cases, antibiotics are given when there is clear evidence of bacterial infection. Some clients, however, receive antibiotics to prevent an infection, a practice called *prophylactic use,* or chemoprophylaxis. Examples of clients who might receive prophylactic antibiotics include those who have a suppressed immune system, those who have experienced deep puncture wounds such as those from dog bites, or those clients who have prosthetic heart valves, prior to receiving medical or dental surgery.

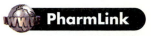

PharmLink

VETERINARY ANTIBIOTICS AND HUMAN HEALTH

21.6 Careful selection of the correct antibiotic is essential for effective pharmacotherapy and to limit adverse effects.

Some antiinfectives are effective against a wide variety of microorganisms. These are called broad-spectrum antibiotics. If the medication is effective against only one or a restricted group of microorganisms, it is referred to as a narrow-spectrum antibiotic.

Selection of an antibiotic that will be effective against a specific organism is an important task of the healthcare practitioner. Selecting the incorrect drug will not only delay proper treatment and give the microorganism more time to infect, but may cause unnecessary side effects in the client as well.

Ideally, laboratory tests should be conducted to identify the organism prior to beginning antiinfective therapy. Lab tests may include examination of body specimens such as urine, sputum, blood, or pus for microorganisms. Organisms isolated from the specimens are grown in the laboratory so that they may be identified. After identification, the laboratory may test several different antibiotics to determine which is most effective against the infecting microorganism. This process of growing the organism and identifying the effective antibiotic is called culture and sensitivity testing.

Proper testing and identification of bacteria may take several days and, in the case of viruses, several weeks. Indeed, some organisms simply cannot be cultured at all. If the infection is severe, the healthcare practitioner will likely begin therapy with a broad-spectrum antibiotic. After the results of the culture and sensitivity tests are known, therapy may be changed to include the antibiotic found to be most effective against the microbe.

In most cases, antiinfective therapy is conducted with a single drug. This is because combining two antibiotics may actually decrease each drug's efficacy, a phenomenon known as antagonism. Use of multiple antibiotics also has the potential to promote resistance. Multi-drug therapy may be warranted, however, if the client's infection is caused by several different organisms or if therapy must be started before culture and sensitivity testing has been completed. Multi-drug therapy is common in the treatment of tuberculosis and infection with HIV.

One common side effect of antiinfective therapy is the creation of secondary infections, called superinfections, that occur when microorganisms normally present in the body are killed by the drug. These normal microorganisms, called host flora, inhabit the skin and the upper respiratory, genitourinary, and intestinal tracts. Some of these organisms serve a useful purpose by producing antibacterial substances and by competing for nutrients with pathogenic organisms. Removal of normal flora by an antibiotic gives pathogenic microorganisms space to grow, or allows for overgrowth of non-affected normal flora. Appearance of a new infection while receiving antiinfective therapy is suspicious of a superinfection. Signs and symptoms of a superinfection may include

NATURAL ALTERNATIVES

The Antibacterial Properties of Goldenseal

Goldenseal (*Hydrastis canadensis*) was once a common plant found in woods in the eastern and midwestern United States. As word spread of its medicinal properties, the plant was harvested to near extinction. In particular, goldenseal was reported to mask the appearance of drugs in the urine of clients wanting to hide their drug abuse. This claim has been proven false.

The roots and leaves of goldenseal are dried and available as capsules, tablets, salves, and tinctures. One of the primary ingredients in goldenseal is hydrastine, which is reported to have antibacterial and antifungal properties. When used topically or locally, it is purported to be of value in treating bacterial and fungal skin infections and oral conditions such as gingivitis and thrush. Other possible indications include hypertension, duodenal ulcers, and conjunctivitis. ■

diarrhea, bladder pain, painful urination, or abnormal vaginal discharges. Broad-spectrum antibiotics are more likely to cause superinfections because they kill so many different species of microorganisms. Figure 21.2 illustrates the production of a superinfection.

PENICILLINS

The penicillins are one of the oldest and safest classes of antibiotics. While not the first antiinfective discovered, penicillin was the first mass-produced antibiotic. Isolated from the fungus *Penicillium* in 1941, penicillin quickly became a miracle drug by preventing thousands of deaths from what are now considered to be minor infections.

21.7 The penicillins are one of the oldest and safest groups of antiinfectives.

Penicillins kill bacteria by disrupting their cell walls. The portion of the chemical structure of penicillin that is responsible for its antibacterial activity is called the beta-lactam ring. Some bacteria secrete an enzyme, called beta-lactamase or penicillinase, which splits the beta-lactam ring. These bacteria are resistant to the effects of most penicillins. The action of penicillinase is illustrated in Figure 21.4. Large numbers of resistant bacterial strains limit the therapeutic usefulness of the penicillins.

Chemical modifications to the original molecule have produced drugs offering several advantages over the first penicillin. Oxacillin (Prostaphlin and others) and cloxacillin (Tegopen) are effective against penicillinase-producing bacteria and are thus called *penicillinase-resistant* penicillins. Although the original penicillin is effective against a narrow range of organisms, some in this class such as ampicillin (Polycillin and others) are effective against a wider range of microorganisms, and are called broad-spectrum penicillins. Commonly prescribed penicillins are listed in Table 21.2 (page 325).

In general, the adverse effects of penicillins are minor and this has contributed to their widespread use for over 50 years. Allergy is the most common adverse effect. Symptoms of penicillin allergy may include rash, fever, and anaphylaxis. The incidence of anaphylaxis is quite low, ranging from 0.04% to 2%. Allergy to one penicillin increases the risk of allergy to other drugs in the same class.

Concept review 21.1

■ Why does antibiotic resistance become more of a problem when antibiotics are prescribed too often?

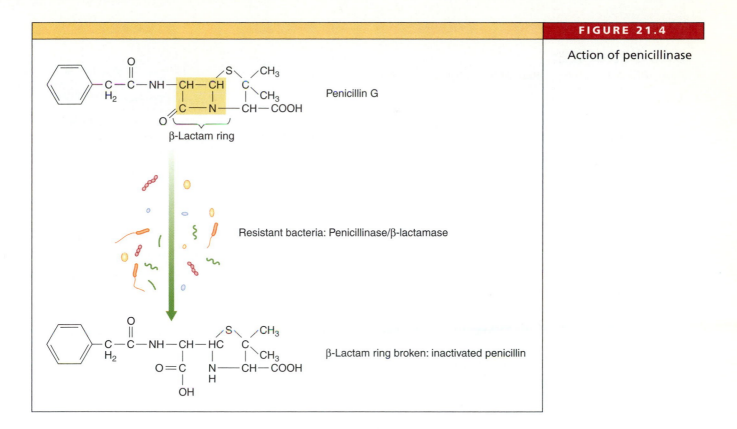

FIGURE 21.4

Action of penicillinase

Penicillin G

β-Lactam ring

Resistant bacteria: Penicillinase/β-lactamase

β-Lactam ring broken: inactivated penicillin

CEPHALOSPORINS

Isolated shortly after the penicillins, the four generations of cephalosporins comprise one of the largest antibiotic classes. Like the penicillins, the cephalosporins contain a beta-lactam ring that is primarily responsible for their antimicrobial activity.

21.8 The cephalosporins are similar in structure and function to the penicillins and are one of the most widely prescribed antiinfective classes.

The cephalosporins are bacteriocidal and inhibit cell wall synthesis. Over 20 cephalosporins are available, and they are classified by their "generation." The first-generation drugs contain a beta-lactam ring and bacteria producing beta-lactamase will normally be resistant to these cephalosporins. The second-generation cephalosporins are more potent, more resistant to beta-lactamase, and exhibit a broader spectrum than the first-generation drugs. The third-generation cephalosporins generally have a longer duration of action, an even broader spectrum, and are resistant to beta-lactamases. Third-generation cephalosporins are sometimes the drugs of first choice against infections by *Pseudomonas, Klebsiella, Neisseria, Salmonella, Proteus,* and *H. influenza.* Newer, fourth-generation drugs are more effective against organisms that have developed resistance to earlier cephalosporins. There are not always clear distinctions among the generations.

The primary therapeutic use of the cephalosporins is for gram-negative infections and for clients who cannot tolerate the less-expensive penicillins. Like the penicillins, allergic reactions are the most common adverse effect. Earlier-generation cephalosporins exhibit kidney toxicity, but this is diminished with the newer drugs. The healthcare provider must be alert that some clients who are allergic to penicillin will also be allergic to the cephalosporins. Despite this small incidence of cross-allergy, the cephalosporins offer a reasonable alternative for clients who are unable to take penicillin. Table 21.3 (page 326) lists selected cephalosporins and their dosages.

DRUG PROFILE:
Penicillin G Potassium (Pentids)

Actions:

Similar to penicillin V, penicillin G is a drug of first choice against *streptococci, pneumococci,* and *staphylococci* organisms that do not produce penicillinase. It is also a drug of first choice for gonorrhea and syphilis caused by susceptible strains. Penicillin V is more acid stable; over 70% is absorbed after an oral dose compared to the 15 to 30% from penicillin G. Because of its low oral absorption, penicillin G is often given by the IV or IM routes. Penicillinase-producing organisms inactivate both penicillin G and penicillin V.

Adverse Effects:

Penicillin G has few side effects. Although not serious, diarrhea, nausea, and vomiting are the most common adverse effects. Anaphylaxis is the most serious adverse effect, though its incidence is very low. Pain at the injection site may occur and superinfections are possible.

Mechanism in Action:

Penicillin G is a narrow spectrum antibiotic that attaches to the penicillin binding protein (PBP) at the active site of selected bacterial cell walls. Following attachment, penicillin G prevents the synthesis of new peptide bridges causing fragmentation of the peptidoglycan cell wall matrix. Death of the bacteria soon follows.

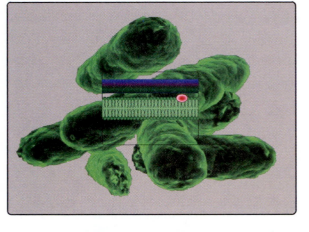

TETRACYCLINES

The first tetracyclines were extracted from *Streptomyces* soil microorganisms in 1948. Their widespread use in the 1950s and 1960s has resulted in a large number of resistant bacterial strains that now limits their therapeutic usefulness.

21.9 The tetracycline class has one of the broadest spectrums, but they are drugs of choice for relatively few diseases.

Tetracyclines exert a bacteriostatic effect by inhibiting bacterial protein synthesis. They are effective against a wide range of gram-negative and gram-positive organisms and have one of the broadest spectrums of any class of antibiotics. Considerable bacterial resistance to the tetracyclines has limited their usefulness. They are drugs of first choice for relatively few diseases: Rocky Mountain spotted fever, typhus, cholera, Lyme disease, and *Chlamydial* infections. Because of their ability to bind calcium molecules, tetracyclines should not be taken with milk because the drug's absorption may be decreased as much as 50%. They may also cause yellow-brown tooth discoloration in young children. Some clients experience photosensitivity during therapy, making their skin particularly susceptible to sunburn. Table 21.4 (page 327) lists the tetracyclines and their dosages.

TABLE 21.2	The Penicillins	
DRUG	**ROUTE AND ADULT DOSE**	**REMARKS**
ampicillin (Polycillin, Omnipen)	PO; 250–500 mg qid.	Broad-spectrum; IM and IV forms available.
amoxicillin (Amoxil, Trimox, Wymox)	PO; 250–500 mg tid.	Broad-spectrum; IV form available; amoxicillin plus clavulanate is called Augmentin.
bacampicillin hydrochloride (Spectrobid)	PO; 400–800 mg bid.	Broad-spectrum
carbenicillin indanylna (Geocillin, Geopen)	PO; 382–764 mg qid.	Extended-spectrum; IM and IV forms available.
cloxacillin (Tegopen)	PO; 250–500 mg qid.	Penicillinase-resistant.
dicloxacillin sodium (Dynapen)	PO; 125–500 mg qid.	Penicillinase-resistant.
mezlocillin sodium (Mezlin)	IM; 1.5–2 g qid (max 24 g/day).	Extended-spectrum; IV form available.
nafcillin sodium (Nafcin, Unipen)	PO; 250 mg – 1 g qid (max 12 g/day).	Penicillinase-resistant; IM and IV forms available.
oxacillin sodium (Prostaphlin, Bactocil)	PO; 250 mg – 1 g qid (max 12 g/day).	Penicillinase-resistant; IV and IM forms available.
Pr penicillin G sodium/potassium (Pentids)	PO; 400,000–800,000 units qid.	IM and IV forms available; ineffective against most forms of *staph aureus*.
penicillin G benzathine (Bicillin)	IM; 1.2 million units as a single dose.	Prolonged duration of action.
penicillin G procaine (Crysticillin, Wycillin)	IM; 600,000–1.2 million units qd.	Prolonged duration of action.
penicillin V (PenVee K, Veetids, Betapen VK)	PO; 125–250 mg qid.	Acid-stable.
pirperacillin sodium (Pipracil)	IM; 2–4 g tid – qid (max 24 g/day).	Extended-spectrum.
piperacillin/tazobactam (Zosyn)	IV; 3.375 g qid over 30 minutes.	Extended-spectrum.
ticarcillin disodium (Ticar)	IM; 1–2 g qid (max 40 g/day).	Extended-spectrum.

MACROLIDES

Erythromycin (E-mycin, Erythrocin), the first macrolide antibiotic, was isolated from *Streptomyces* in a soil sample in 1952. Macrolides are prescribed for infections that are resistant to penicillins.

21.10 The macrolides are safe alternatives to penicillin for many diseases.

The macrolide antibiotics inhibit bacterial protein synthesis and may be either bacteriocidal or bacteriostatic, depending upon the dose and the target organism. Macrolides are considered very safe alternatives to penicillin, although they are drugs of first choice for relatively few diseases. Common uses of macrolides include the treatment of whooping cough, legionnaire's disease, and infections by *Streptococcus*, *Haemophilus influenza*, *Mycoplasma pneumoniae*, and *Chlamydia*.

DRUG PROFILE:
Cefotaxime (Claforan)

Actions:

Cefotaxime is a third-generation cephalosporin with a broad spectrum of activity against gram-negative organisms. It is effective against many organisms that have developed resistance to earlier generation cephalosporins and to other classes of antiinfectives. Cefotaxime exhibits bacteriocidal activity by inhibiting cell wall synthesis. It is prescribed for serious infections of the lower respiratory tract, CNS, genitourinary system, bones, and joints. It may also be used for blood infections such as bacteremia or septicemia. Like many of the cephalosporins, cefotaxime is not absorbed from the GI tract and must be given by the IM or IV routes.

Adverse Effects:

For most clients, cefotaxime and the other cephalosporins are very safe medications. Hypersensitivity is the most common adverse effect, although symptoms may include only a minor rash and itching. Anaphylaxis is possible; thus the healthcare provider should be alert for this reaction. GI-related side effects such as diarrhea, vomiting, and nausea may occur. Some patients experience considerable pain at the injection site.

TABLE 21.3   **The Cephalosporins**

DRUG	ROUTE AND ADULT DOSE	REMARKS
First Generation		
cefadroxil (Duricef, Ultracef)	PO; 500 mg -1 g qd-bid (max 2 g/day).	Binds to bacterial cell walls; bacteriocidal.
cefazolin Sodium (Ancef, Kefzol)	IM; 250 mg-2 g tid (max 12 g/day).	IV form available.
cephalexin (Keflex)	PO; 250–500 mg qid.	Binds to bacterial cell walls; bacteriocidal; broad-spectrum.
Second Generation		
cefonicid sodium (Monocid) second-generation	IM; 1 g qd (max 2 g/day).	IV form available.
cefaclor (Ceclor)	PO; 250–500 mg tid.	Binds to bacterial cell walls; extended-release form available; bacteriocidal.
cefamandole nafate (Mandol)	IM; 500 mg-1g tid-qid (max 12 g/day).	IV form available.
cefprozil (Cefzil)	PO; 250–500 mg qd-bid.	Binds to bacterial cell walls; bacteriocidal.
cefuroxime sodium (Ceftin, Kefurox, Zinacef)	PO; 250–500 mg bid.	Binds to bacterial cell walls; IM and IV forms available; bacteriocidal.
Third and Fourth Generations		
Pr cefotaxime sodium (Claforan)	IM; 1–2 g bid-tid (max 12 g/day).	Third-generation; binds to bacterial cell walls; bacteriocidal; IV form available.
cefdinir (Omnicef)	PO; 300 mg bid.	Third-generation; broad-spectrum.
cefixime (Suprax)	PO; 400 mg qd or 200 mg bid.	Third-generation; binds to bacterial cell walls; bacteriocidal.
cefepime (Maxipime)	IM 0.5–1 g bid (max 3 g/day).	Fourth-generation; IV form available.
ceftriaxone sodium (Rocephin)	IM; 1–2 g qd-bid (max 4 g/day).	Third-generation; binds to bacterial cell walls IV form also available; bacteriocidal.

DRUG PROFILE:
Tetracycline HCl (Achromycin and Others)

Actions:

Tetracycline is effective against a large number of different microorganisms, including some protozoans. It is given orally and has a short half-life. A topical preparation is available for treating acne. It should be administered one to two hours before or after meals to avoid drug interactions.

Adverse Effects:

As a broad-spectrum antibiotic, tetracycline has a tendency to affect intestinal flora and cause superinfections. Diarrhea may be severe enough to cause discontinuation of therapy. Other common side effects include nausea, vomiting, and photosensitivity.

TABLE 21.4	The Tetracyclines	
DRUG	**ROUTE AND ADULT DOSE**	**REMARKS**
Pr tetracycline hydrochloride (Achromycin, Panmycin, Sumycin)	PO; 250–500 mg bid-qid (max 2 g/day).	Short-acting; inhibits protein synthesis; bacteriostatic; IM and topical forms available.
demeclocycline hydrochloride (Declomycin)	PO; 150–300 mg bid-qid (max 2.4 g/day).	Intermediate duration of action; broad-spectrum.
doxycycline hyclate (Doryx. Doxy, Monodox, Vibramycin)	PO; 100 mg bid on day 1, then 100 mg qd (max 200 mg/day).	Long duration of action; IV form available.
minocycline hydrochloride (Dynacin, Minocin, Vectrin)	PO; 200 mg as one dose followed by 100 mg bid.	Long duration of action; IV form available; inhibits protein synthesis; bacteriostatic.
oxytetracycline (Terramycin)	PO; 250–500 mg bid-qid.	Short-acting; IM and IV forms available; broad-spectrum.

The newer macrolides have a longer half-life and cause less GI irritation than erythromycin. For example, azithromycin (Zithromax) has such an extended half-life that it can be administered for only four days, rather the 10 days required for most antibiotics. The shorter duration of therapy could increase client compliance. Commonly prescribed macrolides are shown in Table 21.5.

Concept review 21.2

■ If penicillins are inexpensive, why might a physician prescribe a more expensive cephalosporin or macrolide antibiotic?

AMINOGLYCOSIDES

The aminoglycosides, first isolated from soil organisms in 1942, share a common chemical structure of an amino group (NH_2) and a sugar group. Although more toxic than most other antibiotic classes, they have important therapeutic applications for the treatment of a number of aerobic gram-negative bacteria, mycobacteria, and some protozoans.

DRUG PROFILE:

Erythromycin (E-mycin, Erythrocin)

Actions:

Erythromycin is inactivated by stomach acid and is thus administered as coated tablets or capsules that are intended to dissolve in the small intestine. The drug's main application is for clients who are allergic to penicillins or who may have a penicillin-resistant infection.

Adverse Effects:

The most common side effects from erythromycin are nausea, abdominal cramping, and vomiting, although these are rarely serious enough to cause discontinuation of therapy. Concurrent administration with food reduces this irritation. Its spectrum of activity is similar to that of the penicillins.

TABLE 21.5	The Macrolides	
DRUG	**ROUTE AND ADULT DOSE**	**REMARKS**
Pr erythromycin (E-mycin, Erythrocin)	PO; 250–500 mg qid or 333 mg tid.	Bacteriostatic or bacteriocidal, depending on nature of organism and drug concentration; IV form available.
azithromycin (Zithromax)	PO; 500 mg for one dose, then 250 mg qd for 4 days.	Inhibits protein synthesis; bacteriostatic; IV form available.
clarithromycin (Biaxin)	PO; 250–500 mg bid.	Inhibits protein synthesis; bacteriostatic.
dirithromycin (Dynabac)	PO; 500 mg qd.	Should be taken with food to enhance its activity.

21.11 The aminoglycosides are narrow-spectrum drugs that have the potential to cause serious toxicity.

The first aminoglycoside, streptomycin, was named after *Streptomyces griseus,* the soil organism from which it was isolated. Once widely used, streptomycin is now usually restricted to the treatment of tuberculosis, because of the development of a large number of resistant species. A number of other aminoglycosides sharing similar properties have since been isolated.

ON THE JOB

Periodontal Disease in the Dentist's Office

Periodontal disease is the second most common infectious disease after the common cold, afflicting over 50 million Americans. Beginning as a painless infection, bacteria can build up to separate the teeth from the gums and destroy the soft tissue and bone holding teeth in place.

Periodontal disease has traditionally been treated with oral antibiotics and extensive root planing and scaling by the dental hygienist. Recently, a novel delivery method has been developed, called Atridox, to deliver the antibiotic doxycycline directly to the site where it is needed. The dentist places the Atridox gel in the periodontal pocket. The gel solidifies and releases the antibiotic over a seven-day period. As treatment progresses, the dental hygienist monitors the progress of the disease by measuring the depth of the pocket. A second type of implant, called the Periochip, is also available to deliver the antibacterial chemical chlorhexidine to the periodontal pocket. These implants are tolerated well, usually producing only minor tooth sensitivity or gum pain. ■

DRUG PROFILE:
Gentamicin (Garamycin)

Actions:

Gentamicin is a broad-spectrum, bacteriocidal antibiotic usually prescribed for serious urinary, respiratory, nervous, or GI infections when less toxic antibiotics are contraindicated. It is often used in combination with other antibiotics or when other antibiotics have proven ineffective. It is used parenterally, or as drops, in the case of eye infections.

Adverse Effects:

As with other aminoglycosides, adverse effects from gentamicin may be severe. Loss of hearing or balance, known as ototoxicity, is possible and may become permanent with continued use. Frequent hearing tests should be conducted so that gentamicin may be discontinued if early signs of ototoxicity are detected. The healthcare provider must also be alert for signs nephrotoxicity, as this may limit drug therapy with gentamicin.

oto = *ear*
toxicity = *poison*

nephron = *kidney*

TABLE 21.6	The Aminoglycosides	
DRUG	**ROUTE AND ADULT DOSE**	**REMARKS**
Pr gentamicin sulfate (Garamycin, G-mycin, Jenamicin)	IM; 1.5–2 mg/kg as a loading dose, then 1–2 mg/kg bid-tid.	IV, topical, and ophthalmic forms available.
amikacin sulfate (Amikin)	IM; 5–7.5 mg/kg as a loading dose, then 7.5 mg/kg bid.	Broader spectrum than others in this class; usually bacteriocidal; IV form available.
kanamycin (Kantrex)	IM; 5–7.5 mg/kg bid-tid.	Also used to sterilize the bowel prior to colon surgery; oral, inhalation, and IV forms available.
neomycin sulfate (Mycifradin)	IM; 1.3–2.6 mg/kg qid.	Oral, topical, and IV forms available.
netilmicin sulfate (Netromycin)	IM; 1.3–2.2 mg/kg tid or 2–3.25 mg/kg bid.	Also effective against gentimicin-resistant bacteria; IV form available.
paromomycin sulfate (Humatin)	PO; 7.5–12.5 mg/kg tid.	For parasitic infections of the intestine; also used to treat hepatic coma.
streptomycin sulfate	IM; 15 mg/kg up to 1 g as a single dose.	For tuberculosis, tularemia, and plague.
tobramycin sulfate (Nebcin)	IM; 1 mg/kg tid (max 5 mg/kg/day).	Most effective against *Pseudomonas aeruginosa*; IV form available.

Aminoglycosides are bacteriocidal and act by inhibiting bacterial protein synthesis. They are normally reserved for serious aerobic gram-negative infections, including those caused by *E.coli, Serratia, Proteus, Klebsiella,* and *Pseudomonas*. When used for systemic bacterial infections, they are given parenterally, as they are poorly absorbed from the GI tract. Neomycin is available for topical infections of the skin, eyes, and ears. They are occasionally given orally to sterilize the bowel prior to intestinal surgery. One aminoglycoside, paromomycin (Humatin), is given orally for the treatment of parasitic infections. The student should note the differences in spelling of some of these drugs, from *–mycin* to *–micin,* which reflects the different organisms from which the drugs were originally isolated. Table 21.6 lists selected aminoglycosides and their dosages.

21.12 A number of additional antiinfectives have specific indications.

Some antiinfectives cannot be grouped into classes, or the class is too small to warrant separate discussion. That is not to diminish their importance in medicine; some of these miscellaneous antiinfectives are critically important drugs in certain situations. For example, the drugs in the fluoroquinolone group are quite effective against *Pseudomonas* organisms. The combined antibiotics of sulfamethoxazole and trimethoprim, marketed as Bactrim or Septra, is used extensively for a number of urinary tract infections. Clindamycin (Cleocin) is sometimes the drug of choice for oral infections caused by *Bacteroides* species. Table 21.7 lists some of these miscellaneous antibiotics and their dosages.

DRUG PROFILE:
Vancomycin (Vancocin)

Actions:

Vancomycin is an antibiotic usually reserved for severe infections from gram-positive organisms such as *Staphylococcus aureus* and *Streptococcus pneumoniae*. It is often used after bacteria have become resistant to other, safer antibiotics. It is bacteriocidal, inhibiting bacterial cell wall synthesis. Because vancomycin was not used very frequently during the first 30 years following its discovery, the incidence of vancomycin-resistant organisms is smaller than with other antibiotics. Vancomycin is the most effective drug for treating methicillin-resistant *S. aureus* infections, which have become a major problem in the United States. Vancomycin-resistant strains of *S.aureus,* however, have begun to appear in recent years. Vancomycin is normally given intravenously because it is not absorbed from the GI tract.

Adverse Effects:

Frequent, minor side effects include flushing, hypotension, and rash on the upper body, sometimes called red-man syndrome. More serious adverse effects are possible with higher doses, including nephrotoxicity and ototoxicity. Some clients experience an acute allergic reaction and even anaphylaxis.

TABLE 21.7	Fluoroquinolones and Miscellaneous Antiinfectives	
DRUG	**ROUTE AND ADULT DOSE**	**REMARKS**
Fluroquinolones		
Ciprofloxacin (Cipro)	PO: 250–750 mg bid.	Bacteriostatic; IV and ophthalmic forms available; broad-spectrum; for the treatment of lung, skin, bone, and joint infections.
cinoxacin (Cinobac)	PO; 250–500 mg bid-qid.	Bacteriostatic; for the treatment of UTI.
enoxacin (Penetrex)	PO; 200–400 mg bid.	Bacteriostatic; for the treatment of UTI and gonorrhea.
gatifloxacin (Tequin)	PO; 400 mg qd.	Bacteriostatic; for the treatment of URI, gonorrhea, and UTI; IV form available.
levofloxacin (Levaquin)	PO; 250–500 mg/day qd.	Bacteriostatic; for the treatment of respiratory tract and skin infections; IV form available.

continues

TABLE 21.7	Fluoroquinolones and Miscellaneous Antiinfectives *continued*

DRUG	ROUTE AND ADULT DOSE	REMARKS
lomefloxacin (Maxaquin)	PO; 400 mg qd.	Bacteriostatic; for the treatment of respiratory and urinary tract infections.
moxifloxacin (Avelox)	PO; 400 mg qd.	Bacteriostatic; for the treatment of sinus and respiratory tract infections.
norfloxacin (Noroxin)	PO; 400 mg bid.	Bacteriostatic; for the treatment of UTI; ophthalmic form available.
ofloxacin (Floxin)	PO; 200–400 mg bid.	Bacteriostatic; for the treatment of respiratory and urinary tract infections and gonorrhea; IV and ophthalmic forms available.
sparfloxacin (Zagam)	PO; 400 mg on day one then 200 mg qd.	Bacteriostatic; for the treatment of lung infections.
trovafloxacin/ alatrovafloxacin (Trovan)	PO; 100–300 mg qd.	Bacteriostatic; IV form available; for the treatment of lung infections, gonorrhea, sinusitis.
Miscellaneous Agents		
aztreonam (Azactam)	IM; 0.5–2 g bid-qid (max 8 g/day).	Monobactam class; narrow-spectrum; gram-negative aerobic bacteria; IV form available.
chloramphenicol (Chlorofair, Chloromycetin, Chloroptic, Fenicol)	PO; 12.5 mg/kg qid.	Broad-spectrum; for the treatment of typhoid fever and meningitis; IV form available.
clindamycin hydrochloride (Cleocin)	PO; 150–450 mg qid.	Bacteriostatic; effective against anaerobic organisms; topical, IM, and IV forms available.
imipenem-cilastatin (Primaxin)	IV; 250–500 mg tid-qid (max 4 g/day).	Carbapenum class; combination drug; IM form available; one of the broadest spectrums of any antiinfective.
lincomycin hydrochloride (Lincocin)	PO; 500 mg tid-qid (max 8 g/day).	Bacteriostatic; effective against anaerobic organisms; IM form available.
linezolid (Zyvox)	PO; 600 mg bid.	For vancomycin-resistant *Enterococcus;* IV form available.
meropenum (Merrem IV)	IV; 1–2 g tid.	Carbapenum class; for the treatment of intra-abdominal infections, bacterial meningitis.
methenamine hippurate or mandelate (Mandelamine, Hiprex, Urex)	PO; Hippurate 1 g bid Mandelate 1 g qid.	For the treatment of chronic UTI; broad-spectrum.
nitrofurantoin (Furadantin, Furalan, Furantoin, Marobid, Macrodantin)	PO; 50–100 mg qid.	For the treatment of UTI; extended release form available; interferes with bacterial enzymes; may be bacteriostatic or bacteriocidal.
sulfisoxazole (Gantrisin) sulfonamide	PO; 2–4 g initially followed by 1–2 g qid.	Short-acting sulfonamide; vaginal form available; for the treatment of UTI.
sulfamethoxazole (Gantanol)	PO; 2 g initially followed by 1 g bid-tid.	Intermediate-acting sulfonamide; for the treatment of UTI.
trimethoprim-sulfamethoxazole (TMP-SMZ, Bactrim, Septa)	PO; 160 mgTMP/800 mg SMZ bid.	Combination drug; for the treatment of UTI, *pneumocystis carinii,* and ear infections; IV form available.
Pr vancomycin hydrochloride (Vancocin)	IV; 500 mg qid-1 g bid.	For the treatment of *Staph*-resistant infections.

TUBERCULOSIS

Tuberculosis (TB) is a highly contagious infection caused by the organism *Mycobacterium tuberculosis.* While the microorganisms typically invade the lung, they may also enter other body systems, particularly bone. The slow-growing mycobacteria activate cells of the immune system, which attempt to isolate the microorganisms by creating a wall around them. The mycobacteria usually become dormant, lying inside cavities called tubercles. They may remain dormant during an entire lifetime, or they may become reactivated if the client's immune system becomes suppressed. When active, tuberculosis can be quite infectious, being spread by contaminated sputum. With the immune suppression characteristic of AIDS, the incidence of TB has greatly increased: as many as 20% of all AIDS clients develop active tuberculosis. Infection by a different species of mycobacterium, *M.leprae,* is responsible for the disease known as leprosy.

ANTITUBERCULAR AGENTS

21.13 Pharmacotherapy of tuberculosis requires unique sets of specific drugs because of the slow-growing, complex microbes.

Drug therapy of tuberculosis differs from that of most other infections. *Mycobacteria* have a cell wall that is quite resistant to penetration by antiinfective drugs. In order for the medications to reach the isolated microorganisms in the tubercles, therapy must continue for 6 to 12 months. Although the client may not be infectious this entire time and, indeed, may have no symptoms, it is critical that therapy continue the entire period. Some clients develop multidrug-resistant infections and require therapy for as long as 24 months.

A second difference in the therapy of tuberculosis is that at least two—and sometimes four or more—antibiotics are administered concurrently. During the 6 to 24 months of the treatment period, different combinations of drugs may be used. Multi-drug therapy is necessary because the mycobacterium grows very slowly and resistance is common. The use of multiple drugs and switching the combinations during the long treatment period lowers the potential for resistance and increases the success of the therapy. Table 21.8 lists drugs used in the first-line therapy of tuberculosis. A second group of drugs are more toxic and less effective than the first-line agents and are used when resistance develops.

A third difference is that antituberculosis drugs are used extensively for preventing the disease in addition to treating it. Chemoprophylaxis is common for close contacts or family members of recently infected tuberculosis clients. Therapy usually begins immediately after a client

---

DRUG PROFILE:
Isoniazid (INH)

Actions:

Isoniazid has been a drug of choice for the treatment of *M. tuberculosis* for many years. It is bacteriocidal for actively growing organisms, but bacteriostatic for dormant mycobacteria. It is selective for *M. tuberculosis.* Isoniazid is used alone for chemoprophylaxis, or in combination with other antitubercular drugs for treating active disease.

hepato = liver
toxicity = poison

Adverse Effects:

The most common side effects of isoniazid are numbness of the hand and feet, rash, and fever. Although rare, liver toxicity is a serious adverse effect; thus the healthcare provider should be alert for signs of jaundice, fatigue, elevated hepatic enzymes, or loss of appetite. Liver enzyme tests are usually performed monthly during therapy in order to identify early hepatotoxicity.

TABLE 21.8	First-line Antitubercular Drugs	
DRUG	**ROUTE AND ADULT DOSE**	**REMARKS**
Pr isoniazid (INH, Laniazid, Nydrazid, Teebaconin)	PO: 15 mg/kg qd.	Used in combination with other antituberculars; IM form available.
ethambutol (Myambutol)	PO; 15–25 mg/kg qd.	Used in combination with other antituberculars.
pyrazinamide	PO; 5–15 mg/kg tid-qid (max 2 g/day).	Rifater is a fixed-dose combination of pyrazinamide with isoniazid and rifampin.
rifampin (Rifidin, Rimactane)	PO; 600 mg qd.	Used in combination with other antituberculars; IV form available; also for leprosy, *H. Influenza*, and meningococcus infections.
rifapentine (Priftin)	PO; 600 mg twice a week × 2 months then once a week × 4 months.	Used in combination with other antituberculars.
streptomycin	IM; 15 mg/kg-1 g qd.	Used in combination with other antituberculars; also for several other serious bacterial infections.

receives a positive tuberculin test. Clients with immunosuppression, such as those with AIDS or those receiving immunosuppressant drugs, may receive preventative treatment with antituberculosis drugs. A short-term therapy of two months, consisting of a combination treatment with isoniazid (INH) and pyrazinamide, is approved for tuberculosis prophylaxis in HIV-positive clients.

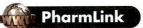

PharmLink

THE REEMERGENCE OF TUBERCULOSIS

Concept review 21.3

▪ How does drug therapy of tuberculosis differ from conventional antiinfective chemotherapy? What are the rationales for these differences?

CLIENT TEACHING

Clients treated for bacterial infections need to know the following:

1. Be certain to take the entire prescription of antiinfective medication exactly as directed. Partial doses, skipped doses, and shortened length of treatment encourage the development of resistant organisms.

2. Your healthcare practitioner may require you to stay in the office for at least 30 minutes after you receive an injection of penicillin to monitor for possible allergic reactions.

3. Avoid intake of caffeinated beverages, citrus fruits, and fruit juices for at least one hour before and two hours after taking oral penicillin to maximize the drug's absorption.

4. To decrease gastrointestinal upset, take oral cephalosporins and oral lincomycin with food, and oral sulfonamides with food or milk.

5. Drink a glass of water with each dose of sulfonamide, tetracycline, lincomycin, or fluoroquinolone, and drink a total of two to three liters of fluid a day.

6. Antacids, dairy products, iron, baking soda, and kaolin-pectin bind and inactivate tetracycline. Separate intake by two to three hours for full antibiotic effectiveness.

7. Sulfonamides, tetracycline, and other antibiotics may interfere with the effectiveness of oral contraceptives. Ask your healthcare provider about the advisability of using an additional form of contraception.

8. Eating active-culture yogurt or buttermilk may decrease the risks for diarrhea and vaginitis associated with antibiotic destruction of normal flora.

9. Avoid sun/tanning exposure while taking sulfonamides and tetracyclines because of photosensitivity.

10. Antibiotics are most effective if taken around the clock, rather than just during normal waking hours. This is especially important with vancomycin. ▪

CHAPTER REVIEW

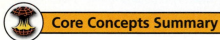 **Core Concepts Summary**

21.1 Pathogens are described by their virulence, pathogenicity, and mechanism of action.

Pathogens are microorganisms that can cause disease. Pathogens can overwhelm natural immune defenses by growing extremely rapidly and invading normal tissues or by producing potent toxins that disrupt normal cellular functions.

21.2 Bacteria are described by their shape, their ability to utilize oxygen, and by their staining characteristics.

Bacteria are organized on the basis of their staining ability and structural and functional characteristics. Certain drugs are effective against gram-positive bacteria and others against gram-negative. Furthermore, some are more effective against aerobic organisms and others against anaerobic organisms.

21.3 Antiinfective drugs are classified by their chemical structure or by their mechanism of action.

Antiinfective drugs are classified based upon similarities in their chemical structure or by their mechanism of action. Because of the large number of antiinfectives available, it is advantageous for the student to understand how to classify these drugs, as medications in the same class exhibit similar pharmacologic activity.

21.4 Antiinfective drugs act by affecting the target organism's metabolism or life cycle.

Bacteria multiply rapidly and drugs have been designed to take advantage of this characteristic. Antiinfectives may be bacteriocidal, bacteriostatic, or both, depending upon the organism and dose.

21.5 Acquired resistance is a major problem with antiinfective drugs.

Errors during replication result in random mutations of the bacterial DNA. Although rare, an occasional mutation may confer antibiotic resistance to a bacterium. Therapy with antibiotics kills the affected bacteria, leaving the resistant ones to multiply and infect the client. To limit this problem, antibiotics should only be prescribed when medically warranted.

21.6 Careful selection of the correct antibiotic is essential for effective pharmacotherapy and to limit adverse effects.

Culture and sensitivity tests are used to identify the type of bacteria present and to determine which antibiotics are most effective. Until test results are obtained, the client may be started on a broad-spectrum antibiotic. Because broad-spectrum drugs are more likely to affect the client's normal flora, a narrow-spectrum drug may be prescribed after the organism is identified.

21.7 The penicillins are one of the oldest and safest groups of antiinfectives.

Penicillins have been widely used because of their high margin of safety and effectiveness. Some clients are allergic to this class of drugs and many bacterial species have become resistant to penicillins, thus limiting their use.

21.8 The cephalosporins are similar in structure and function to the penicillins and are one of the most widely prescribed antiinfective classes.

The cephalosporins consist of a large class of antibiotics, classified by generation, that are considered alternatives to penicillin. In general, they are used for serious gram-negative infections and for clients who are resistant to or cannot tolerate the penicillins.

21.9 The tetracycline class has one of the broadest spectrums, but they are drugs of choice for relatively few diseases.

The tetracyclines have a broader spectrum of action and produce more side effects than the penicillins. Their use is limited to a small number of diseases such as Rocky Mountain spotted fever, typhus, cholera, Lyme disease, and Chlamydial infections.

21.10 The macrolides are safe alternatives to penicillin for many diseases.

The macrolides are generally prescribed when a client is allergic to penicillin or has a penicillin-resistant infection. They produce few side effects.

21.11 **The aminoglycosides are narrow spectrum drugs that have the potential to cause serious toxicity.**

The aminoglycosides are usually reserved for severe gram-negative infections of the urinary tract because they have the potential to cause serious side effects. Most of them are poorly absorbed from the GI tract and must be given parenterally.

21.12 **A number of additional antiinfectives have specific indications.**

A number of important antibiotics do not belong to any of the above classes. The sulfonamides and fluoroquinolones are small groups of drugs having specific applications. Vancomycin is known as the "last chance" antibiotic to be used when resistance has developed to most other antiinfectives.

21.13 **Pharmacotherapy of tuberculosis requires a unique set of specific drugs because of the slow-growing, complex microbes.**

Drug therapy of tuberculosis involves taking multiple drugs for prolonged periods of time. Clients exhibiting a new, positive TB test are often given these drugs prophylactically, even if no signs of the disease are apparent.

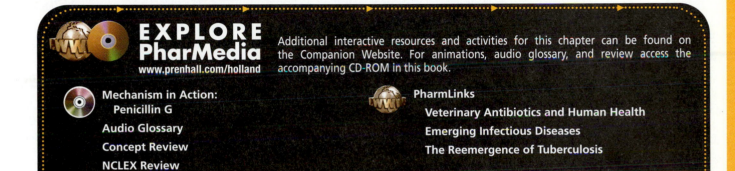

EXPLORE PharMedia
www.prenhall.com/holland

Additional interactive resources and activities for this chapter can be found on the Companion Website. For animations, audio glossary, and review access the accompanying CD-ROM in this book.

Mechanism in Action:
  Penicillin G
Audio Glossary
Concept Review
NCLEX Review

PharmLinks
  Veterinary Antibiotics and Human Health
  Emerging Infectious Diseases
  The Reemergence of Tuberculosis

22 Drugs for Fungal, Viral, and Parasitic Diseases

CORE CONCEPTS

22.1 Fungi are more complex than bacteria and require a different approach to antiinfective therapy.

Systemic Antifungal Agents

22.2 Systemic antifungal drugs are used for serious infections of internal organs.

Superficial Antifungal Agents

22.3 Superficial antifungal drugs are safe and effective in treating infections of the skin, nails, and mucous membranes.

22.4 Viruses are non-living parasites that require a host in order to replicate.

Antiviral Agents

22.5 Antiretroviral drugs used in the treatment of HIV-AIDS do not cure the disease, but they do help many clients live longer.

22.6 A small number of antiviral drugs are available to treat herpes simplex and influenza infections.

Antiparasitic Agents

22.7 While not common in the United States, infections caused by helminths and protozoans cause significant disease worldwide.

OBJECTIVES

After reading this chapter, the student should be able to:

1. Compare and contrast the pharmacotherapy of superficial and systemic fungal infections.
2. Identify the types of clients most likely to acquire serious fungal infections.
3. Describe the basic structure of a virus.
4. Identify viral diseases that may benefit from pharmacotherapy.
5. Explain the purpose and expected outcomes of HIV pharmacotherapy.
6. Define HAART and explain why it is commonly used in the pharmacotherapy of HIV infection.
7. Identify protozoan and helminth infections that may benefit from pharmacotherapy.
8. For each of the following classes, identify representative drugs, explain the mechanism of drug action, primary actions, and important adverse effects.
   a. systemic antifungal agents
   b. superficial antifungal agents
   c. antiretroviral and antiviral agents
   d. antiprotozoan agents
   e. antihelminthic agents
9. Categorize drugs used in the treatment of fungal, viral, protozoan, and helminth infections based on their classification and mechanism of action.

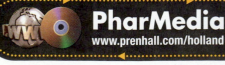

PharMedia
www.prenhall.com/holland

Additional interactive resources and activities for this chapter can be found on the Companion Website. For animations, audio glossary, and review access the accompanying CD-ROM in this book.

acquired immune deficiency syndrome (AIDS): disease caused by the human immunodeficiency virus (HIV) / *page 344*

anemia (ah-NEE-mee-ah): shortage of functional red blood cells / *page 346*

antiretroviral (an-tie-RET-roh-veye-ral): type of drug effective against retroviruses / *page 344*

capsid (CAP-sid): protein coat that surrounds a virus / *page 341*

dermatophytic (der-MAT-oh-FIT-ik): superficial fungal infection / *page 338*

dysentery (DISS-en-tare-ee): severe diarrhea that may include bleeding / *page 349*

fungi (FUN-jeye): kingdom of organisms that includes mushrooms, yeasts, and molds / *page 338*

HAART: highly active antiretroviral therapy; type of drug therapy for HIV infection that includes high doses of multiple medications that are given concurrently / *page 344*

helminth (HELL-minth): type of flat, round, or segmented worm / *page 349*

host: an organism that is being infected by a microbe / *page 341*

influenza (in-flew-EN-zah): common viral infection; often called *flu* / *page 346*

intracellular parasite: an infectious microbe that lives inside host cells / *page 341*

leukopenia (lew-koh-PEE-nee-ah): abnormally low number of white blood cells / *page 346*

malaria (mah-LARE-ee-ah): tropical disease characterized by severe fever and chills caused by the protozoan *Plasmodium* / *page 349*

mycoses (my-KOH-sees): diseases caused by fungi / *page 338*

phlebitis (flee-BITE-iss): inflammation of veins / *page 339*

protozoan (PRO-toh-ZOH-en): single-celled microorganism / *page 347*

reverse transcriptase (ree-VERS trans-CRIP-tace): viral enzyme that converts RNA to DNA / *page 344*

superficial mycoses: fungal diseases of the hair, skin, nails, and mucous membranes / *page 338*

systemic mycoses: fungal diseases affecting internal organs / *page 338*

virus: non-living particle containing nucleic acid that is able to cause disease / *page 341*

yeast (YEEST): type of fungus that is unicellular and divides by budding / *page 338*

Fungi, protozoans, and multicellular parasites are exceedingly more complex than bacteria. Most antibacterial drugs are ineffective against these organisms because their structure and biochemistry are so different from that of bacteria. Although there are fewer medications to treat these diseases, the available medications are usually effective.

Viruses, on the other hand, are not living organisms. A virus infects by entering a host cell and using the host's internal machinery to replicate itself. Antiviral drugs are the least effective of all the antiinfective classes. The number of antiviral medications has increased dramatically in recent years as a result of research into the AIDS epidemic.

Fast Facts Fungal, Viral, and Parasitic Diseases

- About 45 million Americans are infected with genital herpes—one out of every five of the total adolescent and adult population.
- Genital herpes is more common in women than in men, and in blacks over other ethnic groups.
- About 900,000 Americans are currently living with HIV infections; about 40,000 new infections occur each year.
- Seventy percent of new HIV infections occur in men, with the largest risk category being men who have sex with other men.
- Seventy-five percent of the new HIV infections in woman are acquired through heterosexual contact.
- Since the beginning of the AIDS epidemic, over 450,000 Americans have died of AIDS.
- Three hundred to five hundred million cases of malaria occur worldwide each year, with an estimated 2.7 million deaths resulting from the disease.
- Of the more than 200,000 known species of fungi, fewer than 200 are known to infect humans. Ninety percent of these infections are caused by just a few dozen species.

22.1 Fungi are more complex than bacteria and require a different approach to antiinfective therapy.

myc = fungus
oses = conditions

derma = skin
phyto = something that grows

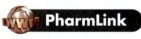

FUNGI IN THE WORLD

Fungi are single-celled or multicellular organisms that are much more complex than bacteria. Many species of fungi normally grow on skin and mucosal surfaces and are part of the normal host flora. The human body is remarkably resistant to infection by these organisms; clients with healthy immune systems experience few serious fungal diseases. Clients who have a suppressed immune system, however, such as those infected with HIV, may experience frequent fungal infections, some of which may require intensive drug therapy. Fungal diseases are called mycoses. Yeasts, which include the common pathogen *Candida albicans,* are types of fungi. Table 22.1 lists the most common fungi that cause disease in humans.

A simple and useful method of classifying fungal infections is to consider them as either superficial or systemic. Superficial mycoses typically affect the scalp, skin, nails, and mucous membranes such as the oral cavity and vagina. Mycoses of this type are often treated with topical agents because the incidence of side effects is much lower by using this route of administration. Superficial fungal infections are sometimes called dermatophytic.

Systemic mycoses are those affecting internal organs such as the lungs, brain, and digestive organs. Although less common than superficial mycoses, systemic fungal infections may be quite serious and affect multiple body systems. Indeed, systemic mycoses are sometimes fatal to clients with suppressed immune systems. Mycoses of this type often require aggressive oral or parenteral medications that produce more side effects than the topical agents.

TABLE 22.1	Fungal Pathogens
NAME OF FUNGUS	**DESCRIPTION**
Systemic	
Aspergillus fumigatus and others	Aspergillosis: opportunistic; most commonly affects lung, but can spread to other organs.
Blastomyces dematitidus	Blastomycosis: begins in the lungs and spreads to other organs.
Candida albicans and others	Candidiasis: most common opportunistic fungal infection; may occur in mucous membranes and nearly any organ.
Coccidioides immitis	Coccidioidomycosis: begins in the lungs and spreads to the skin and other organs.
Cryptococcus neoformans	Cryptococcosis: opportunistic; begins in lungs, but is the most common cause of meningitis in AIDS patients.
Histoplasma capsulatum	Histoplasmosis: begins in the lungs and spreads to other organs.
Mucorales (various species)	Mucormycosis: opportunistic; affects blood vessels; causes sinus infections, stomach ulcers, and others.
Pneumocystis carinii	Pneumocystis pneumonia: opportunistic; primarily pneumonia of the lung, but can spread to other organs.
Topical	
Candida albicans and others	Candidiasis: affects skin, nails, oral cavity (thrush), vagina.
Epidermophyton floccosum	Causes athlete's foot (tinea pedis), jock itch (tinea cruris), and other skin disorders.
Microsporum audouini and others	Causes ringworm of scalp (tinea capitus).
Sporothrix schenckii	Sporotrichosis: affects primarily skin and superficial lymph nodes.
Trichophyton (various species)	Affects scalp, skin, and nails.

SYSTEMIC ANTIFUNGAL AGENTS

Systemic fungal disease may require intensive pharmacotherapy for extended periods of time. Amphoteracin B and fluconazole are drugs of choice.

22.2 Systemic antifungal drugs are used for serious infections of internal organs.

A number of drugs have become available for systemic fungal infections in the past 15 years, due largely to the development of medications for opportunistic fungal disease in AIDS clients. Other clients who may experience systemic infections include those receiving prolonged therapy with corticosteroids (Chapters 20 and 28 ⬭), those experiencing extensive burns, those receiving anticancer drugs (Chapter 23 ⬭), and those who have recently received organ transplants (Chapter 20 ⬭). Systemic antifungal medications have little or no antibacterial activity. Drug therapy is often prolonged.

Amphoteracin B (Fungizone) has been the drug of choice for systemic fungal infections for many years. However, the newer *azole* drugs such as fluconazole (Diflucan), itraconazole, (Sporonox), and ketoconazole (Nizoral) are coming into widespread use. Ketoconazole has become a drug of choice for less severe systemic mycoses or for the prophylaxis of fungal infections. The *azole* drugs have a spectrum of activity similar to that of amphoteracin B, are considerably less toxic, and have the major advantage that they can be administered orally. Several are available for both superficial and systemic mycoses. Table 22.2 lists the primary antifungal drugs.

phleb = vein
itis = inflammation

Concept review 22.1

▪ Why have the number of antifungal and antiviral drugs increased significantly over the past 15 years?

SUPERFICIAL ANTIFUNGAL AGENTS

Superficial fungal infections are generally not severe. Topical antifungal agents are safe and many are available OTC.

DRUG PROFILE:
Amphotericin B (Fungizone)

Actions:

Amphotericin B has a wide spectrum of activity that includes most of the fungi pathogenic to humans; thus, it is a drug of choice for severe systemic mycoses. It acts by binding to fungal cell membranes and causing them to become permeable or leaky. Because it is not absorbed from the GI tract, it is given by intravenous infusion. Treatment may continue for several months. Unlike antibiotics, resistance to amphotericin B is not common.

Adverse Effects:

Amphotericin B can cause a number of serious side effects. Many clients develop fever and chills at the beginning of therapy, which subside as treatment continues. Phlebitis, or inflammation of the veins, is common during IV therapy. Some degree of nephrotoxicity is observed in most clients and laboratory tests of kidney function are normally performed throughout the treatment period.

TABLE 22.2	Antifungal Drugs	
DRUG	**ROUTE AND ADULT DOSE**	**REMARKS**
Pr amphotericin B (Fungizone, Abelcet, Amphotec, Ambisome)	IV; 0.25 mg/kg qd; may increase to1 mg/kg qd or 1.5 mg/kg qod (max 1.5 mg/kg/day).	Cream, lotion, and PO suspension forms available for topical mycoses; must infuse a test dose first; has severe adverse effects.
butenafine hydrochloride (Mentax)	Topical: apply qd x 4 weeks.	For athlete's foot.
butaconazole (Femstat)	Topical: 1 applicatorful intravaginally hs × 3 days.	For vaginal mycoses.
ciclopiroxolamine (Loprox)	Topical: apply bid × 4 weeks.	For skin mycoses.
clotrimazole (Gyne-Lotrimin, Mycelex, Femizole)	Topical: for skin mycoses apply bid × 4 weeks; for vaginal mycoses, insert 1 applicatorful intravaginally hs for 7 days.	For vaginal and skin mycoses, athlete's foot, and candidiasis; vaginal tablet form also available.
econazole nitrate (Spectazole)	Topical: apply bid × 4 weeks.	For skin mycoses.
fluconazole (Diflucan)	PO; 200–400 mg on day one, then 100–200 mg qd × 2–4 weeks.	For both systemic and superficial mycoses; 1% cream available for topical infections; IV form available.
flucytosine (Ancobon)	PO; 50–150 mg/kg in divided doses.	For severe systemic infections such as candidiasis or cryptococcosis; IV form available.
griseofulvin (Fulvicin)	PO; 500 mg microsize or 330–375 mg ultramicrosize qd.	For ringworm and other skin and nail infections.
haloprogin (Halotex)	Topical: apply bid × 2–3 weeks.	For skin mycoses.
itraconazole (Sporonox)	PO; 200 mg qd; may increase to 200 mg bid (max 400 mg/day).	For severe systemic lung mycoses and superficial nail mycoses.
ketoconazole (Nizoral)	PO; 200–400 mg qd.	For severe systemic mycoses; topical form available for superficial mycoses.
miconazole nitrate (Micatin, Monistat)	Topical; apply bid × 2–4 weeks.	For vaginal and skin mycoses; also available as vaginal suppositories and tampons.
naftifine (Naftin)	Topical; apply cream qd or gel bid × 4 weeks.	For skin mycoses.
Pr nystatin (Mycostatin, Nilstat, Nystex)	PO; 500,000–1,000,000 units tid.	For candidiasis; also available as tablets for vaginal mycoses.
oxiconazole nitrate (Oxistat)	Topical; apply qd in the evening × 2 months.	For skin mycoses.
terbinafine hydrochloride (Lamisil)	Topical; apply qd or bid × 7 weeks PO; 250 mg qd × 6–13 weeks.	For skin and nail mycoses.
terconazole (Terazol)	Topical; insert one applicatorful intravaginally at hs × 3–7 days.	For vulvovaginal candidiasis; vaginal suppository form available.
tioconazole (Vagistat)	Topical; insert one applicator ful intravaginally at hs × 1 day.	For vulvovaginal candidiasis.
tolnaftate (Aftate, Tinactin)	Topical; apply bid × 4–6 weeks.	For skin mycoses, ringworm, athlete's foot.
undecylenic acid (Cruex, Desenex)	Topical; apply qd-bid.	For athlete's foot, diaper rash.

DRUG PROFILE:
Nystatin (Fungizone)

Actions:

Although it belongs to the same chemical class as amphoteracin B, nystatin is available in a wider variety of formulations, including cream, ointment, powder, tablets, and lozenges. It is used as a topical agent against *Candida* infections of the vagina, skin, and mouth. It may also be used orally to treat candidiasis of the intestine because it travels through the GI tract without being absorbed.

Adverse Effects:

When given topically, nystatin produces few adverse effects other than minor skin irritation. When given orally, it may cause diarrhea, nausea, and vomiting.

22.3 Superficial antifungal drugs are safe and effective in treating infections of the skin, nails, and mucous membranes.

Superficial fungal infections of the hair, scalp, nails, and the mucous membranes of the mouth and vagina are rarely medical emergencies. Infections of the nails and skin, for example, may be ongoing for months or even years before a client seeks treatment. Unlike systemic fungal infections, topical infections may occur in any client, not just those who have suppressed immune systems.

Superficial antifungal medications are much safer than their systemic counterparts because only very small amounts are absorbed into the blood. Many are available as OTC creams, gels, solutions, and ointments. Although a fungal infection may be diagnosed as superficial, oral antifungal drugs are occasionally prescribed along with the topical agents to be certain that the infection is completely eliminated.

22.4 Viruses are non-living parasites that require a host in order to replicate.

Viruses are non-living particles that infect bacteria, plants, and animals. Viruses contain none of the cell machinery necessary for self-survival that is present in living organisms. In fact, the structure of viruses is quite primitive compared to even the simplest living cell. Surrounded by a protein coat or capsid, a virus contains only a few dozen genes, either in the form of ribonucleic acid (RNA) or deoxyribonucleic acid (DNA), that contain the necessary information needed for viral replication. Figure 22.1 shows the basic structure of the human immunodeficiency virus (HIV).

Although non-living and structurally simple, viruses are capable of remarkable feats. They infect an organism, called the host, by entering a target cell and using the machinery inside that cell to replicate. Thus viruses are called intracellular parasites, meaning that they must be inside a host cell in order to cause infection. The viral host is often very specific: it may be a single species of plant, bacteria, or animal, or even a single type of cell within that species. Most often, viruses that affect one species do not affect others, although cases have been documented where viruses can mutate and cross species, as is likely the case for HIV.

intra = within
cellular = cell

Many viral infections, such as the rhinoviruses that cause the common cold, are self-limiting and require no medical treatment. While symptoms may be annoying, the virus disappears in seven to ten days and causes no permanent damage, if the client is otherwise healthy. Other viruses, such as HIV, can cause serious and even fatal disease and require aggressive

FIGURE 22.1

Structure of the human immunodeficiency virus (HIV)

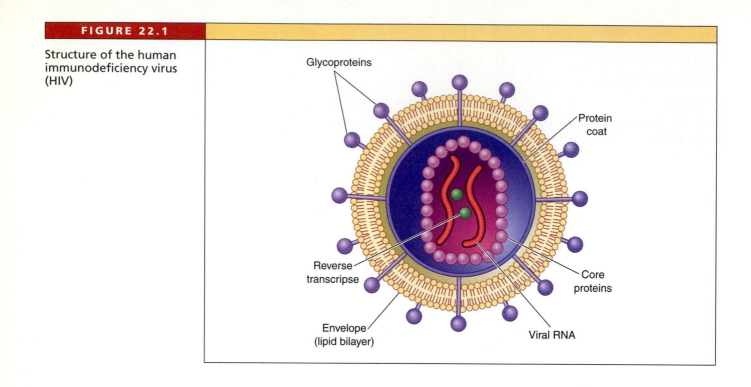

drug therapy. Antiviral therapy is extremely challenging because of the rapid mutation rate of viruses, which can quickly render drugs ineffective. Also complicating therapy is the intracellular nature of the virus, which makes it difficult for medications to find their targets without injuring normal cells. Each of the antiviral drugs is specific to one particular virus. The antiviral medications are shown in Table 22.3.

TABLE 22.3	Antiviral Drugs	
DRUG	**ROUTE AND ADULT DOSE**	**REMARKS**
HIV-AIDS DRUGS		
Non-nucleoside Reverse Transcriptase Inhibitors (NNRTI)		
nevirapine (Viramune)	PO; 200 mg qd × 14 days, then increase to bid.	Used in combination with other antivirals.
delavirdine mesylate (Rescriptor)	PO; 400 mg tid.	Used in combination with other antivirals.
efavirenz (Sustiva)	PO; 600 mg qd.	Used in combination with other antivirals; a once-daily form is available.
Nucleoside Reverse Transcriptase Inhibitors (NRTI)		
Pr zidovudine (Retrovir, AZT)	PO; 200 mg q4h × 1 month then 100 mg q 4 h.	For symptomatic or asymptomatic HIV; unlabeled use; postexposure chemoprophylaxis; IV form available.
abacavir sulfate (Ziagen)	PO; 300 mg bid.	
didanosine (Videx)	PO; 125–300 mg bid.	For use in clients who are intolerant to AZT.
lamivudine (Epivir, 3TC)	PO; 150 mg bid.	Usually given in combination with AZT.
stavudine (Zerit, D4T)	PO; 40 mg bid.	For advanced HIV disease.
zalcitabine (Hivid, ddC)	PO; 0.75 mg tid.	To be given in combination with AZT.

continues

TABLE 22.3	Antiviral Drugs (continued)	
DRUG	**ROUTE AND ADULT DOSE**	**REMARKS**
Protease Inhibitors		
saquinavir mesylate (Invirase, Fortovase)	PO; 600 mg tid.	
amprenavir (Agenerase)	PO; 1200 mg bid.	
idinavir sulfate (Crixivan)	PO; 800 mg tid.	Give 1 hour before or 2 hours after a meal.
nelfinavir mesylate (Viracept)	PO; 750 mg tid.	Give with food.
ritonavir (Norvir)	PO; 600 mg bid.	Give 1 hour before or 2 hours after a meal.
Herpes Virus Drugs		
Pr acyclovir (Zovirax)	PO; 400 mg tid.	For herpes viruses.
cidofovir (Vistide)	IV; 5 mg/kg q week × 2 weeks, then once q week.	For cytomegalovirus retinitis in clients with AIDS; must give probenecid before and after infusion.
famciclovir (Famvir)	PO; 500 mg tid × 7 days.	For herpes viruses.
foscarnet (Foscavir)	IV; 40–60 mg/kg infused over 1–2 hours tid.	For cytomegalovirus retinitis; for the treatment of acyclovir-resistant herpes virus.
ganciclovir (DHPG) (Cytovene)	IV; 5 mg/kg infused over 1 hour bid.	Drug of choice for cytomegalovirus; oral form available.
idoxuridine (IDU) (Herplex)	Topical; 1 drop in each eye q 1 hour during the day and q 2 hours at night.	For herpes eye infections.
trifluridine (Viroptic)	Topical; 1 drop in each eye q2hours during waking hours (max 9 drops/day).	For herpes eye infections.
valacyclovir hydrochloride (Valtrex)	PO; 1.0 g tid.	For herpes viruses.
vidarabine (Vira-A)	Topical; 0.5 inch of ointment in each eye q3h, not to exceed 5 applications/day.	For herpes eye infections.
Influenza Drugs		
amantadine hydrochloride (Symmetrel)	PO; 100 mg bid.	For treatment and prevention of influenza; also for Parkinson's disease.
oseltamivir phosphate (Tamiflu)	PO; 75 mg bid × 5 days.	For treatment of influenza.
rimantadine (Flumadine)	PO: 100 mg bid.	For treatment and prevention of influenza.
zanamivir (Relenza)	Inhalation; 2 inhalations × 5 days.	For treatment of influenza in clients with symptoms of fewer than 2 days.

ANTIVIRAL AGENTS

Antiviral medications for HIV-AIDS have been developed that slow the growth of HIV by three different mechanisms. Resistance develops to these drugs and a cure is not yet obtainable.

22.5 Antiretroviral drugs used in the treatment of HIV-AIDS do not cure the disease, but they do help many clients live longer.

The widespread appearance of HIV infection in 1981 created enormous challenges for public health and for the development of new antiviral drugs. **HIV-AIDS** is unlike any other infectious disease because it is uniformly fatal and demands a continuous supply of new drugs for client survival. The challenges of HIV-AIDS have been met by the development of over 16 new antiviral drugs, with many others currently undergoing clinical trials. Unfortunately, the initial hope of curing HIV-AIDS through antiviral therapy or vaccines has not been realized; none of these medications produce a cure for this disease. HIV mutates extremely rapidly and resistant strains develop so quickly that the creation of new, novel approaches to antiviral drug therapy is an ongoing process.

While drug therapy for HIV-AIDS has not produced a cure, it has resulted in a number of therapeutic successes. For example, many clients infected with HIV are able to live symptom-free with their disease for a much longer time because of antiviral therapy. Furthermore, the transmission of the virus from an HIV-infected mother to her newborn has been reduced dramatically due to drug therapy of the mother prior to delivery and of the baby immediately following birth. These two factors have resulted in a significant decline in the death rate due to HIV-AIDS in the United States. Unfortunately, this decline has not been observed in African countries, where antiviral drugs are not as readily available, largely because of their high cost.

Antiviral medications used for HIV-AIDS are called **antiretrovirals** because they block some component of the replication cycle of HIV, which is classified as a retrovirus. The standard treatment for HIV-AIDS includes aggressive treatment with three to four drugs at a time, a regimen called **highly active antiretroviral therapy (HAART)**. The goal of HAART is to reduce the amount of HIV in the plasma to its lowest possible level. It must be understood, however, that HIV is harbored in locations other than the blood, such as in lymph nodes; therefore, elimination of the virus from the blood is not a cure.

The replication of HIV is illustrated in Figure 22.2. Antiretroviral drugs are classified into three groups, based upon how they inhibit HIV replication.

- Nucleoside Reverse Transcriptase Inhibitors (NRTIs): The oldest antiretroviral drug, Zidovudine (see page 346) belongs to the NRTI class. Drugs in this class are structurally similar to nucleosides, the building blocks of DNA. NRTIs inhibit the action of the viral enzyme **reverse transcriptase**, which converts the viral RNA into DNA.

- Non-nucleoside Reverse Transcriptase Inhibitors (NNRTIs): This class also inhibits the viral enzyme reverse transcriptase, but these drugs are not structurally similar to the building blocks of DNA. Instead, these agents bind directly to the reverse transcriptase molecule and inhibit its function.

- Protease Inhibitors: The newest class of antiretrovirals, these drugs block the final assembly of the HIV particle. They are quite effective at reducing plasma HIV to very low levels, although resistance develops quickly.

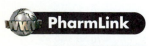

HIV-AIDS ON THE WEB

Concept review 22.2

- Why are viral infections very difficult to treat with current drugs?

22.6 A small number of antiviral drugs are available to treat herpes simplex and influenza infections.

Antiviral drugs can lower the frequency of herpes episodes and diminish the intensity of acute disease (see page 347). Antivirals may also be used to prevent influenza or decrease the severity of influenza symptoms.

FIGURE 22.2

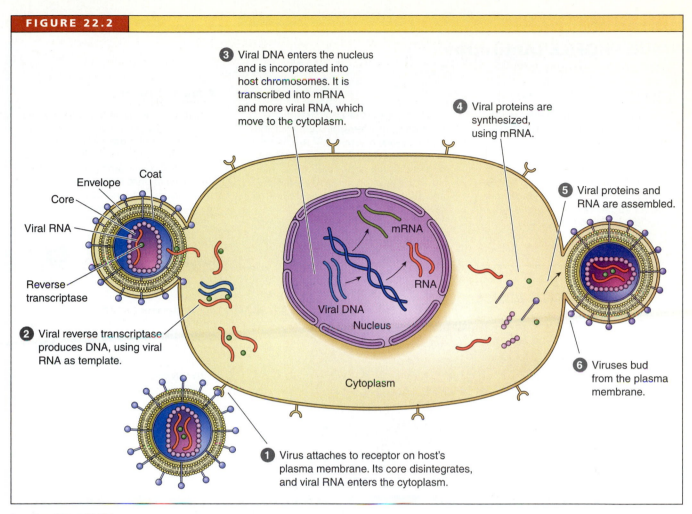

③ Viral DNA enters the nucleus and is incorporated into host chromosomes. It is transcribed into mRNA and more viral RNA, which move to the cytoplasm.

④ Viral proteins are synthesized, using mRNA.

⑤ Viral proteins and RNA are assembled.

Envelope
Coat
Core
Viral RNA
Reverse transcriptase

mRNA
RNA
Viral DNA
Nucleus
Cytoplasm

② Viral reverse transcriptase produces DNA, using viral RNA as template.

⑥ Viruses bud from the plasma membrane.

① Virus attaches to receptor on host's plasma membrane. Its core disintegrates, and viral RNA enters the cytoplasm.

Replication of HIV

Herpes simplex viruses (HSV) are a family of viruses that cause repeated, blister-like lesions on the skin, genitals, and other mucosal surfaces. Some of these viruses remain in latency for many years until physical or emotional stress cause the characteristic lesions to reappear. Types of herpes simplex virus include the following.

- HSV-type 1—non-genital infections of the eye, mouth, and lips
- HSV-type 2—genital infections
- cytomegalovirus (CMV)—affects multiple body systems in immunosuppressed clients

NATURAL ALTERNATIVES

The Antiviral Activity of Hyssop

Hyssop (*Hyssopus officianalis*) is a member of the mint family that originated from the Mediterranean region. The leaves of the plant are dried and available as capsules, tincture, or tea. Hyssop contains a number of substances purported to have antiviral activity, including tannins and a polysaccharide called MR-10. It also contains a number of volatile oils, which give hyssop a strong, pleasant odor and which are occasionally used as flavorings and scents.

Extracts of hyssop are sometimes used topically to treat skin lesions due to herpes virus. It can be used as a gargle for sore throats. It is purported to have an expectorant action that may be of value in bronchitis and viral pneumonia. ▪

DRUG PROFILE (Antiretroviral):
Zidovudine (Retrovir, AZT)

Actions:

Zidovudine was first discovered in the 1960s and its antiviral activity was demonstrated prior to the AIDS epidemic. Structurally, it resembles thymidine, one of the four building blocks of DNA. As the reverse transcriptase enzyme begins to synthesize viral DNA, it mistakenly uses zidvudine as one of the building blocks, thus creating a defective DNA strand. Because of its widespread use over the past 20 years, resistant HIV strains are common. It is usually used in combination with other antiretrovirals, as this slows the development of resistance and allows HIV to be attacked by several different mechanisms.

Adverse Effects:

Zidovudine can result in severe toxicity to blood cells at high doses. Reduced numbers of red blood cells **(anemia)** and white blood cells **(leukopenia)** are common and may limit therapy. Many clients experience GI symptoms such as anorexia, nausea, and diarrhea. Clients may experience fatigue and report generalized weakness.

Mechanism in Action:

Zidovudine resembles the chemical structure of thymidine and with the help of reverse transcriptase becomes incorporated into the infective strand of viral DNA. Once incorporated, zidovudine slows synthesis of HIV, thereby reducing symptoms associated with this disease.

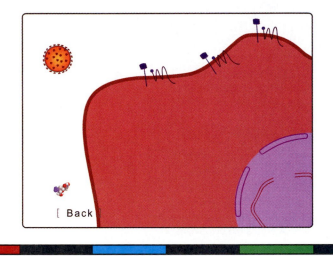

[Back

- varicella-zoster virus—shingles (zoster) and chicken pox (varicella)
- Epstein-Barr virus—mononucleosis and Burkitt's lymphoma, a form of cancer

Influenza is another viral infection that may warrant drug therapy. Influenza produces acute symptoms that include sore throat, sneezing, coughing, fever, and chills. In immunosuppressed clients, an influenza infection may be fatal. For those who are in ill health or who have weak im-

ON THE JOB

Public Health Nurse

The role of the public health nurse is to assist the physician in recognizing and treating diseases that pose a potential threat to the population. The nurse providing care in an HIV-AIDS clinic is one such example.

Clients who suspect that they have HIV infections are often reluctant to seek medical attention because of distrust of the medical establishment and fear of the consequences of their disease. If the nurse is to achieve his/her goals of public protection, an atmosphere of trust and compassion must be quickly established. Clients are unlikely to discuss their intimate sexual history or reveal their sexual partners without a relationship of mutual trust. The nurse must feel free to discuss such intimate details, often using a "street" language that the client will understand. The nurse must somehow convince the client to consider the welfare of others as important as his or her own. The nurse must convince reluctant clients to seek medical attention and to abstain from sexual activity. Although the job is often frustrating, the nurse in such a clinic can save many lives by his/her skill in communication and by showing a non-judgmental acceptance of the client. ■

DRUG PROFILE (Antiviral):
Acyclovir (Zovirax)

Actions:

The antiviral activity of acyclovir is limited to the herpes viruses, for which it is the drug of choice. It is most effective against HSV-1 and HSV-2 and effective only at high doses against CMV and varicella-zoster. Acyclovir acts by inhibiting viral DNA synthesis. Resistance has developed to the drug, particularly in clients with HIV-AIDS. Acyclovir decreases the duration and severity of herpes episodes. When given for prophylaxis, it may decrease the frequency of active herpes episodes, but it does not cure the client. It is available in topical form for placing directly on active lesions, in oral form for prophylaxis, and as an IV for particularly severe disease.

Adverse Effects:

There are few adverse effects to acyclovir when administered topically or orally. When given IV, the drug may cause painful inflammation of vessels at the site of infusion. Because nephrotoxicity is possible, frequent laboratory tests may be performed to monitor kidney function.

---

mune systems, the best approach to this disease is prevention through annual vaccinations (Chapter 20 ⊂▭⊃). The drug amantadine (Symmetrel) has been available to prevent and treat influenza for many years. A new class of drugs called the *neuroamidase inhibitors* was introduced in 1999 to treat active infections. If given within 48 hours of the onset of symptoms, osteltamivir (Tamiflu) and zanamivir (Relenza) are reported to shorten the normal seven-day duration of influenza symptoms to five days. Because all the influenza antivirals produce only modest effects on an active infection, prevention through vaccination remains the best alternative.

ANTIPARASITIC AGENTS

Antiinfectives are used to treat diseases caused by protozoans, worms, and ticks. In general, drugs used to treat these diseases are different from those used to treat bacterial or fungal infections.

22.7 While not common in the United States, infections caused by helminths and protozoans cause significant disease worldwide.

A number of pathogens other than bacteria and fungi may infect humans. These parasites include single-celled animals called protozoans and multicellular organisms such as mites, ticks, and worms. With a few exceptions, antibiotics, antifungal, and antiviral drugs are ineffective against these complex organisms. Drugs prescribed for parasitic diseases may be classified as antimalarials, antiprotozoans (other than the antimalarial agents), antihelminthics, and scabicides/pediculicides. Table 22.4 lists selected antiparasitics. Scabicides and pediculocides are covered in Chapter 30 ⊂▭⊃ .

Protozoans are single-celled organisms that cause significant disease in Africa, South America, and Asia. Travelers to these continents may acquire these infections overseas and bring them back to the United States and Canada. One such protozoan infection is amebiasis, a disease caused by *Entamoeba histolytica*. Infection by *E. histolytica* is common in Africa, Latin America, and Asia, where it frequently causes serious disease. Although primarily an intestinal disease, *E. histolytica* can invade the liver, where it causes abscesses. The primary symptom of amebiasis is a

dys = difficult or painful
enter = intestine

TABLE 22.4	Drugs Used to Treat Helminth and Protozoan Infections	
DRUG	**ROUTE AND ADULT DOSE**	**REMARKS**
Amebicides		
paromomycin sulfate (Humatin)	PO; 25–35 mg/kg divided in 3 doses for 5–10 days.	For acute and chronic amebiasis.
iodoquinol (Yodoxin)	PO; 630–650 mg tid × 20 days (Max 2 g/day).	For intestinal amebiasis.
doxycycline hyclate (Vibramycin)	PO; 100 mg qd.	For traveler's diarrhea.
Antihelminthics		
mebendazole (Vermox)	PO; 100 mg × 1 dose or 100 mg bid × 3 days.	For the treatment of whipworm, roundworm, hookworm, and pinworm.
albendazole (Albenza)	PO; 400 mg bid with meals (max 800 mg/day).	Only antihelminthic drug active against all stages of the helminth life cycle.
ivermectin (Stromectol)	PO; 150–200 μg/kg × 1 dose.	
praziquantel (Biltricide)	PO; 5 mg/kg as a single dose or 25 mg/kg tid.	For all stages of schistomsomasis.
pyrantel pamoate (Antiminith)	PO; 11 mg/kg as asingle dose (max 1 g).	For the treatment of hookworm and roundworm.
Antimalarials		
chloroquine (Aralen)	PO; 600 mg initial dose, then 300 mg weekly.	A drug of choice for malaria; also for amebiasis and rheumatoid arthritis; IM form available.
atovaquone (Mepron)	PO; 750 mg bid × 21 days.	Also for pneumocystis.
hydroxychloroquine sulfate (Plaquenil)	PO; 620 mg initial dose, then 310 mg weekly.	Also for rheumatoid arthritis and lupus erythrematosus.
mefloquine hydrochloride (Lariam)	PO; Prevention: begin with 250 mg once a week × 4 weeks, then 250 mg every other week; Treatment: 1250 mg as a single dose.	For prevention and treatment of malaria.
primaquine phosphate (PRIM-ah-kwin)	PO; 15 mg qd × 2 weeks.	Removes *P.vivax* from its liver reservoir.
pyrimethamine (Daraprim)	PO; 25 mg once per week × 10 weeks.	Also antiprotozoan; drug of choice for toxoplasmosis.
quinine sulfate (Quinamm)	PO; 260–650 mg tid for 3 days.	Largely replaced by other antimalarials; also for nocturnal leg cramps.
Antiprotozoans		
🅟 metronidazole (Flagyl)	PO; 250–750 mg tid.	For many parasitic infections; IV form available.
eflornithine (Ornidyl)	Topical; apply bid × 2 months.	For the reduction of unwanted facial hair in women.
melarsoprol (Arsobal)	IV; 2–3.6 mg/kg for three days, then repeated on day 7 and days 10–21.	Drug of choice for later stages of African trypanosomiasis.

TABLE 22.4	Drugs Used to Treat Helminth and Protozoan Infections *(continued)*	
DRUG	**ROUTE AND ADULT DOSE**	**REMARKS**
nifurtimox (Lampit)	PO; 2–2.5 mg/kg q6h.	Drug of choice for American trypanosomiasis.
pentamidine isothionate (Pentam 300, Nebupent)	IV; 4 mg/kg qd × 14–21 days; infuse over 60 min.	For *Pneumocystis carinii* active infections and prophylaxis; IM and inhalation forms available.
sodium stibogluconate (Pentostam)	IM; 20 mg/kg/day.	For leishmaniasis.
suramin (Germanin)	IV; 1 g on days 1, 3, 7, 14, and 21.	Drug of choice for early stages of African trypanosomiasis.
trimetrexate (Neutrexin)	IV; 45 mg/m^2 qd.	Alternate therapy for *pneumocystis carinii* pneumonia

severe form of diarrhea known as amebic dysentery. Drugs used to treat amebiasis include those that act directly on amebas in the intestine and those that are administered for their systemic effects on the liver and other organs.

Malaria is a disease caused by four species of the protozoan *Plasmodium*. Although rare in the United States and Canada, malaria is the second most common fatal infectious disease in the world, with 300 to 500 million cases occurring annually. The Center for Disease Control (CDC) recommends that travelers to infested areas receive prophylactic antimalarial drugs prior to and during their visit, and for one week after leaving. Drug therapy of malaria interrupts the complex life cycle of the protozoan, which includes transmission by a bite from the female *Anopheles* mosquito. Once inside the body, *Plasmodium* grows in the liver and eventually infects red blood cells. Rupture of infected red blood cells causes severe fever and chills. Drug therapy is successful early in the course of the disease but becomes increasingly difficult because *Plasmodium* enters different stages of its life cycle in the body. Dormant parasites may remain in the liver for years and become resistant to medications. Although chloroquine (Aralen) is the drug of choice for malaria, many other agents are available, because resistance to chloroquine is common.

Helminths consist of various species of parasitic worms, including hookworms, pinworms, roundworms, tapeworms, and flukes. Many of these worms attach to the mucosa of the human intestinal tract. Helminth diseases are quite common in areas of the world lacking high standards of sanitation. Helminth infections in the United States and Canada are generally neither common nor fatal, although drug therapy may be indicated. The most common helminth disease worldwide is caused by the roundworm *Ascaris;* however, infection by the pinworm *Enterobius* is more common in the United States.

proto = *first*
zoans = *animals*

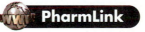

AVOIDING DISEASE WHILE
TRAVELING ABROAD

DRUG PROFILE:
Metronidazole (Flagyl)

Actions:

Metronidazole is the drug of choice for most forms of amebiasis, being effective against amebas in the intestine and in other organs. The drug is somewhat unique among antiparasitic drugs in that it also has antibiotic activity against anaerobic bacteria and thus is used to treat a number of respiratory, bone, skin, and CNS infections. Metronidazole is also a drug of choice for two other protozoan infections: giardiasis from *Giardia lamblia* and trichonomiasis due to *Trichomonas vaginalis.*

Adverse Effects:

The most common side effects of metronidazole are anorexia, nausea, diarrhea, dizziness, and headache. Dryness of the mouth and an unpleasant metallic taste may be experienced. Although side effects are relatively common, most are not serious enough to cause discontinuation of therapy.

Concept review 22.3

■ How do most clients in the United States and Canada acquire protozoan infections?

CLIENT TEACHING

Clients treated for fungal, viral, or parasitic infections need to know the following:

1. Avoid alcohol and other drugs toxic to the liver while taking azole-type antifungals.

2. Griseofulvin, used to treat superficial mycoses, can decrease the effectiveness of oral contraceptives. An alternative method of contraception is advised.

3. Older children and adult clients should swish oral antifungal drugs around in their mouths and swallow them. Caregivers should swab the mouths of infants and toddlers. Wait at least 10 minutes after antifungal treatment to put anything else in the mouth.

4. Rinse the mouth after use of glucocorticoid inhalers to avoid a decrease in local immune defenses against oral candidiasis.

5. Refrain from sexual intercourse while taking antifungal drugs for a vaginal infection until the infection is resolved.

6. When taking antivirals, report bleeding and bruising as well as decreased resistance to infection. These are indications of possible bone marrow suppression that may require dosage adjustment or change of medication.

8. When taking antivirals, do not take any other medications or dietary supplements without consulting your healthcare practitioner because of the risk for interactions.

9. Apply topical antivirals with a glove to prevent infection with additional organisms and to avoid transmission to others. Use a fresh glove for each application. ■

CHAPTER REVIEW

Core Concepts Summary

22.1 Fungi are more complex than bacteria and require a different approach to antiinfective therapy.

Fungi are multicellular organisms. Because most are unaffected by antibiotics, they require different classes of medications. Fungal infections, or mycoses, are only a serious problem in clients with compromised immune systems. Mycoses are classified as superficial or systemic.

22.2 Systemic antifungal drugs are used for serious infections of internal organs.

Systemic mycoses affect the internal organs and may require prolonged and aggressive drug therapy.

Systemic antifungal agents may cause serious adverse effects.

22.3 Superficial antifungal drugs are safe and effective in treating infections of the skin, nails and mucous membranes.

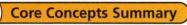

Superficial mycoses of the hair, skin, nails, and mucous membranes are very common, though rarely serious. Antifungals given topically as powders and lotions produce few adverse effects.

22.4 Viruses are non-living parasites that require a host in order to replicate.

Viruses take over the cellular machinery of their host and use it to replicate. While most viral infections require no pharmacotherapy, clients with infections by HIV, herpesviruses, and the influenza virus may benefit from drug treatment.

22.5 Antiretroviral drugs used in the treatment of HIV-AIDS do not cure the disease, but they do help many clients live longer.

Drugs used to treat HIV infections include the nucleoside and non-nucleoside reverse transcriptase inhibitors and protease inhibitors. These drugs may produce significant toxicity. While none are able to cure clients, they may extend the symptom-free period of their lives.

22.6 A small number of antiviral drugs are available to treat herpes simplex and influenza infections.

Drug therapy is used to prolong the latent period of genital herpes and to speed the recovery from active

lesions. A few antivirals are available to prevent influenza and these are most useful when combined with vaccines. New drugs have been developed to shorten the discomfort period for influenza symptoms, although these have limited efficacy.

22.7 While not common in the United States, infections caused by helminths and protozoans cause significant disease worldwide.

Malaria is one of the most common infections in the world and a significant number of drugs are available to disrupt the *Plasmodium* life cycle. Similarly, amebiasis is a common protozoan disease requiring intensive drug treatment. Diseases caused by helminths are common in areas of the world lacking adequate sanitation.

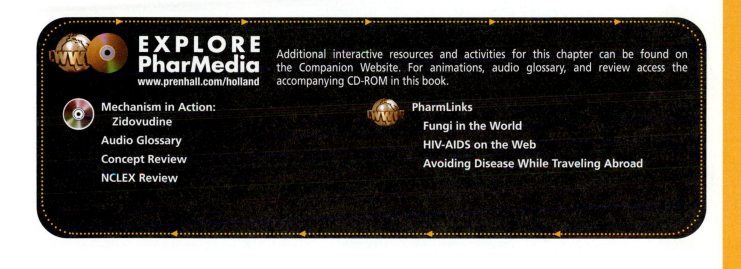

EXPLORE PharMedia
www.prenhall.com/holland

Additional interactive resources and activities for this chapter can be found on the Companion Website. For animations, audio glossary, and review access the accompanying CD-ROM in this book.

Mechanism in Action:
  Zidovudine
Audio Glossary
Concept Review
NCLEX Review

PharmLinks
Fungi in the World
HIV-AIDS on the Web
Avoiding Disease While Traveling Abroad

23 Drugs for Neoplasia

CORE CONCEPTS

23.1 Cancer is characterized by rapid, uncontrolled growth of cells.

23.2 The causes of cancer may be chemical, physical, or biological.

23.3 Personal risk of cancer may be prevented by a number of lifestyle factors.

23.4 Tumors are classified as benign or malignant and named according to their origin.

23.5 Cancer may be treated using surgery, radiation therapy, and drugs.

23.6 To achieve a total cure, every malignant cell must be removed or killed.

23.7 Use of multiple drugs and special dosing schedules are strategies used to improve the success of chemotherapy.

23.8 Serious toxicity limits most of the antineoplastic agents.

Alkylating Agents

23.9 Alkylating agents act by changing the structure of DNA in cancer cells.

Antimetabolites

23.10 Antimetabolites act by disrupting critical cell pathways in cancer cells.

Antitumor Antibiotics

23.11 Because of their cytotoxicity, a few antibiotics are used to treat cancer rather than infections.

Plant Extracts/Alkaloids

23.12 Some plant extracts have been isolated that kill cancer cells by preventing cell division.

Hormones

23.13 Some hormones and hormone antagonists have been found to be effective against certain tumors.

Biologic Response Modifiers

23.14 Biologic response modifiers and some additional antineoplastic drugs have been found to be effective against tumors.

OBJECTIVES

After reading this chapter, the student should be able to:

1. Explain differences between normal cells and cancer cells.

2. Identify the primary causes of cancer.

3. Describe how clients can reduce their probability of acquiring cancer by adopting certain changes to their lifestyle.

4. Differentiate among the terms neoplasm, benign, malignant, carcinoma, and sarcoma.

5. Identify the three primary treatments for cancer.

6. Explain why cancer is difficult to cure.

7. Explain why multiple drugs and special dosing schedules increase the effectiveness of chemotherapy.

8. List the general adverse effects of chemotherapeutic agents.

9. For each of the following, explain the mechanism of drug action, primary actions, and important adverse effects.

   a. alkylating agents
   b. antimetabolites
   c. antitumor antibiotics
   d. hormones and hormone antagonists with antineoplastic activity
   e. plant extracts with antineoplastic activity
   f. biologic response modifiers and miscellaneous anticancer drugs

10. Categorize anticancer drugs based on their classification and mechanism of action.

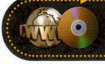

PharMedia
www.prenhall.com/holland

Additional interactive resources and activities for this chapter can be found on the Companion Website. For animations, audio glossary, and review access the accompanying CD-ROM in this book.

adenoma (AH-den-OH-mah): benign tumor of glandular tissue / *page 356*

alopecia (AL-oh-PEESH-ee-uh): hair loss / *page 360*

alkylation (AL-kill-AYE-shun): process by which certain chemicals attach to DNA and change its structure and function / *page 361*

anemia (ah-NEE-mee-ah): shortage of functional red blood cells / *page 360*

angiosarcoma (AN-gee-OH-sar-KOH-mah): cancer of blood vessels / *page 356*

benign (bee-NINE): neither life-threatening nor fatal / *page 356*

biologic response modifiers: natural substances that are able to enhance or stimulate the immune system / *page 371*

cancer (KAN-sir): malignant disease characterized by rapidly growing, invasive cells that spread to other regions of the body and eventually kill the host / *page 354*

carcinogen (kar-SIN-oh-jen): any physical, chemical, or biological factor that causes or promotes cancer / *page 355*

carcinoma (KAR-sin-OH-mah): a malignant tumor / *page 357*

chemotherapy: drug treatment of cancer / *page 357*

folic acid (FOH-lik): water soluble vitamin that is part of a coenzyme essential to the synthesis of nucleic acids / *page 364*

glioma (glee-OH-muh): malignant tumor of the brain / *page 356*

hepatocellular carcinoma: cancer of the liver / *page 357*

Kaposi's sarcoma (kah-POH-sees): vascular cancer that first appears on the skin and then invades internal organs; frequently occurs in AIDS clients / *page 366*

leukemia (lew-KEE-mee-ah): cancer of the blood characterized by overproduction of white blood cells / *page 356*

leukopenia (lew-koh-PEE-nee-ah): shortage of white blood cells / *page 360*

lipoma (lip-OH-mah): benign tumor of fat tissue / *page 356*

liposomes (LIP-oh-sohms): small sacs of lipids designed to carry drugs inside them / *page 366*

lymphoma (lim-FOH-mah): cancer of lymphatic tissue / *page 356*

malignant (mah-LIG-nent): life-threatening or fatal / *page 356*

malignant melanoma: type of skin cancer that metastasizes very quickly / *page 357*

metastasis (mah-TAS-tah-sis): travel of cancer cells from their original site to a distant tissue / *page 355*

nitrogen mustards: class of chemicals that are alkylating agents / *page 361*

neoplasm (NEE-oh-PLAZ-um): same as *tumor;* an abnormal swelling or mass / *page 356*

oncogenes (ON-koh-jeans): genes responsible for the conversion of normal cells into cancer cells / *page 355*

osteogenic sarcoma (OS-tee-oh-JEN-ik): cancer of bone / *page 356*

palliation (PAL-ee-AYE-shun): form of chemotherapy intended to alleviate symptoms rather than cure the disease / *page 357*

purine (PYUR-een): building block of DNA and RNA, either adenine or guanine / *page 363*

pyrimidine (peer-IM-uh-deen): building block of DNA and RNA, either thymine or cytosine in DNA and cytosine and uracil in RNA / *page 363*

radiation therapy: the delivery of high-dose radiation with the intent of killing tumor cells / *page 357*

sarcoma (sar-KOH-mah): cancer of connective tissue such as bone, muscle, or cartilage / *page 356*

taxoids (TAKS-oids): antineoplastic drugs obtained from the Pacific Yew tree / *page 367*

thrombocytopenia (THROM-boh-SEYE-toh-PEE-nee-ah): deficiency of platelets / *page 360*

topoisomerase (TOH-poh-eye-SOM-er-ase): enzyme that assists in the repair of DNA damage / *page 367*

tumor (TOO-more): abnormal swelling or mass / *page 356*

tumor suppressor genes: genes that inhibit the transformation of normal cells into cancer cells / *page 355*

vinca alkaloids (VIN-ka AL-kah-loids): chemicals obtained from the periwinkle plant / *page 365*

Cancer is one of the most feared diseases for a number of valid reasons. It may be silent, producing no symptoms until it is too large to cure. It sometimes requires painful and disfiguring surgery. It may occur at an early age—even during childhood—depriving clients of a normal lifespan. Perhaps worst of all, the medical treatment of cancer often cannot offer a cure, and progression to death is sometimes slow, painful, and psychologically difficult for the client and his or her loved ones.

Many advances have been made in the diagnosis, understanding, and treatment of cancer. Some types of cancer are now curable and therapy may give the client a longer, symptom-free life. This chapter examines the role of drugs in the treatment of cancer. Medications used to treat this disease are called anticancer drugs, antineoplastics, or cancer chemotherapeutic agents.

Fast Facts Cancer

- In 2001, 1,268,000 new cancer cases were projected, and 553,400 deaths occurred.
- Since 1990, over 13 million new cancer cases have been diagnosed.
- Cancer is the leading cause of death in children under 15.
- Colorectal cancer is the third most common cancer in both men and women.

- Leukemia is the most common childhood cancer and is responsible for one quarter of all cancers occurring before age 20.
- Lung cancer accounts for 28% of all cancer deaths.
- Prostrate cancer is the second leading cause of death in men.
- In the year 2000, the following cancer cases were reported.

182,800 new breast cancers (1,400 were in men), with 42,000 deaths
8,600 new cancer cases in children ages 0–14, with 1,600 deaths
130,000 new colon/rectal cancers, with 56,300 deaths
30,800 new leukemias (28,200 adults, 2,600 children), with 21,700 deaths
164,000 new lung cancers, with 159,000 deaths
180,400 new prostate cancers, with 31,900 deaths
1.3 million new skin cancers, with 9,600 deaths (7,700 from melanoma, 1,900 from others)
12,800 cervical cancers, with 4,600 deaths
28,300 new pancreatic cancers, with 28,200 deaths

23.1 Cancer is characterized by rapid, uncontrolled growth of cells.

Cancer is a disease characterized by abnormal, uncontrolled cell division. Cell division is a normal process occurring extensively in most body tissues from conception to late childhood. At some point in time, however, cells suppress this rapid division by repressing the genes responsible for cell growth. This may result in a total lack of division in the case of muscle cells and, perhaps, brain cells. In other cells, the genes controlling division may be reactivated whenever it is necessary to replace worn-out cells, as in the case of blood cells and the lining of the digestive tract.

Cancer is thought to result from damage to the genes controlling cell growth. Once damaged, the cell is no longer responsive to normal chemical signals checking its growth. The cancer cells

FIGURE 23.1

Invasion and metastasis by cancer cells

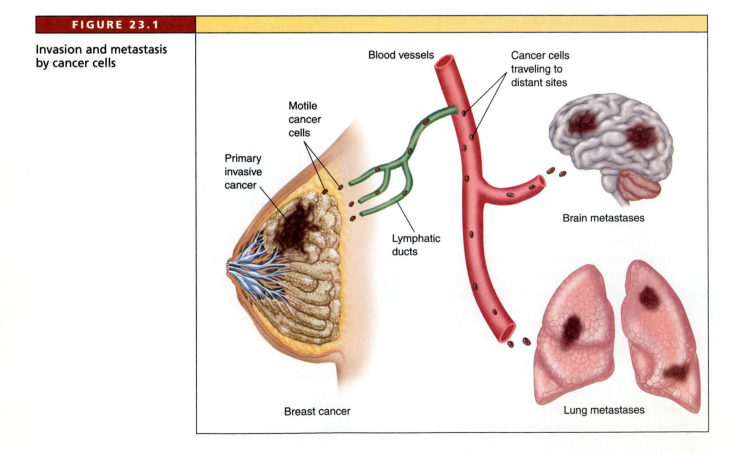

lose their normal functions, divide rapidly, and invade surrounding cells. Indeed, the abnormal cells may travel to distant sites where they populate new tumors, a process called metastasis. Figure 23.1 illustrates some characteristics of cancer cells.

23.2 The causes of cancer may be chemical, physical, or biological.

A large number of factors have been found to cause cancer or to be associated with a higher risk for acquiring the disease. These factors are known as carcinogens.

A large number of chemical carcinogens have been identified. Some of these carcinogens, such as asbestos and benzene have been associated with a higher incidence of cancer in the workplace. Chemicals in tobacco smoke are thought to be responsible for about one-third of all cancer in the United States. The actual site of the cancer may be distant from the entry location, as is the case of bladder cancer caused by the inhalation of certain industrial chemicals. Some of the known chemical carcinogens are listed in Table 23.1.

A number of physical factors are also associated with cancer. For example, exposure to large amounts of X-rays is associated with a higher risk of leukemia. Ultraviolet (UV) light from the sun is a known cause of skin cancer.

Viruses are associated with about 15% of all human cancers. Examples include herpes simplex viruses types I and II, Epstein-Barr virus, papillomavirus, cytomegalovirus, and human T-lymphotrophic viruses. Factors that suppress the immune system, such as the human immunodeficiency virus or drugs given after transplant surgery, may encourage the growth of pre-existing cancer cells, as discussed in Chapter 20 ⌾ .

It is widely known that some cancers have a strong genetic component. The fact that close relatives may acquire the same type of cancer suggests that the client may have certain genes, called oncogenes, that predispose him or her to the condition. These abnormal genes somehow interact with chemical, physical, and biological agents to promote cancer formation in the client. Other genes, called tumor suppressor genes, may inhibit the formation of tumors. If these suppressor genes are damaged, cancer may result. Damage to the suppressor gene known as p53 is associated with cancers of the breast, lung, brain, colon, and bone.

Concept review 23.1

■ What is the fundamental feature that makes a cancer cell different from a normal cell?

TABLE 23.1	Chemicals Associated With an Increased Risk of Cancer
CHEMICAL	TYPE OF CANCER
arsenic	skin and lung
nickel	lung and nasal
asbestos	lung
vinyl chloride	liver
benzene	leukemia
alcohol	liver
polycyclic aromatic hydrocarbons	lung and skin
tobacco substances	lung

23.3 Personal risk of cancer may be prevented by a number of lifestyle factors.

Fortunately, adopting healthy lifestyle habits such as those shown in the following list may reduce the risk of acquiring cancer. Eliminating tobacco use is the most important means of reducing cancer risk. Limiting exposure to exhaled, or second-hand, smoke is also thought to be important. Intake of alcoholic beverages and saturated fats should be limited and body weight kept within medically recommended ranges. The following list shows ways health-care providers can help their clients reduce their risk of cancer.

- Limit or eliminate alcoholic beverage intake.
- Reduce fat in the diet, particularly that from animal sources.
- Choose most of the foods from plant sources; increase fiber in the diet.
- Exercise regularly and keep body weight within optimum guidelines.
- Eliminate tobacco use.
- Reduce or eliminate exposure to second-hand tobacco smoke.
- Self-examine the body monthly for abnormal lumps.
- Examine the skin for abnormal lesions or changes in moles.
- When exposed to direct sun, use skin lotions with the highest SPF (Sun Protection Factor) value.
- Women should have an annual mammogram after age 40.
- Men should have a digital rectal prostate examination and a prostate-specific antigen test annually after age 50.
- For colorectal screening, a fecal occult blood test (FOBT) and flexible sigmoidoscopy should be performed at age 50 with FOBT annually following age 50.
- Women who are sexually active or who have reached age 18 should have an annual Pap test and pelvic examination.

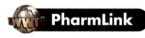

CANCERNET

Certain foods are thought to exert protective effects. These include cold-water fish, such as cod, that contain a high concentration of omega-6 fatty acids. Increased fiber intake in the form of fresh fruits, vegetables, and grains may reduce cancer risk. Regular self-examination of the skin, breasts, or testicles can help identify suspicious lumps or other lesions.

23.4 Tumors are classified as benign or malignant and named according to their origin.

neo = new
plasm = thing formed

The word **tumor** means swelling, abnormal enlargement, or mass. The word **neoplasm** is often used interchangeably with tumor. The suffix *–oma* signifies tumor. Tumors may be either benign or malignant.

 Benign tumors grow slowly, do not metastasize, and rarely require drug treatment. Although they do not kill clients, their growth may result in pressure on nerves, blood vessels, or other tissues. When this occurs, they may be surgically removed; they do not normally grow back. Examples include **adenomas**, which are benign tumors of glandular tissue, and **lipomas**, which are tumors of adipose tissue.

adeno = gland
oma = tumor
lip = fat

 Malignant tumors are called *cancer*. The word **malignant** refers to a disease that grows rapidly worse, becomes resistant to treatment, and normally results in death. The two major divisions of malignant neoplasms are carcinomas and sarcomas. Other types include cancer of the blood-forming cells in bone marrow (**leukemia**), lymphatic tissue (**lymphomas**), and the central nervous system (**gliomas**).

leuk = white
emia = condition
sarc = flesh
angio = blood
osteo = bone
gen = formation

 Sarcomas arise from connective tissue such as bone, muscle, and cartilage. Although less common than carcinomas, they grow extremely rapidly and metastasize early in the progression of the disease. Examples include **osteogenic sarcoma**, a bone cancer, and **angiosarcoma**, a cancer of blood vessels.

Carcinomas are the most common type of malignant neoplasm. Carcinomas grow rapidly, metastasize, and are fatal if left untreated. Examples of carcinomas include **malignant melanoma**, a skin cancer, and **hepatocellular carcinoma**, a cancer of the liver.

melan = *black/pigmented*

23.5 Cancer may be treated using surgery, radiation therapy, and drugs.

There is a much greater possibility for cure if the cancer is treated in its early stages, when the tumor is small and localized to a single area. Once the cancer has spread to distant sites, cure is much more difficult. Thus, it is important to diagnose the disease as early as possible. In an attempt to remove every cancer cell, three treatment approaches are utilized: surgery, radiation therapy, and drug therapy.

Surgery is performed to remove a tumor that is localized to one area, or when the tumor is pressing on nerves, the airways, or other vital tissues. Surgery lowers the number of cancer cells in the body so that radiation and drug therapy can be more successful. Surgery is not an option for tumors of blood cells or when it would not be expected to extend a client's lifespan or to improve the quality of his or her life.

Radiation therapy is an effective way to kill tumor cells through non-surgical means. High doses of ionizing radiation are aimed directly at the tumor and confined to this area, to the maximum extent possible. Radiation treatments may follow surgery in order to kill any cancer cells that were left behind following the operation. Radiation is sometimes given as **palliation** for inoperable cancers to shrink the size of a tumor that may be pressing on vital organs in order to relieve pain or difficulty in breathing or swallowing.

Drug therapy of cancer is sometimes called **chemotherapy**. When these drugs are transported through the blood, they have the potential to reach cancer cells in virtually any location. Some medications are even available to pass across the blood-brain barrier in order to treat brain tumors. Some are instilled directly into body cavities, such as the bladder, in order to bring the highest dose possible to the cancer cells without producing systemic side effects. Anticancer drugs may be given to attempt cure, for palliation, or occasionally as prophylaxis to prevent cancer from occurring. Chemotherapeutic medications are often combined with surgery and radiation in order to increase the probability of a cure.

23.6 To achieve a total cure, every malignant cell must be removed or killed.

In order to cure a client, it is thought that every single cancer cell must be destroyed or removed from the body. Even one malignant cell may produce enough offspring to kill a client. Unlike antiinfective therapy, in which the client's immune system is an active partner in eliminating massive

NATURAL ALTERNATIVES

Green Tea as an Antioxidant

Green tea is prepared from the dried leaves from plants grown in China, Ceylon, and India. Green tea—and to a lesser extent, black tea—have a number of chemicals shown to possess antioxidant activity. Antioxidants are thought to offer a protective effect against cancer by their ability to eliminate free radicals, reactive substances that damage cells. Antioxidants in green tea include polyphenols, epigallocatechin gallate, and catechins.

Other than water, green tea is the world's most widely consumed liquid. The health effects of green tea have been reported since antiquity: the Chinese believed the beverage increased longevity and protected against cancer. The caffeine in green tea also increases mental alertness and provides a mild diuretic effect. Green tea is reported to boost immune function and enhance cardiovascular health by inhibiting the production of low-density lipoproteins. ▪

numbers of microorganisms, the immune system is able to eliminate only a small number of cancer cells. Consider that a 1-cm breast tumor may contain 1,000,000,000 (10^9) cancer cells before it is detected. A drug killing 99% of these cells would be considered a very effective drug indeed. Yet even with this fantastic achievement, 10,000,000 cancer cells would still remain, any one of which could cause the tumor to return and kill the client. The relationship between cell kill and chemotherapy is shown in Figure 23.2. This example illustrates the need to treat tumors at an early stage with multiple drugs and using several methods such as chemotherapy, radiation, and surgery, whenever possible.

23.7 Use of multiple drugs and special dosing schedules are strategies used to improve the success of chemotherapy.

Many cancers are very difficult to treat using medications. While cancer cells are clearly abnormal in many ways, much of their physiology is identical to that of normal cells. It is thus difficult to

FIGURE 23.2

Cell kill and chemotherapy

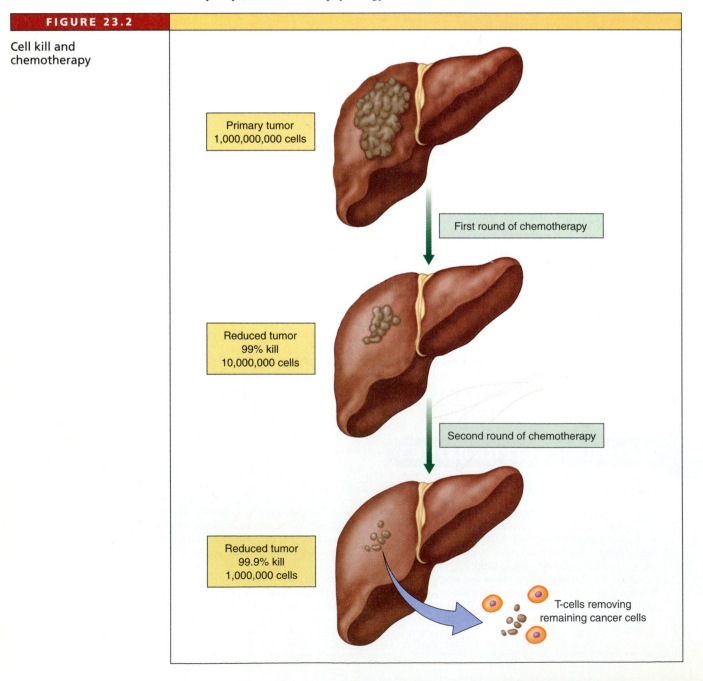

Primary tumor
1,000,000,000 cells

First round of chemotherapy

Reduced tumor
99% kill
10,000,000 cells

Second round of chemotherapy

Reduced tumor
99.9% kill
1,000,000 cells

T-cells removing
remaining cancer cells

FIGURE 23.3

Antineoplastic agents
and the cell cycle

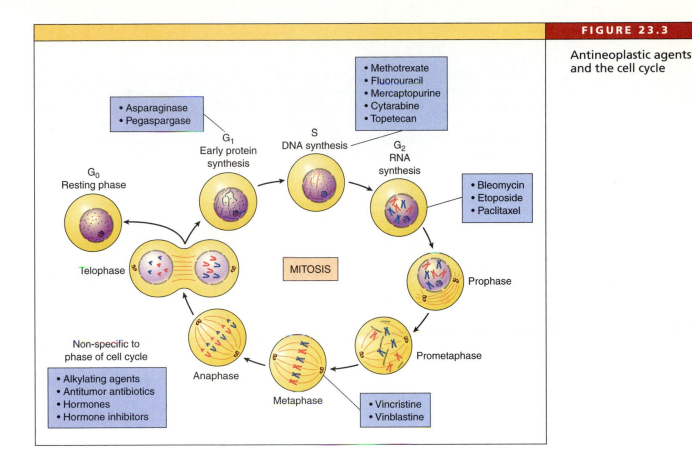

kill cancer cells selectively without profoundly affecting normal cells. Complicating the chance for a pharmacologic cure is the fact that cancer cells often develop resistance to antineoplastic drugs.

A number of treatment strategies have been found to increase the effectiveness of anticancer drugs. In most cases, multiple medications from different antineoplastic classes are given during a course of chemotherapy. These different classes affect different stages of the cancer cell's life cycle, as illustrated in Figure 23.3. This permits the tumor to be attacked from several mechanisms

ON THE JOB

Interventional Radiology

Radiography is primarily a diagnostic field, using ionizing radiation to identify diseases. A branch of the field known as *interventional radiography,* however, treats diseases such as cancer. Radiographers, nurses, and cardiovascular technologists are important members of the interventional radiology team.

Solid tumors often establish their own blood supply, a process known as *angiogenesis.* These tumor vessels can become quite large as the tumor uses them to bring nutrients to its rapidly growing mass.

Under the guidance of X-rays, a very thin plastic tube, or catheter, is placed into the vascular system through a small nick in the skin. The catheter is guided to the site of the tumor vessel and the physician injects antineoplastic drugs directly into the tumor. Immediately following the drug injection, a gel-like substance is sometimes injected to completely occlude the tumor vessel, a process called *chemoembolization.* The occlusion not only starves the tumor, but also allows the injected drugs to remain in the tumor for as long as a month. Higher doses of antineoplastics can be used, as they are injected directly into the tumor. In another interventional radiology procedure known as *tumor ablation,* heat, cold, or substances such as alcohol may be injected into a tumor to kill the cancer cells.

Although these procedures do not effect a cure, a majority of clients experience pain relief and tumor shrinkage. Procedures may be repeated as needed. Interventional radiography offers a nonsurgical, less painful approach to cancer treatment. ▪

of action, thus increasing the percentage of cell kill. Using multiple drugs also allows the dosages of each individual agent to be lowered, thus reducing toxicity and slowing the development of resistance.

Specific dosing schedules or cycles have been found to increase the effectiveness of the antineoplastic agents. For example, some anticancer drugs are given as single doses or perhaps a couple doses over a few days. Several weeks may pass before the next series of doses. This gives normal cells time to recover from the adverse effects of the drugs. It also allows tumor cells that may not have been replicating at the time of the first dose to begin dividing, and thus become more sensitive to the next round of chemotherapy.

Concept review 23.2

■ Why is it important to kill or remove 100% of the cancer cells in order to effect a cure?

23.8 Serious toxicity limits most of the antineoplastic agents.

All anticancer drugs have the potential to cause serious toxicity. These drugs are often pushed to their maximum possible dosages so that the greatest tumor kill can be obtained. Such high dosages always result in adverse effects in the client. Because these drugs primarily affect rapidly growing cells, those tissues that are still dividing in the adult are most susceptible to adverse effects. Hair follicles are damaged, resulting in hair loss or **alopecia**. The lining of the digestive tract is affected, sometimes resulting in severe diarrhea. The vomiting center in the medulla is triggered by many antineoplastics, resulting in severe nausea and vomiting. Blood cells in the bone marrow may be destroyed, causing a reduction in the number of red blood cells (**anemia**), white blood cells (**leukopenia**), and platelets (**thrombocytopenia**). A list of typical adverse effects of anticancer drugs is given in Table 23.2.

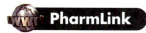

CURRENT INDICATIONS FOR ANTINEOPLASTICS

Antineoplastic drugs act by a wide variety of mechanisms, most of which involve cell killing or cytotoxicity. Classification is quite variable because a drug may kill cells by several different mechanisms and have characteristics from more than one class. Furthermore, the mechanisms by which some medications act is not yet understood. A simple method of classifying this complex group of drugs includes six groups.

- alkylating agents
- antimetabolites
- antitumor antibiotics
- hormones and hormone antagonists having antineoplastic activity
- plant extracts having antineoplastic activity
- miscellaneous anticancer drugs

TABLE 23.2	Adverse Effects of Anticancer Drugs	
CHANGES TO THE BLOOD	**CHANGES TO THE GI TRACT**	**OTHER EFFECTS**
anemia (low red blood cells)	nausea	fatigue
thrombocytopenia	vomiting	opportunistic infections
(low platelets)	diarrhea	ulceration and bleeding of the lips and gums
leukopenia (low white blood cells)	anorexia (loss of appetite)	alopecia (loss of hair)

FIGURE 23.4

Mechanism of action of the alkylating agents

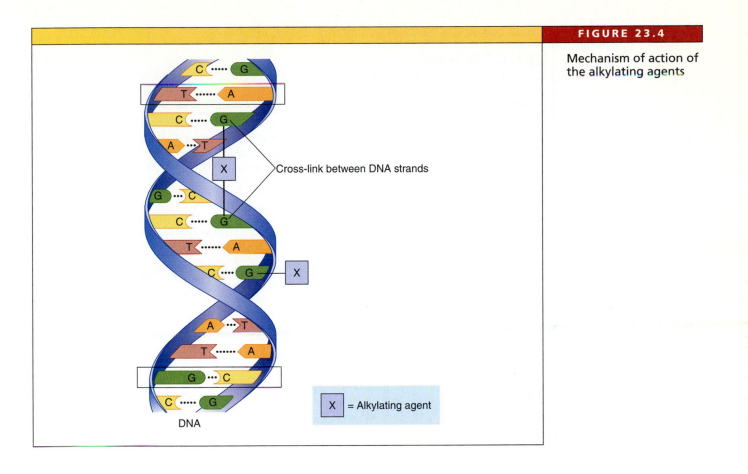

Cross-link between DNA strands

X = Alkylating agent

DNA

ALKYLATING AGENTS

Alkylating agents act by chemically binding to nucleic acids and inhibiting cell division. They are some of the most widely used antineoplastic drugs.

23.9 Alkylating agents act by changing the structure of DNA in cancer cells.

The first alkylating agents, the nitrogen mustards, were developed in secrecy as chemical warfare agents during World War II. Although the drugs in this class have quite different chemical structures, all have the common characteristic of being able to form bonds or linkages with DNA. These agents physically attach to DNA, a process called alkylation. Alkylation changes the shape of DNA and prevents it from functioning normally. Although each alkylating agent attaches to DNA in a different manner, collectively they have the effect of killing—or at least slowing—the replication of tumor cells. The alkylation may occur in any cancer cell; however, the killing action does not occur until the cell begins to divide. Figure 23.4 illustrates the process of alkylation. Table 23.3 lists the alkylating agents and their dosages.

Blood cells are particularly sensitive to alkylating agents, and bone marrow suppression is the most important adverse effect of this class. Within days after administration, declines in red blood cells, white blood cells, and platelets may be measured. Damaging effects on the epithelial cells lining of the GI tract are also common with this class of drugs.

DRUG PROFILE:
Cyclophosphamide (Cytoxan)

Actions:

Cyclophosphamide is a commonly prescribed nitrogen mustard. It is used alone or in combination with other drugs against a wide variety of cancers, including Hodgkin's disease, lymphoma, multiple myeloma, breast cancer, and ovarian cancer. Cyclophosphamide acts by attaching to DNA and disrupting cell division, particularly in rapidly dividing cells. It is one of only a few anticancer drugs that may be given orally.

Adverse Effects:

Cyclophosphamide exerts a powerful immuno-suppressant effect that peaks one to two days after administration. Thrombocytopenia is common, and thus bleeding and bruising may be observed. Nausea, vomiting, and diarrhea are frequently experienced. Cyclophosphamide damages hair follicles, causing alopecia, although this effect is usually reversible. Unlike other nitrogen mustards, cyclophosphamide exhibits very little neurotoxicity.

TABLE 23.3	Alkylating Agents	
DRUG	**ROUTE AND ADULT DOSE**	**REMARKS**
nitrogen mustards		
Pr cyclophosphamide (Cytoxan, Neosar)	PO; initial dose 1–5 mg/kg qd; maintenance dose 1–5 mg/kg q 7–10 days.	For Hodgkin's disease, non-Hodgkin's lymphoma, leukemias, multiple myeloma, cancer of the breast, ovary, and lung; IV form available.
chlorambucil (Leukeran)	PO; initial dose 0.1–0.2 mg/kg qd; maintenance dose 4–10 mg qd.	For chronic lymphocyic leukemia, non-Hodgkin's lymphoma, cancer of the breast and ovary.
estramustine phosphate sodium (Emcyt)	PO; 5 mg/kg tid-qid.	For palliative treatment of advanced prostate cancer.
ifosfamide (Ifex)	IV; 1.2 g/m^2 qd for 5 consecutive days.	For testicular cancer.
mechloroethamine hydrochloride (Mustargen)	IV; 6 mg/m^2 on day 1 and 8 of a 28 day cycle.	For Hodgkin's disease, non-Hodgkin's lymphoma, lung cancer.
melphalan (Alkeran)	PO; 6 mg qd for 2–3 weeks.	For multiple myeloma.
Nitrosoureas		
carmustine (BiCNU, Gliadel)	IV; 200 mg/m^2 q 6 weeks.	For Hodgkin's disease, malignant melanoma, multiple myeloma, brain cancer; topical form for mycosis fungoides.
lomustine (CeeNU)	PO; 130 mg/m^2 as a single dose.	For Hodgkin's disease and brain cancer.
streptozocin (Zanosar)	IV; 500 mg/m^2 for 5 consecutive days.	For pancreatic cancer.
Miscellaneous Alkylating Agents		
busulfan (Myleran)	PO; 4–8 mg qd.	For chronic myelogenous leukemia.
carboplatin (Paraplatin)	IV; 360 mg/m^2 q 4 weeks.	For cancer of the ovary.
cisplatin (Platinol)	IV; 20 mg/m^2 qd for 5 days.	For testicular, bladder, ovarian, uterine, head, and neck carcinomas.
dacarbazine (DTIC-Dome)	IV; 2–4.5 mg/kg qd for 10 days.	For Hodgkin's disease and malignant melanoma.
temozolomide (Temodar)	PO; 150 mg/m^2 qd × 5 consecutive days.	For brain cancer.

ANTIMETABOLITES

Antimetabolites are structurally similar to certain critical cell molecules. They interfere with aspects of the nutrient or nucleic acid metabolism of rapidly growing tumor cells.

23.10 Antimetabolites act by disrupting critical cell pathways in cancer cells.

Rapidly growing cancer cells require large amounts of nutrients and other chemicals to build proteins and nucleic acids. Antimetabolites are drugs that are chemically similar to essential building blocks of the cell. When cancer cells attempt to construct proteins or DNA, they use the antimetabolites instead of the normal building blocks. By disrupting metabolic pathways in this manner, antimetabolites can kill cancer cells or slow their growth.

Several of these antimetabolites resemble **purines** and **pyrimidines**, chemicals that are the building blocks of DNA and RNA. These antimetabolites are called *purine* or *pyrimidine analogs*. For example, floxuridine (FUDR) and fluorouracil (Adrucil) are able to block the formation of thymidylate, an essential chemical needed to make DNA. After becoming activated and incorporated into DNA, cytarabine (Cytosar) blocks DNA synthesis. Figure 23.5 illustrates the similarities of some of these analogs to their natural counterparts. The antimetabolite drugs are shown in Table 23.4 (page 365).

ANTITUMOR ANTIBIOTICS

This class contains antibiotics obtained from bacteria that have the ability to kill cancer cells. They are not widely prescribed, but are very effective against certain tumors.

FIGURE 23.5

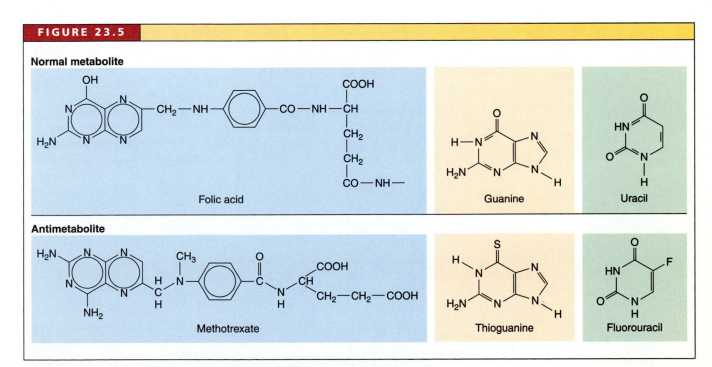

Structural similarities between antimetabolites and their natural counterparts

DRUG PROFILE (Antimetabolite):
Methotrexate (Mexate)

Actions:

Methotrexate is classified as an antifolate because it inhibits folic acid metabolism. Folic acid is a water-soluble vitamin found in eggs, veal, liver, whole grains, and dark green vegetables. Folic acid is part of a coenzyme essential to the synthesis of nucleic acids. By blocking the synthesis of folic acid, methotrexate is able to inhibit replication, particularly in rapidly dividing cells.

Methotrexate is prescribed alone or in combination with other drugs for choriocarcinoma, osteogenic sarcoma, leukemias, head and neck cancers, breast carcinoma, and lung carcinoma. It is occasionally used to treat non-neoplastic disorders such as severe psoriasis and rheumatoid arthritis that has not responded to other medications.

Adverse Effects:

Like many antineoplastics, methotrexate is a potent immunosuppressant. Hemorrhage and bruising are often observed due to low platelet counts. Nausea, vomiting, and anorexia are common. Although rare, pulmonary toxicity may develop and be quite serious. Methotrexate is a pregnancy category X drug.

Mechanism in Action:

Methotrexate interferes with the synthesis of folate by inhibiting three enzymes, thymidylate, dihydrofolate reductase (DHFR), and transformylase. Folate is necessary for the synthesis of DNA, RNA, and protein in rapidly dividing cancer cells.

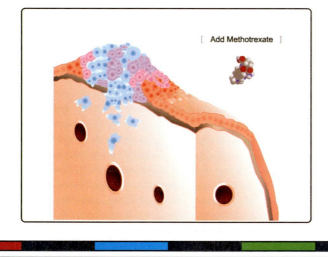

[Add Methotrexate]

23.11 Because of their cytotoxicity, a few antibiotics are used to treat cancer rather than infections.

A number of substances isolated from bacteria have been found to have antitumor properties. These chemicals are more toxic than the traditional antibiotics; thus, their use is restricted to treating specific cancers. All the antitumor antibiotics interact with DNA in a manner similar to the alkylating agents. Because of this, their general actions and side effects are similar to those of the alkylating agents. Unlike the alkylating agents, however, all the antitumor antibiotics must be administered intravenously or through direct instillation into a body cavity using a catheter. Table 23.5 lists the primary antitumor antibiotics.

PLANT EXTRACTS/ALKALOIDS

Plants have been a valuable source for antineoplastic agents. These agents act by preventing cell division.

TABLE 23.4	Antimetabolites	
DRUG	**ROUTE AND ADULT DOSE**	**REMARKS**
Folic Acid Antagonist		
Pr methotrexate (Amethopterin, Folex, Rheumatrx)	IV; 15–30 mg qd × 5 days.	For acute lymphoblastic leukemia, choriocarcinoma, lymphoma, head and neck cancer, testicular cancer, osteogenic sarcoma; oral and IM forms available.
Pyrimidine Analogs		
fluorouracil (5-FU, Adrucil, Efudex, Fluorodex)	IV; 12 mg/kg qd for 4 consecutive days.	For cancer of the breast, colon, rectum, stomach, and pancreas; topical form available for basal cell carcinoma.
capecitabine (Xeloda)	PO; 2500 mg/m^2 qd for 2 weeks.	For breast cancer.
cytarabine (ARA-C, Cytosar-U, Tarabine, DepoCyt)	IV; 200 mg/m^2 as a continuous infusion over 24 hours.	For acute myelogenous leukemia; SC and intrathecal forms available.
floxuridine (FUDR)	Intra-arterial; 0.1–0.6 mg/kg qd as a continuous infusion.	For GI metastasis to the liver.
gemcitabine hydrochloride (Gemzar)	IV; 1000 mg/m^2 q week.	For cancer of the pancreas and lung.
Purine Analogs		
cladribine (Leustatin)	IV; 0.09 mg/m^2 qd as a continuous infusion.	For hairy cell leukemia.
fludarabine (Fludara)	IV; 25 mg/m^2 qd for 5 consecutive days.	For chronic lymphocytic leukemia.
mercaptopurine (6-MP, Purinsthol)	PO; 2.5 mg/kg qd.	For childhood acute leukemia.
pentostatin (Nipent)	IV; 4 mg/m^2 q other week.	For hairy cell leukemia.
thioguanine (TG)	PO; 2 mg/kg qd.	For remission induction in adult acute leukemia.

23.12 Some plant extracts have been isolated that kill cancer cells by preventing cell division.

Chemicals with antineoplastic activity have been isolated from a number of plants, including the common periwinkle (*Vinca rosea*), the Pacific yew, the mandrake plant (May apple) and the shrub *Campothecus accuminata*. Although structurally very different, drugs in this class have the common ability to arrest cell division; thus they are sometimes called *mitotic inhibitors*. The primary plant extracts, or alkaloids, used as antineoplastics are shown in Table 23.6.

The vinca alkaloids, Vincristine (Oncovin) and Vinblastine (Velban), are older medications derived from the periwinkle plant. Their biological properties were described in folklore for many years in various parts of the world prior to their use as anticancer drugs. Similarly, American Indians described uses of the May apple long before teniposide (Vumon) and etoposide (VePesid) were isolated from this plant and used for chemotherapy.

DRUG PROFILE:

Doxorubicin (Adriamycin)

Actions:

Doxorubicin attaches to DNA, causing the DNA strands to break and thus resulting in cellular death. It is prescribed for solid tumors of the lung, breast, ovary, and bladder, and for various leukemias and lymphomas. It is structurally very similar to daunorubicin (Cerubidine).

A novel delivery method has been developed for both doxorubicin and daunorubicin. The drug is enclosed in small sacs, or vesicles, of lipids called liposomes. The liposomal vesicle is designed to open and release the antitumor antibiotic when it reaches a cancer cell. The goal is to deliver a higher concentration of drug to the cancer cells, thus sparing normal cells. The primary indication for this delivery method is AIDS-related Kaposi's sarcoma.

Adverse Effects:

Like many of the anticancer medications, doxorubicin may profoundly lower blood cell counts. Leaking from an injection site can cause severe pain and tissue damage. The most serious concern is delayed cardiac toxicity that may result in irreversible heart failure. Nausea, vomiting, diarrhea, and hair loss are common.

TABLE 23.5	Antitumor Antibiotics	
DRUG	**ROUTE AND ADULT DOSE**	**REMARKS**
Pr doxorubicin (Adriamycin, Rubex)	IV; 60–75 mg/m^2 as a single dose.	For lymphomas, sarcomas, acute leukemia, cancer of the breast, lung, testes, thyroid, and ovary.
bleomycin sulfate (Blenoxane)	IV; 0.25–0.5 units/kg q 4–7 days.	For squamous cell carcinoma, Hodgkin's disease, lymphomas, and testicular cancer.
dactinomycin (Actinomycin D, Cosmegan)	IV; 500 μg qd for a maximum of 5 days.	For Wilm's tumor and rhabdomyosarcoma.
daunorubicin (Cerubidine)	IV; 30–60 mg/m^2 qd for 3–5 days.	For leukemias and lymphomas.
daunorubicin – liposomal formulation (DaunoXsome)	IV; 40 mg/m^2 q 2 weeks.	For Kaposi's sarcoma.
doxorubicin – liposome (Doxil)	IV; 20 mg/m^2 q 3 weeks.	For Kaposi's sarcoma.
epirubicin (Ellence)	IV; 100–120 mg/m^2 as a single dose.	For breast cancer.
idarubicin (Idamycin)	IV; 8–12 mg/m^2 qd × 3 days.	For acute myelogenous leukemia.
mitomycin (Mutamycin)	IV; 2 mg/m^2 as a single dose.	For cancer of the colon, stomach, lung, head and neck, rectum, bladder, pancreatic, and breast; also for malignant melanoma.
mitoxantrone hydrochloride (Novantrone)	IV; 12 mg/m^2 qd × 3 days.	For acute non-lymphocytic leukemia.
plicamycin (Mithramycin, Mithracin)	IV; 25–30 ;μ/kg qd × 8–10 days.	For testicular cancer; also used to manage hypercalcemia.
valrubicin (Valstar)	Intrabladder instillation; 800 mg q week × 6 weeks.	For bladder cancer.

DRUG PROFILE:
Vincristine (Oncovin)

Actions:

Vincristine affects rapidly growing cells by inhibiting their ability to complete mitosis. Although it must be given intravenously, a major advantage of vincristine is that it causes minimal immunosuppression. It is usually prescribed in combination with other antineo-plastics for the treatment of lymphoma, leukemias, Kaposi's sarcoma, Wilm's tumor, bladder carcinoma, and breast carcinoma.

Adverse Effects:

The most serious limiting adverse effects of vincristine relate to nervous system toxicity. Symptoms include numbness and tingling in the limbs, muscular weakness, loss of neural reflexes, and pain. Severe constipation is common. Immunosuppression may occur, though it is less serious than with vinblastine, the other vinca alkaloid. Alopecia is common.

TABLE 23.6 | **Plant Extracts with Antineoplastic Activity**

DRUG	ROUTE AND ADULT DOSE	REMARKS
Mitotic Inhibitors		
Pr vincristine sulfate (Oncovin)	IV; 1.4 mg/m² q week (max 2 mg/m²).	For lymphomas, Hodgkin's disease, Wilm's tumor, and childhood acute leukemia.
vinblastine sulfate (Velban)	IV; 3.7–18.5 mg/m² q week.	For cancer of the breast and testicles; Hodgkin's disease.
vinorelbine tartrate (Navelbine)	IV; 30 mg/m² q week.	For lung cancer.
Taxoids		
docetaxel (Taxotere)	IV; 60–100 mg/m² q 3 weeks.	For breast cancer.
paclitaxel (Taxol)	IV; 135–175 mg/m² q 3 weeks.	For ovarian and breast cancer.
Topoisomerase Inhibitors		
topotecan hydrochloride (Hycamtin)	IV; 1.5 mg/m² qd × 5 days.	For ovarian cancer.
etoposide (VePesid)	IV; 50–100 mg/m² qd × 5 days.	For testicular and lung cancer; choriocarciomas; PO form available.
teniposide (Vumon)	IV; 165 mg/m² q 3–4 days × 4 weeks.	For acute lymphocytic leukemia.
irinotecan hydrochloride (Camptosar)	IV; 125 mg/m² q week × 4 weeks.	For colo-rectal cancer.

The taxoids, which include pacitaxel (Taxol) and docetaxel (Taxotere), have been isolated relatively recently from the Pacific yew. Other recently isolated chemotherapeutic agents include topetecan (Hycamtin) and irinotecan (Camptosar). These agents are called topoisomerase inhibitors because they block the enzyme topoisomerase that helps repair DNA damage.

HORMONES

Hormones significantly affect the growth of some tumors. Use of natural or synthetic hormones or their antagonists as antineoplastic agents is a strategy used to slow the growth of hormone-dependent tumors.

23.13 Some hormones and hormone antagonists have been found to be effective against certain tumors.

A number of hormones are used in cancer chemotherapy, including corticosteroids, estrogens, and androgens. In addition, several hormone antagonists have been found to exhibit antitumor activity. The mechanism of hormone antineoplastic activity is largely unknown. It is likely, however, that these antitumor properties are independent of their normal hormone mechanisms because the doses utilized in cancer chemotherapy are magnitudes larger than the amount naturally present in the body. Other aspects of hormonal therapy are presented in Chapters 28 and 29 ⬤⬤.

In general, hormones and hormone antagonists produce few of the cytotoxic side effects seen with other antineoplastics. They can, however, produce serious side effects when given at high does for prolonged periods. They are normally given for palliation, as they rarely produce cancer cures when used singly. The major hormone and hormone antagonists prescribed for cancer are given in Table 23.7.

BIOLOGIC RESPONSE MODIFIERS

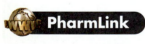

CLINICAL TRIALS

Biologic response modifiers approach cancer treatment from a different perspective than other chemotherapeutic agents. Rather than being cytotoxic to cancer cells, they stimulate the client's own immune system to fight the cancer cells.

DRUG PROFILE:
Tamoxifen (Nolvadex)

Actions:

Because it blocks estrogen receptors in cancer cells, tamoxifen is sometimes classified as an antiestrogenic agent. Tamoxifen is effective against breast tumors that require estrogen for their growth. These susceptible cancer cells are known as ER (estrogen receptor) positive cells. The drug is unique among antineoplastics because it is not only given to clients with breast cancer, it is also given to high-risk clients to prevent the disease. Few if any other antineoplastics are given prophylactically because of their toxicity. Tamoxifen is given orally and is a drug of choice for treating breast cancer.

Adverse Effects:

Other than nausea and vomiting, tamoxifen produces little of the serious toxicity observed with other antineoplastics. Of concern, however, is the association of tamoxifen therapy with an increased risk of uterine cancer. Hot flashes, fluid retention, venous blood clots, and vaginal discharge are relatively common.

TABLE 23.7	Hormone and Hormone Inhibitors Used for Neoplasia	
DRUG	**ROUTE AND ADULT DOSE**	**REMARKS**
Hormones		
diethylstilbestrol (DES, Stilbestrol)	PO; for treatment of prostate cancer, 500 mg tid; for palliation, 1–15 mg qd.	For cancer of the prostate and breast.
ethinyl estradiol (Estinyl)	PO; for treatment of breast cancer, 1 mg tid × 2–3 mos; for palliation of prostate cancer, 0.15–3 mg/day.	For cancer of the prostate and breast.
fluoxymesterone (Halotestin)	PO; 10 mg tid.	For breast cancer.
medroxyprogesterone acetate (Provera, Depo-Provera)	IM; 400–1000 mg q week.	For uterine and renal cancer.
megestrol acetate (Megace)	PO; 40–160 mg bid-qid.	For advanced cancer of the prostate and breast.
prednisone (Deltasone and others)	PO; 20–100 mg/m^2 qd.	For acute leukemia, Hodgkin's disease, lymphomas.
testolactone (Teslac)	PO; 250 mg qid.	For breast cancer.
testosterone (Andro 100, Histerone, Testred, Delatest)	IM; 200–400 mg q 2–4 weeks.	For breast cancer.
Hormone Inhibitors		
Pr tamoxifen citrate (Nolvadex)	PO; 10–20 mg bid.	For breast cancer.
aminoglutethimide (Cytadren)	PO; 250 mg bid-qid.	For prostate, breast, adrenal cancer; must administer hydrocortisone in conjunction with this drug.
anastrozole (Arimidex)	PO; 1 mg qd.	For advanced breast cancer.
bicalutamide (Casodex)	PO; 50 mg qd.	For advanced prostate cancer.
exemestane (Aromasin)	PO; 25 mg qd after a meal.	For advanced breast cancer.
flutamide (Eulexin)	PO; 250 mg tid.	For prostate cancer.
goserelin acetate (Zoladex)	SC; 3.6 mg q 28 days.	For cancer of the prostate and breast.
letrozole (Femara)	PO; 2.5 mg qd.	For advanced breast cancer.
leuprolide acetate (Lupron)	SC; 1 mg qd.	For advanced prostate cancer.
nilutamide (Nilandron)	PO; 300 mg d × 30 days, then 150 mg qd.	For metastatic prostate cancer.
toremifene citrate (Fareston)	PO; 60 mg qd.	For metastatic breast cancer.

23.14 Biologic response modifiers and some additional antineoplastic drugs have been found to be effective against tumors.

A number of anticancer drugs act through mechanisms other than those previously described. For example, asparaginase deprives cancer cells of an essential amino acid. Mitotane (Lysodren) is

DRUG PROFILE:
Interferon alpha-2 (Roferon A, Intron A)

Actions:

Interferon alfa-2 is a biologic response modifier that consists of two very similar drugs; interferon alfa-2A (Roferon A) and interferon alpha-2b (Intron A). Interferon alpha-2b is a natural protein that is produced by human lymphocytes four to six hours after viral stimulation. Large amounts of this drug are obtained through recombinant DNA technology in which the human gene for interferon alpha-2b has been spliced into the bacterium *E. coli*. Interferon alpha-2b affects cancer cells by two mechanisms. First, it enhances or stimulates the immune system to remove more antigens. Second, the drug suppresses the growth of cancer cells. As expected from its origin, interferon alfa-2 also has antiviral activity.

Adverse Effects:

Like most biologic response modifiers, the most common side effect is a flu-like syndrome of fever, chills, dizziness, and fatigue that usually diminishes as therapy progresses. Nausea, vomiting, diarrhea, and anorexia are relatively common. With prolonged therapy, more serious toxicity such as immunosuppression, hepatotoxicity, and neurotoxicity may be observed.

TABLE 23.8	Miscellaneous Anticancer Drugs	
DRUG	**ROUTE AND ADULT DOSE**	**REMARKS**
Pr interferon alfa-2 (Roferon A, Intron A)	SC/IM; 2–3 million units qd for leukemia; increased to 36 million units qd for Kaposi's sarcoma.	For hairy cell leukemia and Kaposi's sarcoma; also for hepatitis and other viral disorders.
altretamine hexamethylmelamine (Hexalen)	PO; 65 mg/m^2 qid.	For ovarian cancer.
asparaginase (Elspar)	IV; 200 IU/kg qd.	For acute lymphocytic leukemia.
hydroxyurea (Hydrea)	PO; 20–30 mg/kg qd.	For palliative treatment of malignant melanoma and chronic granulocytic leukemia.
imatinib (Gleevec)	PO; 400–600 mg qd.	For chronic myeloid leukemia after failure with interferon alfa therapy.
levamisole (Ergamisol)	PO; 50 mg tid × 3 days.	For colon cancer.
mitotane (Lysodren)	PO; 3–4 mg tid-qid.	For adrenal cortex cancer.
pegaspargase (Oncaspar, PEG-L-asparaginase)	IV; 2500 IU/m^2 q 14 days.	For acute lymphocytic leukemia; IM form available.
procarbazine hydrochloride (Matulane)	PO; 2–4 mg/kg qd.	For Hodgkin's disease.
rituximab (Rituxan)	IV; 375 mg/m^2 qd as a continuous infusion.	For non-Hodgkin's lymphomas.
trastuzumab (Herceptin)	IV; 4 mg/kg as a single dose, then 2 mg/kg q week.	For metastatic breast cancer.

similar to the insecticide DDT and poisons cancer cells by forming links to proteins. The uses of these miscellaneous antineoplastics are given in Table 23.8.

Biologic response modifiers are a relatively new class of drugs. Agents in this class do not kill tumor cells directly but instead stimulate the body's immune system. When given concurrently with other antineoplastics, biologic response modifiers help to limit the severe immunosuppressive effects of other anticancer drugs.

Concept review 23.3

■ Why are the biologic response modifiers less toxic to normal body cells than other antineoplastics?

CLIENT TEACHING

Clients treated for cancer need to know the following:

1. If hair loss is expected, cut long hair and be fitted for a wig or hairpiece before starting treatment. Select hats, scarves, and/or turbans. Use mild shampoo and conditioner.

2. When hair is lost, protect the scalp from sunburn with sunscreen or a hat.

3. If appetite is decreased, eat foods that appeal in small amounts at frequent intervals. Your practitioner may order an appetite stimulant such as megestrol acetate (Megace).

4. If nausea is a problem, discuss drugs to control nausea with your practitioner. Drink liquids between meals rather than with food.

5. If your mouth becomes irritated or ulcerated, avoid alcohol-based mouthwash and use plain water or mild salt solution instead. Use a soft toothbrush. Avoid spicy foods and very hot or very cold food and drink. Ask about a mouth rinse to coat, soothe, and numb, such as BMX (Benadryl, Maalox, and xylocaine).

6. Because chemotherapy may decrease sperm production or increase the risk of genetic damage to sperm, men may consider sperm banking prior to receiving chemotherapy.

7. Increase fluid intake to decrease the risk of kidney damage and uric acid crystal formation.

8. Avoid exposure to crowds and individuals with infections or recent vaccinations, as your immune system may be less able to protect you. Report temperatures of 101° or higher.

9. If your white blood count is significantly reduced, you should follow a neutropenic diet to reduce risk of infection from foods. This means you should avoid raw fruits and vegetables, peppercorns, and raw fish and meat.

10. Report easy bruising, blood in the stool or urine, and difficulty clotting. Many chemotherapeutic agents reduce platelet production needed for clot formation. ■

CHAPTER REVIEW

 Core Concepts Summary

23.1 Cancer is characterized by rapid, uncontrolled growth of cells.

Cancer cells grow rapidly, seemingly unaffected by their host surroundings. Cancer cells continue dividing until they invade normal tissues and eventually metastasize.

23.2 The causes of cancer may be chemical, physical, or biological.

A large number of factors have been found to cause or promote cancer. These include many industrial chemicals, X-rays, UV light, and viruses. The genetic make-up of the client plays an important role in whether or not cancer will develop after exposure to carcinogens.

23.3 Personal risk of cancer may be prevented by a number of lifestyle factors.

Eliminating tobacco use and limiting the intake of saturated fats and alcohol are important factors in reducing the risk of contracting cancer. Periodic self-examinations and physician check-ups are important in catching cancer at an early, more treatable stage.

23.4 Tumors are classified as benign or malignant and named according to their origin.

Benign neoplasms grow slowly and rarely result in death. Malignant neoplasms, also known as cancer, are fast-growing and often fatal. Sarcomas and carcinomas are the two major categories of malignant neoplasms.

23.5 Cancer may be treated using surgery, radiation therapy, and drugs.

Drugs are only one means of treating cancer. If the tumor is solid and located in a single area, surgical removal is sometimes warranted. Radiation therapy may be used to kill microscopic cancer cells left behind following surgery or to shrink the size of inoperable tumors.

23.6 To achieve a total cure, every malignant cell must be removed or killed.

It is possible that a single cancer cell may be able to clone itself and kill its host. Therefore, in order to achieve a complete cure, every single cancer cell must be eliminated through surgery, radiation, drugs, or by the client's own immune system.

23.7 Use of multiple drugs and special dosing schedules are strategies used to improve the success of chemotherapy.

Combinations of antineoplastic drugs are often used to attack cancer cells from several different mechanisms and to allow lower doses than if a single agent were used. The schedule of drug administration is critical to the success of the chemotherapy.

23.8 Serious toxicity limits most of the antineoplastic agents.

Antineoplastic drugs are the most toxic medications used for pharmacotherapy. Adverse effects are expected and may be severe. While each agent has somewhat different toxicity, common adverse effects include thrombocytopenia, anemia, leukopenia, alopecia, severe nausea, vomiting, and diarrhea.

23.9 Alkylating agents act by changing the structure of DNA in cancer cells.

Alkylating agents are some of the oldest and most reliable of the antineoplastic drugs. By attaching to DNA, they prevent the cancer cell from replicating.

23.10 Antimetabolites act by disrupting critical cell pathways in cancer cells.

Antimetabolites act by blocking some aspect of cancer cell metabolism. By blocking the synthesis of critical cellular molecules, the drugs can slow the growth of cancer cells.

23.11 Because of their cytotoxicity, a few antibiotics are used to treat cancer rather than infections.

Antitumor antibiotics attach to the DNA of cancer cells, thus inhibiting their growth. Their properties and side effects resemble those of the alkylating agents.

23.12 Some plant extracts have been isolated that kill cancer cells by preventing cell division.

Natural extracts of the periwinkle plant and the Pacific yew have provided several important antineoplastic agents. Drugs in this class include the vinca alkaloids, the taxoids, and the topoisomerase inhibitors.

23.13 Some hormones and hormone antagonists have been found to be effective against certain tumors.

A number of estrogens, androgens, corticosteroids, and hormone inhibitors have antitumor activity. They have very specific uses, usually for tumors of reproductive-related organs such as the breast, prostate, or uterus.

21.14 Biologic response modifiers and some additional antineoplastic drugs have been found to be effective against tumors.

Biologic response modifiers are a small group of chemicals used to stimulate the client's immune system. While much research has focused on this approach to chemotherapy, these drugs have only limited success.

EXPLORE
PharMedia
www.prenhall.com/holland

Additional interactive resources and activities for this chapter can be found on the Companion Website. For animations, audio glossary, and review access the accompanying CD-ROM in this book.

Mechanism in Action:
  Methotrexate
Audio Glossary
Concept Review
NCLEX Review

PharmLinks
CancerNet
Current Indications for Antineoplastics
Clinical Trials

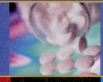

5   THE RESPIRATORY, DIGESTIVE, AND RENAL SYSTEMS

24 Drugs for Pulmonary Disorders

CORE CONCEPTS

24.1 The physiology of the respiratory system involves two main processes: ventilation and respiration.

24.2 Bronchioles are lined with smooth muscle that controls the amount of air entering the lungs.

24.3 Inhalation is an effective route of administration for pulmonary drugs because it delivers medications directly to their sites of action.

ASTHMA

24.4 Asthma is a chronic inflammatory disease characterized by bronchospasm.

Beta-adrenergic Agonists

24.5 Beta-adrenergic agonists are the most effective drugs for relieving acute bronchospasm; methylxanthines and anticholinergics are alternatives.

Glucocorticoids

24.6 Glucocorticoids are very effective for the long-term prophylaxis of asthma.

Mast Cell Inhibitors

24.7 Cromolyn is one of the safest medications for the prophylaxis of asthma, but it is not effective at relieving acute bronchospasm.

Antitussives, Expectorants, and Mucolytics

24.8 Several drugs are effective at loosening bronchial secretions and relieving cough.

CHRONIC OBSTRUCTIVE PULMONARY DISEASE (COPD)

24.9 Chronic obstructive pulmonary disease is a disorder treated with multiple drugs.

OBJECTIVES

After reading this chapter, the student should be able to:

1. Identify basic anatomical structures associated with the respiratory system.

2. Explain how the autonomic nervous system controls airflow in the bronchial tree.

3. Explain why the inhalation route is an effective route of drug administration for pulmonary medicines.

4. Describe the types of devices used to deliver medications via the inhalation route.

5. Describe some common causes and symptoms of asthma, chronic bronchitis, and emphysema.

6. For each of the following classes, identify representative drugs, explain the mechanism of drug action, primary actions on the respiratory system, and important adverse effects.
   a. beta-adrenergic agonists/sympathomimetics
   b. glucocorticoids
   c. anticholinergics
   d. mast-cell stabilizers
   e. expectorants
   f. antitussives
   g. mucolytics

7. Categorize drugs used in the treatment of pulmonary disorders based on their classification and mechanism of action.

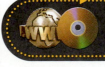

PharMedia
www.prenhall.com/holland

Additional interactive resources and activities for this chapter can be found on the Companion Website. For animations, audio glossary, and review access the accompanying CD-ROM in this book.

alveoli (al-VEE-oh-lie): dilated sacs at the end of the bronchial tree where gas exchange occurs / *page 378*

antitussive (anti-TUSS-ive): drug used to suppress cough / *page 386*

asthma (AZ-muh): chronic inflammatory disease of the airways / *page 380*

bronchi: (BRON-ky): primary passageway of the bronchial tree that contains smooth muscle / *page 378*

bronchioles (BRON-key-oles): very small bronchi / *page 378*

bronchoconstriction (BRON-koh-kun-STRIK-shun): decrease in diameter of the airway due to contraction of bronchial smooth muscle / *page 379*

bronchodilation (BRON-koh-dye-LAY-shun): increase in diameter of the airway due to relaxation of bronchial smooth muscle / *page 378*

bronchospasm (bron-koh-SPAZ-um): rapid constriction of the airways / *page 379*

chronic bronchitis (KRON-ik bron-KEYE-tis): chronic disease of the lungs characterized by excess mucous production and inflammation / *page 387*

dry powder inhaler (DPI): device used to convert a solid drug to a fine powder for the purpose of inhalation / *page 379*

dyspnea (DISP-nee-uh): shortness of breath / *page 380*

emphysema (em-fuss-EE-muh): terminal lung disease characterized by dilation of the alveoli / *page 387*

expectorant (eks-PEK-tor-ent): drug used to increase bronchial secretions / *page 386*

expiration (ex-purr-AY-shun): movement of air out of the lungs / *page 377*

inspiration (in-spurr-AY-shun): movement of air into the lungs / *page 377*

metered dose inhaler (MDIS): device used to deliver a precise amount of drug to the respiratory system / *page 379*

mucolytic: drug used to loosen thick mucous / *page 387*

nebulizer (NEB-you-lyes-ur): device used to convert liquid drugs into a fine mist for the purpose of inhalation / *page 379*

perfusion (purr-FEW-shun): blood flow through a tissue or organ / *page 378*

pharynx (FAIR-inks): passageway for food from the mouth to the esophagus and for air from the nose to the larynx / *page 378*

respiration (res-purr-AY-shun): exchange of oxygen and carbon dioxide / *page 377*

status asthmaticus (STAT-us az-MAT-ik-us): acute form of asthma requiring immediate medical attention / *page 380*

trachea (TRAY-kee-ah): passageway for air from the pharynx to the bronchi / *page 378*

ventilation (ven-tah-LAY-shun): process by which air is moved into and out of the lungs / *page 377*

The respiratory system is one of the most important organ systems; a mere five to six minutes without breathing may result in death. When functioning properly, the respiratory system provides the body with the oxygen critical for all cells to function. Measurement of respiration rate and depth and listening to chest sounds with a stethoscope provide the healthcare provider with valuable clues as to what may be happening internally. The respiratory system also provides a means by which the body can rid itself of excess acids and bases, a topic that is covered in Chapter 27 ⊂⊃ .

This chapter examines medications used in the therapy of asthma, a disease characterized by inflammation and acute constriction of the airway. Drugs used for seasonal allergies are covered in Chapter 20 ⊂⊃ *. Antiinfectives used in the treatment of lung infections such as pneumonia and tuberculosis were covered in Chapters 21 and 22* ⊂⊃ *.*

24.1 The physiology of the respiratory system involves two main processes: ventilation and respiration.

The primary function of the respiratory system is to bring oxygen into the body and to remove carbon dioxide. The process by which gasses are exchanged is called **respiration**. The basic structures of the respiratory system are shown in Figure 24.1a.

Ventilation is the process of moving air into and out of the lungs. As the muscular diaphragm contracts and lowers in position, it creates a negative pressure that draws air into the lungs. This process, known as **inspiration**, requires energy to produce the contraction. During **expiration**, the diaphragm relaxes and air leaves the lung passively, with no energy expenditure required. Ventilation is a purely mechanical process that occurs approximately 12–18 times per minute in adults, a rate determined by neurons in the brain stem. This rate may be modified by a number of factors, including emotions, fever, stress, and the pH of the blood.

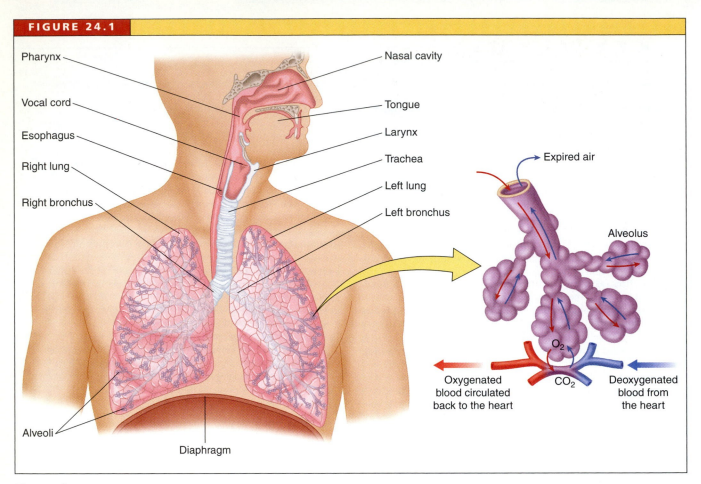

FIGURE 24.1

The respiratory system

Air entering the respiratory system travels through the nose, the pharynx, and the trachea and into the bronchi, which divide into smaller and smaller passages called bronchioles. The bronchial tree ends in dilated sacs called alveoli. Although they have no smooth muscle, the alveoli are abundantly rich in capillaries. An extremely thin membrane in the alveoli separates the airway from the pulmonary capillaries, allowing gasses to readily move between the internal environment of the blood and the inspired air. As oxygen crosses this membrane, it is exchanged for carbon dioxide, a cellular waste product that travels from the blood to the air. The lung is richly supplied with blood. Blood flow through the lung is called perfusion. The process of gas exchange is shown in Figure 24.1.

Concept review 24.1

■ What is the difference between ventilation and perfusion?

24.2 Bronchioles are lined with smooth muscle that controls the amount of air entering the lungs.

Bronchioles are elastic structures that are able to vary the size of their diameter, or *lumen,* with the specific needs of the body. Changes in the diameter of the bronchiolar lumen are made possible by smooth muscle lining the bronchial tree. This smooth muscle is controlled by the autonomic nervous system. During the fight-or-flight response, beta$_2$ adrenergic receptors of the sympathetic nervous system are stimulated, the bronchiolar smooth muscle relaxes, and bronchodilation results. This allows more air to enter the alveoli, thus increasing the oxygen supply to the body during periods of stress or exercise.

During periods of rest, nerves from the parasympathetic nervous system are activated, causing the bronchiolar smooth muscle to contract and the lumen to narrow, resulting in bronchoconstriction. Parasympathetic stimulation also has the effect of slowing respiration rate; sympathetic stimulation has the opposite effect. Autonomic nerves serving bronchiolar smooth muscle are frequent targets for medications.

24.3 Inhalation is an effective route of administration for pulmonary drugs because it delivers medications directly to their sites of action.

Oxygen and carbon dioxide are not the only gasses that can be easily exchanged in the alveoli. Anesthetics such as nitrous oxide and halothane (Fluothane) are delivered via the respiratory route and enter the blood extremely rapidly to cause CNS depression, as discussed in Chapter 12 ⊂▭ . Solvents such as paint thinners and glues are sometimes intentionally inhaled and cause serious adverse effects to the nervous system and even death. The onset of action of inhaled substances is almost instantaneous.

Medications are often given via the inhalation route for their local effects. Inhaled drugs can give immediate relief for bronchospasm, a condition during which the bronchiolar smooth muscle rapidly contracts, leaving the client gasping for breath. Drugs may also be given to loosen thick mucous in the bronchial tree. An advantage of delivering medications via inhalation is that they are delivered directly to the sites where they are needed, thus reducing the potential for systemic side effects.

Several devices are used to deliver medications via the inhalation route. Nebulizers are small machines that vaporize a liquid drug into a fine mist that can be inhaled, often using a facemask. If the drug is a solid, it may be administered using a dry powder inhaler (DPI). A DPI is a small device that is activated by the process of inhalation to deliver a fine powder directly to the bronchial tree. Turbohalers and rotahalers are types of DPIs. Metered dose inhalers (MDIs) are a third type of device commonly used to deliver respiratory medicines. MDIs use a propellant to deliver a measured dose of drugs to the lungs during each inhalation. The client times his or her inhalation to the puffs of drug emitted from the MDI. Clients must be carefully instructed on the correct use of these devices because drug dose is dependent upon their correct use. Two devices used to deliver respiratory agents are shown in Figure 24.2.

FIGURE 24.2

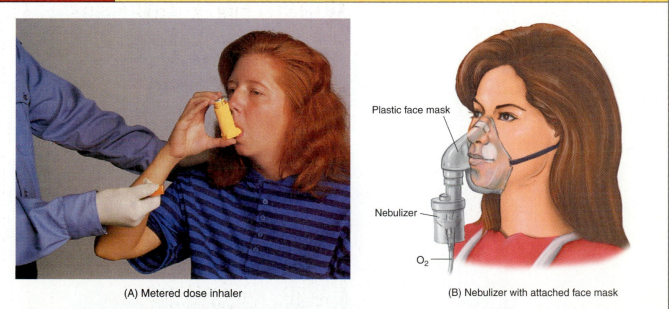

(A) Metered dose inhaler

(B) Nebulizer with attached face mask

Devices used to deliver respiratory drugs *SOURCE: Pearson Education/PH College.*

Concept review 24.2

▪ Name the three types of devices used to deliver drugs by the inhalation route. What are the differences among them?

ASTHMA

Asthma is a chronic disease with both inflammatory and bronchospasm components. Drugs are given to either decrease the frequency of asthmatic attacks or to terminate attacks in progress.

24.4 Asthma is a chronic inflammatory disease characterized by bronchospasm.

dys = painful or difficult
pnea = breathing

Asthma is one of the most common chronic conditions in the United States, affecting almost 15 million Americans. The disease is characterized by acute bronchospasm, which causes intense breathlessness, or dyspnea, coughing, and gasping for air. Along with bronchoconstriction, the acute inflammatory response is initiated, stimulating mucous secretion and edema of the airway. These conditions are illustrated in Figure 24.3. Status asthmaticus is a severe, prolonged form of asthma that is unresponsive to drug treatment and may lead to respiratory failure. Typical causes of asthmatic attacks are shown in Table 24.1.

Although the exact cause of asthma is sometimes unknown, it is believed to be the result of chronic airway inflammation. Because asthma has both a bronchoconstriction component and an

FIGURE 24.3

Changes in bronchioles during an asthma attack: (a) normal bronchiole; and (b) in asthma attack   *SOURCE: Pearson Education/PH College.*

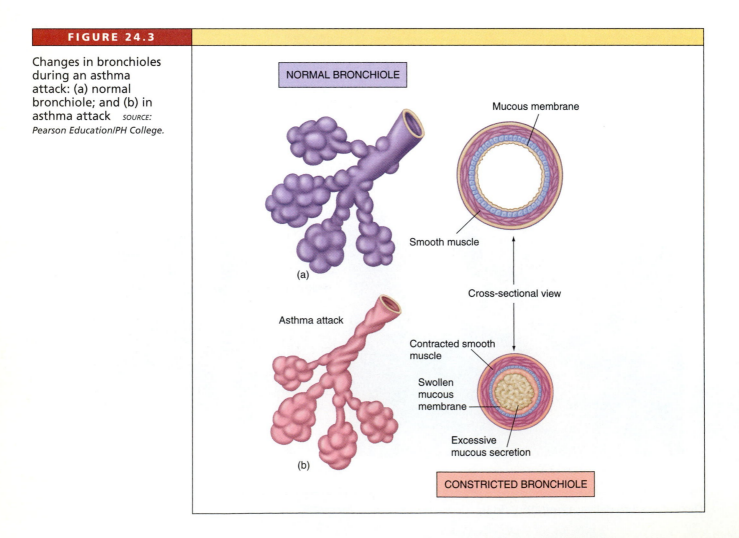

TABLE 24.1	Some Common Causes of Asthma
allergens	pollen from trees, grasses, and weeds animal dander household dust mold
air pollutants	tobacco smoke ozone nitrous and sulfur oxides fumes from cleaning fluids or solvents burning leaves
respiratory infections	bacterial, fungal, and viral
stress	emotional stress or anxiety exercise in dry, cold climates
chemicals and food	drugs such as aspirin, ibuprofen, and beta-blockers sulfite preservatives food such as nuts, monosodium glutamate (MSG), shellfish, and dairy products

inflammatory component, drug therapy of the disease focuses on one or both of these mechanisms. The goals of drug therapy are twofold: to terminate acute bronchospasms in progress and to reduce the frequency of acute asthma attacks. Different drugs are usually needed to achieve each of these goals. A summary of the various drugs used to treat respiratory diseases is presented in Figure 24.4.

FIGURE 24.4

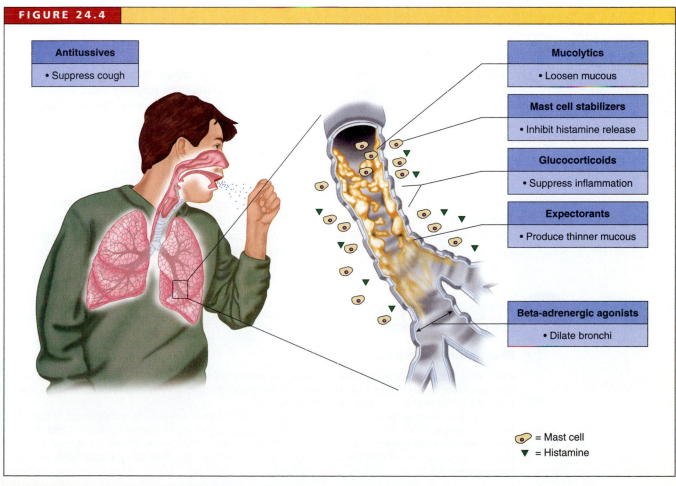

Antitussives
• Suppress cough

Mucolytics
• Loosen mucous

Mast cell stabilizers
• Inhibit histamine release

Glucocorticoids
• Suppress inflammation

Expectorants
• Produce thinner mucous

Beta-adrenergic agonists
• Dilate bronchi

= Mast cell
= Histamine

Drugs used to treat respiratory disorders

Fast Facts Asthma

- Over 15 million people have asthma.
- Asthma is responsible for over 1.5 million emergency room visits and over 500,000 hospitalizations each year.
- Over 5,500 clients die of asthma each year.
- Estimated direct and indirect costs for asthma total more than $12 billion each year.
- The incidence of asthma has been dramatically increasing each year since 1980 in all age, sex, and ethnic groups. The highest rate of increase has been among blacks.
- The highest incidence of asthma is in clients under the age of 18. From 7 to 10% of children have the disease.
- In adults, asthma is slightly more common in females than in males. In children, however, the disease affects twice as many boys as girls.

BETA-ADRENERGIC AGONISTS

Selective beta$_2$-agonists are effective at relieving acute bronchospasm. They are some of the most common agents used in the pharmacotherapy of asthma and other pulmonary diseases.

24.5 Beta-adrenergic agonists are the most effective drugs for relieving acute bronchospasm; methylxanthines and anticholinergics are alternatives.

Beta-adrenergic agonists, or sympathomimetics, are drugs of choice in the treatment of acute bronchoconstriction. In most cases, the agents used for pulmonary disease are selective for beta$_2$ receptors in the lung, thus they produce fewer cardiac side effects than the non-selective beta-agonists. When inhaled, they produce rapid bronchodilation by relaxing bronchiolar smooth muscle. Inhaled beta-adrenergic agonists produce little systemic toxicity because only small amounts of the drugs are absorbed. When given orally, a longer duration of action is achieved, but systemic side effects such as tachycardia and tremor are more frequently experienced. Tolerance may develop to the therapeutic effects of the beta-agonists; therefore the client must be instructed to seek medical attention should the drugs prove to become less effective with continued use.

Blocking the parasympathetic nervous system produces similar effects to stimulation of the sympathetic nervous system. It is predictable, then, that anticholinergic drugs would cause bronchodilation and thus have potential use in the pharmacotherapy of asthma and other pulmonary diseases. The most widely used drug in this class, ipratropium (Atrovert, Combivent), is taken via

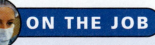

ON THE JOB

Respiratory Therapists

Respiratory therapists are an essential part of the healthcare team. In addition to assisting in the diagnosis of respiratory diseases by obtaining and analyzing sputum, breath, and blood specimens, the respiratory therapist plays a key role in drug therapy.

Respiratory therapists are responsible for giving clients drug treatments with aerosol forms of bronchodilators, antibiotics, and mucolytics. They monitor highly sophisticated equipment and chart clients' responses to therapy. Education is an important part of the job, as the therapist must teach clients the correct use of inhalers and oxygen apparati so that they may be operated safely in the home environment. ■

DRUG PROFILE:
Salmeterol (Serevent)

Actions:

Salmeterol acts by selectively binding to beta$_2$-adrenergic receptors in bronchiolar smooth muscle to cause bronchodilation. Its 12-hour duration of action is longer than that of many other bronchodilators. It has been shown to be of benefit in preventing exercise-induced bronchospasm. Because salmeterol takes 10–25 minutes to act, it should not be used for the termination of acute bronchospasm.

Adverse Effects:

Serious adverse effects from salmeterol are uncommon. Like other beta-agonists, some clients experience headaches, nervousness, and restlessness. Because of its potential to cause tachycardia, clients with heart disease should be monitored regularly.

Mechanism in Action:

Salmeterol relieves bronchospasm by binding selectively with beta$_2$ receptors located on the cellular membranes of bronchiolar smooth muscle. Since salmeterol is a selective beta$_2$ agonist, there is less potential for activating beta$_1$ cardiac receptors, especially if administered as an aerosol. It is primarily used to treat asthma.

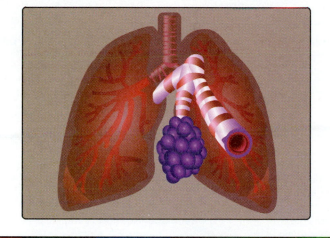

inhalation to rapidly relieve bronchospasm. Because it is not readily absorbed from the lungs, it produces few systemic side effects, although it is considered less effective than beta-agonists. Inhaled anticholinergics are generally not sufficiently efficacious when used alone, but are beneficial when combined with beta-agonists or glucocorticoids.

The third group of drugs prescribed for their bronchodilation effect is the methylxanthines. Chemically related to caffeine, theophylline (Theo-dur and others) and aminophylline (Somophylline) were considered drugs of choice for bronchoconstriction twenty years ago. Theophylline, however, has a narrow margin of safety and interacts with a large number of other drugs. Side effects such as nausea, vomiting, and CNS stimulation are relatively common, and dysrhythmias may be observed at high doses. Having been largely replaced by safer and more effective drugs, the current use of theophylline is primarily for the long-term oral prophylaxis of persistent asthma. Bronchodilators used for asthma are shown in Table 24.2.

GLUCOCORTICOIDS

Inhaled glucocorticoids are used for the long-term prevention of asthmatic attacks. Oral glucocorticoids may be used for the short-term management of acute asthma.

24.6 Glucocorticoids are very effective for the long-term prophylaxis of asthma.

Glucocorticoids are the most effective drugs available for the prevention of acute asthmatic episodes. When inhaled on a daily schedule, glucocorticoids suppress inflammation without producing major side effects. Clients should be informed that inhaled glucocorticoids must be taken

TABLE 24.2	Bronchodilators Used for Asthma	
DRUG	**ROUTE AND ADULT DOSE**	**REMARKS**
albuterol (Proventil, Salbutamol)	PO; 2–4 mg tid-qid.	Beta$_2$-agonist; relaxes smooth muscle of the bronchial tree; nebulizer form available.
epinephrine (Adrenalin, Bronkaid, Primatene)	SC; 0.1–0.5 ml of 1:1000 q 20 min-4 hours.	Non-selective alpha and beta-agonist; SC and IV forms are given for emergency situations; available via inhalation to terminate asthmatic attacks.
bitolterol mesylate (Tornalate)	MDI; 2 inhalations tid-qid.	Beta$_2$-agonist; short acting; nebulizer form available.
isoetharine (Bronkosol, Bronkometer)	MDI; 1–2 inhalations q4h up to 5 days.	Beta$_2$-agonist; increases vital capacity and decreases airway resistance; nebulizer form available.
isoproteronol (Isuprel, Medihaler-Iso)	MDI; 1–2 inhalations q4 hours-qid.	Non-selective beta$_1$ and beta$_2$-agonist; IV and SC forms available.
levalbuterol hydrochloride (Xopenex)	Nebulizer; 0.63 mg tid-qid.	Beta$_2$-agonist; short acting; facilitates mucous drainage; increases vital capacity.
metaproterenol sulfate (Alupent, Metaprel)	MDI; 2–3 inhalations q3–4h (max 12 inhalations/day).	Beta$_2$-agonist; short acting; relaxes smooth muscle of bronchi; nebulizer form available.
pirbuterol acetate (Maxair)	MDI; 2 inhalations qid (max 12 inhalations/day).	Beta$_2$-agonist; short acting.
(Pr) salmeterol xinafoate (Serevent)	MDI; 2 inhalations bid.	Beta$_2$-agonist; long acting; facilitates mucous drainage and decreases reaction to allergens; DPI form available.
terbutaline sulfate (Brethaire, Brethine)	PO; 2.5–5 mg tid.	Beta$_2$-agonist; extended-release form available.
theophylline (Theo-dur)	PO; 0.4–0.6 mg/kg/hr divided tid-qid.	Methylxanthine; IV and extended-release form available.
aminophylline (Truphylline)	PO; 0.25–0.75 mg/kg/hr divided qid.	Methylxanthine; IV form available.
ipratropium bromide (Atrovert, Combivent)	MDI; 2 inhalations qid (max 12 inhalations/day).	Anticholinergic; combivent is a combination of ipratropium plus albuterol.

daily to produce their therapeutic effect and that these medications are not effective at terminating episodes in progress. For some clients, a beta-adrenergic agonist may be prescribed along with an inhaled glucocorticoid, as this permits the dose of the glucocorticoid to be reduced as much as fifty percent. Selected glucocorticoids used in the pharmacotherapy of asthma are shown in Table 24.3.

For severe, persistent asthma that is unresponsive to other treatments, oral glucocorticoids may be prescribed. If taken for longer than 10 days, oral glucocorticoids may produce significant adverse effects such as adrenal gland suppression, peptic ulcers, and hyperglycemia. Other uses and adverse effects of glucocorticoids are presented in Chapters 20 and 28 ⊂⊃.

DRUG PROFILE:
Beclomethasone (Beclovent, Beconase, Vancenase, Vanceril)

Actions:

Beclomethasone is a glucocorticoid available through aerosol inhalation for asthma or as a nasal spray for allergic rhinitis. Beclomethasone acts by reducing inflammation, thus decreasing the frequency of asthma attacks. It is not a bronchodilator and should not be used to terminate asthma attacks in progress.

Adverse Effects:

Inhaled beclomethasone produces few systemic side effects. Because small amounts may be swallowed with each dose, the client should be observed for signs of glucocorticoid toxicity when taking the drug for prolonged periods. Local effects may include hoarseness in the voice. Like all glucocorticoids, the anti-inflammatory properties of beclamethasone can mask infections. A large percentage of clients taking beclomethasone on a long-term basis will develop Candidiasis, a fungal infection in the throat, due to the constant deposits of drug in the oral cavity. The treatment of fungal infections was discussed in Chapter 22 ⚭ .

TABLE 24.3	Glucocorticoids Used for Asthma	
DRUG	**ROUTE AND ADULT DOSE**	**REMARKS**
Pr beclomethasone dipropionate (Beclovent, Vanceril)	MDI; 1–2 inhalations tid or qid (max 20 inhalations/day).	Intranasal form available for allergic rhinitis.
budesonide (Pulmicort Turbohaler)	DPI; 1–2 inhalations (200 ;µg/inhalation) qd (max 800 ;µg/day).	Intranasal form available for allergic rhinitis.
flunisolide (AeroBid)	MDI; 2–3 inhalations bid or tid (max 12 inhalations/day).	Intranasal form available for allergic rhinitis.
fluticasone (Flovent)	MDI (44 mcg); 2 inhalations bid (max 10 inhalations/day).	Intranasal form available for allergic rhinitis; also available in 110 and 120 mcg inhalers.
methylprednisolone (Depo-Medrol, Medrol)	PO; 4–48 mg qd.	Available in IM, IV forms; also for neoplasia and adrenal insufficiency.
prednisone (Deltasone, Meticorten)	PO; 5–60 mg qd.	Only available in oral form; also for neoplasia.
triamcinolone (Azmacort)	MDI; 2 inhalations tid or qid (max 16 inhalations/day).	Also available in IM, SC, intradermal, topical, and oral forms.

MAST CELL INHIBITORS

Two mast cell inhibitors play a limited though important role in the prophylaxis of asthma. These drugs act by inhibiting the release of histamine from mast cells.

24.7 Cromolyn is one of the safest medications for the prophylaxis of asthma, but it is not effective at relieving acute bronchospasm.

Cromolyn (Intal) is an anti-inflammatory drug that is useful in preventing asthma attacks. When administered via an MDI or a nebulizer, cromolyn is a safe alternative to the glucocorticoids. Maximum therapeutic benefit may take several weeks. Like the glucocorticoids, clients must be informed that cromolyn should be taken on a daily basis and should not be used to terminate acute attacks. An intranasal form of cromolyn (Nasalcrom) is used in the treatment of seasonal allergies.

Nedocromil (Tilade) is an anti-inflammatory drug that has actions and uses similar to cromolyn. The drug has few adverse effects when administered with an MDI, although some clients experience an unpleasant taste. Cromolyn and nedocromil are sometimes called mast cell stabilizers because their action serves to inhibit mast cells from releasing histamine and other chemical mediators of inflammation.

Concept review 24.3

■ Distinguish the classes of drugs that prevent asthma attacks from those that can terminate an attack in progress. Name at least one drug in each class.

ANTITUSSIVES, EXPECTORANTS, AND MUCOLYTICS

A small number of drugs are available to suppress cough and control excess mucous production. Antitussives reduce the cough reflex and expectorants and mucolytics help the client to remove thick bronchial secretions.

24.8 Several drugs are effective at loosening bronchial secretions and relieving cough.

Cough is a normal reflex mechanism that serves to forcibly remove excess secretions and foreign material from the bronchial tree. In diseases such as emphysema and bronchitis, or when liquids have been aspirated into the bronchi, it is not desirable to suppress the normal cough reflex. Dry, hacking, non-productive cough, however, can be quite irritating to the membranes of the throat and can deprive a client of much needed rest. It is these types of conditions in which therapy with

anti = *against*
tussive = *pertaining to a cough*

drugs that control cough, known as antitussives, may be warranted.

Narcotic analgesics are the most efficacious class of antitussives. Codeine is the most frequently used opioid antitussive. Doses needed to suppress the cough reflex are very low, thus there is minimal potential for dependence. Most codeine cough mixtures are classified as Schedule V drugs, and are reserved for more serious cough conditions.

The most frequently used OTC antitussive is dextromethorphan. This medication is included in most severe cold and flu preparations. Side effects are very rare. Though not as efficacious as codeine, there is no risk of dependence with dextromethorphan, as it is not an opioid.

Expectorants are drugs that increase bronchial secretions. Expectorants act by reducing the thickness or viscosity of bronchial secretions, thus increasing mucous flow that can then be removed more easily by coughing. The most effective OTC expectorant is guaifenesin. Like dex-

NATURAL ALTERNATIVES

Horehound for Respiratory Disorders

Horehound has been used as herbal remedy since the ancient Egyptians and was popular with American Indians. In folklore, it was reported to aid in a number of respiratory disorders including asthma, bronchitis, whooping cough, and infections such as tuberculosis. Non-respiratory uses include bowel disorders, jaundice, and wound healing.

Active ingredients of horehound are found throughout the flowering plant. The chief constituent is a bitter substance called *marrubium* that stimulates secretions. Formulations include tea, dried or fresh leaves and liquid extracts. Horehound has an expectorant action when treating colds and is also available as cough drops. It is purported to restore normal secretions to the lung and other organs. ▪

tromethorphan, guaifenesin produces few adverse effects and is a common ingredient in many OTC cold and flu preparations. Higher doses of guaifensin are available by prescription.

Acetylcysteine (Mucomyst) is one of the few drugs available to directly loosen thick, viscous bronchial secretions. Drugs of this type are called mucolytics. Acetylcysteine is delivered by the inhalation route and is not available OTC. It is used in clients who have cystic fibrosis or other diseases that produce large amounts of thick bronchial secretions.

muco = *mucous*
lytic = *destruction or disintegration*

CANADIAN LUNG ASSOCIATION

CHRONIC OBSTRUCTIVE PULMONARY DISEASE (COPD)

COPDs are progressive lung disorders primarily caused by tobacco smoking. Drugs may bring symptomatic relief but do not cure the disorders.

24.9 Chronic obstructive pulmonary disease is a progressive disorder treated with multiple drugs.

Chronic obstructive pulmonary disease (COPD) is a major cause of death and disability. The two primary disorders classified as COPDs are chronic bronchitis and emphysema. Both are strongly associated with smoking tobacco products and, secondarily, air pollutants. In chronic bronchitis, excess mucous is produced in the bronchial tree due to inflammation and irritation from smoke or pollutants. The airway becomes partially obstructed with mucous, thus giving the classic signs of dyspnea and coughing. Because microbes enjoy the mucous-rich environment, pulmonary infections are common. Gas exchange may be impaired.

COPD is a progressive disease, with the terminal stage being emphysema. After years of chronic inflammation, the bronchioles lose their elasticity and the alveoli dilate to maximum size in order to get more air into the lungs. The client suffers from extreme dyspnea caused by even the slightest physical activity.

bronch = *bronchus*
itis = *inflammation*

Clients with COPD may receive a number of pulmonary drugs for symptomatic relief of their disorder. The goals of pharmacologic therapy are to treat infections and to control cough and bronchospasm. Most clients receive bronchodilators such as ipratropium, beta$_2$ agonists, or inhaled glucocorticoids. Mucolytics and expectorants are sometimes indicated to reduce the viscosity of the bronchial mucous and to aid in its removal. Oxygen therapy may be used in clients with emphysema. Clients should be taught to avoid taking any drugs that have beta-blocking activity or that otherwise cause bronchoconstriction. Respiratory depressants should be avoided. It is important to note that none of the pharmacologic therapies offer a cure for COPD; they only treat the symptoms of a progressively worsening disease.

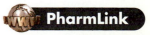

AMERICAN LUNG ASSOCIATION

CLIENT TEACHING

Clients treated for pulmonary disorders need to know the following:

1. When using MDIs or DPIs, an interval of at least one minute should elapse between puffs.
2. When taking more than one respiratory medicine, take the bronchodilator first. This opens the airways and increases the effectiveness of the second medication.
3. To reduce the oral absorption of inhaled medicines, rinse the mouth thoroughly following inhaler use.
4. If you find that the same amount of medication is not effective any longer, report this tolerance to your physician or nurse practitioner. Do not take extra medication without notifying your health provider.
5. Inhaled glucocorticoids must be taken on a regular basis to be effective—not as needed. They should not be taken to stop acute asthma attacks.
6. If taking theophylline, avoid caffeine-containing foods and beverages.
7. When taking beta-adrenergic agonists, any abnormalities in pulse rate, changes in blood pressure, or sensations of palpitations should be reported immediately.
8. If taking antihistamines for the first time, avoid operating machinery or performing other tasks requiring alertness, as drowsiness may occur.
9. Hard candies, chewing gum, or ice chips may be used to reduce the dry mouth caused by some decongestants and antihistamines.
10. Do not use decongestant nasal sprays for more than two to three days, unless instructed to do so by your healthcare practitioner. ■

CHAPTER REVIEW

Core Concepts Summary

24.1 **The physiology of the respiratory system involves two main processes: ventilation and respiration.**

The respiratory system brings needed oxygen into the body through inspiration and removes carbon dioxide through expiration. The process of moving air in and out of the lungs, or ventilation, is distinct from the process of gas exchange across the alveoli, a process known as respiration.

24.2 **Bronchioles are lined with smooth muscle that controls the amount of air entering the lungs.**

The autonomic nervous system affects the amount of air entering the bronchial tree by constricting or relaxing bronchial smooth muscle.

24.3 **Inhalation is an effective route of administration for pulmonary drugs because it delivers medications directly to their sites of action.**

Inhalation is frequently used as a route of drug administration for those medications targeted for the respiratory system. Nebulizers, DPIs, and MDIs are used to deliver drugs via the inhalation route.

24.4 **Asthma is a chronic inflammatory disease characterized by bronchospasm.**

Asthma is a common disease characterized by chronic airway inflammation. Exposure to a number of factors, including allergens, can cause an acute episode.

24.5 **Beta-adrenergic agonists are the most effective drugs for relieving acute bronchospasm; methylxanthines and anticholinergics are alternatives.**

Inhaled beta$_2$ adrenergic agonists are the drugs of choice for relieving bronchhospasm. Anticholinergics are sometimes used for their bronchoconstriction properties, but fewer are available due to their incidence of side effects. Methylxanthines, once widely used in pulmonary medicine, are now second-choice drugs in relieving bronchospasm due to their higher potential for side effects.

24.6 **Glucocorticoids are very effective for the long-term prophylaxis of asthma.**

Inhaled glucocorticoids are the drugs of choice for asthma prophylaxis. The inhaled glucocorticoids, even when used on a long-term basis, produce few side effects compared to oral glucocorticoids.

24.7 **Cromolyn is one of the safest medications for the prophylaxis of asthma, but it is not effective at relieving acute bronchospasm.**

Cromolyn and nedocromil belong to a small group of drugs called mast cell stabilizers. Although not as effective as the glucocorticoids for asthma prophylaxis, they are still frequently prescribed.

24.8 **Several drugs are effective at loosening bronchial secretions and relieving cough.**

Antitussives are effective at inhibiting the cough reflex. Although opioids are the most effective, there is some risk of physical dependence. Guanifensin is an OTC drug used to increase bronchial secretions so that cough may be more productive. Mucolytics loosen mucous so that it may be more easily removed from the bronchial tree.

24.9 **Chronic obstructive pulmonary disease is a progressive disorder treated with multiple drugs.**

Chronic bronchitis and emphysema are two COPDs that often require multiple drug therapy. Bronchodilators, expectorants, mucolytics, antibiotics, and oxygen may offer symptomatic relief.

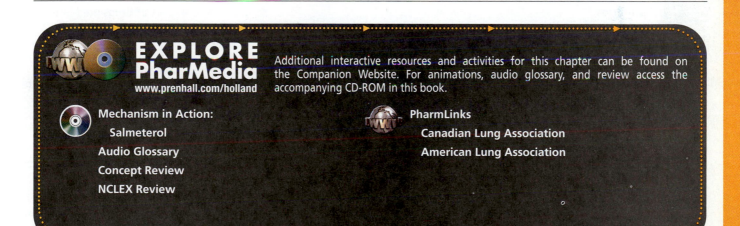

EXPLORE PharMedia
www.prenhall.com/holland

Additional interactive resources and activities for this chapter can be found on the Companion Website. For animations, audio glossary, and review access the accompanying CD-ROM in this book.

Mechanism in Action:
   Salmeterol
Audio Glossary
Concept Review
NCLEX Review

PharmLinks
   Canadian Lung Association
   American Lung Association

CORE CONCEPTS

25.1 The digestive system is responsible for breaking down food, absorbing nutrients, and eliminating wastes.

PEPTIC ULCER DISEASE AND GASTROESOPHAGEAL REFLUX DISEASE

25.2 Peptic ulcer disease is caused by an erosion of the mucosal layer of the stomach or duodenum.

25.3 Peptic ulcer disease is best treated by a combination of lifestyle changes and pharmacotherapy.

H₂-Receptor Antagonists

25.4 H₂-receptor blockers are often drugs of first choice in treating peptic ulcers.

Proton Pump Inhibitors

25.5 Proton pump inhibitors are effective at reducing gastric acid secretion.

Antacids

25.6 Antacids are effective at neutralizing stomach acid and reducing the symptoms of reflux disease.

Antibiotics for *H. Pylori*

25.7 Antibiotics are administered to eliminate *Helicobacter pylori,* the cause of many peptic ulcers.

25.8 Several miscellaneous drugs are also beneficial in treating peptic ulcer disease.

CONSTIPATION

Laxatives

25.9 Laxatives are used to promote defecation.

DIARRHEA

Antidiarrheals

25.10 Opioids are the most effective drugs for controlling diarrhea.

NAUSEA AND VOMITING

Antiemetics

25.11 Several drugs are available to treat nausea, vomiting, and motion sickness.

WEIGHT LOSS

Anorexiants

25.12 Anorexiants are drugs used for the short-term management of obesity.

OBJECTIVES

After reading this chapter, the student should be able to:

1. Describe the major anatomical structures of the digestive system.

2. Identify common causes, signs, and symptoms of peptic ulcer disease.

3. Identify the four major classes of drugs used to treat peptic ulcer disease.

4. Explain why two or more antibiotics are used concurrently in the treatment of *H. pylori.*

5. Explain conditions when the drug treatment of constipation is warranted.

6. Identify the four major classes of laxatives.

7. Explain conditions when the drug treatment of diarrhea is warranted.

8. Identify the four major classes of antiemetics.

9. Describe the types of drugs used in the short-term management of obesity.

10. For each of the following classes identify representative drugs, explain the mechanism of drug action, primary actions related the digestive system, and important adverse effects.
    a. H₂-receptor antagonists
    b. proton pump inhibitors
    c. antacids
    d. antibiotics for *H. pylori*
    e. laxatives
    f. antidiarrheals
    g. antiemetics
    h. anorexiants

11. Categorize drugs used in the treatment of digestive system disorders based on their classification and mechanism of action.

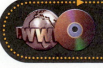

PharMedia
www.prenhall.com / holland

Additional interactive resources and activities for this chapter can be found on the Companion Website. For animations, audio glossary, and review access the accompanying CD-ROM in this book.

alimentary canal (AL-uh-MEN-tare-ee): the hollow tube in the digestive system that starts in the mouth and includes the esophagus, stomach, small intestine, and large intestine / *page 392*

anorexia (AN-oh-REX-ee-uh): loss of appetite / *page 394*

anorexiant (AN-oh-REX-ee-ant): drug used to suppress appetite / *page 407*

antacid (an-TASS-id): drug that neutralizes stomach acid / *page 397*

antiemetic (AN-tie-ee-MET-ik): drug that prevents vomiting / *page 403*

cathartic (kah-THAR-tik): drug that causes complete evacuation of the bowel / *page 401*

constipation (kon-stah-PAY-shun): infrequent passage of abnormally hard and dry stools / *page 401*

Crohn's disease (KROHNS): chronic inflammatory bowel disease affecting the ileum and sometimes the colon / *page 394*

defecation (def-ah-KAY-shun): evacuation of the colon; bowel movement / *page 401*

diarrhea: abnormal frequency and liquidity of bowel movements / *page 401*

dietary fiber: substance neither digested nor absorbed that contributes to the fecal mass / *page 401*

digestion (dye-JES-chun): process by which the body breaks down ingested food into small molecules that can be absorbed / *page 392*

emesis (EM-eh-sis): vomiting / *page 403*

emetic (ee-MET-ik): drug used to induce vomiting / *page 406*

gastoesophageal reflux disease (GERD) (GAS-troh-ee-SOF-ah-JEEL REE-flux): the regurgitation of stomach contents into the esophagus / *page 394*

H^+, K^+-ATPase: enzyme responsible for pumping acid onto the mucosal surface of the stomach / *page 397*

H_2-receptor antagonist: drug that inhibits the effects of histamine at its receptors in the GI tract / *page 397*

Helicobacter pylori (hee-lick-oh-BAK-tur py-LOR-eye): bacterium associated with a large percentage of peptic ulcer disease / *page 394*

parietal cells (par-EYE-it-al): cells in the stomach mucosa that secrete hydrochloric acid / *page 393*

peptic ulcer: erosion of the mucosa in the alimentary canal, most commonly in the stomach and duodenum / *page 393*

peristalsis (pair-ih-STAL-sis): involuntary wave-like contraction that occurs in the alimentary canal / *page 392*

proton-pump inhibitors: drugs that inhibit the enzyme H^+, K^+-ATPase / *page 397*

ulcerative colitis (UL-sir-ah-tiv koh-LIE-tuss): inflammatory bowel disease of the colon / *page 394*

vestibular apparatus (vest-IB-you-lar): portion of the inner ear responsible for the sense of position / *page 404*

Zollinger-Ellison syndrome (ZOLL-in-jer ELL-ih-sun): disorder of having excess acid secretion in the stomach / *page 399*

Very little of the food we eat is directly available to body cells. Food must be broken down, absorbed, and chemically modified before it is in a form useful to cells. The digestive system performs these functions and more. Some disorders of the digestive system are mechanical in nature, slowing or accelerating the transit of food through the gastrointestinal tract. Other disorders are metabolic in nature, affecting the secretion of digestive fluids or the absorption of essential nutrients. Many signs and symptoms are non-specific and may be caused by any number of different disorders. Drug therapy is also non-specific, often treating symptoms rather than curing the disorder. This chapter examines the common diseases of the digestive system for which drug therapy is effective.

Fast Facts Digestive Disorders

- Sixty to seventy million Americans are affected by a digestive disease.
- Thirteen percent of all hospitalizations are for digestive disorders.
- Ulcers are responsible for about 40,000 sugeries annually.
- Over 400,000 new cases of peptic ulcer disease are diagnosed each year.
- Colorectal cancer is the second leading cause of cancer deaths, killing more than 55,000 Americans annually.
- About 140,000 new cases of colorectal cancer occur each year.
- Irritable bowel syndrome affects 10–20% of adults.
- Americans spend over 33 billion annually on weight reduction products and services.
- The incidence of motion sickness peaks from ages four to ten, then begins to decline.

25.1 The digestive system is responsible for breaking down food, absorbing nutrients, and eliminating wastes.

The digestive system consists of two basic anatomical divisions: the alimentary canal and the accessory organs. The **alimentary canal**, also called the gastrointestinal (GI) tract, is a long, continuous, hollow tube that extends from the mouth to the anus. The accessory organs of digestion include the liver, gallbladder, and pancreas. The structure of the digestive system is shown in Figure 25.1.

Digestion is the process by which the body breaks down ingested food into small molecules that can be absorbed. The primary functions of the GI tract are to physically transport ingested food and to provide the necessary enzymes and surface area for chemical digestion and absorption. The inner surface is lined with a mucosa layer that secretes acids, bases, mucous, and enzymes important to digestion. The mucosa of the small intestine is lined with tiny projections called *villi* and *microvilli* that provide a huge surface area for the absorption of food and medications.

peri = around
stalsis = contraction

Substances are propelled along the GI tract by the contractions of several layers of smooth muscle, a process known as **peristalsis**. The speed of transit is critical to the absorption of nutrients and water and for the removal of wastes. If peristalsis is too fast, substances will not have sufficient contact with the mucosa to be absorbed. In addition, the large intestine will not have enough time to absorb water, and diarrhea may result. Abnormally slow transit times may result in constipation or even obstructions in the small or large intestine.

In order to chemically break down ingested food, a large number of enzymes and other substances are required. Digestive enzymes are secreted by the salivary glands, stomach, small in-

FIGURE 25.1

The digestive system
SOURCE: *Pearson Education/PH College.*

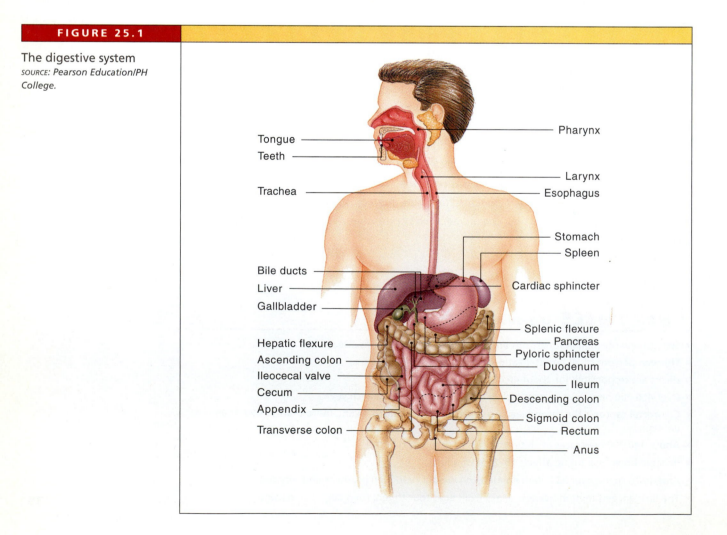

testine, and pancreas. The liver makes bile, which is stored in the gallbladder, until needed for lipid digestion. Because these digestive substances are not common targets for drug therapy, their discussion in this chapter is limited, and the student should refer to anatomy and physiology texts for additional information.

PEPTIC ULCER DISEASE AND GASTROESOPHAGEAL REFLUX DISEASE

An ulcer is a sore or erosion of the mucosal layer of the GI tract. Although ulcers may occur in any portion of the GI tract, the duodenum is the most common site.

25.2 Peptic ulcer disease is caused by an erosion of the mucosal layer of the stomach or duodenum.

pept = to digest
ic = pertaining to

The term **peptic ulcer** refers to a lesion located in either the stomach (gastric) or small intestine (duodenal). The disorder is associated with a number of risk factors, which are presented in the following list.

- close family history of peptic ulcer disease
- blood group O
- tobacco smoking
- consumption of alcoholic beverages
- consumption of beverages and food containing caffeine
- ingestion of drugs, including corticosteroids, aspirin, and NSAIDS
- excessive psychological stress levels
- infection with *Helicobacter pylori*

One to three liters of hydrochloric acid are secreted each day by **parietal cells** in the stomach mucosa. Although this strong acid aids in the chemical breakdown of food and helps to protect the body from ingested microbes, it may be quite damaging to stomach cells. A number of natural defenses protect the stomach mucosa against this extremely acidic chemical. Certain cells lining the GI tract secrete mucous and bicarbonate, a basic ion that neutralizes acid. These form a protective layer such that the pH at the mucosal surface is nearly neutral. Once reaching the duodenum, the stomach contents are further neutralized by bicarbonate from pancreatic and biliary secretions. These natural defenses are shown in Figure 25.2.

ON THE JOB

Radiographers and Barium Sulfate

Barium sulfate is the most frequent drug administered by radiographers. Barium sulfate is an inorganic substance that has two properties ideal to imaging the GI tract: it is very dense, and it is not absorbed by the body. The high density of this drug enables it to absorb X-rays so that the outline of the alimentary canal may be visualized. Because it is not absorbed, there are no systemic side effects.

Suspensions of barium given orally are used to visualize the esophagus, stomach, and small intestine. Given rectally as a barium enema, the anatomy of the entire large intestine may be visualized. Some of the disorders that may be diagnosed using barium sulfate include cancer of the esophagus, stomach, or colon, peptic ulcers, narrowing or obstruction of the alimentary canal, diverticula, and polyps. ▪

FIGURE 25.2

FIGURE 25.2

Natural defenses against stomach acid
SOURCE: Pearson Education/PH College.

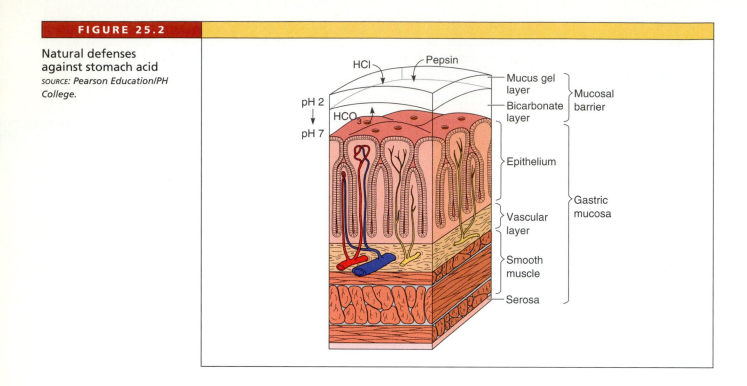

The primary cause of peptic ulcers is infection by the gram-negative bacterium *Helicobacter pylori*. In non-infected clients, duodenal ulcers are commonly caused by therapy with nonsteroidal antiinflammatory drugs (NSAIDS). Secondary factors that contribute to the ulcer and its subsequent inflammation include hypersecretion of acid and hyposecretion of adequate mucous protection. Figure 25.3 illustrates the mechanism of peptic ulcer formation.

The characteristic symptom of duodenal ulcer is a gnawing or burning upper abdominal pain that occurs one to three hours after a meal. The pain often disappears following ingestion of food. Nighttime pain, nausea, and vomiting are uncommon. If the erosion progresses deeper into the mucosa, bleeding will occur and this may be evident as bright red blood in vomit or black, tarry stools. Many duodenal ulcers heal spontaneously, although they often reoccur after months of remission.

an = not or without
orexia = appetite

Gastric ulcers are less common than the duodenal type and have different symptoms. Although relieved by food, pain may continue even after a meal. Loss of appetite, known as anorexia, weight loss, and vomiting are more common. Remissions may be infrequent or absent. Medical follow-up of gastric ulcers sometimes proceeds for many years because a small percentage of the erosions become cancerous. The most severe ulcers may penetrate through the wall of the stomach and cause death. Whereas duodenal ulcers occur most frequently in the 30-to-50 year-old age group, gastric ulcers are more common over age 60.

Ulceration in the lower small intestine is known as Crohn's disease and erosions in the large intestine are called ulcerative colitis. These diseases, together, are categorized as inflammatory bowel disease, and are treated with the anti-inflammatory medications discussed in Chapter 20 ⬚. Particularly severe cases may require immunosuppressant drugs such as cyclosporine (Neoral, Sandimmune) or methotrexate (Amethopterin).

Gastroesophageal reflux disease (GERD) is a condition in which the acidic contents of the stomach move upwards into the esophagus. This causes an intense burning known as *heartburn,* and may lead to ulcers in the esophagus. The cause of GERD is usually a loosening of the sphincter located between the esophagus and the stomach. Many of the drugs prescribed for peptic ulcers are also used to treat GERD.

PharmLink

**DIGESTIVE DISORDER
DIAGNOSIS INFORMATION**

Concept review 25.1

■ What are the similarities and differences between duodenal ulcers and gastric ulcers?

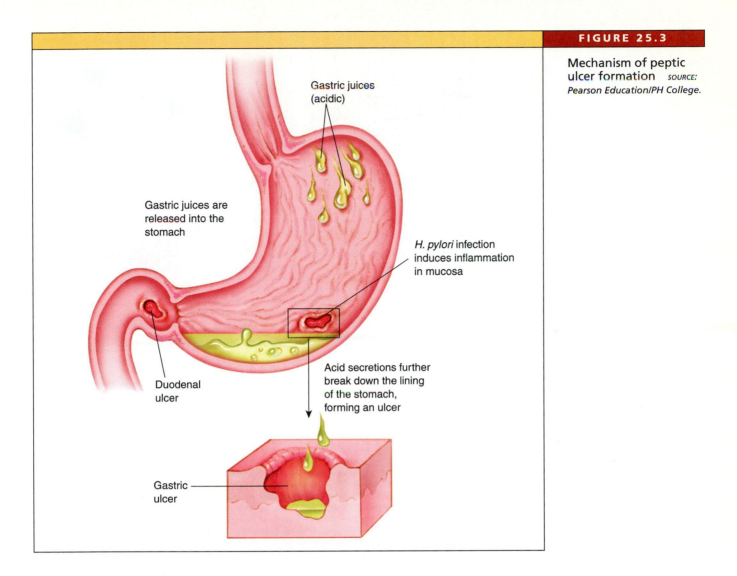

FIGURE 25.3

Mechanism of peptic ulcer formation   *SOURCE: Pearson Education/PH College.*

Gastric juices (acidic)

Gastric juices are released into the stomach

H. pylori infection induces inflammation in mucosa

Duodenal ulcer

Acid secretions further break down the lining of the stomach, forming an ulcer

Gastric ulcer

25.3 Peptic ulcer disease is best treated by a combination of lifestyle changes and pharmacotherapy.

Before starting drug therapy, clients are usually advised to change lifestyle factors that are associated with peptic ulcer disease. For example, eliminating tobacco and alcohol use and reducing stress often cause the ulcer to go into remission.

For clients requiring drug therapy, a wide variety of both prescription and OTC medications are available. These agents fall into four primary classes, plus one miscellaneous group.

- H_2-receptor antagonists
- antibiotics
- proton pump inhibitors
- antacids
- miscellaneous agents

The goals of pharmacotherapy are to provide immediate relief from symptoms, promote healing of the ulcer, and prevent recurrence of the disease. The choice of medication depends upon the source of the disease (infectious versus inflammatory), the severity of symptoms, and the convenience of OTC versus prescription drugs. The mechanisms of action of the four major classes of drugs used to treat peptic ulcer disease are shown in Figure 25.4.

FIGURE 25.4

Mechanisms of action
of antiulcer drugs

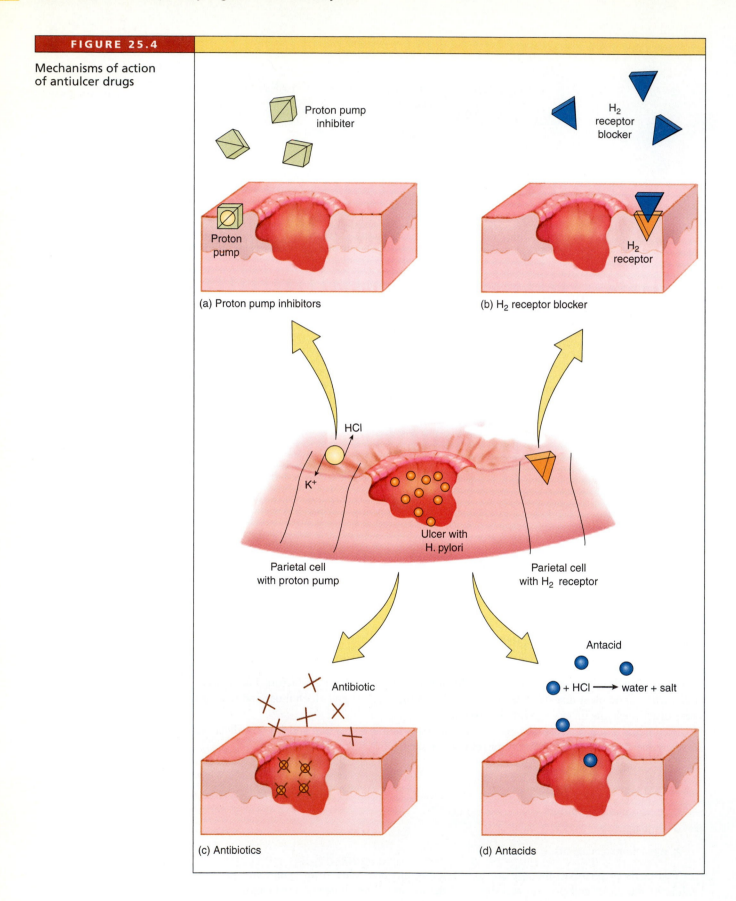

(a) Proton pump inhibitors

Proton pump inhibiter

Proton pump

H$_2$ receptor blocker

(b) H$_2$ receptor blocker

H$_2$ receptor

HCl

K$^+$

Ulcer with H. pylori

Parietal cell with proton pump

Parietal cell with H$_2$ receptor

Antibiotic

(c) Antibiotics

Antacid

+ HCl ⟶ water + salt

(d) Antacids

H₂-RECEPTOR ANTAGONISTS

The discovery of the H₂-receptor antagonists in the 1970s marked a major breakthrough in the treatment of peptic ulcer disease. Since then, they have become available OTC and have become drugs of first choice in the treatment of peptic ulcer disease.

25.4 H₂-receptor blockers are often drugs of first choice in treating peptic ulcers.

As discussed in Chapter 20 , histamine has two types of receptors. While activation of H₁ receptors produces the classic symptoms of allergy, the H₂-receptors are responsible for increasing acid secretion in the stomach. Cimetidine (Tagamet), the first **H₂-receptor antagonist**, and other drugs in this class are quite effective at suppressing the volume and acidity of stomach acid. These medications are also used to treat the symptoms of GERD. Cimetidine is available OTC for the treatment of heartburn. Side effects of the H₂-receptor blockers are minor and rarely cause discontinuation of therapy. Doses of the H₂-receptor antagonists are given in Table 25.1.

Concept review 25.2

- Explain the following statement: All H₂-receptor antagonists are antihistamines, but not all antihistamines are H₂-receptor antagonists.

PROTON PUMP INHIBITORS

Proton pump inhibitors act by blocking the enzyme responsible for secreting hydrochloric acid in the stomach. They are widely used in the short-term therapy of peptic ulcer disease.

25.5 Proton pump inhibitors are effective at reducing gastric acid secretion.

Proton pump inhibitors are relatively new medications widely used in the treatment of peptic ulcer disease and GERD. Drugs in this class reduce acid secretion in the stomach by binding irreversibly to the enzyme **H⁺, K⁺-ATPase**. In the parietal cells of the stomach, this enzyme acts as a pump to release acid (also called H⁺, or protons) onto the surface of the GI mucosa. The proton pump inhibitors reduce acid secretion to a greater extent than the H₂-receptor antagonists and have a longer duration of action. The three proton pump inhibitors are shown in Table 25.2.

ANTACIDS

Antacids are alkaline substances that have been used to neutralize stomach acid for hundreds of years. They are readily available as OTC medications.

25.6 Antacids are effective at neutralizing stomach acid and reducing the symptoms of reflux disease.

Prior to the development of H₂-receptor antagonists and proton pump inhibitors, **antacids** were the mainstay of peptic ulcer and GERD pharmacotherapy. Indeed, many clients still use these

DRUG PROFILE:
Ranitidine (Zantac)

Actions:

Ranitidine has become a drug of choice in this class. It has a higher potency than cimetidine that allows it to be administered once daily, usually at bedtime. Adequate healing of the ulcer takes approximately four to eight weeks. Clients at high risk for the disease may continue on drug maintenance for prolonged periods in order to prevent recurrence. Gastric ulcers heal more slowly than duodenal ulcers, and thus require longer drug therapy. IV and IM forms are available for the treatment of stress-induced bleeding in acute situations.

Adverse Effects:

Ranitidine does not cross the blood-brain barrier to any appreciable extent, so the confusion and CNS depression observed with cimetidine is not expected with ranitidine. Ranitidine has fewer drug-drug interactions than cimetidine. Although rare, severe reductions in the number of red and white blood cells and platelets are possible; thus, periodic laboratory blood counts may be performed. High doses may result in impotence or a loss of libido in men.

Mechanism in Action:

Ranitidine blocks the H_2-receptor and provides relief of pain due to gastric acid secretion in clients with peptic ulcer or gastro-esophageal reflux disease. Because ranitidine does not readily cross the blood-brain-barrier, central side effects such as drowsiness and sedation are less evident.

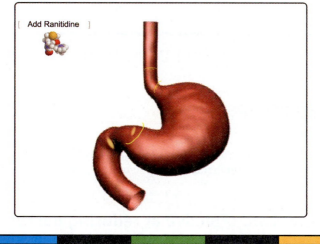

[Add Ranitidine]

TABLE 25.1	H_2-Receptor Antagonists	
DRUG	**ROUTE AND ADULT DOSE**	**REMARKS**
cimetidine (Tagamet)	PO; 300–400 mg bid-qid or 800 mg at hs for active ulcers; 300 mg bid or 400 mg at hs for ulcer prophylaxis.	Intended for short term treatment; decreases the metabolism of many medications; IM and IV forms available.
famotidine (Pepcid)	PO; 20 mg bid or 40 mg at hs for active ulcers; 20 mg at hs for ulcer prophylaxis.	No identified drug interactions; IV form available.
nizatidine (Axid)	PO; 300 mg at hs for active ulcers; 150 mg at hs for ulcer prophylaxis.	
Pr ranitidine (Zantac)	PO; 100–150 mg bid or 300 mg at hs for active ulcers; 150 mg at hs for ulcer prophylaxis.	IM and IV forms available; ranitidine with bismuth citrate is given concurrently with clarithromycin for *Helicobacter* infections

DRUG PROFILE:
Omeprazole (Prilosec)

Actions:

Omeprazole was the first proton pump inhibitor approved for peptic ulcer disease. Although this agent may take two hours to reach therapeutic levels, its effects may last 72 hours. It is used for the short-term, four- to eight-week therapy of peptic ulcers and GERD. Most clients are symptom-free after two weeks of therapy. It is used for longer periods in clients who have chronic hypersecretion of gastric acid, a condition known as Zollinger-Ellison syndrome. It is the most effective drug for this syndrome. Omeprazole is only available in oral form.

Adverse Effects:

Adverse effects are generally minor and include headache, nausea, diarrhea, and abdominal pain. The main concern with proton pump inhibitors is that long-term use has been associated with an increased risk of gastric cancer in laboratory animals. Because of this potential effect, therapy is generally limited to two months.

TABLE 25.2	Proton Pump Inhibitors	
DRUG	**ROUTE AND ADULT DOSE**	**REMARKS**
Pr omeprazole (Prilosec)	PO; 20–60 mg qd-bid.	Often used in combination with antibiotics for *Helicobacter* infections; also for GERD.
lansoprazole (Prevacid)	PO; 15–60 mg qd.	Often used in combination with antibiotics for *Helicobacter* infections; Prevac combines lansoprazole, amoxacillin, and clarithromycin.
rabeprazole sodium (AcipHex)	PO; 20 mg qd × 4–8 weeks.	Also for GERD.

inexpensive and readily available OTC medications. Antacids, however, are no longer recommended as the sole medication for peptic ulcer disease.

Antacids are alkaline, inorganic compounds of aluminum, magnesium, or calcium. Combinations of aluminum hydroxide and magnesium hydroxide are the most common type. Both aluminum hydroxide and magnesium hydroxide are bases, capable of rapidly neutralizing stomach acid. Simethicone is sometimes added to antacid preparations because it reduces gas bubbles that cause bloating and discomfort.

Unless taken in extremely large amounts, antacids are very safe. When given in high doses, aluminum compounds may interfere with phosphate metabolism and cause constipation. Magnesium compounds may cause diarrhea. Common antacids are shown with their trade names in Table 25.3. Doses are not given because they are highly variable. Clients should follow the label instructions very carefully and not take more than the recommended dosages.

ANTIBIOTICS FOR *H. PYLORI*

Most peptic ulcers are associated with the bacterium *H. pylori*. To more rapidly and effectively eliminate peptic ulcers, several antibiotics are used to eradicate this bacterium.

TABLE 25.3	Selected Antacids
BRAND NAME	**CHEMICAL COMPOSITION**
Amphojel	aluminum hydroxide
Tums, Titralac	calcium carbonate
Mylanta Gel-caps, Rolaids	calcium carbonate with magnesium hydroxide
Maalox	magnesium hydroxide and aluminum hydroxide
Mylanta, Maalox Plus, Gelusil, Rulox Plus	magnesium hydroxide and aluminum hydroxide with simethicone
Gaviscon	magnesium trisilicate and aluminum hydroxide
Riopan	magaldrate
Alka Seltzer, Baking soda	sodium bicarbonate

25.7 Antibiotics are administered to eliminate *Helicobacter pylori,* the cause of many peptic ulcers.

H. pylori is associated with 90% of all duodenal ulcers and 75% of all gastric ulcers. This organism has adapted well as a human pathogen by devising ways to neutralize the high acidity surrounding it and by making chemicals called *adhesins* that allow it to stick tightly to the GI mucosa. *H. pylori* infections can remain active for life if not treated appropriately. Elimination of this organism causes ulcers to heal more rapidly and to remain in remission longer. The following antibiotics are commonly used for this purpose.

■ amoxicillin (Amoxil and others)

■ clarithromycin (Biaxin)

■ metronidazole (Flagyl)

■ tetracycline (Achromycin and others)

Two or more antibiotics are given concurrently, as this has been found to increase the effectiveness of therapy and to lower the potential for bacterial resistance. Antibiotic therapy generally continues for 7–14 days. Bismuth compounds are sometimes added to the antibiotic regimen. While not antibiotics, bismuth compounds do inhibit bacterial growth and prevent *H. pylori* from adhering to the surface of the gastric mucosa. Dosages and additional information for these anti-infectives can be found in Chapters 21 and 22 .

25.8 Several miscellaneous drugs are also beneficial in treating peptic ulcer disease.

Three additional drugs are beneficial in treating peptic ulcer disease. Sucralfate (Carafate) consists of sucrose (a sugar) plus aluminum hydroxide (an antacid). The drug produces a thick, gel-like substance that coats the ulcer, protecting it against further erosion and promoting healing. Very little of the drug is absorbed from the GI tract. Other than constipation, side effects are minimal.

Misoprostol (Cytotec) is a prostaglandin-like substance that acts by inhibiting gastric acid secretion and stimulating the production of protective mucous. Its primary use is for the prevention of peptic ulcers in clients taking high doses of NSAIDS or glucocorticoids. Diarrhea and abdominal cramping are relatively common. Classified as a pregnancy Category X drug, misoprostol is contraindicated in pregnant clients. In fact, misoprostal is sometimes used to terminate pregnancies, as discussed in Chapter 29 .

Pirenzepine (Gastozepine) is a cholinergic-blocker (muscarinic) that inhibits the autonomic receptors responsible for gastric acid secretion. Although the action of pirenzepine is somewhat selective to the stomach, other anticholinergic effects such as dry mouth and constipation are possible.

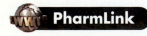

PharmLink

JOHNS HOPKINS' PEPTIC
ULCER DISEASE SITE

Concept review 25.3

■ Why are antibiotics prescribed to treat peptic ulcer disease?

CONSTIPATION

A major function of the large intestine is to reabsorb water from stools. Reabsorption of too much water, however, can lead to small, hard stools. Difficult or infrequent bowel movements, known as constipation, is a common problem with a large number of different causes that include lack of exercise, insufficient food or fluid intake, lack of sufficient insoluble dietary fiber, and certain medications such as opioids. Positive dietary changes and mild exercise should be considered before drugs are utilized. The normal frequency of bowel movements varies widely among individuals, from two to three per day, to as few as one per week.

Occasional constipation is so common as to not warrant drug therapy, but consistently infrequent, painful bowel movements may warrant treatment. Also, pharmacotherapy may be indicated following surgical procedures to prevent the client from straining or bearing down when attempting a bowel movement. Drugs are given to cleanse the bowel prior to surgery or for diagnostic procedures of the colon, such as a colonoscopy or barium enema.

LAXATIVES

Laxatives are drugs that promote bowel movements. Many are available OTC for self-treatment of simple constipation.

25.9 Laxatives are used to promote defecation.

Laxatives are drugs that promote bowel movements or defecation. Cathartic is a related term that implies a strong and complete bowel emptying. When taken in prescribed amounts, laxatives have few side effects. Selected medications used to treat constipation are listed in Table 25.4. These drugs are often classified into four primary groups and a miscellaneous category.

laxat = to loosen
ive = nature of, quality of

- bulk-forming: absorb water, thus adding size to the fecal mass
- stimulant: irritate the bowel to increase peristalsis
- saline/osmotic: cause water to be retained in the fecal mass to cause a more watery stool
- stool softeners/surfactant: bring more water and fat into the stools
- miscellaneous: act by mechanisms other than the above

Concept review 25.4

■ Bismuth compounds are used to treat several digestive disorders. What are they?

DIARRHEA

Occasionally, the colon does not reabsorb enough water from the fecal mass and stools become watery. Diarrhea is an increase in the frequency and fluidity of bowel movements. Like constipation,

dia = through/between
rrhea = flow/discharge

DRUG PROFILE:
Psyllium Mucilloid (Metamucil and Others)

Actions:

Like other bulk-forming laxatives, psyllium is an insoluble fiber that is indigestible and not absorbed from the GI tract. When taken with plenty of water, psyllium swells and increases the size of the fecal mass by drawing water into the intestine. The larger the size of the fecal mass, the more the defecation reflex will be stimulated to promote bowel movements. Several doses of psyllium may be needed to produce a therapeutic effect. More frequent doses of psyllium may cause a small reduction in blood cholesterol level.

Adverse Effects:

Psyllium rarely produces side effects. It generally causes less cramping than the stimulant-type laxatives and produces a more natural bowel movement. If taken with insufficient water, it may cause obstructions in the esophagus or intestine.

TABLE 25.4	**Laxatives**	
DRUG	**ROUTE AND ADULT DOSE**	**REMARKS**
bisacodyl (Dulcolax)	PO; 10–15 mg qd prn.	Stimulant type.
calcium polycarbophil (FiberCon, Fiberall, Mitrolan)	PO 1 g qid prn.	Bulk-forming type.
castor oil (Emulsoil, Neoloid, Purge)	PO; 15–60 ml qd prn.	Stimulant type; the only laxative to act on the small intestine.
docusate (Surfak, Dialose, Colace)	PO; 50–500 mg qd.	Stool softener/surfactant type.
magnesium hydroxide (Milk of Magnesia)	PO; 20–60 ml qd prn.	Saline type.
methylcellulose (Citrocel)	PO; 5–20 ml tid in 8–10 oz water.	Bulk-forming type.
mineral oil	PO; 45 ml bid.	Miscellaneous type; lubricates the stools.
phenolphthalein (Ex-Lax, Feen-A-Mint, Correctol)	PO; 60–240 mg qd prn.	Stimulant type.
Pr psyllium muciloid (Metamucil, Naturcil)	PO 1–2 tsp in 8 oz water qd prn.	Bulk-forming type; also used for diarrhea and as an aid in lowering blood cholesterol.
sodium biphosphate (Fleet Phospho-Soda)	PO; 15–30 ml mixed in water qd prn.	Saline type; available as enema.

occasional diarrhea is a common disorder that does not warrant drug therapy. When prolonged or severe, especially in children, diarrhea can result in significant loss of body fluids and medications may be indicated. Prolonged diarrhea may lead to acid-base or electrolyte disorders, as discussed in Chapter 27 ⬭ .

Diarrhea is not a disease; it is a symptom of an underlying disorder. Diarrhea may be caused by certain medications, infections of the bowel, inflammatory bowel disorders such as Crohn's disease or ulcerative colitis, and chemicals such as lactate. Superinfections occurring during antiinfective therapy are common causes of diarrhea.

Drug therapy of diarrhea depends upon the severity of the condition and whether or not a specific cause can be identified. If the cause is an infectious disease, an antibiotic or antiparasitic drug is indicated. If the cause is inflammatory in nature, antiinflammatory drugs are warranted. If the cause appears to be iatrogenic, the offending medication should be discontinued and another substituted.

ANTIDIARRHEALS

The opioids are used for severe cases of diarrhea because they are the most efficacious of the antidiarrheal agents. Several OTC agents are available for mild cases.

25.10 Opioids are the most effective drugs for controlling diarrhea.

Several opioids are available that slow peristalsis in the colon with only a slight risk of dependence. A few less-effective agents, such as bismuth subsalicylate (Pepto-Bismol), are available OTC for mild diarrhea. The same psyllium preparations that are used to treat constipation may also slow or prevent diarrhea, as they tend to absorb large amounts of fluid and form bulkier stools. Selected agents used to treat diarrhea are shown in Table 25.5.

NAUSEA AND VOMITING

Nausea is an uncomfortable, subjective sensation that is sometimes accompanied by dizziness and an urge to vomit. Vomiting, or emesis, is a reflex primarily controlled by the medulla of the brain. Nausea and vomiting are common symptoms associated with a wide variety of conditions such as food poisoning, early pregnancy, extreme pain, trauma to the head or abdominal organs, inner ear disorders, and emotional disturbances. In treating nausea or vomiting, an important therapeutic goal is to remove the cause, whenever feasible.

ANTIEMETICS

Drugs from several different pharmacologic classes are prescribed to prevent nausea and vomiting. Clients receiving antineoplastic medications may receive three or more antiemetics in order to reduce the nausea and vomiting from the anticancer drugs.

25.11 Several drugs are available to treat nausea, vomiting, and motion sickness.

Many drugs cause nausea or vomiting as a side effect. The most extreme example of this is the antineoplastic agents, almost all of which cause some degree of nausea or vomiting. In fact, therapy with antineoplastic drugs is one of the most common reasons why antiemetic medications are prescribed. When cancer chemotherapy is initiated, it is not uncommon for a client to receive

anti = *against*
emetic = *vomit*

DRUG PROFILE:
Diphenoxylate with Atropine (Lomotil)

Actions:

The primary antidiarrheal ingredient in Lomotil is diphenoxylate. Like other opioids, diphenoxylate slows peristalsis, resulting in additional water being reabsorbed from the colon and more solid stools. It is effective for moderate to severe diarrhea. The atropine in Lomotil is not added for its anticholinergic effect; it is added to discourage clients from taking too much of the drug.

Adverse Effects:

Unlike most opioids, diphenoxylate has no analgesic properties and has an extremely low potential for abuse. Some clients experience dizziness or drowsiness and care should be taken not to operate machinery until the effects of the drug are known. Other CNS depressants, including alcohol, will add to its CNS depressant effect. At higher doses, the anticholinergic effects of atropine may be observed, which include drowsiness, dry mouth, and tachycardia.

TABLE 25.5	Antidiarrheals	
DRUG	**ROUTE AND ADULT DOSE**	**REMARKS**
Pr diphenoxylate hydrochloride with atropine (Lomotil)	PO; 1–2 tabs or 5–10 ml tid-qid.	Opioid; schedule V drug.
bismuth salts (Pepto-bismol)	PO; 2 tabs or 30 ml PRN.	OTC adsorbent.
paregoric (Camphorated opium tincture)	PO; 5–10 ml q 2 hours u to qid prn.	Opioid; schedule III drug.
difenoxin with atropine (Motofen)	PO; 1–2 mg after each diarrhea episode (max 8 mg/day).	Opioid; schedule IV drug.
furazolidone (Furoxone)	PO; 100 mg qid.	For bacterial or protozoal GI infections.
kaolin-pectin (Kaopectate)	PO; 60–120 ml after each diarrhea episode.	OTC adsorbent.
loperamide (Imodium)	PO; 4 mg as a single dose, then 2 mg after each diarrhea episode (max 16 mg/day).	Opioid; abuse is so low, it is not classified as a controlled substance.

three or more antiemetics. Antiemetic drugs belong to a number of different classes, including the following.

- phenothiazines
- antihistamines
- serotonin receptor antagonists
- glucocorticoids
- benzodiazepines

To avoid losing antiemetic medication due to vomiting, many of these agents are available through the IM, IV, and/or suppository routes. The most effective antiemetics are serotonin receptor antagonists. The individual antiemetic drugs are shown in Table 25.6.

Motion sickness is a disorder affecting a portion of the inner ear known as the **vestibular apparatus** that is associated with significant nausea. The most common drug used for motion sick-

TABLE 25.6	Antiemetics	
DRUG	**ROUTE AND ADULT DOSE**	**REMARKS**
cyclizine hydrochloride (Marezine)	PO; 50 mg q4-qid.	Antihistamine; for prevention of motion sickness and post op nausea and vomiting; IM form available.
dexamethasone (Decadron)	IV; 10–20 mg prior to chemotherapy.	Glucocorticoid; IM, inhalation, and IV forms available; also for inflammatory disorders, severe allergies, acute asthma, and neoplasia.
dimenhydrinate (Dramamine)	PO; 50–100 mg q4-qid (max 400 mg/day).	Antihistamine; also used for allergies and cold/flu symptoms; IM and IV forms available.
diphenhydramine (Benadryl)	PO; 25–50 mg tid–qid (max 300 mg/day).	Antihistamine; IM, IV, and topical forms available; also for allergies, Parkinson's disease, and anaphylaxis.
dolasetron mesylate (Anzemet)	PO; 100 mg 1 h prior to chemotherapy.	Serotonin-receptor antagonist; IV form available.
granisetron (Kytril)	IV; 10μg/kg 30 minutes prior to chemotherapy.	Serotonin-receptor antagonist; oral form available.
hydroxyzine (Atarax, Vistaril)	PO; 25–100 mg tid or qid.	Antihistamine; IM form available; also for anxiety and as a pre-op medication.
lorazepam (Ativan)	IV; 1.0–1.5 mg prior to chemotherapy.	Benzodiazepine; IM and IV forms available; also for anxiety, insomnia, and as a pre-op medication.
meclizine (Antivert, Bonine)	PO: 25–50 mg qd, take 1 h before travel.	Antihistamine; for motion sickness and nausea associated with vertigo.
methylprednisolone (Medrol, Solu-medrol)	IV; 2 doses of 125–500 mg 6 hours apart prior to chemotherapy.	Glucocorticoid; IM and IV forms available; also for inflammatory disorders, severe allergies, acute asthma, and neoplasia.
metoclopramide (Reglan)	PO; 2 mg/kg 1 h prior to chemotherapy.	Phenothiazine-like; IV and IM forms available; also for GERD, facilitation of small bowel intubation, and gastric stasis.
ondansetron hydrochloride (Zofran)	IV; 4 mg tid prn.	Serotonin-receptor antagonist; IM and PO forms available.
perphenazine (Phenazine, Trilafon)	PO; 8–16 mg bid–qid.	Phenothiazine; IM and IV forms available; also for psychoses.
Pr prochlorperazine (Compazine)	PO; 5–10 mg tid or qid.	Phenothiazine; IM, IV, and suppository forms available; also for treatment of psychoses.
promethazine (Phenergan)	PO; 12.5–25 mg q4-qid.	Both a phenothiazine and an antihistamine; IM, IV, and suppository forms available; also for allergic disorders and as an adjunct to anesthesia and surgery.
scopolamine (Hyoscine, Transderm Scop)	Transdermal; 0.5 mg q72h.	Anticholinergic; oral, IV, IM, and SC forms available.
thiethylperazine (Torecan)	PO; 10 mg qd-tid.	Phenothiazine; IM form available.

ness is scopolamine, which is administered as a transdermal patch placed behind the ear. Antihistamines such as dimenhydrinate (Dramamine) and meclizine (Antivert) are also effective, but may cause significant drowsiness in some clients. Drugs used to treat motion sickness are most effective when taken 20 to 60 minutes before travel is expected.

DRUG PROFILE: (Antiemetic)
Prochlorperazine (Compazine)

Actions:

Prochlorperazine is a phenothiazine, a class of drugs usually prescribed for psychotic disorders as discussed in Chapter 9 🔗 . The phenothiazines are actually the largest class of medications prescribed for severe nausea and vomiting and prochlorperazine is the most frequently prescribed antiemetic drug in its class. Prochlorperazine depresses the vomiting center in the medulla. It is frequently given by the rectal route, where absorption is rapid.

Adverse Effects:

Prochlorperazine produces dose-related anticholinergic side effects such as dry mouth, constipation, and tachycardia. When used for prolonged periods at higher doses, extrapyramidal symptoms resembling those of Parkinson's disease are a serious concern (Chapters 9 and 10 🔗).

On some occasions, it is desirable to stimulate the vomiting reflex with drugs called **emetics**. Indications for emetics include ingestion of poisons and overdoses of oral drugs. Ipecac syrup, given orally, or apomorphine, given SC, will induce vomiting in about 15 minutes.

WEIGHT LOSS

Hunger occurs when the hypothalamus in the brain recognizes the levels of certain chemicals (glucose) or hormones (insulin) in the blood. Hunger is a normal physiologic response that drives people to seek nourishment. Appetite is somewhat different than hunger. Appetite is a psychological response that drives food intake based upon associations and memory. For example, people often eat not because they are experiencing hunger, but because it is a particular time of day, or because they find the act of eating pleasurable or social.

ANOREXIANTS

Despite the public's desire for effective drugs to induce weight loss, few anorexiants are available. The approved anorexiants used for the treatment of obesity produce only modest effects.

NATURAL ALTERNATIVES

Ginger for Nausea

Ginger is obtained from the roots of the herb *Zingiber officianale* that grows in a wide variety of places across the world. Active ingredients include aromatic oils that give the herb its characteristic scent and antiemetic activity. Because of its widespread use as a spice in Asian cooking, ginger is widely available in a number of forms, including tincture, tea, dried and fresh root, and capsules. Commercial products that use ginger as a flavoring include ginger cookies, gingerbread, and ginger ale. Consumers should check the product ingredients to be certain that the item truly contains ginger extract, rather than artificial ginger flavoring.

Ginger has been used in Chinese medicine for thousands of years. Indications relating to the digestive system include nausea, vomiting, morning sickness, and motion sickness. Studies have shown its effectiveness to be comparable to OTC medications.

Ginger is purported to have other significant benefits. The herb is said to have anti-inflammatory properties that are of benefit to clients with arthritis. It is sometimes given to clients with flu symptoms to help coughs and lower fever. Because of a possible effect on blood clotting, clients taking anticoagulants should avoid ginger unless otherwise directed by a physician or nurse practitioner. ■

DRUG PROFILE: (Anorexiant)
Sibutramine (Meridia)

Actions:

Sibutramine, a serotonin reuptake inhibitor, is the most widely prescribed appetite suppressant for the short-term control of obesity. When combined with a reduced calorie diet, sibutramine may produce a gradual weight loss of at least 10% of initial body weight over a period of a year. Sibutramine therapy is not recommended for longer than one year.

Side Effects:

Headache is the most common complaint reported during sibutramine therapy, although insomnia and dry mouth are also possible. The drug should be used with great care in clients with cardiac disorders, as it may cause tachycardia and raise blood pressure. It is a Schedule IV drug with low potential for dependence.

25.12 Anorexiants are drugs used for the short-term management of obesity.

Obesity may be defined as being more than 20% above the ideal body weight. Because of the prevalence of obesity in our society and the difficulty most clients experience when following weight reduction plans for extended periods of time, drug manufacturers have long sought to develop safe drugs that induce weight loss. In the 1970s, amphetamine and dextroamphetamine (Dexedrine) were widely prescribed as anorexiants to reduce appetite. These drugs, however, are quite addictive and amphetamines are rarely prescribed for this purpose today. In the 1990s, the combination of fenfluramine and phenteramine, known as fen-phen was widely prescribed, until fenfluramine was removed from the market for causing heart valve defects. Attempts to produce drugs that promote weight loss by blocking lipid absorption produced orlistat (Xenical). Orlistat produces only a very small increase in weight reduction compared to placebos.

CLIENT TEACHING

Clients treated for digestive disorders need to know the following:

1. Do not smoke tobacco when taking H₂-receptor antagonists, as this interferes with the drug action.
2. When starting therapy with H₂-receptor antagonists or proton pump inhibitors, drowsiness may occur. Operating equipment or taking alcohol or other CNS drugs should be monitored carefully.
3. When taking medications for peptic ulcer, avoid drugs that may cause stomach irritation such as aspirin or NSAIDS.
4. Shake liquid antacids well before pouring. Chewable tablets should be chewed very well before swallowing.
5. Bulk-forming laxatives and stool softeners may take several days for results. Be patient and do not take more than prescribed.
6. Take bulk-forming laxatives with at least two full glasses of water, as this aids in forming more bulk.
7. Before taking antiemetic medications, try other methods of relieving nausea, such as drinking flat carbonated beverages or weak tea or eating small amounts of crackers or dry toast.
8. When taking phenothiazines or antihistamines as antiemetics, use sugarless candy, gum, or ice chips to minimize dry mouth.
9. If constipation is a frequent problem, try drinking more fluids and adding more fiber to the diet rather than taking laxatives on a continual basis. Foods rich in fiber include all fruits and vegetables, bran cereals, and whole grain breads.
10. Medications taken to suppress hunger produce only modest weight loss and are not effective without a reduced-calorie diet. True, sustained weight loss can only be achieved by modification of dietary habits. ▪

CHAPTER REVIEW

Core Concepts Summary

25.1 The digestive system is responsible for breaking down food, absorbing nutrients, and eliminating wastes.

The alimentary canal provides a large surface area for the absorption of nutrients and drugs. Substances are propelled through the GI tract by peristalsis. Abnormally fast or slow peristalsis can affect nutrient, drug, and water absorption.

25.2 Peptic ulcer disease is caused by an erosion of the mucosal layer of the stomach or duodenum.

Infection with *H. pylori* and therapy with NSAIDS are the most common causes of peptic ulcers. A gnawing pain in the upper abdomen that is relieved by eating is the most common symptom of duodenal ulcer. Though less common, gastric ulcers may be more serious and require longer treatment and follow-up. GERD is a disorder that gives similar symptoms to peptic ulcers and is treated with many of the same medications.

25.3 Peptic ulcer disease is best treated by a combination of lifestyle changes and pharmacotherapy.

Before beginning drug therapy, the client should consider eliminating tobacco and alcohol and reducing stress levels, as these will favor remission of peptic ulcer disease. Goals of drug therapy include relief of symptoms, promotion of ulcer healing, and prevention of recurrences.

25.4 H$_2$-receptor blockers are often drugs of first choice in treating peptic ulcers.

H$_2$-receptor antagonists reduce the volume and acidity of stomach acid. Healing of duodenal ulcers occurs in four to eight weeks, and side effects are uncommon.

25.5 Proton pump inhibitors are effective at reducing gastric acid secretion.

Proton pump inhibitors diminish gastric acid secretion by interfering with the enzyme H$^+$, K$^+$-ATPase, which is present in the parietal cells in the stomach.

Although very effective, use is usually limited to two months due to the possibility of long-term adverse effects.

25.6 Antacids are effective at neutralizing stomach acid and reducing the symptoms of reflux disease.

Once drugs of choice for treating peptic ulcer disease, antacids are now primarily used to give immediate relief for the heartburn associated with GERD or peptic ulcer disease.

25.7 Antibiotics are administered to eliminate *Helicobacter pylori*, the cause of many peptic ulcers.

Elimination of H. pylori using combination therapy with several different antibiotics has been found to promote more rapid ulcer healing and longer remissions.

25.8 Several miscellaneous drugs are also beneficial in treating peptic ulcer disease.

Sucralfate (Carafate) produces a gel-like substance that provides a protective coating for ulcers. Misoprostol (Cytotec) inhibits gastric acid secretion and promotes the secretion of protective mucous. Pirenzepine (Gastozepine) inhibits acid secretion by blocking cholinergic receptors.

25.9 Laxatives are used to promote defecation.

Laxatives are given to promote emptying of the colon. Laxatives act by stimulating peristalsis or by adding more bulk or water to the fecal mass.

25.10 Opioids are the most effective drugs for controlling diarrhea.

Diarrhea is treated by addressing its cause, which may include anti-inflammatory drugs or antiinfectives. Opioids are the most effective drugs for relieving severe diarrhea, but they have some abuse potential. OTC bismuth compounds can help with simple diarrhea.

25.11 **Several drugs are available to treat nausea, vomiting, and motion sickness.**

Symptomatic treatment of nausea and vomiting includes drugs from many different classes, including phenothiazines, antihistamines, corticosteroids, benzodiazepines, and serotonin receptor antagonists. Motion sickness can be controlled through medications such as transdermal scopolamine or dimenhydrinate (Dramamine).

25.12 **Anorexiants are drugs used for the short-term management of obesity.**

Only a few drugs are available for the short-term management of obesity, and these drugs produce only modest effects. The anorexiant sibutramine (Merdia) and the lipid absorption blocker orlistat (Xenical) are used to help obese clients lose weight.

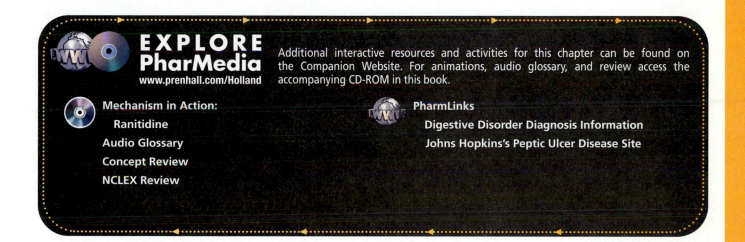

EXPLORE PharMedia
www.prenhall.com/Holland

Additional interactive resources and activities for this chapter can be found on the Companion Website. For animations, audio glossary, and review access the accompanying CD-ROM in this book.

Mechanism in Action:
  Ranitidine
Audio Glossary
Concept Review
NCLEX Review

PharmLinks
  Digestive Disorder Diagnosis Information
  Johns Hopkins's Peptic Ulcer Disease Site

26 Vitamins, Minerals, and Herbs

CORE CONCEPTS

Vitamins

26.1 Vitamins are organic substances that are needed in small amounts to promote growth and maintain health.

26.2 Vitamins are classified as fat-soluble or water-soluble.

26.3 Failure to meet the recommended dietary allowances (RDAs) for vitamins may result in deficiency disorders.

26.4 Vitamin therapy is indicated for only very specific conditions.

Minerals

26.5 Minerals are inorganic substances needed in very small amounts to maintain normal body metabolism.

Herbs and Dietary Supplements

26.6 Natural products obtained from plants have been used as medicines for thousands of years.

26.7 Herbal products are available in a variety of formulations.

26.8 Herbal products and dietary supplements are regulated by the Dietary Supplement Health and Education Act of 1994.

26.9 Herbs may have important pharmacologic actions and result in adverse effects.

OBJECTIVES

After reading this chapter, the student should be able to:

1. Identify characteristics that differentiate a vitamin from other nutrients.

2. Describe the functions of common vitamins and minerals.

3. Explain the rationale behind Recommended Daily Allowances (RDAs).

4. Describe conditions or diseases for which vitamin or mineral therapy may be warranted.

5. Identify several drug-vitamin, drug-mineral, and drug-herbal interactions.

6. Compare and contrast the functions of major minerals and trace minerals.

7. Explain why herbal and dietary supplements have increased in popularity in recent years.

8. Identify the parts of an herb that may contain active ingredients and the types of formulations made from these parts.

9. Describe the strengths and weaknesses of the Dietary Supplement Health and Education Act of 1994 (DSHEA).

10. Describe some adverse effects that may be caused by herbal preparations.

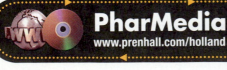

PharMedia
www.prenhall.com/holland

Additional interactive resources and activities for this chapter can be found on the Companion Website. For animations, audio glossary, and review access the accompanying CD-ROM in this book.

![key icon]

K E Y   T E R M S

botanical (boh-TAN-ik-ul): plant extract used to treat or prevent illness / *page 417*

dietary supplement: non-drug substance regulated by the DSHEA / *page 419*

Dietary Supplement Health and Education Act of 1994 (DSHEA): primary law in the United States regulating herb and dietary supplements / *page 419*

folic acid (foh-lik): B vitamin that is a coenzyme in protein and nucleic acid metabolism; also known as *folate* / *page 414*

hemoglobin (HEE-moh-glow-bin): substance in a red blood cell that contains iron and transports oxygen and CO_2 / *page 416*

herb: plant with a soft stem that is used for healing or as a seasoning / *page 417*

hypervitaminosis: excess intake of vitamins / *page 414*

intrinsic factor: chemical secreted by the stomach that is required for absorption of vitamin B_{12} / *page 414*

major mineral (macromineral): inorganic compound needed by the body in amounts of 100 mg or more daily / *page 416*

pernicious (megaloblastic) anemia (pur-NISH-us ah-NEE-mee-ah): type of anemia usually caused by lack of secretion of intrinsic factor / *page 414*

provitamin: an inactive chemical that is converted to a vitamin in the body / *page 412*

Recommended Dietary Allowance (RDA): amount of vitamin or mineral needed daily to avoid a deficiency in a healthy adult / *page 412*

trace mineral: inorganic compound needed by the body in amounts of 20 mg or less daily / *page 416*

vitamins: organic compounds required by the body in small amounts / *page 412*

The vitamin, mineral, and herbal supplement business is a multibillion dollar industry. Although aggresive marketing often leads clients to believe that dietary supplements are essential to maintain health, most people obtain all necessary nutrients through their normal diet. Once the body has obtained the amount of vitamin or mineral it needs to carry on metabolism, the excess is simply excreted or stored. There are some conditions, however, where dietary supplementation is necessary and will benefit the client's health. This chapter will focus on these conditions and explore the role of vitamins, minerals, and herbal supplements in pharmacology.

Fast Facts Vitamins, Minerals, Herbs, and Dietary Supplements

- About 40% of Americans take vitamin supplements daily.
- There is no difference between the chemical structure of a natural vitamin and a synthetic vitamin, yet consumers pay much more for the natural type.
- Vitamin B_{12} is only present in animal products. Vegetarians may find adequate amounts in fortified cereals, nutritional supplements, or yeast.
- Administration of folic acid during pregnancy has been found to reduce birth defects in the nervous system of the baby.
- Clients who never go outside or never receive sun exposure may need vitamin D supplements.
- Heavy menstrual periods may result in considerable iron loss.
- Technically, vitamins and herbs cannot increase a client's energy levels. Energy can only be provided by adding calories in carbohydrates, proteins, and fats.
- "Organic" foods do not necessarily contain a higher concentration of vitamins or minerals than non-organic foods. Read labels and compare the nutritional values of organic and non-organic foods.

VITAMINS

Vitamins are essential substances needed in very small amounts to maintain homeostasis. Clients having a low or unbalanced dietary intake, those who are pregnant, or those experiencing a chronic disease may benefit from vitamin therapy.

26.1 Vitamins are organic substances that are needed in small amounts to promote growth and maintain health.

Vitamins are organic compounds required by the body in very small amounts for growth and for the maintenance of normal metabolic processes. Since the discovery of thiamine in 1911, over a dozen substances have been identified as vitamins. Because scientists did not know the chemical structures of the vitamins when they were discovered, they were assigned letters and numbers such as A, B$_{12}$, and C. These names are still widely used today.

pro = before
vitamin = essential
substance

An important characteristic of vitamins is that, with the exception of vitamin D, human cells cannot synthesize them. They or their precursors—known as **provitamins**—must be supplied in the diet. A second important characteristic is that if the vitamin is not present in adequate amounts, the body's metabolism will be disrupted and disease will result. Furthermore, the symptoms of the deficiency can be reversed by the administration of the missing vitamin.

Vitamins serve diverse and important roles in human physiology. For example, the B complex vitamins are coenzymes essential to many metabolic pathways. Vitamin A is a precursor of retinal, a pigment needed for normal vision. Calcium metabolism is regulated by a hormone that is derived from Vitamin D. Without Vitamin K, abnormal prothrombin is produced and blood clotting is affected.

26.2 Vitamins are classified as fat-soluble or water-soluble.

A simple way to classify vitamins is by their ability to mix with water. Those that dissolve easily in water are called water-soluble vitamins. Examples include vitamin C and the B vitamins. Those that dissolve in lipids are called fat-soluble and include vitamins A, D, E, and K.

The difference in solubility affects the way the vitamins are absorbed by the GI tract and stored in the body. The water-soluble vitamins are absorbed along with water in the digestive tract and easily dissolve in blood and body fluids. When excess water-soluble vitamins are absorbed, they cannot be stored for later use, and are simply excreted in the urine. Because they are not stored to any significant degree, they must be ingested daily, otherwise deficiencies will quickly develop.

Fat-soluble vitamins, on the other hand, cannot be absorbed in sufficient quantity in the small intestine unless they are ingested with other lipids. These vitamins can be stored in large quantities in the liver and fat. Should the client not ingest sufficient quantities, fat-soluble vitamins are removed from storage depots in the body as needed. Unfortunately, this storage can lead to dangerously high levels of the fat-soluble vitamins, if they are taken in excessive amounts.

26.3 Failure to meet the recommended dietary allowances (RDAs) for vitamins may result in deficiency disorders.

Based upon scientific research on humans and animals, the Food and Drug Administration has established levels for the intake of vitamins and minerals called **Recommended Dietary Allowances (RDAs)**. Canada publishes similar data called the Recommended Nutrient Intake (RNI). The RDA values represent the minimum amount of vitamin or mineral needed to prevent a deficiency in a healthy adult. The RDAs are revised periodically to reflect the latest scientific research. Current RDAs are shown in Table 26.1.

It is important that clients and healthcare providers understand that the body's needs for certain vitamins and minerals may vary widely. Clients who are pregnant, have chronic disease, or who exercise vigorously have different nutritional needs than the average adult. Recognizing and adjusting for these nutritional differences are essential to maintaining good health.

Vitamin, mineral, or herbal supplements should never substitute for a balanced diet. Sufficient intake of proteins, carbohydrates, and lipids is needed for proper health. Furthermore, al-

TABLE 26.1	Vitamins			

VITAMIN	FUNCTION(S)	RDA MEN	WOMEN	COMMON CAUSE(S) OF DEFICIENCY
A	visual pigments, epithelial cells	1000 RE[1]	800 RE	Prolonged dietary deprivation, particularly where rice is the main food source; pancreatic disease; cirrhosis.
D	calcium and phosphate metabolism	5 mcg	5 mcg	Low dietary intake; inadequate exposure to sunlight.
E	antioxidant	10 TE[2]	8 TE	Premature infants; malabsorption diseases.
K	cofactor in blood clotting	70 mcg	65 mcg	Newborns; liver disease; long-term parenteral nutrition; certain drugs such as cephalosporins and salicylates.
thiamine B_1	coenzyme in metabolic reactions	1.2 mg	1.1 mg	Prolonged dietary deprivation, particularly where rice is the main food source; hyperthyroidism; pregnancy; liver disease; alcoholism.
riboflavin B_2	coenzyme in metabolic reactions	1.3 mg	1.1 mg	Inadequate consumption of milk or animal products; chronic diarrhea; liver disease; alcoholism.
niacin B_3	coenzyme in metabolic reactions	16 mg	14 mg	Prolonged dietary deprivation, particularly where Indian corn (maize) or millet is the main food source; chronic diarrhea; liver disease; alcoholism.
pyridoxine B_6	coenzyme in amino acid metabolism	1.3 mg	1.3 mg	Alcoholism; oral contraceptive use; malabsorption diseases.
folate	coenzyme in amino acid and nucleic acid metabolism	400 mcg	400 mcg	Pregnancy; alcoholism; cancer; oral contraceptive use.
Pr cobalamin B_{12}	coenzyme in nucleic acid metabolism	2.4 mcg	2.4 mcg	Lack of intrinsic factor, inadequate intake of foods from animal origin.
biotin	coenzyme in metabolic reactions	30 mcg	30 mcg	Deficiencies are rare.
pantothenic acid	coenzyme in metabolic reactions	5 mg	5 mg	Deficiencies are rare.
C	coenzyme and antioxidant	60 mg	60 mg	Inadequate intake of fruits and vegetables; pregnancy; chronic inflammatory disease; burns; diarrhea; alcoholism.

[1] retinoid equivalents
[2] alpha = tocopherol equivalents

though the label on a vitamin supplement may indicate that it contains 100% of the RDA for a particular vitamin, the body may absorb as little as 10 to 15% of the amount ingested. With the exception of vitamins A and D, it is not harmful for most clients to consume two to three times the recommended levels of vitamins.

26.4 Vitamin therapy is indicated for only very specific conditions.

Most clients who eat a normal, balanced diet are able to obtain all the necessary nutrients they need without vitamin supplementation. Indeed, megavitamin therapy is not only expensive, but may be harmful to health if taken for prolonged periods. Hypervitaminosis, or toxic levels of vitamins, has been reported for vitamins A, C, D, E, B_6, niacin, and folic acid.

hyper = above
vitamin = vitamin
osis = condition

Vitamin deficiencies in the United States are most often the result of poverty, fad diets, chronic alcoholism, or prolonged parenteral feeding. Infancy and childhood are times of potential deficiency due to the high growth demands placed on the body. In addition, requirements for all nutrients are increased during pregnancy and lactation. The absorption of food diminishes with age and often the quantity of ingested food is reduced, leading to vitamin deficiencies in elderly clients. Vitamin deficiencies in clients with chronic liver and kidney disease are well documented. Clients with alcohol or serious drug dependency are often deficient in the quality and quantity of their nutritional intake. Table 26.1 shows the functions of the vitamins and some common causes of deficiencies.

Certain drugs affect vitamin metabolism. Alcohol is well known for its ability to inhibit the absorption of thiamine and folic acid; alcohol abuse is the most common cause of thiamine deficiency in the United States. Folic acid levels may be reduced in clients taking phenothiazines, oral contraceptives, phenytoin (Dilantin), or barbiturates. Vitamin D deficiency can be caused by therapy with certain anticonvulsants. Inhibition of vitamin B_{12} absorption has been reported with a number of drugs including trifluoperazine (Stelazine), alcohol, and oral contraceptives.

megalo = large
blastic = embryonic state

The most obvious consequence of B_{12} deficiency is a type of anemia called pernicious or megaloblastic anemia. Insufficient vitamin B_{12} creates a lack of activated folic acid, which is essential for DNA synthesis and cell division. Lack of vitamin B_{12} will also affect the nervous system, causing tingling or numbness in the limbs, mood disturbances, and even hallucinations in severe deficiencies.

Treatment of vitamin B_{12} deficiency is most often accomplished by weekly or biweekly IM or SC injections. Although oral supplements are available, they are only effective in clients who have sufficient intrinsic factor and normal absorption in the small intestine. Parenteral adminis-

DRUG PROFILE:
Cyanocobalamin (Cyanabin and Others)

Actions:

Cyanocobalamin is a purified form of vitamin B_{12} that is administered in deficiency states. Vitamin B_{12} is not synthesized by either plants or animals; only bacteria perform this function. Because only miniscule amounts of vitamin B_{12} are required (3 mcg/day), deficiency of this vitamin is not usually caused by insufficient dietary intake. The most common cause of vitamin B_{12} deficiency is lack of a chemical called intrinsic factor, which is secreted by stomach cells. Intrinsic factor is required for vitamin B_{12} to be absorbed from the intestine. Figure 26.1 illustrates the metabolism of vitamin B_{12}/cyanocobalamin. Inflammatory diseases of the stomach or surgical removal of the stomach (gastrectomy) may result in deficiency of intrinsic factor. Inflammatory diseases of the small intestine that affect food and nutrient absorption may also cause vitamin B_{12} deficiency.

Adverse Effects:

Side effects from cyanocobalamin are uncommon. Hypokalemia is possible and serum potassium levels are monitored periodically.

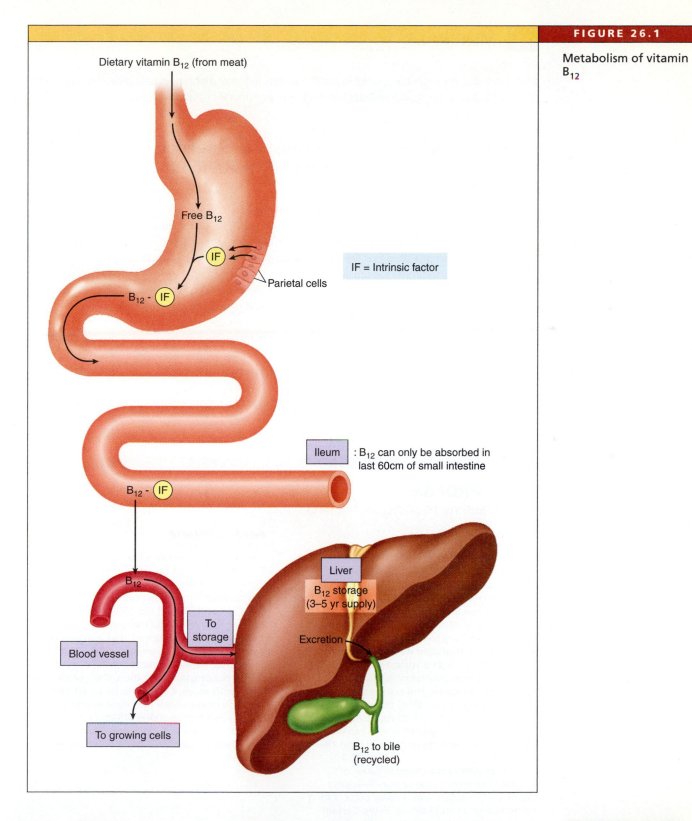

FIGURE 26.1

Metabolism of vitamin B$_{12}$

Dietary vitamin B$_{12}$ (from meat)

Free B$_{12}$

IF

Parietal cells

B$_{12}$ - IF

IF = Intrinsic factor

Ileum : B$_{12}$ can only be absorbed in last 60cm of small intestine

B$_{12}$ - IF

Liver

B$_{12}$ storage (3–5 yr supply)

Excretion

B$_{12}$

To storage

Blood vessel

To growing cells

B$_{12}$ to bile (recycled)

tration rapidly reverses most signs and symptoms of B$_{12}$ deficiency. If the disease has been prolonged, symptoms may take longer to resolve, and some neurological damage may be permanent. Treatment may need to continue for the remainder of the client's life.

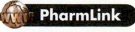

PharmLink

NATIONAL COUNCIL AGAINST HEALTH FRAUD

Concept review 26.1

▪ What are some conditions where the RDA for a vitamin may not be sufficient?

MINERALS

Like vitamins, minerals are needed in small amounts to maintain homeostasis. A normal, balanced diet will provide the proper amounts of the required minerals in most clients.

26.5 Minerals are inorganic substances needed in very small amounts to maintain normal body metabolism.

Minerals are inorganic substances that constitute about 4% of the body weight. Minerals are classified as **major minerals (macrominerals)** or **trace minerals**. The seven major minerals must be obtained daily from dietary sources in amounts of 100 mg or higher. Required daily amounts of the nine trace minerals are 20 mg or less. These minerals are listed in Table 26.2.

Some minerals, such as sodium and magnesium, appear primarily as ions in body fluids. Others, such as iron and cobalt, are usually bound to organic molecules. The functions of many of the minerals in human physiology, such as calcium, sodium, and potassium, are well known. The functions of some of the trace minerals, such as aluminum, silicon, arsenic, and nickel, are less understood.

an = lack of
emia = blood condition
osteo = bone
por = passage
osis = condition

Most minerals are needed in very small amounts for human metabolism; a normal, balanced diet will supply the necessary quantities. Indeed, excess amounts of some minerals can lead to toxicity. For example, arsenic, chromium, and nickel have been implicated as human carcinogens and excess sodium intake can lead to water retention and hypertension.

Mineral supplements are indicated for certain disorders. Iron-deficiency anemia is the most common nutritional deficiency in the world, and is a common indication for iron supplements.

DRUG PROFILE:
Ferrous Sulfate (Ferralyn and Others)

Actions:

Ferrous sulfate is an iron supplement. Iron is a mineral essential to the function of several biological molecules, the most significant of which is **hemoglobin**. Each molecule of hemoglobin in a red blood cell contains four iron atoms, each of which can bind reversibly to an oxygen atom. Sixty to eighty percent of all iron in the body is associated with hemoglobin.

hemo = blood
globin = protein

Because free iron is toxic, the body binds the mineral to protein complexes called ferritin, hemosiderin, and transferrin. After red blood cells die, nearly all of the iron in their hemoglobin is recycled for later use. Because of this recycling, very little iron is excreted; thus, dietary iron requirements in most clients are small.

Iron deficiency is a common cause of anemia. The usual cause of iron-deficiency anemia is blood loss, such as may occur during menstruation or from peptic ulcers. Certain clients have an increased demand for iron, including those who are pregnant and those undergoing intensive athletic training. Ferrous sulfate is available in a wide variety of dosage forms to prevent or rapidly reverse symptoms of iron-deficiency anemia.

Adverse Effects:

The most common side effect of iron sulfate is GI upset. Although taking iron with meals will diminish GI upset, food can decrease the absorption of iron by as much as 70%. Furthermore, antacids should not be taken with iron because they also reduce absorption of the mineral. It is recommended that iron preparations be administered one hour before or two hours after a meal. However, if the client experiences major gastric irritation, the iron may be taken with meals. Clients should be advised that iron preparations may darken stools, and that this is a harmless side effect. Excessive doses of iron are very toxic and clients should be advised to take their medication exactly as directed.

TABLE 26.2	Minerals		
MAJOR MINERALS	**RECOMMENDED DAILY INTAKE**	**TRACE MINERALS**	**RECOMMENDED DAILY INTAKE**
calcium	1–1.2 g	chromium	50–200 mcg
chloride	750 mg	copper	1.5–3 mg
magnesium	men: 420 mg women: 320 mg	fluoride	1.5–4 mg
phosphorous	700 mg	iodide	150 mcg
potassium	2.0 g	iron	men: 10 mg women: 15 mg
sodium	500 mg	manganese	2–5 mg
sulfur	not established	molybdenum	75–250 mg
		selenium	men: 70 mcg women: 55 mcg
		zinc	

Women at high risk of osteoporosis are advised to consume extra calcium, either in their diet or as a supplement.

Certain drugs affect mineral metabolism. For example, clients taking loop or thiazide diuretics are usually advised to add potassium to their diets. Corticosteroids, oral contraceptives, and a number of other drugs can produce sodium retention. The uptake of iodine by the thyroid gland can be impaired by certain oral hypoglycemics and lithium carbonate (Eskalith). Oral contraceptives have been reported to lower the plasma levels of zinc and increase those of copper.

Concept review 26.2

■ What is the difference between a vitamin and a mineral?

HERBS AND DIETARY SUPPLEMENTS

In recent years, the number of people seeking alternatives to conventional medical therapies has increased exponentially. Many herbs possess healing properties and are used by clients as supplements to traditional pharmacotherapy.

26.6 Natural products obtained from plants have been used as medicines for thousands of years.

Technically, an herb is a botanical without any woody tissue such as stems or bark. Over time, the terms *botanical* and *herb* have come to be used interchangeably to refer to any plant product with some useful application either as a food enhancer, such as flavoring, or as a medicine.

The healing properties of botanicals have been recorded for thousands of years. One of the earliest recorded uses of plant products was a prescription for garlic in 3000 BC. Eastern and Western medicine have recorded thousands of herbs and herb combinations reputed to have therapeutic value. Some of the most popular herbal remedies and their primary uses are shown in Table 26.3

TABLE 26.3	Popular Medicinal Herbs	
COMMON NAME	**MEDICINAL PART**	**PRIMARY USE(S)**
aloe	juice from the leaves	Skin ailments (topical); treatment of constipation (oral).
astragalus	roots	Enhance immune function; antioxidant; antiviral; improve cardiac function.
black cohosh	roots	Relief of menopausal symptoms.
dong quai	root, leaves, and fruit	Relief of menstrual and menopausal symptoms.
echinacea	entire plant	Enhance immune system; anti-inflammatory.
feverfew	leaves	Prevent or relieve migraine headaches; arthritis; allergies.
garlic	bulbs	Reduce blood cholesterol; reduce blood pressure; anticoagulation.
ginger	root	Relief of GI upset; motion sickness; anti-inflammatory.
gingko	leaves and seeds	Improve memory; reduce dizziness.
ginseng	root	Relieve stress; enhance immune system; decrease fatigue.
goldenseal	rhizome and roots	Anti-infective; anti-inflammatory.
kava kava	rhizome	Reduce stress; promote sleep.
ma huang (Ephedra)	young shoots, rhizomes, and roots	Reduce bronchospasm; increase energy; antitussive.
saw palmetto	ripe fruit/berries	Relieve urinary problems related to prostate enlargement.
St. John's wort	flowers, leaves, stems	Reduce depression; reduce anxiety; anti-inflammatory.
valerian root	roots	Relieve stress; promote sleep.

With the birth of the pharmaceutical industry in the late 1800s, the interest in herbal medicine began to wane. Synthetic drugs could be standardized and produced more cheaply than natural herbal products. Beginning in the 1970s and continuing to the present, alternative therapies and herbal medicine have experienced a remarkable resurgence, such that the majority adult Americans are either currently taking botanicals on a regular basis or have taken them in the past. This increase in popularity has been the result of a number of factors, including increased availability of herbal products, aggressive marketing by the herbal industry, an increased attention to natural alternatives, and a renewed interest in preventive medicine. In addition, the high cost of prescription medicines has driven clients to seek less expensive alternatives.

26.7 Herbal products are available in a variety of formulations.

The pharmacologically active chemicals in an herbal product may be present in only one specific part of the plant, or in all parts. For example, the active chemicals in chamomile are in the aboveground portion such as the leaves, stems, or flowers. For other herbs, such as ginger, the underground rhizomes and roots are used for their healing properties. In collecting herbs for home use, it is essential to know which portion of the plant contains the active chemicals.

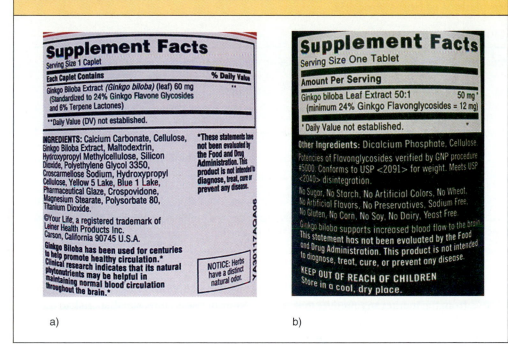

FIGURE 26.2A AND B

Photograph of two Ginkgo biloba labels. Note lack of standardization: a) 60 mg of extract, 24% Ginkgo Flavone Glycosides and 6% terpenes and b) 50:1 Ginkgo Leaf Extract, 24% Ginkgo Flavinoglycosides

Most medications contain only one active chemical. This chemical can be standardized and measured, and the amount of drug received by the client is precisely known. It is a common misunderstanding that herbs also contain one active ingredient, which can be extracted and delivered to clients in precise doses, like drugs. Herbs, however, may contain dozens of active chemicals, many of which have not yet been isolated, studied, or even identified. It is possible that many of these substances work together synergistically and may not have the same activity if isolated. Furthermore, the strength of an herbal preparation may vary depending upon where it was grown and how it was collected and stored. Some attempts have been made to standardize herbal products, using a marker substance such as the percent flavones in ginkgo or the percent lactones in kava kava. An example is shown in Figure 26.2. Until science can better characterize these substances, however, it is best to conceptualize the active ingredient of an herb as being the herb itself.

The two basic formulations of herbal products are solid and liquid. Solid products include pills, tablets, and capsules made from the dried herbs. Sometimes, solid products are salves and ointments that are administered topically. Liquid formulations are made by extracting the active chemicals from the plant using solvents such as water, alcohol, or glycerol. The liquids are then concentrated in various strengths for ingestion. The various liquid formulations of herbal preparations are described in Table 26.4. Figure 26.3 illustrates some of the formulations of ginkgo biloba, one of the most popular herbals.

26.8 Herbal products and dietary supplements are regulated by the Dietary Supplement Health and Education Act of 1994.

Since the passage of the Food, Drug, and Cosmetic Act in 1936, Americans have come to expect that all approved prescription and OTC drugs have passed rigid standards of safety prior to being marketed. Furthermore, it is expected that these drugs have been tested for efficacy and that they truly provide the medical benefits claimed by the manufacturer. Americans cannot and should not expect the same quality standards for herbal products. These products are regulated by a far less rigorous law, the Dietary Supplement Health and Education Act of 1994 (DSHEA).

According to the DSHEA, "dietary supplements" are exempted from the Food, Drug, and Cosmetic Act. Dietary supplements are defined as products intended to enhance or supplement the diet, such as botanicals, vitamins, minerals, or any other extract or metabolite that is not already

TABLE 26.4	Liquid Formulations of Herbal Products
PRODUCT	**DESCRIPTION**
tea	Fresh or dried herbs are soaked in hot water for 5–10 minutes before ingestion; convenient.
infusion	Fresh or dried herbs are soaked in hot water for long periods, at least 15 minutes; stronger than teas.
decoction	Fresh or dried herbs are boiled in water for 30–60 minutes until much of the liquid has boiled off; very concentrated.
tincture	Extraction of active ingredients using alcohol by soaking the herb; alcohol remains as part of the liquid.
extract	Extraction of active ingredients using organic solvents to form a highly concentrated liquid or solid form; solvent may be removed or be part of the final product.

approved as a drug by the FDA. One strength of the legislation is that it gives the FDA the power to remove from the market any product that poses a "significant or unreasonable" risk to the public. It also requires these products to be clearly labeled as "dietary supplements." An example of an herbal label for black cohosh is shown in Figure 26.4

Unfortunately, the DSHEA has several significant flaws that lead to a lack of standardization in the herbal industry and to less protection of the consumer.

- Dietary supplements do not have to be tested prior to marketing.
- Efficacy does not have to be demonstrated by the manufacturer.
- The manufacturer does not have to prove the safety of the dietary supplement. If it is to be removed from the market, the government has to prove that the dietary supplement is unsafe.
- Dietary supplements must state that the product is not intended to diagnose, treat, cure, or prevent any disease. However, the label may make claims about the products effect on body structure and function, such as the following:
  • helps promote healthy immune systems
  • reduces anxiety and stress
  • helps to maintain cardiovascular function
  • may reduce pain and inflammation
- The DSHEA does not regulate the accuracy of the label; the product may or may not contain the product listed, in the amounts claimed.

FIGURE 26.3	
Photograph of three different Ginkgo Formulations: tea bags, liquid extract and tablets	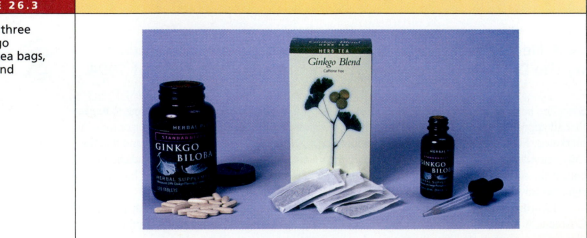

FIGURE 26.4A AND B

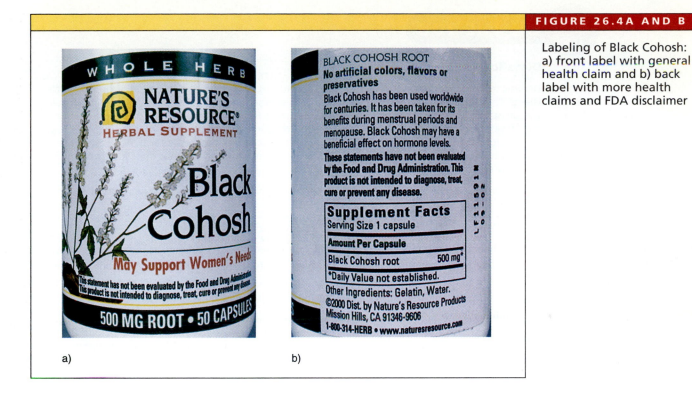

a)

b)

Labeling of Black Cohosh:
a) front label with general
health claim and b) back
label with more health
claims and FDA disclaimer

Concept review 26.3

▪ How does the federal regulation of drugs differ from that of herbal supplements?

26.9 Herbs may have important pharmacologic actions and result in adverse effects.

A key concept to remember when dealing with alternative therapies is that "natural" is not synonymous with "better" or "safe." There is no question that some botanicals contain active chemicals as powerful—and perhaps more effective—than currently approved medications. Thousands of years of experience combined with current medical research have shown that some of these herbal remedies have actions that are therapeutic. Because a substance comes from a natural product, however, does not make it safe or effective. For example, poison ivy is natural but it certainly is neither safe nor therapeutic. Natural products may not offer an improvement over conventional therapy in treating certain disorders and, indeed, may be of no value whatsoever. Furthermore, a client who substitutes an unproven alternative therapy for an established, effective medical treatment may delay healing and suffer irreparable harmful effects.

Some herbal products contain ingredients that can interact with prescription drugs. When obtaining medical histories, healthcare providers should include questions on the use of dietary supplements. Clients taking medications with potentially serious adverse effects such as insulin, warfarin (Coumadin), or digoxin (Lanoxin) should be warned never to take any herbal product without first discussing their needs with a healthcare practitioner.

Another warning that must be heeded with natural products is to beware of allergic reactions. Most herbal products contain a mixture of ingredients, many of which have not been identified. It is not unusual to find dozens of different chemicals in teas and infusions made from the flowers, leaves, or roots of a plant. Clients who have known allergies to food products or medicines should seek medical advice before taking a new herbal product. It is always wise to take the smallest amount possible when starting herbal therapy—even less than the recommended dose—to see if allergies or other adverse effects occur.

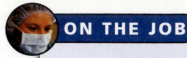

ON THE JOB

Dietetic Technician

Dietetic technicians play an important role in performing nutritional assessment and counseling for clients. They are trained to identify nutritional problems and provide patient education that can help the client deal with her or his disease more effectively. In some environments, dietetic technicians may develop menus, supervise food service personnel, purchase food, and monitor food quality. Typical employment locations include hospitals, long-term care facilities, restaurants, and schools. Educational training for dietetic technicians is usually two years in length and is offered at community and technical colleges. ■

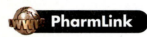

PharmLink

HERB RESEARCH FOUNDATION

All healthcare providers have an obligation to seek the latest medical information on herbal products, as there is a good possibility that their clients are using them to supplement prescription medicines. Clients should be advised to be skeptical of claims on the labels of dietary supplements and to seek their health information from reputable sources. Healthcare providers should never condemn a client's use of alternative medicines, but instead should be supportive and seek to understand the patient's goals for taking the supplements. The healthcare provider will often need to educate the client on the role of alternative therapies in the treatment of his or her disorder and discuss which treatment or combination of treatments will best meet his or her health goals.

CLIENT TEACHING

Clients treated with vitamins, minerals, or herbs need to know the following:

1. Liquid iron preparations can stain teeth. Dilute these solutions with juice or water and rinse the mouth after taking the medication to reduce staining.

2. If you are receiving regular monthly injections of vitamin B_{12}, do not take additional oral supplements of vitamin B_{12} or folic acid without the advice of your healthcare provider.

3. Do not take more than the recommended doses of any vitamin or mineral without first checking with your healthcare provider. While small amounts of these substances are beneficial, large amounts may be dangerous.

4. Rather than self-medicate with expensive vitamin, mineral, or herbal supplements, examine your diet and add foods that naturally supply these substances. See a dietician for advice, particularly if you have special needs such as pregnancy or diabetes.

5. When starting a new herbal supplement, always begin with the lowest possible dose and observe for possible side effects.

6. If you are taking prescription medicines, have chronic illness, or are pregnant, consult with your healthcare provider before initiating herbal therapies.

7. If you are taking calcium supplements, avoid foods with high zinc or oxalate content, as these may interfere with absorption. These foods include nuts, peas, beans, spinach, and soy products.

8. Niacin, or vitamin B_3, is also effective at lowering lipid levels. The dose for lowering cholesterol, however, is two to three grams per day whereas the vitamin dose is only 25 mg per day.

9. When giving a medical or drug history to your physician or dentist, always report vitamins, minerals, herbs, or dietary supplements that you are taking on a regular basis. If you have known allergies to any herbs or dietary supplements, be sure to report these also. ■

CHAPTER REVIEW

 Core Concepts Summary

26.1 Vitamins are organic substances that are needed in small amounts to promote growth and maintain health.

With one exception, vitamins cannot be synthesized by the body and thus must be provided in the diet. Although only very small amounts of vitamins are needed, lack of sufficient quantity will result in disease.

26.2 Vitamins are classified as fat-soluble or water-soluble.

Water-soluble vitamins include vitamin C and the B vitamins. Fat-soluble vitamins include vitamins A, D, E, and K. Water soluble vitamins cannot be stored and must be ingested daily, whereas excess fat-soluble vitamins can be stored for later use.

26.3 Failure to meet the recommended dietary allowances (RDAs) for vitamins may result in deficiency disorders.

RDA values represent the minimum amount of vitamin or mineral needed to prevent a deficiency in a healthy adult. These values must be adjusted for changes in health status, such as athletic training, pregnancy, or chronic disease.

26.4 Vitamin therapy is indicated for only very specific conditions.

Most clients do not need vitamin supplementation and excess intake may lead to hypervitaminosis. Indications for vitamin therapy include alcoholism, pregnancy or breast-feeding, chronic kidney or liver disease, therapy with certain drugs that affect vitamin metabolism, and reduced food intake in elderly clients.

26.5 Minerals are inorganic substances needed in very small amounts to maintain normal body metabolism.

Like vitamins, most clients receive all the minerals they need through a balanced diet. Certain conditions such as osteoporosis or iron-deficiency anemia do warrant mineral therapy.

26.6 Natural products obtained from plants have been used as medicines for thousands of years.

Thousands of herbal therapies are recorded in Eastern and Western history. The popularity of alternative, herbal remedies has increased in recent years.

26.7 Herbal products are available in a variety of formulations.

Unlike drugs, herbs contain a large number of chemicals that may act synergistically to produce a therapeutic effect. The active ingredients may be in the flowers, stems, or roots of an herb. Formulations include tablets, capsules, teas, or extracts.

26.8 Herbal products and dietary supplements are regulated by the Dietary Supplement Health and Education Act of 1994.

The DSHEA loosely regulates herbal and dietary supplements. Dietary supplements and herbal products can be marketed without any proof that they are safe or effective. They do not have to be tested prior to marketing. Their labels may contain statements that are inaccurate.

26.9 Herbs may have important pharmacologic actions and result in adverse effects.

A substance that comes from a natural product is not necessarily safe or effective. Although botanicals may have therapeutic applications, they may not be the best product for the disease and may interact with prescription medicines.

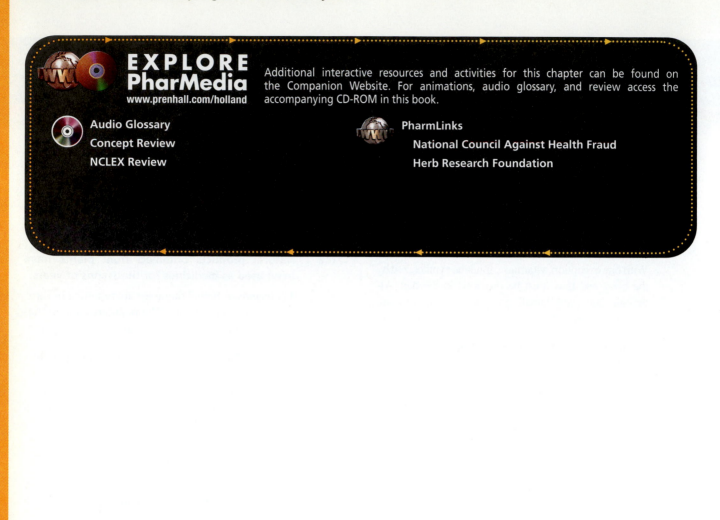

EXPLORE
PharMedia
www.prenhall.com/holland

Additional interactive resources and activities for this chapter can be found on the Companion Website. For animations, audio glossary, and review access the accompanying CD-ROM in this book.

Audio Glossary
Concept Review
NCLEX Review

PharmLinks
National Council Against Health Fraud
Herb Research Foundation

27 Drugs for Kidney, Acid-Base, and Electrolyte Disorders

CORE CONCEPTS

27.1 The kidneys regulate fluid volume, electrolytes, acids, and bases.

27.2 As filtrate travels through the nephron, its composition changes dramatically as a result of the processes of reabsorption and secretion.

Diuretics

27.3 Most diuretics act by blocking sodium reabsorption in the nephron.

27.4 The most efficacious diuretics are those that affect the loop of Henle.

27.5 The thiazides are the most widely prescribed class of diuretics.

27.6 Although less efficacious than the loop diuretics, potassium-sparing diuretics may help prevent hypokalemia.

27.7 Several less commonly prescribed diuretics have specific indications.

Acid-Base Agents

27.8 Acids and bases can be administered to maintain normal body pH.

Electrolytes

27.9 Electrolytes are charged substances that play an important role in body chemistry.

FLUID-EXPANDING AGENTS

27.10 Intravenous fluid therapy using crystalloids and colloids is used to replace lost fluids.

OBJECTIVES

After reading this chapter, the student should be able to:

1. Describe the general structure and functions of the urinary system.

2. Compare and contrast the three major classes of diuretics.

3. Identify common causes of alkalosis and acidosis and the drugs used to treat these disorders.

4. Describe conditions in which therapy with IV fluids may be indicated.

5. Explain the importance of electrolyte balance in the body.

6. Identify causes of potassium imbalance and the drugs used to treat these conditions.

7. Compare and contrast colloids and crystalloids used in IV therapy.

8. For each of the following classes, identify representative drugs, explain the mechanism of drug action, primary actions, and important adverse effects

    a. loop diuretics
    b. thiazide diuretics
    c. potassium-sparing diuretics
    d. acidic agents
    e. basic agents
    f. electrolytes
    g. colloids
    h. crystalloids

9. Categorize drugs used in the treatment of urinary system, acid-base, fluid, and electrolyte disorders based on their classification and mechanism of action.

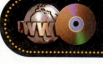

PharMedia
www.prenhall.com/holland

Additional interactive resources and activities for this chapter can be found on the Companion Website. For animations, audio glossary, and review access the accompanying CD-ROM in this book.

acidosis (ah-sid-OH-sis): condition of having too many acids; plasma pH below 7.35 / *page 435*

aldosterone (al-DOH-stair-own): hormone secreted by the adrenal cortex that increases sodium reabsorption in the distal tubule of the kidney / *page 433*

alkalosis (al-kah-LOH-sis): condition of having too many bases; plasma pH above 7.45 / *page 435*

anions (an-EYE-ons): negatively charged ions / *page 436*

Bowman's capsule: portion of the nephron that filters blood and receives the filtrate from the glomerulus / *page 428*

carbonic anhydrase (kar-BON-ik an-HY-drase): enzyme that forms carbonic acid by combining carbon dioxide and water / *page 434*

cations (KAT-eye-ons): positively charged ions / *page 436*

colloids (KAHL-oyds): type of IV solution consisting of large organic molecules that are unable to cross membranes / *page 438*

crystalloids (KRIS-tall-oyds): type of IV solution resembling blood plasma minus proteins that is capable of crossing membranes / *page 438*

distal tubule: portion of the nephron that collects filtrate from the loop of Henle / *page 428*

diuretic (dye-your-ET-ik): drug that increases urine output / *page 430*

electrolytes (ee-LEK-troh-lites): small, charged ions / *page 436*

filtrate (FIL-trate): fluid in the nephron that is filtered at Bowman's capsule / *page 428*

hyperkalemia (HY-purr-kay-LEE-mee-ah): high potassium levels in the blood / *page 433*

hypokalemia (hy-poh-kay-LEE-mee-uh): low potassium levels in the blood / *page 431*

loop of Henle (HEN-lee): portion of the nephron between the proximal and distal tubules / *page 428*

osmotic pressure (oz-MOT-ik): force exerted when there is an imbalance of solutes on each side of a semipermeable membrane / *page 438*

nephron (NEF-ron): functional unit of the kidney / *page 428*

pH: a measure of the acidity or alkalinity of a solution / *page 435*

proximal tubule (PROX-im-al): portion of the nephron that collects filtrate from Bowman's capsule / *page 428*

reabsorption: movement of substances from the kidney tubule back into the blood / *page 430*

secretion: movement of substances from the blood into the kidney tubule after filtration has occurred / *page 430*

Maintaining proper fluid volume, electrolyte composition, and acid-base balance are essential to life. Conditions such as hemorrhage and dehydration must be treated quickly, otherwise fluids and electrolytes will be rapidly depleted. Disorders of acid-base balance may occur quickly as in diabetics or may proceed more slowly, over a period of months. Fortunately, safe, effective drugs are available to rapidly reverse most symptoms of fluid volume, electrolyte, or acid-base imbalance.

Fast Facts Renal Disorders

- Over 12,000 kidney transplants were performed in 1999.
- Over 47,000 people are currently on a waiting list for kidney transplants.
- One out of every 750 people is born with a single kidney. A single kidney is larger and more vulnerable to injury from heavy contact sports.
- Urinary tract infection (UTI) is more common in women: 20–30% of females experience recurrent infections.
- About 260,000 Americans suffer from chronic kidney failure and 50,000 die annually from causes related to the disease.
- Type 2 diabetes is the leading cause of chronic kidney failure, accounting for 30 to 40% of all new cases each year.
- Hypertension is the second leading cause of chronic kidney failure, accounting for about 25% of all new cases each year.

27.1 The kidneys regulate fluid volume, electrolytes, acids, and bases.

When most people think of the kidneys, they think of excretion. While this is certainly true, the kidneys have many other homeostatic functions. The kidneys are the primary organs for regulating fluid balance, electrolyte composition, and acid-base balance of body fluids. They also secrete the enzyme renin, which helps to regulate blood pressure (Chapter 14 ⬤▭) and erythropoietin,

FIGURE 27.1

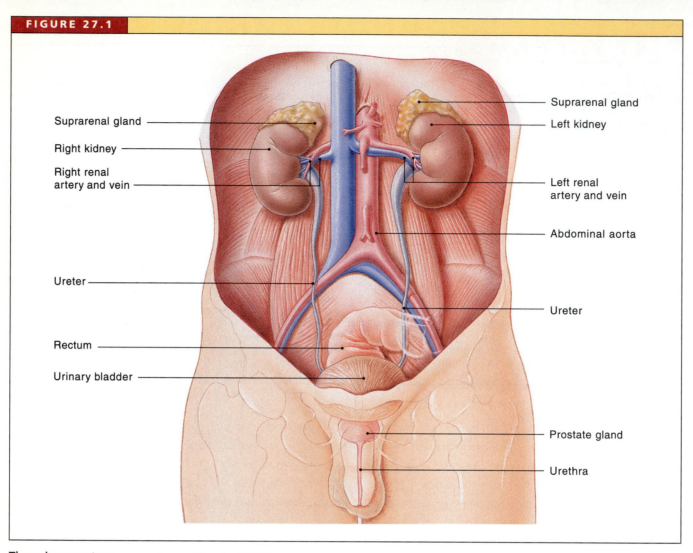

Suprarenal gland

Right kidney

Right renal
artery and vein

Ureter

Rectum

Urinary bladder

Suprarenal gland

Left kidney

Left renal
artery and vein

Abdominal aorta

Ureter

Prostate gland

Urethra

The urinary system   *SOURCE: Pearson Education/PH College.*

a hormone that stimulates red blood cell production. In addition, the kidneys are responsible for the production of calcitriol, the active form of vitamin D, that helps maintain bone homeostasis (Chapter 30 ⌸). It is not surprising that the overall health of the client is strongly dependent upon proper functioning of the kidneys.

The urinary system consists of two kidneys, two ureters, one urinary bladder, and a urethra. These structures are shown in Figure 27.1. Each kidney contains over a million **nephrons**, the functional units of the kidney. As blood enters a nephron, it is filtered through a semipermeable membrane known as **Bowman's capsule**. Water and other small molecules readily pass through Bowman's capsule and enter the first section of the nephron called the **proximal tubule**. Once in the nephron, the fluid is called **filtrate**. After leaving the proximal tubule, the filtrate travels through the **loop of Henle** and, subsequently, the **distal tubule**. Nephrons empty their filtrate into tubes called *common collecting ducts,* and then into larger and larger collecting portions inside the kidney. Fluid leaving the collecting ducts and entering subsequent portions of the kidney is called *urine.* The parts of the nephron are illustrated in Figure 27.2.

Concept review 27.1

■ How does the composition of filtrate differ from that of blood?

FIGURE 27.2

The nephron

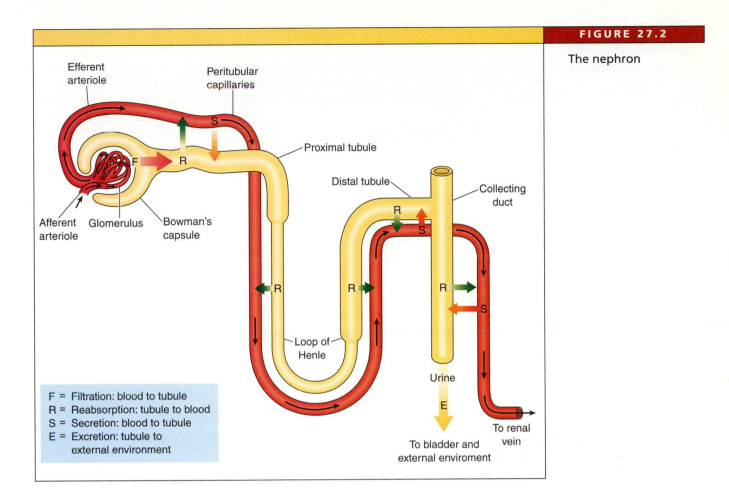

Efferent arteriole

Peritubular capillaries

Proximal tubule

Distal tubule

Collecting duct

Afferent arteriole Glomerulus Bowman's capsule

Loop of Henle

Urine

To renal vein

To bladder and external enviroment

F = Filtration: blood to tubule
R = Reabsorption: tubule to blood
S = Secretion: blood to tubule
E = Excretion: tubule to
    external environment

27.2 As filtrate travels through the nephron, its composition changes dramatically as a result of the processes of reabsorption and secretion.

When filtrate passes through Bowman's capsule, its composition is the same as plasma minus blood proteins, such as albumin, that are too large to pass through the filter. As it travels through

NATURAL ALTERNATIVES

Saw Palmetto for Urinary and Prostate Disorders

Saw palmetto is obtained from the sable palm *Serenoa repens,* which grows in the southeastern United States. The active ingredients come from the ripe berries that contain a number of sterols and alcoholic compounds. Some of these compounds are antiestrogenic, blocking estrogen receptors. Preparations include dried berries, capsules, and tincture. A tea is available but not common, as the taste and smell of saw palmetto is unpleasant.

Saw palmetto has an interesting pharmacologic history. The berries were used by Native Americans as food, not medicines. During the 19th century, saw palmetto berry extract was listed in the National Formulary, an official list of approved treatments, but was removed in 1950. As the population aged and prostate disorders became more widely recognized, saw palmetto gained popularity.

Perhaps the most widespread use of saw palmetto is in the treatment of benign prostatic hypertrophy (BPH). When used in clients with BPH, saw palmetto stimulates urinary flow, reduces painful urination, and decreases nocturia. The extract is purported to reduce swelling of the prostate. Other indications include cold, flu, cough, inflammation, and asthma. ▪

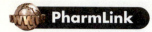

the nephron, the composition of filtrate changes dramatically. Some substances in the filtrate pass across the walls of the nephron to reenter the blood, a process known as reabsorption. Water is the most important molecule reabsorbed in the tubule. For every 47 gallons of water entering the filtrate each day, 45.5 gallons are reabsorbed, leaving only 1.5 liters to be excreted in the urine. Glucose, amino acids, and essential substances such as sodium, chloride, calcium, and bicarbonate are also reabsorbed.

Certain ions and some molecules too large to pass through Bowman's capsule can still enter the urine by crossing from the blood to the filtrate using a process known as secretion. Potassium, phosphate, hydrogen, and ammonium ions and many organic acids enter the filtrate through this mechanism.

Reabsorption and secretion are critical to the pharmacokinetics of many drugs. Some drugs are reabsorbed, whereas others are secreted into the filtrate. For example, approximately 90% of a dose of penicillin G enters the urine through secretion. The processes of reabsorption and secretion are shown in Figure 27.2.

DIURETICS

Diuretics are medications that adjust the volume and/or composition of body fluids. They are of particular value in the treatment of hypertension and for removing edema fluid in clients with heart failure.

27.3 Most diuretics act by blocking sodium reabsorption in the nephron.

dia = thoroughly
uretic = to urinate

A diuretic is a drug that increases urine output. Mobilizing excess fluid in the body for the purpose of excretion is particularly desirable in the following conditions.

- hypertension (Chapter 14 ⬤▬⬤)
- heart failure (Chapter 15 ⬤▬⬤)
- kidney failure
- liver failure or cirrhosis

Most diuretics act by blocking sodium reabsorption in the nephron, thus sending more of this ion to the urine. Chloride ion (Cl⁻) follows sodium. Because water molecules also tend to stay with sodium ions, blocking the reabsorption of sodium will keep more water in the filtrate. The more water retained in the filtrate, the greater the volume of urination, or diuresis. Some drugs, like furosemide (Lasix), act by preventing the reabsorption of sodium in the loop of Henle. Because there is an abundance of sodium in the loop of Henle, furosemide is capable of producing large increases in urine output. Other drugs, such as the thiazides, act on the distal tubule. Because most sodium has already been reabsorbed from the filtrate by the time it reaches this point in the nephron, the thiazides generally produce less diuresis than furosemide. The sites at which the various diuretics act are shown in Figure 27.3.

27.4 The most efficacious diuretics are those that affect the loop of Henle.

The most effective diuretics are called *loop* or *high-ceiling diuretics*. The drugs in this class act by blocking the reabsorption of sodium and chloride in the loop of Henle. When given IV, they have the ability to move large amounts of fluid through the kidney in a very short time

FIGURE 27.3

Sites of action of the diuretics

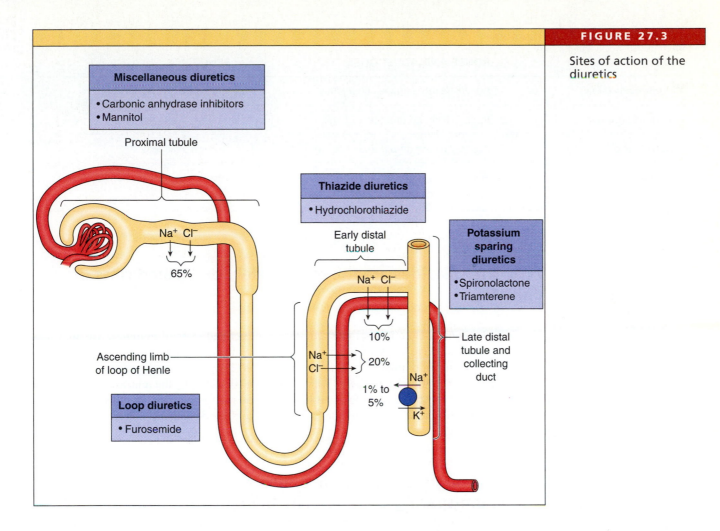

period. Loop diuretics are used to reduce the edema associated with heart failure, hepatic cirrhosis, or chronic renal failure. Furosemide (Lasix) and torsemide (Demadex) are also approved for hypertension.

Furosemide is the most commonly prescribed loop diuretic. A drug profile for furosemide was given in Chapter 15. Unlike the thiazide diuretics, furosemide is able to increase urine output even when blood flow to the kidneys is diminished. Torsemide (Demadex) has a longer half-life than furosemide, which offers the advantage of once-a-day dosing. Bumetamide (Bumex) is 40 times more potent than furosemide, but has a shorter duration of action.

The rapid excretion of large amounts of water may produce a number of adverse effects such as dehydration and electrolyte imbalances. Signs of dehydration include thirst, dry mouth, weight loss, and headache. Hypotension, dizziness, and even fainting can result from the fluid loss. Excess potassium loss, known as hypokalemia, may result in dysrhythmias, and potassium supplements may be indicated. Potassium loss is of particular concern to clients who are also taking digoxin (Lanoxin). Although rare, ototoxicity is possible. Because of the potential for serious side effects, the loop diuretics are normally reserved for clients with moderate to severe fluid retention, or when other diuretics have failed. Information on the loop diuretics is given in Table 27.1.

de = not/without
hydration = water

Concept review 27.2

- Why are drugs that block sodium reabsorption at the loop of Henle more efficacious than those that act on the distal tubule?

TABLE 27.1	Loop Diuretics	
DRUG	**ROUTE AND ADULT DOSE**	**REMARKS**
furosemide (Lasix)	PO; 20–80 mg qd (max 600 mg/day).	IV and IM forms available.
bumetanide (Bumex)	PO; 0.5–2 mg qd (max 10 mg/day).	IV form available.
ethacrynic acid (Edecrin)	PO; 50–100 mg qd-bid (max 400 mg/day).	IV form available.
torsemide (Demadex)	PO; 4–20 mg qd.	Also for hepatic cirrhosis; IV form available.

27.5 The thiazides are the most widely prescribed class of diuretics.

The thiazides comprise the largest, most commonly prescribed class of diuretics. The thiazides act on the distal tubule to block sodium reabsorption and increase water excretion. Their primary use is for the treatment of mild to moderate hypertension. They are less efficacious than the loop diuretics and are not effective in clients with severe renal disease. All the thiazide diuretics have equivalent efficacy. Other than ototoxicity, the side effects of the thiazides are identical to those of the loop diuretics, though their frequency is less. The thiazide and thiazide-like diuretics are listed in Table 27.2.

27.6 Although less efficacious than the loop diuretics, potassium-sparing diuretics may help prevent hypokalemia.

One of the most serious potential adverse effects of the thiazide and loop diuretics is potassium loss. The potassium-sparing diuretics are able to produce a mild diuresis without affecting blood potassium levels.

Normally, sodium and potassium are exchanged in the distal tubule; Na^+ is reabsorbed back into the body and K^+ is secreted into the tubule. Potassium-sparing diuretics block this exchange, caus-

DRUG PROFILE:
Chlorothiazide (Diuril)

Actions:

Chlorothiazide is commonly prescribed for mild to moderate hypertension and may be combined with other antihypertensives in the treatment of severe hypertension. It is also used to treat edema due to heart failure, liver disease, and corticosteroid or estrogen therapy. When given orally, it may take as long as four weeks to obtain the optimum therapeutic effect. When given IV, results are seen in 15 to 30 minutes.

Adverse Effects:

Excess loss of water and electrolytes can occur. Symptoms may include thirst, weakness, lethargy, muscle cramping, hypotension, or tachycardia. Due to the potentially serious consequences of hypokalemia, clients concurrently taking digoxin should be carefully monitored. The intake of potassium-rich foods should be increased and potassium supplements may be indicated.

TABLE 27.2	Thiazide and Thiazide-like Diuretics	
DRUG	**ROUTE AND ADULT DOSE**	**REMARKS**
(Pr) hydrochlorothiazide (Hydrodiuril, HCTZ)	PO; 12.5–100 mg qd-tid.	Short-acting.
bendroflumethiazide (Naturetin)	PO; 2.5–20 mg qd-bid.	Intermediate-acting.
benzthiazide (Aquatag, Exna, Hydrex)	PO; 25–200 mg qd or qod.	Intermediate-acting.
(Pr) chlorothiazide (Diuril)	PO; 250–500 mg qd-bid.	IV form available; short-acting.
chlorthalidone (Hygroton)	PO; 50–100 mg qd.	Thiazide-like; long-acting.
hydroflumethiazide (Diucardin, Saluron)	PO; 25–100 mg qd-bid.	Intermediate-acting.
indapamide (Lozol)	PO; 2.5–5 mg qd.	Thiazide-like; long-acting.
methylclothiazide (Aquatensin, Enduron)	PO; 2.5–10 mg qd.	Long-acting.
metolazone (Zaroxolyn, Mykrox)	PO; 5–20 mg qd.	Thiazide-like; intermediate-acting.
polythiazide (Renese)	PO; 1–4 mg qd.	Long-acting.
quinethazone (Hydromox)	PO; 50–100 mg qd.	Thiazide-like; intermediate-acting.
trichlormethiazide (Metahydrin, Naqua, Niazide, Diurese)	PO; 1–4 mg qd-bid.	Long-acting.

ing sodium to stay in the tubule and ultimately leave through the urine. When sodium is blocked, the body retains more K^+. Because most of the sodium has already been removed by the time the filtrate reaches the distal tubule, potassium-sparing diuretics produce only a mild diuresis and are usually used in combination with thiazide or loop diuretics in order to minimize potassium loss.

Unlike the loop and thiazide diuretics, clients taking potassium-sparing diuretics should not take potassium supplements or be advised to add potassium-rich foods to their diet. Intake of excess potassium when taking these medications may lead to hyperkalemia.

DRUG PROFILE:
Spironolactone (Aldactone)

Actions:

Spironolactone acts by blocking sodium reabsorption in the distal tubule. It accomplishes this by inhibiting **aldosterone**. Aldosterone is a hormone secreted by the adrenal cortex that is responsible for increasing the renal reabsorption of sodium in exchange for potassium, thus causing water retention. When blocked by spironolactone, sodium and water excretion is increased and the body retains more potassium.

Adverse Effects:

Spironolactone does such an efficient job of retaining potassium that **hyperkalemia** may develop. The probability of hyperkalemia is increased if the client takes potassium supplements or is concurrently taking ACE inhibitors, as described in Chapter 14 ⬭ . Signs and symptoms of hyperkalemia include muscle weakness, ventricular tachycardia, or fibrillation. When potassium levels are monitored carefully and maintained within normal values, side effects from spironolactone are uncommon.

TABLE 27.3	Potassium-sparing Diuretics	
DRUG	**ROUTE AND ADULT DOSE**	**REMARKS**
Pr spironolactone (Aldactone)	PO; 25–400 mg qd-bid.	Often used in conjunction with other diuretics to increase the diuretic effect; monitor serum potassium level.
amiloride hydrochloride (Midamor)	PO; 5 mg qd (max 20 mg/day).	Monitor serum potassium level; use with caution in diabetics.
triamterene (Dyrenium)	PO; 100 mg bid (max 300 mg/day).	Monitor serum potassium levels; often causes elevated BUN.

27.7 Several less commonly prescribed diuretics have specific indications.

intra = within
ocular = eye

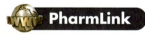

THE FLORIDA HEALTH SITE

A few diuretics cannot be classified as loop, thiazide, or potassium-sparing agents. These diuretics have very limited and specific indications. Three of these drugs inhibit carbonic anhydrase, an enzyme that affects acid-base balance by its ability to form carbonic acid from water and carbon dioxide. For example, acetazolamide (Diamox) is a carbonic anhydrase inhibitor used to decrease intraocular fluid pressure in clients with open-angle glaucoma (Chapter 32 ⬭). Unrelated to its diuretic effect, acetazolamide also has applications as an anticonvulsant and in treating motion sickness.

The osmotic diuretics also have very specific applications. For example, mannitol is used to maintain urine flow in clients with acute renal failure or during prolonged surgery. Mannitol can also be used to lower intraocular pressure in certain types of glaucoma. It is a very potent diuretic that is only given by the IV route. Table 27.4 lists some of the miscellaneous diuretics.

ACID-BASE AGENTS

Unless quickly corrected, acidosis and alkalosis can have serious or fatal consequences. Acidic and basic agents may be given to correct pH imbalances in body fluids.

TABLE 27.4	Miscellaneous Diuretics	
DRUG	**ROUTE AND ADULT DOSE**	**REMARKS**
Pr acetazolamide (Diamox)	PO; 250–375 mg qd in am.	Carbonic anhydrase inhibitor; IV form available.
dichlorphenamide (Daramide, Oratrol)	PO; 25–50 mg qd-tid.	Carbonic anhydrase inhibitor.
mannitol	IV; 100g infused over 2–6h.	Osmotic type.
methazolamide (Neptazane)	PO; 50–100 mg bid or tid.	Carbonic anhydrase inhibitor.
urea (Ureaphil)	IV; 1.0–1.5 g/kg over 1–2.5 hours.	Osmotic type.

TABLE 27.5	Causes of Alkalosis and Acidosis
ACIDOSIS	**ALKALOSIS**
Respiratory origins of acidosis ■ hypoventilation or shallow breathing ■ airway constriction ■ damage to respiratory center in medulla Metabolic origins of acidosis ■ severe diarrhea ■ kidney failure ■ diabetes mellitus ■ excess alcohol ingestion ■ starvation	Respiratory origin of alkalosis ■ hyperventilation due to asthma, anxiety, or high altitude Metabolic origins of alkalosis ■ constipation for prolonged periods ■ ingestion of excess sodium bicarbonate ■ diuretics that cause potassium depletion ■ severe vomiting

27.8 Acids and bases can be administered to maintain normal body pH.

The degree of acidity or alkalinity of a solution is measured by its pH. A pH of 7.0 is defined as neutral, above 7.0 as basic or alkaline, and below 7.0 as acidic. To maintain homeostasis, the pH of plasma and most body fluids must be kept within the very narrow range of 7.35 to 7.45. Nearly all proteins and enzymes in the body function within this range of pH values. At pH values above 7.45, alkalosis develops and symptoms of CNS stimulation occur that include nervousness and convulsions. Acidosis occurs below a pH of 7.35, and symptoms of CNS depression may result in coma. In either alkalosis or acidosis, death may result if large changes in pH are not corrected immediately. Common causes of alkalosis and acidosis are shown in Table 27.5.

alkal = basic
osis = condition

Alkalosis may be reversed by the administration of acidic agents such as IM or IV ammonium chloride. When this drug is metabolized in the liver, acid (H^+) is formed and the pH of body fluids decreases. Ammonium chloride will also acidify the urine, which is beneficial in treating many urinary tract infections and in promoting the excretion of alkaline drugs such as amphetamines. In less severe cases, the alkalosis may be corrected by administering sodium chloride combined with potassium chloride. This combination increases the renal excretion of bicarbonate ion (a base), which indirectly increases the acidity of the blood. The correction of acid-base imbalances is illustrated in Figure 27.4.

DRUG PROFILE:
Sodium Bicarbonate

Actions:

Acidosis is a more common event than alkalosis, occurring during shock, cardiac arrest, or diabetes mellitus. Sodium bicarbonate is the drug of choice for correcting acidosis: the bicarbonate ion (HCO_3) directly raises the pH of body fluids. Sodium bicarbonate may be given orally, if acidosis is mild, or IV, in cases of acute disease. Although sodium bicarbonate neutralizes gastric acid, it is rarely used to treat peptic ulcers due to its tendency to cause gas and gastric distension. After absorption, it makes the urine more basic, which aids in the renal excretion of acidic drugs such as the barbiturates and salicylates.

Adverse Effects:

Most of the side effects of sodium bicarbonate therapy are the result of metabolic alkalosis caused by too much bicarbonate ion. Symptoms may include confusion, irritability, slow respiration rate, and vomiting. Simply discontinuing the sodium bicarbonate infusion often reverses these symptoms; however, potassium chloride or ammonium chloride may be administered to reverse the alkalosis.

FIGURE 27.4

Acid-base imbalances

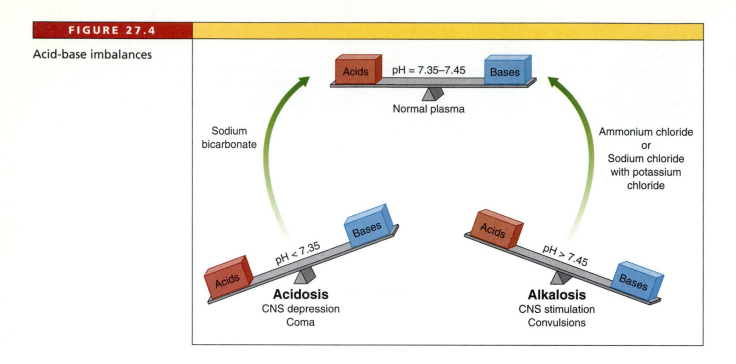

ELECTROLYTES

Electrolytes are small, charged molecules essential to homeostasis. Too little or too much of an electrolyte may result in serious disease and must be quickly corrected.

27.9 Electrolytes are charged substances that play an important role in body chemistry.

electro = *conducts electricity*
lyte = *solution*

In Chapter 26, the role of minerals in human physiology was discussed ⊂⊃. In certain body fluids, some of these minerals become ions and possess a charge. Small, inorganic molecules possessing a positive or negative charge are called electrolytes. Positively charged electrolytes are called cations; those with a negative charge are called anions. They are essential to many body functions, including nerve conduction, muscle contraction, and bone growth and remodeling. Too little or too much of an electrolyte can result in disease. The major body electrolytes and their deficit and excess states are listed in Table 27.6.

The most serious side effects of potassium chloride are related to accumulation of excess potassium. Hyperkalemia may occur if the client takes potassium supplements concurrently with

ON THE JOB

Medical Laboratory Technician

Laboratory tests are essential to the proper diagnosis of kidney, electrolyte, and acid-base disorders. Medical laboratory technicians are trained to perform a wide variety of tests on tissues and body fluids that help the physician make the proper diagnosis and provide the correct treatment to the client. Laboratory technicians learn to perform these tests using various methodologies and advanced computerized instruments. They help ensure that the equipment is properly standardized and functioning properly. Most are employed in hospital or large medical clinic settings. The usual educational preparation is a two-year associate degree. One-year certificate programs are also available. ▪

DRUG PROFILE:
Potassium Chloride

Actions:

Potassium is one of the most important electrolytes in body fluids, and levels must be maintained within a narrow range of values between 3.5 and 5.5 mEq/L. Too much or too little potassium may lead to serious consequences and must be immediately corrected. Neurons and muscle fibers are most sensitive to potassium loss. Muscle weakness, dysrhythmias, and cardiac arrest are possible consequences.

Therapy with loop or thiazide diuretics is the most common cause of potassium loss. Clients taking thiazide or loop diuretics are usually instructed to take oral potassium supplements in order to prevent hypokalemia. Severe vomiting or diarrhea, chronic stress, and lack of sufficient dietary intake may also lead to hypokalemia.

Potassium chloride is the drug of choice for treating or preventing hypokalemia. It is also used to treat mild forms of alkalosis. Dosage forms include oral and IV preparations. Oral forms include tablets, powders, and liquids, usually heavily flavored due to the unpleasant taste of the drug.

Adverse Effects:

Nausea and vomiting are common because potassium chloride irritates the GI mucosa. The drug may be taken with meals or antacids to lessen the gastric distress.

TABLE 27.6	Electrolytes		
	ION	EXCESS	DEFICIENCY
Cations			
calcium	Ca^{++}	hypercalcemia	hypocalcemia
magnesium	Mg^{++}	hypermagnesemia	hypomagnesemia
potassium	K^+	hyperkalemia	hypokalemia
sodium	Na^+	hypernatremia	hypokalemia
Anions			
bicarbonate	HCO_3^{--}	-	-
chloride	Cl^-	hyperchloremia	hypochloremia
phosphate	PO_4^- or HPO_4^{--}	hyperphosphatemia	hypophosphatemia
sulfate	SO_4^{--}	-	-

potassium-sparing diuretics. Some of the signs and symptoms of hyperkalemia are the same as hypokalemia: muscle weakness, dysrhythmias, and cardiac arrest. In mild cases of hyperkalemia, potassium levels may be returned to normal by eliminating the dietary sources of potassium or by reducing the dose of potassium chloride. In severe cases, serum potassium levels may be lowered by administering glucose and insulin, which cause potassium to leave the extracellular fluids and enter cells. Calcium salts may be given to counteract potential potassium toxicity on the heart, and sodium bicarbonate may be infused to correct any acidosis that may be concurrent with the hyperkalemia.

FLUID-EXPANDING AGENTS

Loss of fluids from the body can result in dehydration and shock. Fluid-expanding solutions are used to maintain blood volume and support blood pressure.

CORE CONCEPTS

27.10 Intravenous fluid therapy using crystalloids and colloids is used to replace lost fluids.

Intravenous fluid therapy is the replacement of water and ions that have been lost through hemorrhage, severe burns, diarrhea, vomiting, or inadequate fluid intake. In all these conditions, loss of water from the client has exceeded the intake of water. Shock, dehydration, or electrolyte loss may occur. Large fluid or electrolyte losses may be fatal; thus, IV fluid therapy is often initiated to quickly replace these lost substances.

Intravenous replacement fluids are of two basic types: colloids and crystalloids. **Colloids** are proteins or other large molecules that remain suspended in the blood for a long period of time because they are too large to cross membranes. While circulating, they draw water molecules from the cells and tissues into the blood vessels through their ability to increase **osmotic pressure**. These agents are sometimes called *plasma* or *volume expanders*. Examples of colloids include the following.

- plasma protein fraction (Plasmanate, PlasmaPlex, Plasmatein, PPF, Protenate)
- albumin (Albuminar, Albutein, Buminate, Plasbumin)
- dextran 40 (Gentran 40, Hyskon, Rheomacrodex) or dextran 70 (Macrodex)
- hetastarch (Hespan)

Crystalloids are IV solutions that contain electrolytes in concentrations resembling those of plasma. Unlike colloids, crystalloid solutions leave the blood and enter cells. They are used to replace fluids that have been lost and to promote urine output. Common crystalloids include the following.

- normal saline (0.9% sodium chloride)
- lactated Ringer's
- plasmalyte
- hypertonic saline (3% sodium chloride)
- 5% dextrose in water (D_5W)

Concept review 27.3

- How does a colloid IV fluid differ from a crystalloid?

CLIENT TEACHING

Clients treated for urinary, acid-base, and fluid disorders need to know the following:

1. When taking diuretics, drink plenty of water if dry mouth or thirst develops, unless otherwise directed by your healthcare practitioner.

2. Potassium chloride tablets are irritating to the GI mucosa and should be taken with food. Do not crush or suck the tablets. If nausea or heartburn occurs, take antacids along with the KCl.

3. To avoid nighttime diuresis, take diuretics at least two hours before bedtime.

4. If you are diabetic, monitor your blood sugar levels very closely when taking loop diuretics, as these drugs may elevate blood glucose.

5. Thiazide diuretics should not be taken during pregnancy or breast-feeding.

6. When taking loop or thiazide diuretics, increase your intake of potassium-rich foods such as dark, leafy vegetables, nuts, citrus fruits, bananas, and potatoes. If you are taking a potassium-sparing diuretic, avoid these foods unless otherwise instructed by your healthcare practitioner.

7. When taking diuretics, avoid caffeinated beverages. The diuretic effect of the caffeine combined with your prescription medication may cause dehydration. ■

CHAPTER REVIEW

 Core Concepts Summary

27.1   The kidneys regulate fluid volume, electrolytes, acids, and bases.

The kidneys are essential to the overall health of the client, controlling fluid volume, electrolyte composition, and acid-base balance. The functional unit of the kidney is the nephron.

27.2   As filtrate travels through the nephron, its composition changes dramatically as a result of the processes of reabsorption and secretion.

Filtrate entering the proximal tubule resembles plasma, without proteins. Through the processes of reabsorption and secretion, the filtrate composition changes to produce urine.

27.3   Most diuretics act by blocking sodium reabsorption in the nephron.

Diuretics are drugs that increase urine output, usually by blocking sodium reabsorption. Indications for diuretics include hypertension, heart failure, kidney failure, and liver disease.

27.4   The most efficacious diuretics are those that affect the loop of Henle.

The high-ceiling or loop diuretics such as furosemide act by blocking sodium reabsorption in the loop of Henle. They are the most efficacious diuretics, but may cause dehydration and electrolyte loss.

27.5   The thiazides are the most widely prescribed class of diuretics.

Though less effective than the loop diuretics, the thiazides are more frequently prescribed because of their lower incidence of serious side effects.

27.6   Though less efficacious than the loop diuretics, potassium-sparing diuretics may help prevent hypokalemia.

Potassium-sparing diuretics are less efficacious than the loop diuretics. Their primary advantage is that they do not cause potassium loss.

27.7 **Several less commonly prescribed diuretics have specific indications.**

Carbonic anhydrase inhibitors and osmotic diuretics are not commonly prescribed. They have specific applications, such as decreasing intraocular pressure and maintaining urine flow during renal failure.

27.8 **Acids and bases can be administered to maintain normal body pH.**

Ammonium chloride can be administered to quickly reverse alkalosis. Sodium chloride with potassium chloride can reverse alkalosis indirectly. Sodium bicarbonate is used to reverse acidosis.

27.9 **Electrolytes are charged substances that play an important role in body chemistry.**

Electrolyte imbalances can cause serious disease. Hypokalemia is a serious potential adverse effect of drug therapy with certain diuretics. Oral or IV potassium chloride can reverse symptoms of hypokalemia. Although less common, hyperkalemia may be just as serious and may be reversed by administration of glucose or insulin.

27.10 **Intravenous fluid therapy using crystalloids and colloids is used to replace lost fluids.**

Colloids are solutions such as Dextran and albumin that are used to expand plasma volume and maintain blood pressure. Crystalloids are fluids such as normal saline or lactated Ringer's that replace fluids and electrolytes that have been lost from cells and tissues.

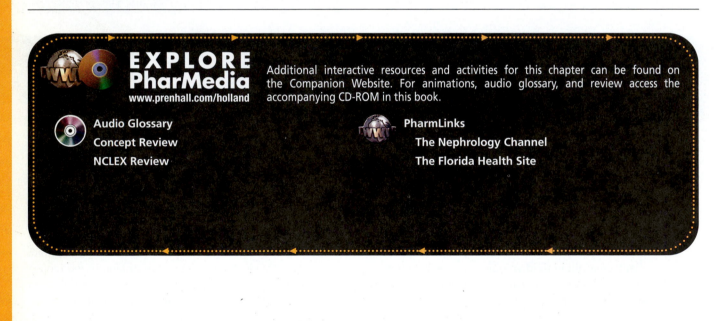

6

THE ENDOCRINE AND REPRODUCTIVE SYSTEMS

28 Drugs for Endocrine Disorders

CORE CONCEPTS

28.1 The endocrine system maintains homeostasis by using hormones as chemical messengers.

28.2 Hormones are used as replacement therapy, as antineoplastics, and for their natural, therapeutic effects.

28.3 The hypothalamus and the pituitary gland secrete hormones that control other endocrine organs.

28.4 Insulin and glucagon are secreted by the pancreas.

TYPE 1 DIABETES MELLITUS

Insulin

28.5 Type 1 diabetes is treated by dietary restrictions and insulin injections.

TYPE 2 DIABETES MELLITUS

Oral Hypoglycemics

28.6 Type 2 diabetes is controlled through lifestyle changes and oral hypoglycemic agents.

28.7 The thyroid gland controls the basal metabolic rate and affects every cell in the body.

THYROID DISORDERS

Thyroid and Antithyroid Agents

28.8 Thyroid disorders may be treated by administering thyroid hormone or by decreasing the activity of the thyroid gland.

28.9 Glucocorticoids are released during periods of stress and influence carbohydrate, lipid, and protein metabolism in most cells.

Glucocorticoids

28.10 Glucocorticoids are prescribed for adrenocortical insufficiency and a wide variety of other conditions.

28.11 Of the many pituitary and hypothalamic hormones, only a few have clinical applications as drugs.

OBJECTIVES

After reading this chapter, the student should be able to:

1. Describe the general structure and functions of the endocrine system.

2. Compare and contrast the functions of the pancreatic hormones.

3. Compare and contrast the causes, signs, symptoms, and treatment of type 1 and type 2 diabetes mellitus.

4. Identify the five types of insulin.

5. Describe the signs and symptoms of insulin overdose and underdose.

6. Explain the primary functions of the thyroid gland.

7. Identify the signs and symptoms of hypothyroidism and hyperthyroidism.

8. Explain the primary functions of the adrenal cortex.

9. Describe the signs and symptoms of Addison's disease and Cushing's syndrome.

10. For each of the following drugs or drug classes identify representative drugs, explain the mechanism of drug action, primary actions, and important adverse effects.

    a. insulin
    b. oral hypoglycemics
    c. thyroid hormone
    d. antithyroid agents
    e. glucocorticoids
    f. growth hormone
    g. antidiuretic hormone

11. Categorize drugs used in the treatment of endocrine disorders based on their classification and mechanism of action.

PharMedia
www.prenhall.com/holland

Additional interactive resources and activities for this chapter can be found on the Companion Website. For animations, audio glossary, and review access the accompanying CD-ROM in this book.

Addison's disease (ADD-iss-uns): hyposecretion of gluco-corticoids and aldosterone by the adrenal cortex / *page 457*

adrenocorticotropic hormone (ACTH) (uh-dreen-oh-kor-tik-o-TRO-pik): hormone secreted by the pituitary that stimulates the release of glucocorticoids by the adrenal cortex / *page 454*

atrophy (AT-troh-fee): shrinkage or wasting away of a tissue / *page 457*

basal metabolic rate: resting rate of metabolism in the body / *page 451*

cretinism (KREE-ten-izm): dwarfism and mental retardation caused by lack of thyroid hormone during infancy / *page 451*

Cushing's syndrome (KUSH-ings): condition caused by excessive corticosteroid secretion by the adrenal glands or by overdosage with corticosteroid medication / *page 457*

diabetes insipidus (die-uh-BEE-tees in-SIP-uh-dus): excessive urination due to lack of secretion of antidiuretic hormone / *page 459*

diabetes mellitus, type 1 (die-uh-BEE-tees MEL-uh-tiss): disease characterized by absent secretion of insulin by the pancreas that usually begins in the early teens / *page 448*

diabetes mellitus, type 2: disease characterized by insufficient secretion of insulin by the pancreas or by lack of sensitivity of insulin receptors that usually begins in middle age / *page 450*

dwarfism: below normal height caused by a deficiency in thyroid hormone or growth hormone / *page 459*

follicular cells (fo-LIK-yu-lur): cells in the thyroid gland that secrete thyroid hormone / *page 451*

glucocorticoid (glu-ko-KORT-ik-oyd): type of hormone secreted by the outer portion of the adrenal gland that includes cortisol / *page 454*

Grave's disease: syndrome caused by hypersecretion of thyroid hormone / *page 453*

hormones: chemicals secreted by endocrine glands that act as chemical messengers to affect homeostasis / *page 443*

hyperglycemia (hi-pur-gli-SEEM-ee-uh): abnormally high level of glucose in the blood / *page 447*

hypoglycemia (hi-po-gli-SEEM-ee-uh): abnormally low level of glucose in the blood / *page 447*

hypothalamus (hi-po-THAL-ih-mus): region of the brain that affects emotions and drives, and that secretes releasing factors that affect the pituitary gland / *page 445*

islets of Langerhans (EYE-lits of LANG-gur-hans): clusters of cells in the pancreas responsible for the secretion of insulin and glucagon; also called the *pancreatic islets* / *page 447*

ketoacids (KEY-to-ass-ids): waste products of lipid metabolism that lower the pH of the blood / *page 448*

myxedema (mix-uh-DEEM-uh): condition caused by insufficient secretion of thyroid hormone / *page 452*

negative feedback: in homeostasis, when the first hormone in a pathway is shut off by the last hormone or product in the pathway / *page 444*

parafollicular cells (pair-uh-fo-LIK-u-lur): cells in the thyroid gland that secrete calcitonin / *page 451*

pituitary gland (pit-TOO-it-air-ee): endocrine gland in the brain responsible for controlling many other endocrine glands / *page 445*

releasing factors: hormones secreted by the hypothalamus that affect secretions in the pituitary gland / *page 445*

somatotropin (so-mat-oh-TROH-pin): another name for growth hormone / *page 459*

vasopressin (vaz-oh-PRESS-in): another name for antidiuretic hormone / *page 459*

Like the nervous system, the endocrine system is a major controller of homeostasis. But while a nerve may exert instantaneous control over a single muscle or gland, a hormone from the endocrine system may affect all body cells and take as long as several days to produce a measureable response. Small amounts of hormones may produce very profound effects on the body. Conversely, deficiencies of small quantities may produce equally as profound physiologic changes. This chapter examines common endocrine disorders and their pharmacotherapy. The reproductive hormones are covered in Chapter 29 ⊂⊃ .

endo = within
crine = to secrete

28.1 The endocrine system maintains homeostasis by using hormones as chemical messengers.

The endocrine system consists of various glands that secrete chemical messengers called hormones. Hormones are released in response to a change in the body's internal environment. For example, when the level of glucose in the blood rises, the pancreas secretes insulin. When blood levels of calcium fall, parathyroid hormone (PTH) is released from the parathyroid gland. The various endocrine glands are illustrated in Figure 28.1.

FIGURE 28.1

The endocrine system
SOURCE: *Pearson Education/PH College.*

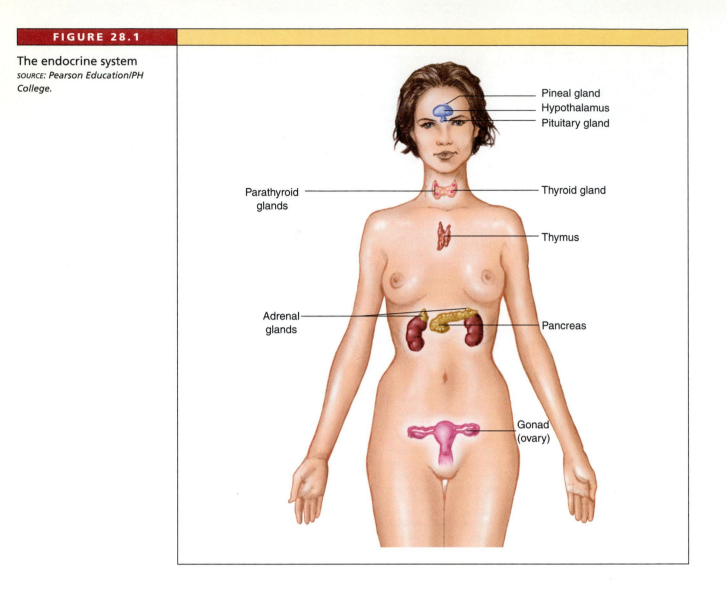

After they are secreted, hormones enter the blood and are transported throughout the body. Some hormones, such as insulin and thyroid hormone, have receptors on nearly every cell in the body and thus produce widespread physiologic changes. Others, such as parathyroid hormone and oxytocin, have receptors on only a few specific types of cells.

In the endocrine system, it is common for one hormone to control the secretion of another hormone. In addition, it is common for the last hormone or action in the pathway to provide feedback to turn off the action of the first hormone. For example, as serum calcium falls, PTH is released. PTH causes an increase in serum calcium, which provides feedback to the parathyroid glands to shut off PTH secretion. This is a common feature of endocrine homeostasis known as negative feedback.

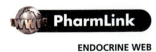

ENDOCRINE WEB

28.2 Hormones are used as replacement therapy, as antineoplastics, and for their natural, therapeutic effects.

The goals of hormone pharmacotherapy vary widely. In many cases, the hormone is administered simply as replacement therapy for clients who are unable to secrete sufficient quantities of their own, endogenous hormones. Examples of replacement therapy include the administration of thyroid hormone after the thyroid gland has been surgically removed, or supplying insulin to clients

TABLE 28.1	Selected Endocrine Disorders and Their Drug Treatment		
GLAND	**HORMONE (S)**	**DISORDER**	**DRUGS**
adrenal cortex	glucocorticoids	hypersecretion: Cushing's syndrome	None
		hyposecretion	glucocorticoids
thyroid	thyroid hormone (T3 and T4)	hypersecretion: Graves disease	propylthiouracil (Propacil)
		hyposecretion: myxedema (adults) and cretinism (children)	thyroid hormone (Synthroid)
pituitary	growth hormone	hyposecretion: dwarfism	somatrem (Protopin) and somatropin (Humatrope and others)
	antidiuretic hormone	hyposecretion: diabetes insipidus	vasopressin (Pitressin), desmopressin (DDAVP, Stimate), and lypressin (Diapid)
pancreas (Islets of Langerhans)	insulin	hyposecretion: diabetes mellitus	insulin

whose pancreas is not functioning. Replacement therapy usually supplies the same, low-level amounts of the hormone that would normally be present in the body. A summary of selected endocrine disorders and their drug therapy is shown in Table 28.1.

Some hormones are used in cancer chemotherapy. Examples include testosterone for breast cancer and estrogen for testicular cancer. The antineoplastic mechanism of action of these hormones is not known. When used as antineoplastics, the doses of the hormones far exceed those levels normally present in the body (Chapter 23 ⬭).

Another goal of hormone therapy may be to produce an exaggerated response that is part of the normal action of the drug in order to achieve some therapeutic advantage. Supplying hydrocortisone to suppress inflammation is an example of taking advantage of the normal action of the glucocorticoids, but at higher amounts than would normally be present in the body. Supplying small amounts of estrogen or progesterone at specific times during the menstrual cycle can prevent ovulation and pregnancy. In this example, the client is supplied natural hormones; however, they are given at a time when levels in the body are normally low.

28.3 The hypothalamus and the pituitary gland secrete hormones that control other endocrine organs.

Two endocrine structures in the brain deserve special recognition because they control many other endocrine glands. The **hypothalamus** secretes chemicals called **releasing factors** or *releasing hormones* that travel via blood vessels a short distance to an area immediately below, called the anterior **pituitary gland**. These releasing factors tell the pituitary which hormone to release. After the pituitary releases the appropriate hormone, it travels to its target organ to cause its effect. For example, the hypothalamus secretes thyrotropin-releasing hormone that travels to the pituitary gland with the message to secrete thyroid-stimulating hormone (TSH). TSH then travels to its target organ—the thyroid gland—to stimulate the release of thyroid hormone. Hormones associated with the pituitary gland are shown in Figure 28.2.

FIGURE 28.2

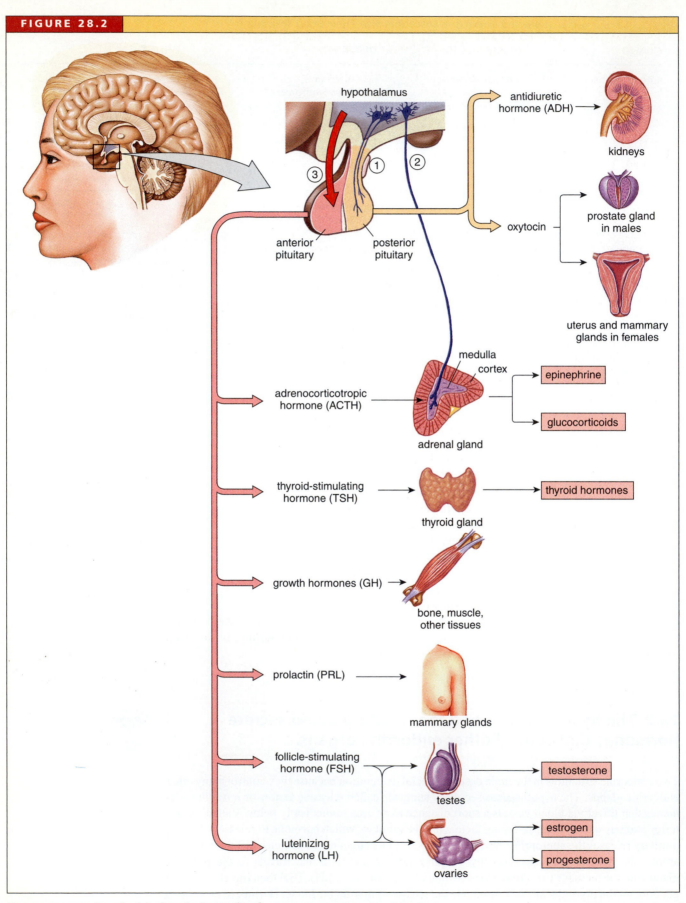

Hormones associated with the pituitary gland   SOURCE: Pearson Education/PH College.

28.4 Insulin and glucagon are secreted by the pancreas.

Located behind the stomach and between the duodenum and spleen, the pancreas is an essential gland to both the digestive and endocrine systems. It is responsible for the secretion of several enzymes into the pancreatic duct that flow into the duodenum to assist in the chemical digestion of nutrients. This is its exocrine function. Certain cells in the pancreas, called **islets of Langerhans**, are responsible for its endocrine function: the secretion of glucagon and insulin. As with other endocrine organs, the pancreas secretes these hormones directly into blood capillaries, where they are available for transport to body tissues.

exo = out/away from
crine = to secrete

Insulin secretion is regulated by a number of chemical, hormonal, and nervous factors. One of the most important regulators is the level of glucose in the blood. After a meal, when glucose levels are high (**hyperglycemia**), the pancreas is stimulated to secrete insulin. The islet cells stop secreting insulin when blood glucose is low (**hypoglycemia**) or when high levels of insulin provide negative feedback to the pancreas.

Insulin affects carbohydrate, lipid, and protein metabolism in most cells of the body. One of its most important actions is to assist in glucose transport. Without insulin, glucose cannot enter cells. A cell may be literally swimming in glucose, but it cannot enter and be used for fuel by the cell without insulin. The brain is an important exception, not requiring insulin for glucose transport. Insulin is said to have a hypoglycemic effect because its presence causes glucose to leave the blood and enter cells.

Islet cells in the pancreas also produce glucagon. Glucagon is best thought of as an antagonist to insulin because its actions are opposite to those of insulin. When levels of glucose are low, glucagon is secreted. Its primary function is to maintain adequate levels of glucose in the blood between meals. It has a hyperglycemic effect, as its presence moves glucose from cells, primarily in the liver, to the blood. Figure 28.3 illustrates the relationships between blood glucose, insulin, and glucagon.

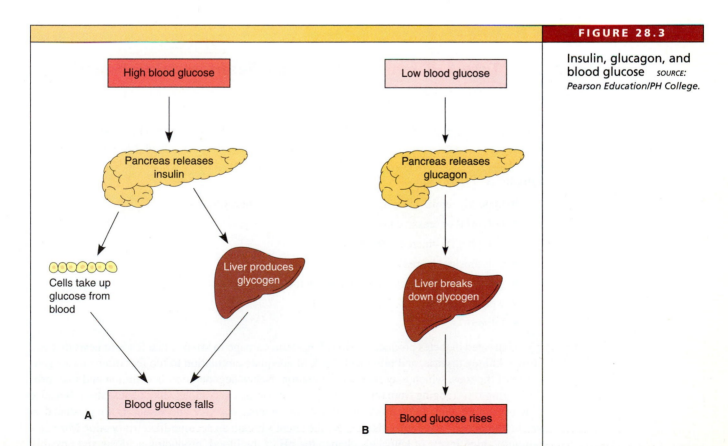

FIGURE 28.3

Insulin, glucagon, and blood glucose *SOURCE: Pearson Education/PH College.*

TYPE 1 DIABETES MELLITUS

dia = through
betes = to go

Type 1 diabetes mellitus is one of the most common diseases of childhood. Sometimes called *juvenile-onset diabetes* because it is often diagnosed between the ages of 11 to 13, the disease results from a lack of insulin secretion by the pancreas. There is a genetic component to type 1 diabetes, and children and siblings of people with the disease have a higher risk of acquiring the disorder.

Fast Facts Diabetes Mellitus

- Of the 16 million Americans who have diabetes, 5 million probably do not know that they have the disease.
- Each day, 2,200 people are diagnosed with diabetes.
- Diabetes causes more than 198,000 deaths each year; it is the sixth leading cause of death.
- Diabetes is the leading cause of blindness in adults; each year 12,000–24,000 people lose their sight because of diabetes.
- Diabetes is responsible for 50% of non-traumatic lower limb amputations; 56,000 amputations are performed each year in diabetics.
- Costs for diabetes treatment exceed $100 billion annually—one in every seven healthcare dollars.
- Diabetes is the leading cause of end-stage renal disease, accounting for about 40% of new cases.

INSULIN

28.5 Type 1 diabetes is treated by dietary restrictions and insulin injections.

The signs and symptoms of type 1 diabetes are consistent from client to client. The most diagnostic sign is a sustained hyperglycemia. Fasting plasma glucose levels of 126 mg/dl or greater on at least two separate occasions is diagnostic for diabetes. Following are the typical signs and symptoms of type 1 diabetes.

- hyperglycemia—fasting blood glucose greater than 126 mg/dl
- polyuria—excessive urination
- polyphagia—increase in hunger
- polydipsia—increased thirst
- glucosuria—high levels of glucose in the urine
- weight loss
- fatigue

Untreated diabetes produces serious long-term damage to arteries that leads to heart disease, stroke, kidney disease, and blindness. Lack of adequate circulation to the feet often causes gangrene of the toes, which may require amputation. Nerve degeneration is common and may produce symptoms ranging from tingling in the fingers or toes to complete loss of sensation. Because glucose cannot enter cells, lipids are utilized as an energy source and ketoacids are produced as waste products. These ketoacids can give the client's breath an acetone-like, fruity odor. More importantly, high levels of ketoacids change the pH of the blood, producing acidosis and possibly coma (Chapter 27 ⬭).

Type 1 diabetes requires drug therapy with insulin or hypoglycemics. Insulin is reserved for the more severe deficiency states, whereas the oral hypoglycemics are given for milder forms of diabetes. Type 1 diabetes is treated with a combination of proper meal planning, exercise, and insulin. Food must be eaten regularly, every four to five hours, as skipping meals can have profound effects on blood glucose. Regular, moderate exercise helps the cellular responsiveness to insulin.

The treatment goal with insulin therapy is to maintain blood glucose levels within strict, normal limits. Five types of insulin are available, differing in their onset and duration of action. Until the 1980s, the source of all insulin was beef or pork pancreas. Most insulin today, however, is human insulin obtained through recombinant DNA technology. The most common route of administration for insulin is SC: the drug cannot be given orally because it is destroyed by digestive enzymes. All insulin preparations produce the same actions and side effects. Doses of insulin are highly individualized for each client; some clients may need two or more injections daily. Occasionally, two different types of insulin are mixed to obtain the desired therapeutic effect. Common insulin preparations are given in Table 28.2.

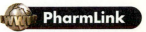 **PharmLink**

AMERICAN DIABETES ASSOCIATION AND HEALTHY LIVING

DRUG PROFILE:
Regular Insulin (Humulin R, Novolin R, Pork Regular Iletin II, Regular Purified Pork Insulin)

Actions:

Regular insulin is prepared from pork pancreas or as human insulin through recombinant DNA technology. It is classified as short-acting insulin, with an onset of 30 to 60 minutes, a peak effect at two to three hours, and a duration of five to seven hours. Its primary action is to promote the entry of glucose into cells. For the emergency treatment of acute ketoacidosis, it may be given SC or IV. Regular insulin is also available as Humulin 70/30 (a mixture of 30% regular insulin and 70% isophane insulin) or as Humulin 50/50 (a mixture of 50% of both regular and isophane insulin).

Adverse Effects:

The most serious adverse effect from insulin therapy is hypoglycemia. Hypoglycemia may result from taking too much insulin, not properly timing the insulin injection with food intake, or skipping a meal. Dietary carbohydrates must be in the blood when insulin is injected, otherwise the drug will remove too much glucose and signs of hypoglycemia—tachycardia, confusion, sweating, and drowsiness—will ensue. If severe hypoglycemia is not quickly treated with glucose, convulsions, coma, and death may follow.

TABLE 28.2	Insulin Preparations		
DRUG	**TYPE**	**ONSET OF ACTION (HR)**	**DURATION OF ACTION (HR)**
Pr regular insulin (Humulin R, Novolin R, Regular Iletin I and II)	short-acting	0.5–1	6–8
lispro insulin (Humalog)	short-acting	0.25	6–8
isophane insulin (NPH Iletin I and II, Humulin N, Novolin N	intermediate-acting	1–2	18–24
lente insulin (Lente Iletin II, Lente L, Humulin L, Novolin L	intermediate-acting	1–2.5	18–24
ultralente insulin (Humulin-U Ultralente)	long-acting	4–8	more than 36

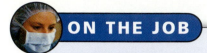

TYPE 2 DIABETES MELLITUS

There are a number of differences between type 1 and type 2 diabetes. Unlike type 1, which begins in the early teens, **type 2 diabetes mellitus** begins in the middle-age group and is sometimes referred to as *age-onset diabetes*. It is more common in overweight clients and those having low HDL-cholesterol and high triglyceride levels. Approximately 90% of all diabetics are type 2.

28.6 Type 2 diabetes is controlled through lifestyle changes and oral hypoglycemic agents.

Unlike type 1 diabetics, type 2 clients are capable of secreting insulin, although in relatively deficient amounts. The fundamental problem in type 2, however, is that insulin receptors in the target tissues have become insensitive or resistant to the hormone. Thus the small amount of insulin present does not bind to its receptors, and no effect is achieved. While type 1 diabetics must take insulin, type 2 diabetes is usually controlled with oral hypoglycemic agents. In severe, unresponsive cases, insulin may also be necessary for type 2 diabetics. The long-term consequences of type 1 and type 2 diabetes are the same.

Another important difference is that proper diet and exercise can sometimes increase the sensitivity of insulin receptors to the point that drug therapy is unnecessary for type 2 diabetics. Many clients with type 2 diabetes are obese and will need a medically supervised plan to reduce weight gradually and exercise safely. This is an important lifestyle change for such clients; they will need to maintain these changes for the remainder of their lives.

ORAL HYPOGLYCEMICS

Oral hypoglycemic medications are prescribed after diet and exercise have failed to bring blood glucose levels to within normal values. The five classes of oral hypoglycemic agents are only used for type 2 diabetes. Classification of these drugs is based upon their chemical structures and mechanisms of action.

All oral hypoglycemics have the common action of lowering blood glucose levels when taken on a regular basis. They all have the potential to cause hypoglycemia; thus, periodic laboratory tests are conducted to monitor blood glucose levels. Type 2 diabetes sometimes progresses such that a combination of two oral hypoglycemics, or an oral hypoglycemic agent with insulin, is required to bring glucose levels to within normal limits. The oral hypoglycemics are shown in Table 28.3.

Concept review 28.1

- Why are oral hypoglycemic drugs ineffective at treating type 1 diabetes?

THYROID DISORDERS

28.7 The thyroid gland controls the basal metabolic rate and affects every cell in the body.

The thyroid gland lies in the neck, just below the larynx and in front of the trachea. Follicular cells in the gland secrete thyroid hormone, which is actually a combination of two different hormones: thyroxine (tetraiodothyronine or T_4) and triiodothyronine (T_3). Iodine is essential for the synthesis of these hormones and is provided through the dietary intake of common iodized salt. Parafollicular cells in the thyroid gland secrete calcitonin, a hormone that is involved with calcium homeostasis (Chapter 30 🔗).

Thyroid function is regulated through multiple levels of hormonal control. Thyroid-releasing hormone (TRH) from the hypothalamus stimulates the pituitary gland to secrete thyroid-stimulating hormone (TSH). TSH then stimulates the thyroid gland to release thyroid hormone. After thyroid hormone has reached a certain level in the blood, it operates in a negative feedback loop to shut off secretion of TRH and TSH. The negative feedback mechanism for the thyroid gland is shown in Figure 28.4.

Thyroid hormone affects nearly every cell in the body by regulating basal metabolic rate, the baseline speed by which cells perform their functions. By increasing cellular metabolism, thyroid hormone increases body temperature. Thyroid hormone is critical to the growth of the nervous system. Deficiency during infancy may result in a combination of dwarfism and severe mental retardation known as cretinism.

Fast Facts Thyroid Disorders

- Hypothyroidism is 10 times more common in women than men; hyperthyroidism is 5–10 times more common in women.
- The two most common thyroid diseases, Grave's disease and Hashimoto's thyroiditis, are autoimmune diseases and may run in families.
- One of every 4,000 babies is born without a working thyroid gland.
- About 15,000 new cases of thyroid cancer are diagnosed each year.
- One of every five women over age 75 has Hashimoto's thyroiditis.

DRUG PROFILE:
Glipizide (Glucotrol)

Actions:

Glipizide belongs to the sulfonylurea group of hypoglycemics. It is a second-generation sulfonylurea that offers the advantages of higher potency, once-a-day dosing, fewer side effects, and fewer drug-drug interactions than the first-generation medications in this class. Glipizide stimulates the pancreas to secrete more insulin and also increases the sensitivity of insulin receptors in target tissues. Some degree of pancreatic function is required for glipizide to lower blood glucose. Maximum effects are achieved if the drug is taken 30 minutes prior to the primary meal of the day.

Adverse Effects:

Hypoglycemia is less frequent with glipizide than with first-generation sulfonylureas. Clients should stay out of the sun, as rashes and photosensitivity are possible. Some clients experience mild, GI-related effects such as nausea, vomiting, or loss of appetite. Glipizide and other sulfonylureas have the potential to interact with a number of drugs; thus, the client should always consult with a healthcare practitioner before adding a new medication or herbal supplement. Ingestion of alcohol will result in distressing symptoms that include headache, flushing, nausea, and abdominal cramping.

Mechanism in Action:

Glipizide, an oral hypoglycemic agent, lowers glucose blood levels by stimulating insulin release from pancreatic cells. This drug is used for the treatment of non-insulin-dependent diabetes mellitus (type 2). Because it is a sulfonylurea drug, sensitivity reactions are possible.

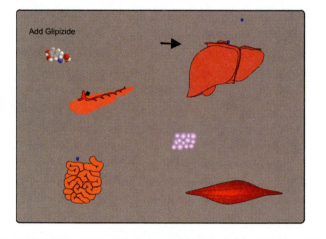

Add Glipizide

- Post-partum thyroiditis occurs in 5% to 9% of women after giving birth, and may recur in future pregnancies.
- Both hyperthyroidism and hypothyroidism can affect a woman's ability to become pregnant; both also can cause miscarriages.

THYROID AND ANTITHYROID AGENTS

Thyroid disorders are quite common and drug therapy is often indicated. The correct dose of thyroid or antithyroid drug is highly individualized and may require periodic adjustment.

28.8 Thyroid disorders may be treated by administering thyroid hormone or by decreasing the activity of the thyroid gland.

Hypothyroidism is a common disease caused by insufficient secretion of either TSH or thyroid hormone. Symptoms of hypothyroidism in adults, also known as myxedema, include slowed body metabolism, slurred speech, bradycardia, weight gain, low body temperature, and intolerance to cold environments. Low or absent thyroid function may be a consequence of autoimmune disease, surgical removal of the gland, or aggressive treatment with antithyroid drugs. Hypothyroidism is treated with natural or synthetic thyroid hormone.

Hypersecretion of thyroid hormone results in symptoms that are the opposite of hypothyroidism: increased body metabolism, tachycardia, weight loss, high body temperature, and anxi-

TABLE 28.3	The Oral Hypoglycemics	
DRUG	**ROUTE AND ADULT DOSE**	**REMARKS**
acarbose (Precose)	PO; 25–100 mg tid (max 300 mg/day).	Alpha-glucosidase inhibitor.
acetohexamide (Dymelor)	PO; 250 mg qd (max 1500 mg/day).	First-generation sulfonylurea.
chlorpropamide (Chloronase, Diabinese, Glucamide)	PO; 100–250 mg qd (max 750 mg/day).	First-generation sulfonylurea.
glimepiride (Amaryl)	PO; 1–4 mg qd (max 8 mg/day).	Second-generation sulfonylurea.
Pr glipizide (Glucotrol)	PO; 2.5–20 mg qd-bid (max 40 mg/day).	Second-generation sulfonylurea; Glucotrol XL is an extended release form.
glyburide (DiaBeta, Micronase, Glynase)	PO; 1.25–10 mg qd-bid (max 20 mg/day).	Second-generation sulfonylurea; Glyburide combined with metformin is Glucovance.
metformin (Glucophage)	PO; 500 mg qd-tid (max 3 g/day).	Biguanide; extended-release form available.
miglitol (Glyset)	PO; 25–100 mg tid (max 300 mg/day).	Alpha-glucosidase inhibitor type.
nateglinide (Starlix)	PO; 60–120 mg tid.	Similar to second-generation sulfonylureas.
pioglitazone (Actos)	PO; 15–30 mg qd (max 45 mg/day).	Glitazone type
repaglinide (Prandin)	PO; 0.5–4 mg bid-qid.	Glitazone type
rosiglitazone (Avandia)	PO; 2–4 mg qd-bid (max 8 mg/day).	Glitazone type
tolazamide (Tolamide, Tolinase)	PO; 100–500 mg qd-bid (max 1 g/day).	First-generation sulfonylurea.
tolbutamide (Orinase)	PO; 250–1500 mg qd-bid (max 3 g/day).	First-generation sulfonylurea.

ety. A particularly severe form of hyperthyroidism is called **Grave's disease**. If the cause of the hypersecretion is found to be a tumor, the disease is corrected through surgical removal of the thyroid gland, or thyroidectomy. In less severe conditions, the client may receive antithyroid medications or ionizing radiation to kill or inactivate some of the hyperactive thyroid cells. Antithyroid agents are sometimes given 10 to 14 days prior to thyroidectomy to decrease bleeding during surgery. The thyroid and antithyroid medications are shown in Table 28.4.

Concept review 28.2

▪ If thyroid hormone is secreted by the thyroid gland, how can a deficiency in this hormone be caused by disease in the hypothalamus or pituitary?

28.9 Glucocorticoids are released during periods of stress and influence carbohydrate, lipid, and protein metabolism in most cells.

The adrenal glands lie on top of each kidney. Although small in size, they secrete several essential classes of steroid hormones, called glucocorticoids, mineralocorticoids, and androgens. Collectively, these hormones are referred to as *corticosteroids* or *adrenocortical hormones*.

ad = *toward*
ren = *kidney*
al = *pertaining to*

FIGURE 28.4

Feedback mechanisms
of the thyroid gland

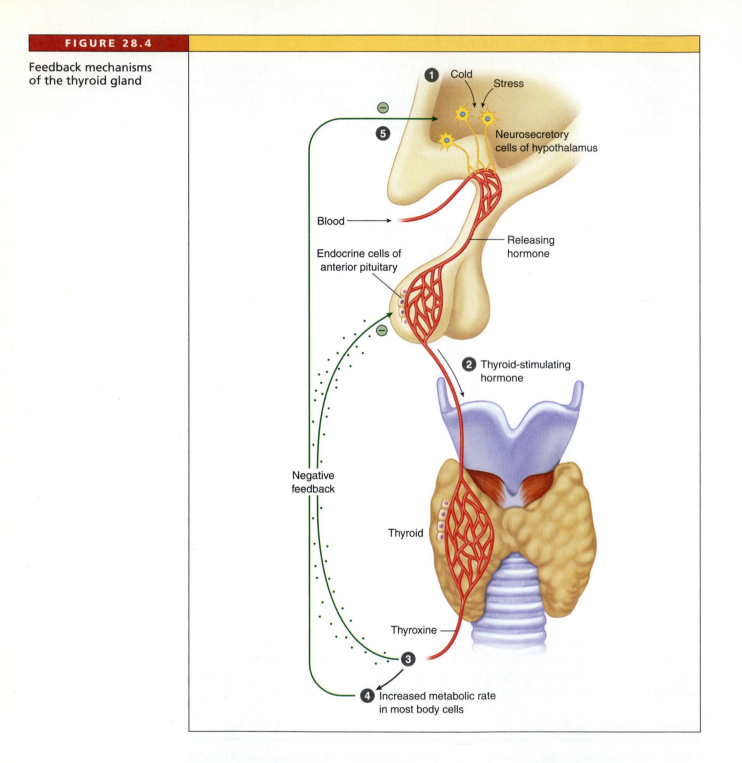

1 Cold | Stress

Neurosecretory
cells of hypothalamus

5

Blood

Endocrine cells of
anterior pituitary

Releasing
hormone

2 Thyroid-stimulating
hormone

Negative
feedback

Thyroid

Thyroxine

3

4 Increased metabolic rate
in most body cells

gluco = sweet/sugar
corti = cortex
oid = resemble

Cortisol is one of about 30 glucocorticoids secreted from the outer portion, or cortex, of the adrenal gland. Glucocorticoids affect the metabolism of nearly every cell in the body. During long-term stress, these hormones mobilize the formation of glucose and increase the breakdown and utilization of proteins and lipids. They have a potent anti-inflammatory effect that was discussed in Chapters 20 and 24 ⬭ . They also serve to promote homeostasis of the cardiovascular, nervous, and musculoskeletal systems.

Control of glucocorticoid levels begins with corticotropin releasing factor (CRF), secreted by the hypothalamus. CRF travels to the pituitary, where it causes the release of **adrenocorticotropic hormone (ACTH).** ACTH travels through the blood and reaches the adrenal cortex, causing it to release cortisol and other glucocorticoids. When the level of cortisol in the blood rises, it provides negative feedback to the hypothalamus and pituitary to shut off further re-

DRUG PROFILE (Thyroid):
Levothyroxine (Synthroid)

Actions:

Levothyroxine is a synthetic form of thyroxine (T_4) used for replacement therapy in clients with low thyroid function. Actions are those of thyroid hormone, and include loss of weight, improved tolerance to environmental temperature, increased activity, and increased pulse rate. Blood levels of thyroid hormone are monitored carefully until the client's symptoms stabilize. To achieve the proper level of thyroid function, doses may require periodic adjustments for several months or longer.

Adverse Effects:

The difference between a therapeutic dose of levothyroxine and one that produces adverse effects is quite narrow. Adverse effects of levothyroxine resemble symptoms of hyperthyroidism and include tachycardia, anxiety, insomnia, weight loss, and heat intolerance. Menstrual irregularities may occur in females. Long-term use of levothyroxine has been associated with osteoporosis in women.

TABLE 28.4	Thyroid and Antithyroid Medications	
DRUG	**ROUTE AND ADULT DOSE**	**REMARKS**
Thyroid Preparations		
Pr levothyroxine (Levothyroid, Synthroid, Eltroxin, Levoxyl, Levo-T)	PO; 100–400 µg/day.	Synthetic T_4; IV form available.
liothyronine (Cytomel)	PO; 25–75 µg qd.	Synthetic T_3
liotrix (Euthroid, Thyrolar)	PO; 12.5–30 µg qd.	Mix of synthetic T_3 and synthetic T_4 in a 1:4 ratio.
thyroid (S-P-T, Thyrar, Thyroid USP)	PO; 60–100 mg qd.	Animal thyroid glands.
Antithyroid Preparations		
Pr propylthiouracil (PTU)	PO; 100–150 mg tid.	
potassium iodide and iodine (Lugol's solution, Thyro-block)	PO; 0.1–1.0 ml tid.	IV form available; Lugol's is a mixture of 5% elemental iodine and 10% potassium iodide.
radioactive iodide (^{131}I, Iodotope)	PO; 0.8–150 mCi (based on radiation quantity).	May take 2–3 months for full therapeutic effect.
methimazole (Tapazole)	PO; 5–15 mg tid.	10 × more potent than propylthioruacil.

lease of glucocorticoids from the adrenal gland. This negative feedback mechanism is shown in Figure 28.5.

GLUCOCORTICOIDS

The glucocorticoids are used as medications in replacement therapy for clients with adrenocortical insufficiency and to dampen inflammatory and immune responses. They are one of the most widely prescribed drug classes.

DRUG PROFILE (Antithyroid):
Propylthiouracil (Propacil)

Actions:

Propylthiouracil is administered to clients with hyperthyroidism, sometimes prior to surgery. It acts by interfering with the synthesis of T_3 and T_4. Because it does not affect thyroid hormone that has already been secreted, its action may be delayed from several days to as long as six to twelve weeks. Effects include a return to normal thyroid function: weight gain, reduction in anxiety, less insomnia, and slower pulse rate.

Adverse Effects:

Overtreatment with propylthiouracil produces symptoms of hypothyroidism. In addition, a small percentage of clients display blood changes such as decreased platelet and white blood cell counts. Periodic laboratory blood counts and thyroid hormone values are necessary to establish the proper dosage.

FIGURE 28.5

Feedback control of the adrenal cortex

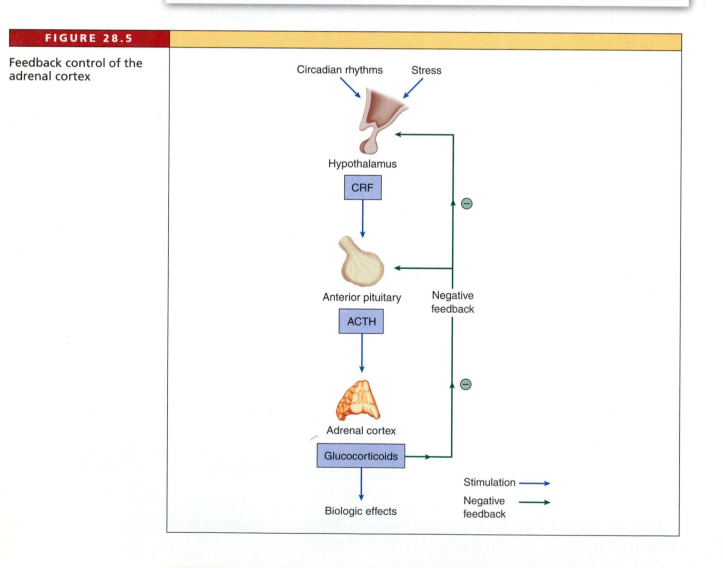

28.10 Glucocorticoids are prescribed for adrenocortical insufficiency and a wide variety of other conditions.

Lack of adequate corticosteroid production, known as *adrenocortical insufficiency,* may be caused by hyposecretion by the adrenal cortex or by inadequate secretion of ACTH from the pituitary. Symptoms include hypoglycemia, fatigue, hypotension, and GI disturbances such as anorexia, vomiting, and diarrhea. Primary adrenocortical insufficiency, known as **Addison's disease**, is quite rare and includes a deficiency of both glucocorticoids and mineralocorticoids.

Secondary adrenocortical insufficiency is relatively common and may result from long-term therapy with glucocorticoids. When glucocorticoids are taken as medications for prolonged periods, the pituitary receives a message through the negative feedback mechanism to stop secreting ACTH. Without stimulation from ACTH, the adrenal cortex shrinks in size and stops secreting endogenous glucocorticoids, a condition known as adrenal **atrophy**. If a client abruptly discontinues the glucocorticoid medication, the shrunken adrenal glands will not be able to secrete sufficient glucocorticoids for a period of time and symptoms of adrenocortical insufficiency will appear.

a = without
***trophy** = nourishment*

The goal of replacement therapy is to achieve the same physiologic level of glucocorticoids in the blood that would be present if the adrenal glands were functioning properly. Clients requiring replacement therapy may need to take glucocorticoids their entire lives.

Many glucocorticoid preparations are available via the topical, oral, IM, IV, and other routes to treat a variety of disorders. The role of corticosteroids in the treatment of inflammation and allergic rhinitis was presented in Chapters 20 and 24, respectively ⊂▭⊃ . Following is a list of the various disorders that may be treated with corticosteroids.

- allergies
- asthma
- seasonal rhinitis
- skin disorders such as contact dermatitis and rashes
- neoplastic disease such as Hodgkins disease, leukemias, and lymphomas
- shock
- rheumatic disorders such as rheumatoid arthritis, ankylosing spondylitis, and bursitis
- post-transplant surgery to suppress the immune system
- chronic inflammatory bowel disease such as ulcerative colitis and Crohn's disease
- adrenal insufficiency
- hepatic, neurological, and renal disorders characterized by edema

Significant adverse effects can occur during long-term therapy with corticosteroids. An array of signs and symptoms known as **Cushing's syndrome** includes adrenal atrophy, osteoporosis, increased risk of infections, delayed wound healing, peptic ulcers, and a redistribution of fat around the shoulders and neck. Mood and personality changes may occur, with the client becoming psychologically dependent upon the therapeutic effects of the drug. Some of the glucocorticoids, such as hydrocortisone, also have mineralocorticoid activity and thus can cause retention of sodium and water. Alternate-day dosing, whereby the drug is administered every other day, is sometimes used to limit adrenal atrophy. Clients taking inhaled or topical corticosteroids, or who receive the drugs for two weeks or less, exhibit few adverse effects. Some of the glucocorticoids used in replacement therapy are shown in Table 28.5.

Concept review 28.3

- Why does administration of glucocorticoids for extended periods result in adrenal atrophy?

28.11 Of the many pituitary and hypothalamic hormones, only a few have clinical applications as drugs.

Of the 15 different hormones secreted by the pituitary and hypothalamus, only a few are used for drug therapy. This is because some of these hormones can only be obtained from natural sources and it is usually easier to give drugs affecting the target organs, rather than from the pituitary or hypothalamus. Two pituitary hormones, prolactin and oxytocin, affect the reproductive system and will be discussed in Chapter 29 ⊂▭⊃ . Of those remaining, growth hormone and antidiuretic hormone have some clinical utility.

DRUG PROFILE:
Hydrocortisone (Cortef, Hydrocortone)

Actions:

Structurally identical to the natural hormone cortisol, hydrocortisone is a synthetic corticosteroid that is the drug of choice for treating adrenocortical insufficiency. When used for replacement therapy, it is given at physiologic doses. Once proper dosing is achieved, its therapeutic effects should mimic those of natural corticosteroids. Hydrocortisone is also available for the treatment of inflammation, allergic disorders, and many other conditions. Intraarticular injections may be given to decrease severe inflammation in affected joints.

Adverse Effects:

When used at physiologic doses for replacement therapy, adverse effects of hydrocortisone should not be evident. The client and the healthcare professional must be vigilant, however, in observing for signs of Cushing's syndrome, which can develop with high doses. If taken for longer than two weeks, hydrocortisone should be discontinued gradually.

TABLE 28.5	Selected Corticosteroids	
DRUG	**ROUTE AND ADULT DOSE**	**REMARKS**
cortisone acetate (Cortistan, Cortone)	PO; 20–300 mg qd.	Short-acting; IM form available; also has mineralocorticoid activity.
Pr hydrocortisone (Solu-cortef)	PO; 2–80 mg tid-qid.	Short-acting; IV, topical, and IM forms available; also has mineralocorticoid activity.
methylprednisolone (Solu-medrol, Medrol)	PO; 2–60 mg qd-qid.	Intermediate-acting; IV and IM forms available; has little mineralocorticoid activity.
prednisolone (Delta-Cortef)	PO; 5–60 mg qd-qid.	Intermediate-acting; IV and IM forms available; has little mineralocorticoid activity.
prednisone (Deltasone, Meticorten, Orasone, Panasol)	PO; 5–60 mg qd-qid.	Intermediate-acting; has little mineralocorticoid activity.
triamcinolone (Aristocort, Atolone, Kenacort, Kenalog-E)	PO; 4–48 mg qd-qid.	Intermediate-acting; IV, intra-articular, SC, topical, inhalation and IM forms available; has little mineralocorticoid activity.
betamethasone (Celestone)	PO; 0.6–7.2 mg qd.	Long-acting; IV, topical, and IM forms available; has little mineralocorticoid activity.
dexamethasone (Decadron, Dexasone, Hexadrol, Maxidex)	PO; 0.25–4 mg bid-qid.	Long-acting; IV, ophthalmic, topical, intranasal, inhalation, and IM forms available; has little mineralocorticoid activity.
fludrocortisone (Florinef)	PO; 0.1–0.2 mg qd.	Long-acting; also has strong mineralocorticoid activity.

Growth hormone, known as somatotropin, stimulates the growth of nearly every cell in the body. Deficiency of this hormone in children results in dwarfism. Unlike a deficiency of thyroid hormone, however, growth hormone deficiency usually does not cause mental impairment. Two preparations of human growth hormone, somatrem (Protopin) and somatropin (Humatrope and others), are available as replacement therapy in children. If therapy is begun early in life, as much as six inches of growth may be achieved. Growth hormone is not very effective at promoting growth in short children who have no growth hormone deficiency. It is not approved for this purpose.

As its name implies, antidiuretic hormone (ADH) conserves water in the body. ADH is secreted from the posterior pituitary gland and acts on the collecting ducts in the kidney to increase water reabsorption. A deficiency of ADH, known as diabetes insipidus, causes the client to lose large volumes of water. ADH is also called vasopressin because it has the capability to raise blood pressure when secreted in large amounts. Three preparations of ADH are available for the treatment of diabetes insipidus: vasopressin (Pitressin), desmopressin (DDAVP, Stimate), and Lypressin (Diapid). Desmopressin is occasionally used by the intranasal route for enuresis (bedwetting).

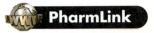

RESEARCH ON GROWTH DISORDERS

CLIENT TEACHING

Clients treated for endocrine disorders need to know the following:

1. When taking oral corticosteroids for more than two weeks, do not miss doses or discontinue the drug without consulting your healthcare provider.

2. When taking oral corticosteroids, see your physician if any infections, cuts, or injuries appear to be healing abnormally slowly.

3. If taking hydrocortisone for replacement therapy, take the medication between 6:00 AM and 9:00 AM, as this is the time when natural corticosteroids are released.

4. When taking insulin or oral hypoglycemics, report any signs of hypoglycemia such as weakness, sweating, dizziness, tremor, anxiety, or tachycardia to your healthcare provider immediately. Mild symptoms may be treated with small amounts of sugar in the form of candy or fruit juice.

5. Insulin and oral hypoglycemics should always be taken at the same time each day.

6. When self-monitoring blood glucose, normal values are 80 to 120 mg/dl before meals and 100 to 140 mg/dl before bedtime.

7. Store unopened vials of insulin in the refrigerator. Do not use after the expiration date.

8. If taking insulin or oral hypoglycemics, read the directions to all medications very carefully because many drug-drug interactions are possible. Medications such as corticosteroids, thiazide diuretics, and sympathomimetics can raise blood glucose levels and inhibit the effects of insulin.

9. If you are diabetic, check with your healthcare provider if you intend to begin a vigorous exercise program. Often, insulin doses should be reduced or extra food ingested just prior to intense exercise.

10. If self-injecting insulin, carefully follow all instructions provided by your healthcare practitioner to avoid injury or infection.

11. When taking thyroid medication, your pulse rate is a good indicator of drug effectiveness. Contact your healthcare practitioner if your pulse rate consistently exceeds 100 or if you notice any other significant change.

12. Finding the correct dosage of thyroid hormone often takes several months. Do not change your dose without being advised to do so by your healthcare practitioner. ▪

CHAPTER REVIEW

 Core Concepts Summary

28.1 The endocrine system maintains homeostasis by using hormones as chemical messengers.

Hormones are secreted by endocrine glands in response to changes in the internal environment. The hormones act on their target cells to return the body to homeostasis. Negative feedback prevents the body from over-responding to internal changes.

28.2 Hormones are used as replacement therapy, as antineoplastics, and for their natural, therapeutic effects.

Hormones are often given as replacement therapy to clients who are not able to secrete sufficient quantities of endogenous hormones. In high doses, several hormones may be used as antineoplastics. Hormones may also be used therapeutically to take advantage of their natural physiologic effects.

28.3 The hypothalamus and the pituitary gland secrete hormones that control other endocrine organs.

The hypothalamus secretes releasing hormones that signal the anterior pituitary gland to release its hormones. Pituitary hormones travel throughout the body to affect many other organs.

28.4 Insulin and glucagon are secreted by the pancreas.

The pancreas secretes insulin after a meal, when blood glucose levels are high. Insulin permits glucose to leave the blood and enter cells. Glucagon has effects opposite to those of insulin, causing glucose to leave tissues and enter the blood.

28.5 Type 1 diabetes is treated by dietary restrictions and insulin injections.

Type 1 diabetes is diagnosed in late childhood and is caused by a lack of insulin secretion by the pancreas. Parenteral insulin is provided and must be

carefully timed to coincide with meals. Taking too much insulin or skipping meals may result in acute hypoglycemia. Untreated diabetes leads to serious long-term consequences.

28.6 Type 2 diabetes is controlled through lifestyle changes and oral hypoglycemic agents.

Type 2 diabetes is more common than type 1, occurs in older clients, and is primarily due to a lack of sensitivity of insulin receptors. Drug therapy starts with oral hypoglycemics and may proceed to insulin injections if the disease is not controlled appropriately.

28.7 The thyroid gland controls the basal metabolic rate and affects every cell in the body.

The thyroid gland secretes thyroid hormone, which is essential for the growth and metabolism of all cells. Thyroid hormone is a combination of two different hormones, thyroxine and triiodothyronine, both of which require iodine for their synthesis.

28.8 Thyroid disorders may be treated by administering thyroid hormone or by decreasing the activity of the thyroid gland.

Hypothyroidism produces symptoms such as slowed body metabolism, slurred speech, bradycardia, weight gain, low body temperature, and intolerance to cold environments. Administration of thyroid hormone reverses these symptoms. Hyperthyroid clients exhibit the opposite symptoms. Hyperthyroidism may be treated with drugs that kill or inactivate thyroid cells.

28.9 Glucocorticoids are released during periods of stress and influence carbohydrate, lipid, and protein metabolism in most cells.

The adrenal cortex secretes glucocorticoids in response to stimulation by ACTH from the pituitary.

Glucocorticoids affect the metabolism of nearly every cell in the body and have a potent anti-inflammatory effect.

28.10 Glucocorticoids are prescribed for adrenocortical insufficiency and a wide variety of other conditions.

Glucocorticoids are given to clients whose adrenal glands are unable to produce adequate amounts of these hormones, and for a wide variety of other conditions. When used at high doses, oral therapy is often limited to two weeks because of the potential for producing Cushing's syndrome and adrenal atrophy.

28.11 Of the many pituitary and hypothalamic hormones, only a few have clinical applications as drugs.

Growth hormone, or somatotropin, is used to increase the height in children with growth hormone deficiencies. ADH, or vasopressin, increases water reabsorption in the kidney and is used to treat diabetes insipidus.

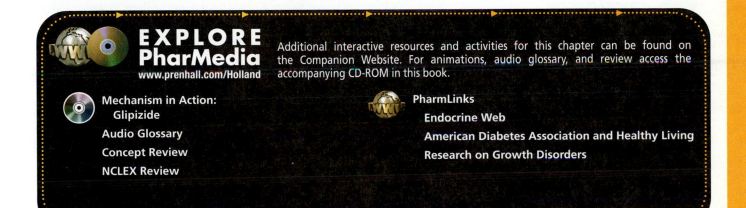

EXPLORE PharMedia
www.prenhall.com/Holland

Additional interactive resources and activities for this chapter can be found on the Companion Website. For animations, audio glossary, and review access the accompanying CD-ROM in this book.

Mechanism in Action:
Glipizide
Audio Glossary
Concept Review
NCLEX Review

PharmLinks
Endocrine Web
American Diabetes Association and Healthy Living
Research on Growth Disorders

29 Drugs for Disorders and Conditions of the Reproductive System

CORE CONCEPTS

29.1 Testosterone, estrogen, and progesterone are the primary hormones contributing to the growth, health, and maintenance of the reproductive system.

CONTRACEPTION

Oral Contraceptives

29.2 Low doses of estrogens and progestins are used for contraception.

MENOPAUSE

Estrogens

29.3 Estrogens are used for replacement therapy and in the treatment of prostate cancer.

UTERINE ABNORMALITIES

Progestins

29.4 Progestins are prescribed for dysfunctional uterine bleeding.

LABOR AND BREASTFEEDING

Oxytocin and Tocolytics

29.5 Oxytocin and tocolytics are drugs used to influence uterine contractions.

HYPOGONADISM

Androgens

29.6 Androgens are used to treat hypogonadism or delayed puberty in males and breast cancer in females.

ERECTILE DYSFUNCTION

Erectile Dysfunction Agents

29.7 Erectile dysfunction is a common disorder that may be successfully treated with drug therapy.

BENIGN PROSTATIC HYPERPLASIA (BPH)

Antiprostatic Agents

29.8 In its early stages, benign prostatic hyperplasia may be treated successfully with drug therapy.

OBJECTIVES

After reading this chapter, the student should be able to:

1. Identify and describe the primary functions of the steroid sex hormones.
2. Explain the mechanisms by which estrogen and progestins prevent conception.
3. Describe the role of drug therapy in the treatment of menopausal and postmenopausal symptoms.
4. Identify the role of the steroid sex hormones in the chemotherapy of cancer.
5. Describe the uses of progestins in the therapy of dysfunctional uterine bleeding.
6. Compare and contrast oxytocin and tocolytics in antepartum and postpartum treatment.
7. Explain the role of androgens in the treatment of hypogonadism.
8. Describe the role of drug therapy in the treament of erectile dysfunction and benign prostatic hyperplasia (BPH).
9. For each of the following drugs or drug classes, identify representative drugs, explain the mechanism of drug action, primary actions, and important adverse effects.
   a. oral contraceptive preparations
   b. estrogens
   c. progestins
   d. oxytocin
   e. tocolytics
   f. androgens
   g. drugs for erectile dysfunction
   h. drugs for BPH
10. Categorize drugs used in the treatment of reproductive disorders and conditions based on their classification and mechanism of action.

PharMedia
www.prenhall.com/holland

Additional interactive resources and activities for this chapter can be found on the Companion Website. For animations, audio glossary, and review access the accompanying CD-ROM in this book.

amenorrhea (ah-men-oh-REE-ah): lack of normal menstrual periods / **page 469**

androgens (AN-droh-jens): steroid sex hormones that promote the appearance of masculine characteristics / **page 464**

antepartum (an-teh-PART-um): prior to the onset of labor / **page 473**

benign prostatic hyperplasia (BPH) (bee-NINE pros-TAT-ik hy-purr-PLAY-shuh): non-malignant enlargement of the prostate gland / **page 476**

breakthrough bleeding: bleeding at abnormal times during the menstrual cycle / **page 468**

corpus cavernosum (KORP-us kav-ver-NOH-sum): tissue in the penis that fills with blood during an erection / **page 476**

dysfunctional uterine bleeding: hemorrhage that occurs at abnormal times or in abnormal quantity during the menstrual cycle / **page 469**

endometrium (en-doh-MEE-tree-um): inner lining of the uterus / **page 464**

estrogen (ES-troh-jen): class of steroid sex hormones produced by the ovary / **page 464**

follicle-stimulating hormone (FSH): hormone secreted by the pituitary gland that regulates sperm or egg production / **page 464**

hypogonadism (hy-poh-GO-nad-izm): below normal secretion of the steroid sex hormones / **page 474**

hysterectomy (hiss-ter-EK-toh-mee): surgical removal of the uterus / **page 469**

impotence (IM-poh-tense): inability to obtain or sustain an erection; also called erectile dysfunction / **page 474**

leutinizing hormone (LH) (LEW-ten-iz-ing): hormone secreted by the pituitary gland that triggers ovulation in the female and stimulates sperm production in the male / **page 464**

libido (lih-BEE-do): interest in sexual activity / **page 475**

menopause (MEN-oh-paws): period of time when females stop secreting estrogen and menstrual cycles cease / **page 467**

menorrhea (men-oh-REE-uh): prolonged or excessive menstruation / **page 469**

oligomenorrhea (ol-ego-men-oh-REE-uh): infrequent menstruation / **page 469**

ovulation (ov-you-LAY-shun): release of an egg by the ovary / **page 464**

oxytocin (ox-ee-TOH-sin): hormone secreted by the pituitary gland that stimulates uterine contractions and milk ejection / **page 471**

postpartum (post-PART-um): occurring after childbirth / **page 473**

progesterone (pro-JESS-ter-own): hormone responsible for building up the uterine lining in the second half of the menstrual cycle and during pregnancy / **page 464**

prolactin (pro-LAK-tin): hormone secreted by the pituitary gland that stimulates milk production in the mammary glands / **page 472**

tocolytic (toh-koh-LIT-ik): drug used to inhibit uterine contractions / **page 472**

virulization (veer-you-lih-ZAY-shun): appearance of masculine secondary sex characteristics / **page 475**

The male and female reproductive systems are regulated by a small number of hormones that are responsible for the growth and maintenance of the reproductive organs. These hormones can be supplemented with natural or synthetic hormones to achieve a variety of therapeutic goals, ranging from replacement therapy, to prevention of pregnancy, to milk production. This chapter examines drugs used to treat disorders and conditions of the reproductive system.

Fast Facts Reproductive Conditions and Disorders

- Erectile dysfunction affects 10 to 15 million Americans—about one in four men over age 65.
- BPH affects 50% of men over age 60, and 90% of men over age 80.
- There is a wide range of ages when women reach menopause: 8 of 100 women will stop menstruating before age 40, and 5 of 100 will continue beyond age 60.
- About half the cases of dysfunctional uterine bleeding are diagnosed in women over 45 years of age; however, 20% of cases occur under the age of 20.
- Compared to just ten years ago, oral contraceptives now contain two to four times less estrogen.
- The primary reason why a woman may become pregnant while on oral contraceptives is skipping a dose.
- A non-smoking woman aged 25 to 29 has a 2 in 100,000 chance of dying from complications due to oral contraceptives. The risk of a woman in this age group dying in an automobile accident is 74 in 100,000.
- Oral contraceptives have more benefits than simply contraception. It is estimated that each year they prevent the following.

  51,000 cases of pelvic inflammatory disease
  9,900 hospitalizations for ectopic pregnancy
  27,000 cases of iron-deficiency anemia
  20,000 hospitalizations for certain types of non-malignant breast disease

29.1 Testosterone, estrogen, and progesterone are the primary hormones contributing to the growth, health, and maintenance of the reproductive system.

The sex hormones are steroids synthesized from cholesterol. While the male and female gonads produce the vast majority of sex hormones, the adrenal cortex also secretes small amounts. Male and female hormones are present in both sexes.

estro = desire
gen = producing/forming

The ovaries synthesize the female sex hormones estrogen and progesterone. Estrogen is actually a generic term for three different female sex hormones: estradiol, estrone, and estriol. Estrogen is responsible for the maturation of the reproductive organs and for the appearance of the secondary sex characteristics in the female. Estrogen also has numerous metabolic effects on nonreproductive tissues, including the brain, kidneys, blood vessels, and skin. For example, estrogen helps to maintain low blood cholesterol levels and facilitates calcium uptake by bones to help maintain proper bone density (Chapter 30). At about age 50–55, the ovaries stop secreting estrogen as women enter menopause.

The ovaries also secrete a class of hormones called *progestins,* the most common of which is progesterone. Progesterone, in combination with estrogen, promotes breast development and the monthly changes in the ovaries and uterus known as the menstrual cycle. When progesterone levels fall sharply at the end of the cycle, a portion of the inner lining of the uterus, the endometrium, is shed and menstrual bleeding occurs. During pregnancy, progesterone secreted by the placenta maintains a healthy endometrium for the fetus and prevents premature labor contractions.

andro = male
gen = producing/forming

Androgens are male sex hormones. The testes secrete testosterone, the primary androgen responsible for maturation of the male sex organs and the secondary sex characteristics of the male. Unlike the cyclic secretion of estrogen and progesterone in the female, the secretion of testosterone is relatively constant in the adult male. Like estrogen, testosterone has metabolic effects in tissues outside the reproductive system. Of particular note is its ability to build muscle mass, which contributes to the difference in muscle strength and body composition between males and females.

The ovaries and testes are regulated by the pituitary hormones: follicle-stimulating hormone (FSH) and leutinizing hormone (LH). FSH regulates sperm or egg production. LH in the female triggers the release of the egg, a process known as ovulation, and promotes the secretion of estrogen and progesterone by the ovary. In males, LH—sometimes called *interstitial cell-stimulating hormone*—regulates the production of testosterone. The relationship between the hypothalamus, pituitary, and the reproductive hormones is illustrated in Figure 29.1.

NATURAL ALTERNATIVES

Dong Quai for Premenstrual Syndrome

Since antiquity, Dong quai has been recognized as an important herb for women's health in Chinese medicine. Obtained from *Angelica sinensis,* a small plant that grows in China, Dong quai contains a number of active substances that are said to exert analgesic, antipyretic, anti-inflammatory, and antispasmodic activity. The dried root is available as capsules, tablets, teas, and tinctures.

The reproductive effects of Dong quai may be due to active substances that have estrogenic activity. These estrogenic ingredients act as a "uterine tonic" to improve the overall hormonal balance of the female reproductive system. Dong quai is used to treat the symptoms of premenstrual syndrome as well as other disorders such as irregular menstrual periods or painful menstruation.

Dong quai has also been used for its cardiovascular effects. It is purported to increase circulation by dilating blood vessels. Because some of the active ingredients of Dong quai may have anticoagulant activity, clients taking warfarin (Coumadin) or high doses of aspirin should not take the herb without notifying their healthcare practitioner. ■

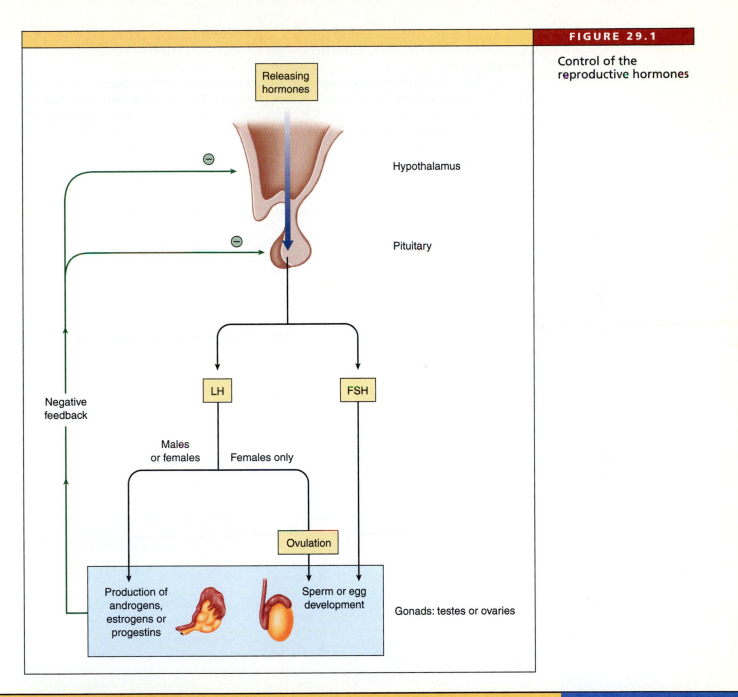

FIGURE 29.1

Control of the reproductive hormones

CONTRACEPTION

ORAL CONTRACEPTIVES

Oral contraceptives are medications used to prevent pregnancy. Most oral contraceptives are composed of a combination of estrogens and progestins. In small doses, they are able to inhibit ovulation.

29.2 Low doses of estrogens and progestins are used for contraception.

The most widespread pharmacological use of the female sex hormones is for the prevention of pregnancy. When used appropriately, they are nearly 100% effective. Most oral contraceptives contain a combination of estrogen and progestin, although a few contain only progestin. The most common estrogen used in these preparations is ethinyl estradiol, and the most common progestin is norethindrone.

A wide variety of different oral contraceptive preparations are available, differing in dose and type of estrogen and progestin. Selection of a specific formulation is individualized to each client, and determined by which drug gives the best contraceptive protection with the fewest side effects. Table 29.1 lists some of the oral contraceptives and their compositions. As shown in Figure 29.2, special packaging assists the client in taking this medication on a daily basis.

The estrogen-progestin oral contraceptives prevent ovulation, which is required for conception to occur. These hormones act by providing negative feedback to the pituitary that shuts down secretion of LH and FSH. Without these pituitary hormones, the egg cannot mature and ovulation is prevented. The estrogen-progestin agents also make the lining of the uterus less favorable to receive an embryo.

There are three basic estrogen-progestin formulations: monophasic, biphasic, and triphasic. The most common is the monophasic, which delivers a constant amount of estrogen and progestin

TABLE 29.1 — **Selected Oral Contraceptives**

TRADE NAME	TYPE	ESTROGEN	PROGESTIN
Alesse	monophasic	ethinyl estradiol; 20 µg	levonorgestrel; 0.1 mg
Desogen	monophasic	ethinyl estradiol; 30 µg	desogestrel; 0.15 mg
Lo-Ovral	monophasic	ethinyl estradiol; 30 µg	norgestrel; 0.3 mg
Loestrin Fe 1.5/30	monophasic	ethinyl estradiol; 30 µg	norethindrone; 1.5 mg
Ortho-Cept	monophasic	ethinyl estradiol; 30 µg	desogestrel; 0.15 mg
Ortho-Cyclen	monophasic	ethinyl estradiol; 35 µg	norgestimate; 0.25 mg
Pr Ortho-Novum 7/7/7	triphasic	ethinyl estradiol; 35 µg ethinyl estradiol; 35 µg ethinyl estradiol; 35 µg	norethindrone; 0.5 mg (Phase 1) norethindrone; 0.75 mg (Phase 2) norethindrone; 1.0 mg (Phase 3)
Ortho-Tri-Cyclen	triphasic	ethinyl estradiol; 35 µg ethinyl estradiol; 35 µg ethinyl estradiol; 35 µg	norgestimate; 0.5 mg (Phase 1) norgestimate; 0.75 mg (Phase 2) norgestimate; 1.0 mg (Phase 3)
Tri-Levlen	triphasic	ethinyl estradiol; 30 µg ethinyl estradiol; 40 µg ethinyl estradiol; 30 µg	levonorgestrel; 0.05 mg (Phase 1) levonorgestrel; 0.075 mg (Phase 2) levonorgestrel; 0.125 mg (Phase 3)
Triphasil	triphasic	ethinyl estradiol; 30 µg ethinyl estradiol; 40 µg ethinyl estradiol; 30 µg	norgestrel; 0.05 mg (Phase 1) norgestrel; 0.075 mg (Phase 2) norgestrel; 1.25 mg (Phase 3)
Micronor	progestin-only	none	norethindrone; 0.35 mg
Nor-Q.D.	progestin-only	none	norethindrone; 0.35 mg
Ovrette	progestin-only	none	norgestrel; 0.075 mg

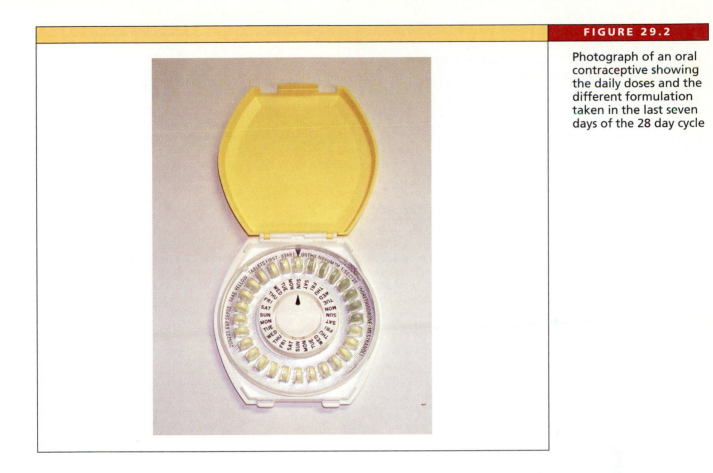

FIGURE 29.2

Photograph of an oral contraceptive showing the daily doses and the different formulation taken in the last seven days of the 28 day cycle

throughout the menstrual cycle. In biphasic agents, the amount of estrogen in each pill remains constant, but the amount of progestin is increased toward the end of the menstrual cycle in order to better nourish the uterine lining. In triphasic formulations, the amount of both estrogen and progestin vary in three distinct phases during the 28-day cycle.

The progestin-only oral contraceptives prevent pregnancy primarily by producing a thick, viscous mucous at the entrance to the uterus that prevents penetration by sperm. Progestin-only agents are less effective than estrogen-progestin combinations, and produce a higher incidence of menstrual irregularities. Because of this, they are generally reserved for clients who are at high risk to side effects from estrogen.

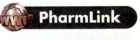

THE HISTORY OF CONTRACEPTION

MENOPAUSE

meno = month
pause = cessation

Menopause is the permanent cessation of menses, resulting in a lack of estrogen secretion by the ovaries. Menopause is neither a disease nor a disorder, but is a natural consequence of aging that is often accompanied by number of unpleasant symptoms.

ESTROGENS

In addition to their application as oral contraceptives, estrogens are widely used to reduce unpleasant symptoms associated with menopause and to treat certain cancers. Higher doses are used for these conditions, thus more side effects are observed.

DRUG PROFILE:
Ortho-Novum 1/35 (Ethinyl Estradiol)

Actions:

Ortho-Novum is typical of the monophasic oral contraceptives, containing fixed amounts of estrogen and progesterone for 21 days, followed by placebo tablets for seven days. It is nearly 100% effective at preventing conception. If a dose is missed, the client should take the dose as soon as possible, or take two tablets the next day. If two consecutive doses are missed, conception is possible and the client should use other birth control methods until the regular dosing schedule is reestablished. Ortho-Novum should not be continued if the client misses two consecutive menstrual periods or otherwise suspects she is pregnant. Ortho-Novum is also available as a biphasic and triphasic preparation.

Adverse Effects:

Like most oral contraceptives, Ortho-Novum can increase the risk of thromboembolic disease: the potential for blood clots, hemorrhage, pulmonary embolism, or stroke. This is particularly true in smokers, who carry a five times greater risk of a fatal myocardial infarction than non-smokers. Because of this risk, Ortho-Novum is contraindicated in clients with a history of stroke, MI, or other serious vascular disease. It should be used with caution in clients with hypertension, as it has the potential to raise blood pressure. Bleeding in the early or mid-menstrual cycle, known as **breakthrough bleeding**, is relatively common and may be severe enough to require a medication change in some clients. Any unusual breast lumps should be reported immediately to the healthcare practitioner; estrogen stimulates certain types of pre-existing breast cancer.

Mechanism in Action:

Ethinyl estradiol with norethindrone is a monophasic oral contraceptive. This preparation prevents ovulation by negative feedback control targeted at the hypothalamic-pituitary axis. When the right combination of estrogens and progestins are present in the bloodstream, the release of follicle stimulating hormone (FSH) and luteinizing hormone (LH) is inhibited. LH is the hormone responsible for ovulation.

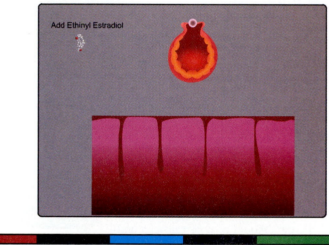

Add Ethinyl Estradiol

29.3 Estrogens are used for replacement therapy and in the treatment of prostate cancer.

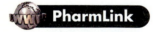

PSYCHOLOGICAL AND PHARMACOLOGICAL ASPECTS OF MENOPAUSE

When estrogen secretion becomes deficient, irregular or painful menstrual cycles may result, thus providing an indication for replacement drug therapy. In addition, surgical removal of the ovaries usually requires estrogen supplementation because the adrenal glands cannot supply sufficient quantities of estrogen.

Estrogen replacement therapy offers relief from many menopausal symptoms and from the potential, long-term consequences of estrogen loss that are listed in Table 29.2. In postmenopausal women, estrogen replacement therapy has been found to significantly reduce the incidence of cardiovascular disease. In addition, estrogen helps to prevent osteoporosis and debilitating bone fractures in these clients, as discussed in Chapter 30.

When used as replacement therapy, estrogen is usually combined with a progestin. The purpose of the progestin is to counteract some of the adverse effects that estrogen has on the uterus. Some of the estrogen and estrogen-progesterone combinations used for replacement therapy are shown in Table 29.3.

High doses of estrogens are sometimes used to treat prostate and breast cancer. Prostate cancer is usually dependent on androgens for growth, and administration of estrogens will suppress androgen secretion. As an antineoplastic hormone, estrogen is rarely used alone: it is one of many agents used in combination for the chemotherapy of cancer, as discussed in Chapter 23.

TABLE 29.2	Potential Consequences of Estrogen Loss Related to Menopause
Early menopausal symptoms	mood disturbances, depression, irritability
	insomnia
	hot flashes
	irregular menstrual cycles
	headaches
Mid-menopausal symptoms	vaginal atrophy, increased infections, painful intercourse
	skin atrophy
	stress urinary incontinence
	sexual disinterest
Post-menopausal conditions	cardiovascular disease
	osteoporosis
	Alzheimer's-like dementia
	colon cancer

UTERINE ABNORMALITIES

Dysfunctional uterine bleeding is a condition in which hemorrhage occurs on a non-cyclic basis or in abnormal amounts. It is the health problem most frequently reported by women and a common reason for hysterectomy, or surgical removal of the uterus. Types of dysfunctional uterine bleeding include the following conditions.

hyster = *womb/uterus*
ectomy = *excision*
a = *lack of*
meno = *month*
rhea = *flow*
oligo = *scanty*

- amenorrhea—absence of menstruation
- oligomenorrhea—infrequent menstruation
- menorrhea—prolonged or excessive menstruation
- breakthrough bleeding—hemorrhage between menstrual periods
- postmenopausal bleeding—uterine hemorrhage after menopause

DRUG PROFILE:
Conjugated Estrogens (Premarin) and Conjugated Estrogens with Medroxyprogesterone (Prempro)

Actions:

Premarin contains a mixture of different estrogens. It exerts several positive metabolic effects, including an increase in bone mass and a reduction in LDL cholesterol. It may also lower the risk of coronary artery disease and colon cancer. When used as post-menopausal replacement therapy, it is typically combined with a progestin, as in Prempro.

Adverse Effects:

Adverse effects from Prempro or Premarin include nausea, fluid retention, breast tenderness, and weight gain. As with oral contraceptives, estrogens are contraindicated in clients with a history of thromboembolic disease. Estrogens, when used alone, have been associated with a higher risk of uterine cancer. Adding a progestin exerts a protective effect by lowering the risk of uterine cancer. Unfortunately, recent studies have suggested that while the progestin protects against uterine cancer, it may increase the risk of breast cancer following long-term use. The risks of adverse effects increase in clients over age 35. Conjugated estrogens are a category X drug and should not be taken during a known or suspected pregnancy.

TABLE 29.3	Selected Estrogens and Progestins Used for Replacement Therapy		
DRUG	**ROUTE AND ADULT DOSE**		**REMARKS**
Estrogens			
estradiol (Estraderm, Estrace)	PO; 1–2 mg qd.		Available as vaginal cream and as a transdermal patch; also for breast and prostate cancer and to relieve postpartum breast engorgement.
(Pr) estrogen, conjugated (Premarin)	PO: 0.3–1.25 mg qd × 21 days each month.		Also for postcoital contraception and breast cancer.
estropipate (Ogen)	PO: 0.75–6 mg qd × 21 days each month.		Also for female hypogonadism and palliative treatment of postate cancer; available as a vaginal cream.
estradiol cypionate (depGynogen, Depogen)	IM; 1–5 mg q 3–4 weeks.		
estradiol valerate (Delestrogen, Duragen-10, Valergen)	IM; 10–20 mg q 4 weeks.		Also for breast cancer and to relieve postpartum breast engorgement.
ethinyl estradiol (Estinyl, Feminone)	PO: 0.02–0.05 mg qd × 21 days each month.		Also for breast and prostate cancer and as a postcoital contraceptive.
Progestins			
progesterone micronized (Prometrium)	PO; 400 mg at hs × 10 days.		IM and rectal forms available; intrauterine insert available for contraception.
(Pr) medroxyprogesterone (Provera, Cycrin)	PO: 5–10 mg qd on days 1–12 of menstrual cycle.		Also for endometrial and renal carcinoma; IM form available.
norethindrone acetate	PO: 5 mg qd × 2 weeks; increase by 2.5 mg/d q2 weeks (max 15 mg/day).		Also for endometriosis.
norethindrone (Micronor, Nor-Q.D.)	PO: 0.35 mg qd beginning on day 1 of menstrual cycle.		Also for endometriosis.

PROGESTINS

Besides being used in oral contraceptives, progestins are prescribed for various uterine abnormalities. They are occasionally used for specific cancers in combination with other antineoplastics.

29.4 Progestins are prescribed for dysfunctional uterine bleeding.

The function of natural progesterone is to prepare the uterus for implantation of the embryo and pregnancy. If implantation does not occur, levels of progesterone fall dramatically and menses begins. If pregnancy occurs, the ovary continues to secrete progesterone until the placenta develops sufficiently to begin producing the hormone.

The non-contraceptive indications for progesterone include the treatment of various uterine disorders. Dysfunctional uterine bleeding is often caused by a hormonal imbalance between estrogen and progesterone. While estrogen increases the thickness of the endometrium, bleeding occurs sporadically unless balanced by an adequate amount of progesterone secretion. Administration of a progestin in a pattern starting five days after the onset of menses and continuing for the next 20 days

DRUG PROFILE:
Medroxyprogesterone (Provera)

Actions:

Medroxyprogesterone is a synthetic progestin with a prolonged duration of action. Like its natural counterpart, the primary target tissue for medroxyprogesterone is the endometrium of the uterus. It inhibits the negative effect of estrogen on the uterus, thus restoring normal hormonal balance. When used for dysfunctional uterine bleeding, it is typically administered for 5 to 10 days. Three to seven days after discontinuation of the drug, withdrawal bleeding occurs. The medication is often timed so that the withdrawal bleeding occurs during the estimated normal menses time. Several cycles of drug administration may be required to restore normal cyclic function. Medroxyprogesterone may also be given IM for the palliation of metastatic uterine or renal carcinoma.

Adverse Effects:

Medroxyprogesterone is a category X drug and should be discontinued if pregnancy is suspected or confirmed. The most common side effects are breakthrough bleeding and breast tenderness. The most serious side effects relate to thromboembolic disease.

can sometimes help to establish a normal, monthly cyclic pattern. Oral contraceptives may also be prescribed for this disorder.

Progestins are occasionally prescribed for the treatment of metastatic endometrial carcinoma. In these cases, it is used for palliation, usually in combination with other antineoplastics. Selected progestins and their dosages are shown in Table 29.3.

Concept review 29.1

▪ Why is a progestin usually prescribed along with estrogen in oral contraceptives and when treating postmenopausal symptoms?

LABOR AND BREASTFEEDING

OXYTOCIN AND TOCOLYTICS

Oxytocin is natural hormone that has two primary functions: to stimulate uterine contractions during childbirth and to eject milk from the mammary glands following delivery. Other drugs, known as *tocolytics,* are used to inhibit uterine contractions during premature labor.

29.5 Oxytocin and tocolytics are drugs used to influence uterine contractions.

Oxytocin is a hormone secreted by the posterior portion of the pituitary gland, whose target organs are the uterus and the breast. It is secreted in larger and larger amounts as the growing fetus distends the uterus. This is an example of positive feedback: as distension increases, oxytocin secretion increases. As blood levels of oxytocin rise, the uterus is stimulated to contract, thus

FIGURE 29.3

Oxytocin and breastfeeding

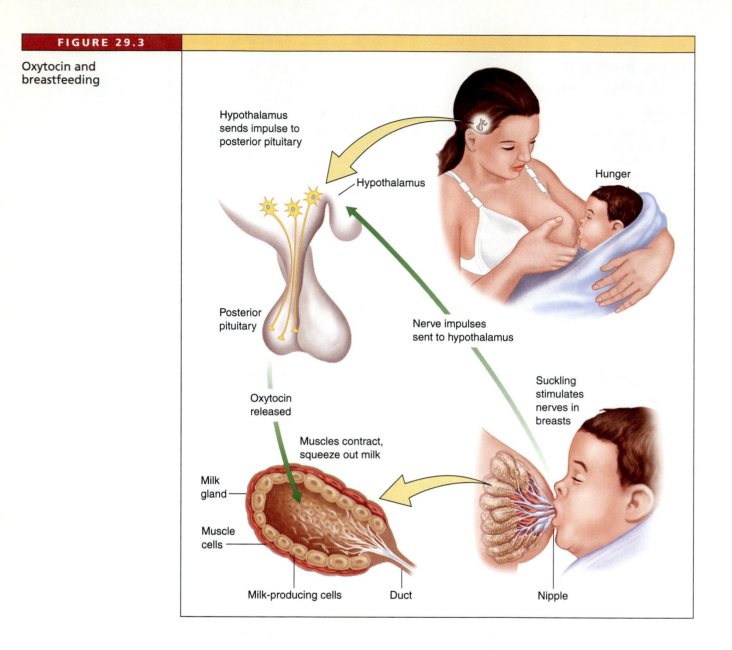

Hypothalamus sends impulse to posterior pituitary

Hypothalamus

Hunger

Posterior pituitary

Nerve impulses sent to hypothalamus

Oxytocin released

Suckling stimulates nerves in breasts

Muscles contract, squeeze out milk

Milk gland

Muscle cells

Milk-producing cells   Duct   Nipple

assisting in labor and the delivery of the fetus and the placenta. In postpartum clients, oxytocin is also released in response to suckling, whereby it causes milk to be ejected from the mammary glands following delivery. Oxytocin does not increase the volume of milk production. This function is provided by the pituitary hormone **prolactin**, which increases the synthesis of milk. The actions of oxytocin during breastfeeding are illustrated in Figure 29.3.

Several other drugs may be used to promote uterine contractions. Dinoprostone (Cervidil and others) is used to initiate labor or to expel a fetus that has died. Mifepristone (RU 486) is used for the emergency prevention of pregnancy, and is nearly 100% effective if taken within three days following unprotected intercourse. Given from weeks three to seven following conception, the combination of mifepristone with misoprostal (Cytotec) is 80–90% effective at terminating pregnancy.

There are certain clinical situations in which it is desirable to slow uterine contractions. **Tocolytics** are drugs used to inhibit the uterine contractions experienced in premature labor. Terminating premature labor allows additional time for the fetus to develop and may permit the pregnancy to reach normal term. Typically, the mother is given a monitor with a sensor that records uterine contractions. This information is used to determine the doses and timing of tocolytic medications. The drugs used as uterine stimulants and tocolytics are shown in Table 29.4.

toco = childbirth
lytic = destructive

DRUG PROFILE:
Oxytocin (Pitocin, Syntocinon)

Actions:

Oxytocin is given by several different routes depending upon its intended action. Given IV immediately prior to birth, or antepartum, oxytocin induces labor by stimulating contractions of the smooth muscle in the uterus. It is timed to the final stage of pregnancy, after the cervix is dilated and presentation of the fetus has occurred. Oxytocin may also be infused after delivery, or postpartum, to reduce hemorrhage after expulsion of the placenta and to aid in returning normal muscular tone to the uterus.

A second route of administration is intranasally. This route is used to promote the ejection of milk from the mammary glands, a process known as *milk letdown*. Milk letdown is an immediate response that occurs within minutes after applying spray or drops to the nostril during breast-feeding.

Adverse Effects:

Adverse effects of oxytocin are uncommon in the mother or fetus. When given IV, vital signs of the fetus and mother are monitored continuously to avoid complications in the fetus, such as dysrhythmias or intracranial hemorrhage. Serious complications in the mother may include uterine rupture, seizures, or coma.

ante = before
partum = labor

post = after
partum = labor

TABLE 29.4	Uterine Stimulants and Tocolytics	
DRUG	**ROUTE AND ADULT DOSE**	**REMARKS**
Stimulants		
Pr oxytocin (Pitocin, Syntocinon)	IV (antepartum); 1 mU/min starting dose to a maximum of 20 mU/min.	Nasal spray form used for milk ejection.
dinoprostone (Cervidil, Prepidil, Prostin E$_2$)	Intravaginal; 10 mg.	For terminating pregnancy through second trimester or following fetal death; or cervial ripening prior to induction of labor.
methylergonovine maleate (Methergine)	PO; 0.2–0.4 mg bid-qid.	IV and IM forms available; usually for postpartum delivery of the placenta.
mifepristone (RU 486)	PO; 600 mg as a single dose.	For termination of early pregnancy in combination with misoprostol.
misoprostol (Cytotec)	PO; 400 μg as a single dose.	For termination of early pregnancy in combination with mifepristone; also for peptic ulcers.
Tocolytics		
ritodrine hydrochloride (Yutopar)	IV; 50–100 μg/min starting dose, increased by 50 μg/min q 10 min.	Selective for beta$_2$-adrenergic-receptors; oral form available.
terbutaline sulfate (Brethine)	IV; 10 μg/min (max 80 μg/min).	Selective for beta$_2$-adrenergic-receptors; also available in oral and inhalation form for bronchodilation.
magnesium sulfate	IV; 1–4 g in 5% dextrose by slow infusion.	Also used as an anticonvulsant in preeclampsia; IM form available.
nifedipine (Procardia)	PO; 10 mg as a single dose (max 40 mg in 1 hr).	Calcium channel blocker also used for cardiovascular disorders.

Concept review 29.2

■ What is the difference between the effects of prolactin and oxytocin on the breast?

HYPOGONADISM

ANDROGENS

Androgens are male sex hormones that affect male sex characteristics and promote the maturation of the sex organs. Therapeutically they are used to treat hypogonadism and certain cancers.

29.6 Androgens are used to treat hypogonadism or delayed puberty in males and breast cancer in females.

Deficiency of testosterone in pre-pubertal males can result in a lack of maturation of the sex organs, a condition called hypogonadism. In adult males, lack of testosterone can lead to impotence and low sperm counts. Failure of the testes to produce adequate amounts of testosterone may be the result of pituitary disease, hereditary disorders, or unknown causes. Drug therapy with testosterone or other androgens promotes normal gonadal development and may restore normal reproductive function. Some of the androgens used therapeutically are shown in Table 29.5.

High doses of androgens are occasionally used to treat certain types of breast cancer. Androgens are normally used as a palliative measure in combination with other antineoplastics.

Anabolic steroids are testosterone-like compounds with hormonal activity. They are frequently taken inappropriately by athletes who hope to build muscle mass and strength, thereby obtaining a competitive edge. When taken in large doses for prolonged periods, anabolic steroids can produce significant adverse effects, some of which may persist for many months after discontinuation of the drugs. These drugs tend to raise cholesterol levels and may cause low sperm counts and impotence in men. In women, menstrual irregularities are likely, with an obvious increase in masculine characteristics. Permanent liver damage may result. Behavioral changes include aggression and psychological dependence. The use of anabolic steroids is illegal and strongly discouraged by physicians and athletic associations.

ERECTILE DYSFUNCTION

Erectile dysfunction, or impotence, is a common disorder in men. The defining characteristic of this condition is the inability to either obtain an erection or to sustain an erection long enough to achieve successful intercourse.

ERECTILE DYSFUNCTION AGENTS

29.7 Erectile dysfunction is a common disorder that may be successfully treated with drug therapy.

The incidence of erectile dysfunction increases with advancing age, although it may occur in an adult male of any age. Certain diseases, most notably atherosclerosis, diabetes, stroke, and hypertension, are associated with a higher incidence of the condition. Psychogenic causes may in-

DRUG PROFILE:
Testosterone Base (Andro and Others)

Actions:

The primary therapeutic use of testosterone is for the treatment of hypogonadism in males. The administration of testosterone to young males who have an abnormally delayed puberty will stimulate normal secondary sex characteristics to appear, including enlargement of the sexual organs, facial hair, and a deepening of the voice. In adult males, testosterone administration will increase interest in sexual activity, or libido, and restore masculine characteristics that may be deficient. Long duration IM injections are available that last up to two weeks, in addition to transdermal patches.

Adverse Effects:

An obvious side effect of testosterone therapy is virilization or appearance of masculine characteristics, which is usually only of concern when the drug is taken by female clients. Salt and water are often retained, causing edema. Liver damage is rare although potentially serious adverse effect. Acne and skin irritation is common during therapy. Testosterone is a category X drug and thus should not be taken if pregnancy is confirmed or suspected.

TABLE 29.5	**Selected Androgens**	
DRUG	**ROUTE AND ADULT DOSE**	**REMARKS**
Pr testosterone (Andro 100, Histerone, Testoderm)	PO; 10–25 mg q 2–3 days.	IM, topical, and buccal forms available; for hypogonadism and breast cancer; also for postpartum breast engorgement.
danazol (Danocrine)	PO; 200–400 mg bid × 3–6 months.	For endometriosis, fibrocystic breast disease, and hereditary angioedema.
fluoxymesterone (Halotestin)	PO; 2.5–20 mg qd for replacement therapy.	For hypogonadism, breast cancer, and postpartum breast engorgement.
methyltestosterone (Android, Testred)	PO; 10–50 mg qd.	For hypogonadism, breast cancer, and postpartum breast engorgement.
nandrolone phenproprionate (Durabolin, Hybolin)	IM; 50–100 mg q week.	For breast cancer only.
testosterone cypionate (Depotest, Andro-Cyp, Depo-testosterone)	IM; 50–400 mg q2–4 wk.	For hypogonadism, breast cancer, and postpartum breast engorgement.
testosterone enanthate (Andro LA, Delatest, Delatestryl)	IM; 50–400 mg q2–4 wk.	For hypogonadism and breast cancer.
testolactone (Teslac)	PO; 250 mg qid.	For breast cancer only.

clude depression, fatigue, guilt, or fear of sexual failure. A number of common drugs cause impotence as a side effect, including the thiazide diuretics, phenothiazines, serotonin reuptake inhibitors, tricyclic antidepressants, propranolol (Inderal), and diazepam (Valium).

The marketing of sildenafil (Viagra) has revolutionized the medical therapy of erectile dysfunction. The drug is the most effective treatment for this disorder.

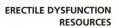 **PharmLink**

ERECTILE DYSFUNCTION RESOURCES

Concept review 29.3

■ Why do you think that sildenafil is used to treat erectile dysfunction rather than testosterone?

DRUG PROFILE:
Sildenafil (Viagra)

Actions:

When sildenafil was approved as the first pharmacologic treatment for erectile dysfunction in 1998, it set a record for pharmaceutical sales for any new drug in U.S. history. Sildenafil acts by relaxing the erectile tissues in the penis called the corpus cavernosa, which allows increased blood flow into the organ. The increased blood flow results in a firmer and longer-lasting erection in about 70% of men taking the drug. The onset of action is relatively rapid, usually less than an hour, and its effects last two to four hours. Despite considerable research interest, no effects of sildenafil have been shown on female sexual function, and this drug is not approved for use by women.

Adverse Effects:

The most serious adverse effects with sildenafil occur in men who are concurrently taking organic nitrates, common drugs used in the therapy of angina (Chapter 17). Because life-threatening hypotension has been reported, sildenafil is contraindicated for clients taking organic nitrates. Minor side effects include headache, flushing, and nasal congestion. Sildenafil should not be taken more than once per day.

Mechanism in Action:

Sildenafil (Viagra) causes dilation of blood vessels emptying blood directly into the corpora cavernosa of the penis. This results in engorgement of the corpora cavernosa leading to an erection and improved sexual performance. Sexual performance is prolonged by occlusion of penile blood vessels.

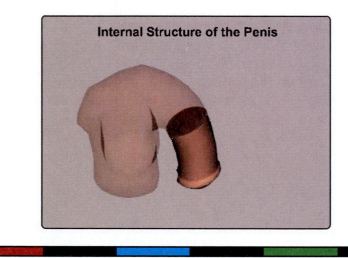

Internal Structure of the Penis

BENIGN PROSTATIC HYPERPLASIA (BPH)

hyper = above
plasia = growth

Benign prostatic hyperplasia (BPH) is an enlargement of the prostate gland that occurs in most men of advanced age. It is a non-malignant disorder that progressively decreases the outflow of urine by obstructing the urethra, causing difficult urination. Common symptoms include increased urinary frequency (usually with small amounts of urine), increased urgency to urinate, excessive nighttime urination, decreased force of the urinary stream, and a sensation that the bladder did not empty completely. In severe cases, surgery is needed to restore the patency of the urethra. In milder cases, drug therapy may be of benefit. BPH is illustrated in Figure 29.4.

ANTIPROSTATIC AGENTS

A few drugs are available to treat benign enlargement of the prostate. Although the drugs have limited efficacy, they have some value in treating mild disease. Because drug therapy alleviates the symptoms but does not cure the disease, these medications must be taken the remainder of the client's life, or until surgery is indicated.

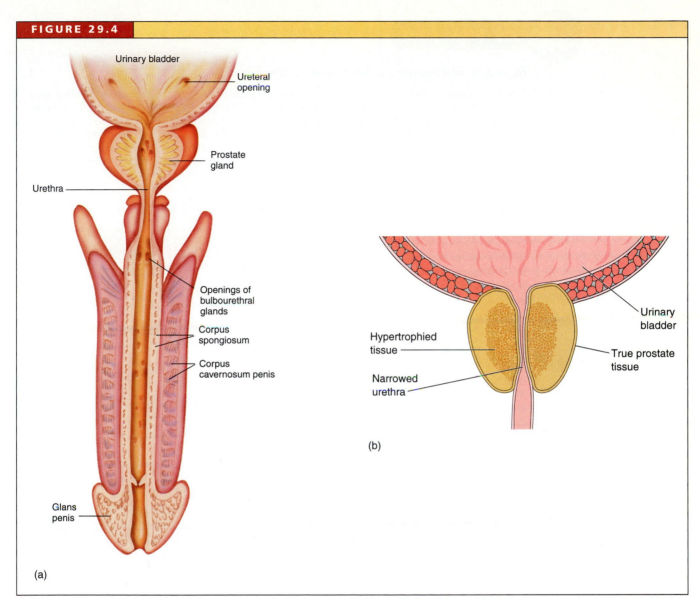

FIGURE 29.4

Benign prostatic hyperplasia: (a) normal prostate with penis; (b) benign prostatic hyperplasia
SOURCE: Pearson Education/PH College.

29.8 In its early stages, benign prostatic hyperplasia may be treated successfully with drug therapy.

Although primarily used for hypertension, several alpha$_1$-adrenergic blockers have been approved for BPH. Alpha-blockers relax smooth muscle in the prostate gland, thus easing the urinary obstruction. Doxazocin (Cardura) and terazocin (Hytrin) are of particular value to clients who have both hypertension and BPH. A third alpha$_1$-blocker, tamsulosin (Flomax), has no effect on blood pressure and its only indication is BPH. Additional information on the alpha-blockers is presented in Chapter 14 ⬭ .

Finasteride (Proscar) is also used to promote shrinkage of enlarged prostates and to help restore urinary function in clients with BPH. Finasteride acts by inhibiting an enzyme responsible for converting testosterone to one of its metabolites, 5-alpha-dihydrotestosterone. This drug is also marketed as Propecia, which is prescribed to promote hair regrowth in clients with male-pattern

ON THE JOB

Marriage and Family Health Counselor/Therapist

Many counseling-related professions are available to those who desire an occupation dealing very closely with clients and their problems. The marriage and family health counselor assists clients seeking information and advice related to reproductive and family health. The counselor provides support for the client that helps lead them to rational and informed decisions. Typical issues may include pregnancy, substance abuse, and career counseling. Related professions include community counselor, mental health counselor, and school counselor. Potential employment locations include hospitals, schools, mental health agencies, and correctional institutions. The length of the educational program varies from a minimum of two years to graduate-level study. ■

baldness. Doses of finasteride are five times higher when prescribed for BPH than when prescribed for baldness. Finasteride is a category X drug, and women who are pregnant or who may become pregnant should avoid the semen of men taking the drug.

CLIENT TEACHING

Clients treated for reproductive disorders need to know the following:

1. If taking oral contraceptives, schedule frequent medical checkups. Take your blood pressure periodically and report any persistent changes to your healthcare practitioner.

2. Discontinue oral contraceptives, estrogen, or progestins immediately if pregnancy is suspected. Continued use may injure the fetus.

3. Be certain to inform your healthcare provider if you are taking oral contraceptives. Some drugs decrease the effectiveness of oral contraceptives and could result in pregnancy. These drugs include several common antibiotics and anticonvulsants.

4. A balanced diet is important when taking oral contraceptives, as these drugs may lower levels of folic acid and vitamin B_6.

5. If taking antihypertensive drugs, monitor your blood pressure carefully when taking sildenafil. An increased risk of hypotension is possible.

6. Before beginning hormone replacement therapy, a baseline mammogram should be performed. Monthly breast self-examinations should be conducted in addition to an annual exam by a healthcare provider.

7. When taking androgens, expect virilization to occur. Prolonged erections, known as *priapism*, should be reported to your healthcare provider immediately. This is a sign of overdose and permanent damage to the penis may result. ■

CHAPTER REVIEW

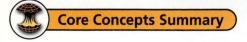

Core Concepts Summary

29.1 Testosterone, estrogen, and progesterone are the primary hormones contributing to the growth, health, and maintenance of the reproductive system.

Estrogen and progesterone are secreted by the ovary and are responsible for reproductive health in females. Testosterone is secreted by the testes and is responsible for the growth and maintenance of the male reproductive system. The sex hormones are controlled by FSH and LH from the pituitary.

29.2 **Low doses of estrogens and progestins are used for contraception.**

The most common oral contraceptives contain low doses of an estrogen combined with a progestin. Nearly 100% effective, these drugs act by preventing ovulation. Thromboembolic disease is a potentially serious adverse effect in some clients.

29.3 **Estrogens are used for replacement therapy and in the treatment of prostate cancer.**

Estrogens are often used to reduce the symptoms and consequences of estrogen loss in menopausal and post-menopausal women. A progestin is sometimes added to reduce the adverse effects of estrogen. Thromboembolic disease is a contraindication for estrogen therapy.

29.4 **Progestins are prescribed for dysfunctional uterine bleeding.**

Abnormal uterine bleeding may be the result of an imbalance between progesterone and estrogen secretion. Administration of progestins can often reestablish a normal, cyclic menstrual pattern. High doses of progestins are also used as antineoplastics.

29.5 **Oxytocin and tocolytics are drugs used to influence uterine contractions.**

Oxytocin is administered to stimulate uterine contractions to aid in labor and delivery. Intranasally, it assists in milk letdown. Mifepristone is a uterine stimulant that is used to prevent and terminate pregnancy. Tocolytics are used to relax uterine smooth muscle so that pregnancy may reach term.

29.6 **Androgens are used to treat hypogonadism or delayed puberty in males and breast cancer in females.**

Administration of testosterone promotes the appearance of masculine characteristics, a desirable action in males with hypogonadism. Anabolic steroids are testosterone-like drugs taken illegally to increase athletic performance, which may produce serious, permanent adverse effects in both males and females.

29.7 **Erectile dysfunction is a common disorder that may be successfully treated with drug therapy.**

Erectile dysfunction is a common disorder with many possible physiologic and psychogenic causes. Sildenafil is effective at promoting more rigid and longer-lasting erections. It is contraindicated in clients taking organic nitrates.

29.8 **In its early stages, benign prostatic hyperplasia may be treated successfully with drug therapy.**

BPH results in urinary difficulties that may be treated by drug therapy or surgery. $Alpha_1$-blockers relax smooth muscle in the prostate to promote urine flow. Finasteride shrinks the prostate to improve urinary function. Drugs are effective only in mild cases of BPH.

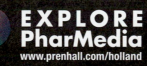

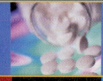

7

THE MUSCULOSKELETAL SYSTEM, INTEGUMENTARY SYSTEM, AND EYES AND EARS

30 Drugs for Muscle Spasms and Bone Disorders

CORE CONCEPTS

MUSCLE SPASMS

30.1 Muscle spasms occur for a variety of reasons.

Antispasmodic Drugs

30.2 The purpose of antispasmodic drugs is to improve mobility.

30.3 Many antispasmodic drugs treat spasticity at the level of the central nervous system.

30.4 Some antispasmodic drugs act directly on muscle tissue.

HYPOCALCEMIA

30.5 Proper functioning of nerves, muscles, and bones depends on calcium and vitamin D.

Calcium Supplements and Vitamin D Therapy

30.6 Calcium supplements and vitamin D therapy are useful in treating osteomalacia, rickets, and hypocalcemia.

WEAK AND FRAGILE BONES

30.7 Osteoporosis is a disorder characterized by weak and fragile bones.

Inhibitors of Bone Resorption

30.8 Weak and fragile bones are improved by drugs that inhibit bone resorption.

PAGET'S DISEASE

30.9 Paget's disease is treated by drug therapies similar to those used for weak and fragile bones.

ARTHRITIC DISORDERS AND GOUT

30.10 Arthritis is one of the major problems affecting mobility.

Antiarthritic Drugs

30.11 Drug therapy for arthritis depends upon the nature of the disorder.

Uric Acid-Inhibitors

30.12 Gout is treated by medications that prevent a buildup of uric acid.

OBJECTIVES

After reading this chapter, the student should be able to:

1. Explain the spinal neural circuitry that underlies muscle spasms.

2. Explain the goal of antispasmodic drug therapy.

3. Compare and contrast the roles of the following drug categories in treating muscle spasticity: centrally acting drugs and drugs acting directly on muscle tissue.

4. Identify important symptoms or disorders associated with an imbalance of calcium, vitamin D, parathyroid hormone, and calcitonin.

5. Discuss drug treatments for hypocalcemia, osteomalacia, and rickets.

6. Identify important disorders characterized by weak, fragile, or abnormal bones.

7. For each of the following drugs classes, know representative drugs, explain their mechanisms of action, primary actions, and/or important adverse effects.
    a. calcium supplements and vitamin D therapy
    b. estrogen replacement therapy
    c. estrogen receptor modulator drugs
    d. statins
    e. slow-release sodium fluoride
    f. biphosphonates
    g. calcitonin

8. Identify common musculoskeletal/joint disorders and the drugs used to treat them.

PharMedia
www.prenhall.com/holland

Additional interactive resources and activities for this chapter can be found on the Companion Website. For animations, audio glossary, and review access the accompanying CD-ROM in this book.

acute gouty arthritis (ah-CUTE GOW-ty are-THRYE-tis): condition where uric acid crystals quickly accumulate in the joints of the big toes, heels, ankles, wrists, fingers, knees, or elbows, resulting in red, swollen, or inflamed tissue / *page 501*

antispasmodic (ANN-tie-spaz-MOD-ik) **drugs**: medications that relieve symptoms of abnormal muscle tension and muscle spasticity / *page 484*

autoantibodies (AW-tow-ANN-tee-BAH-dees): proteins called rheumatoid factors released by B lymphocytes; these tear down the body's own tissue / *page 498*

biphosphonates (bye-FOSS-foh-nayts): family of drugs that block bone resorption by inhibiting osteoclast activity / *page 495*

bone deposition: the opposite of bone resorption; the process of depositing mineral components into bone / *page 489*

bone resorption (ree-SORP-shun): process of bone demineralization or the breaking down of bone into mineral components / *page 489*

calcifediol (kal-SIF-eh-DYE-ol): intermediate form of Vitamin D / *page 489*

calcitonin (kal-sih-TOH-nin) **therapy**: treatment typically administered to women who cannot take estrogen or biphosphonate therapy or for clients with Paget's disease / *page 495*

calcitriol (kal-si-TRY-ol): substance that is transformed in the kidneys during the second step of the conversion of Vitamin D to its active form / *page 489*

cholecalciferol (KOH-lee-kal-SIF-er-ol): inactive form of Vitamin D / *page 489*

dystonia (diss-TONE-ee-ah): muscle spasm characterized by abnormal tension starting in one area of the body and progressing to other areas / *page 484*

estrogen (ESS-troh-jen) **replacement therapy** (ERT): course of treatment involving the administration of reproductive hormones to postmenopausal women / *page 495*

gout (GOWT): metabolic disorder characterized by the accumulation of uric acid in the bloodstream or joint cavities / *page 498*

osteoarthritis (OSS-tee-oh-are-THRYE-tis): disorder characterized by degeneration of joints such as the fingers, spine, hips, and knees / *page 498*

osteomalacia (OSS-tee-oh-muh-LAY-shee-uh): rickets in children; disease characterized by softening of the bones without alteration of basic bone structure / *page 491*

osteoporosis (OSS-tee-oh-poh-ROH-sis): condition where bones become brittle and susceptible to fracture / *page 492*

Paget's (PAH-jets) **disease**: disorder characterized by weak, enlarged, and abnormal bones / *page 492*

rheumatoid arthritis (ROO-mah-toyd are-THRYE-tis): systemic autoimmune disorder characterized by inflammation of multiple joints / *page 498*

selective estrogen receptor modulators (SERMs): drugs that directly produce an action similar to estrogen in body tissues; used for the treatment of osteoporosis in postmenopausal women / *page 495*

spasticity (spas-TISS-ih-tee): inability of opposing muscle groups to move in a coordinated manner / *page 484*

tetany (TET-ah-nee): disorder characterized by prolonged muscle spasms, cramps, and twitches / *page 490*

Disorders associated with movement are some of the most difficult conditions to treat because the mechanisms underlying them span at least four important systems in the body: the nervous system, muscular system, endocrine system, and skeletal system. Proper body movement depends not only upon intact neural pathways, but also on proper functioning of muscles, which, in turn, depend on circulating minerals like sodium, potassium, and calcium in the bloodstream. The balance of calcium in addition to hormones like estrogen, parathyroid hormone, and calcitonin is critical to the proper functioning of these body systems. The skeletal system and joints are at the core of body movement and must be free of any defect that could affect stability of the other systems.

This chapter focuses on the pharmacotherapy of important musculoskeletal disorders. The first part deals with spasticity, and the second part deals with a range of bone disorders including osteomalacia and rickets, osteoporosis, and Paget's disease. The importance of calcium balance and the action of vitamin D are stressed as they relate to proper functioning of nerves, muscles, and bones. Drugs used to treat muscle spasms and important bone disorders are discussed. Finally, important joint disorders and the medications used to treat them are mentioned in view of the major mobility problems that would occur without medical intervention.

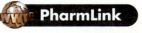

PharmLink

THE NATIONAL INSTITUTE OF ARTHRITIS AND MUSCULOSKELETAL AND SKIN DISEASES

MUSCLE SPASMS

Muscle spasms occur when muscles become tightened and develop a fixed pattern of resistance. Clients with muscle spasms may experience loss of coordination, pain, and reduced mobility.

30.1 Muscle spasms occur for a variety of reasons.

Muscle spasms develop for several reasons including overmedication with antipsychotic drugs (Chapter 9 ⬤▭) and progressive brain disorders (Chapter 10 ⬤▭). When muscle spasms occur, however, it is often because of neurological damage to pathways responsible for muscle contraction. This damage may be associated with brain or spinal cord injury, stroke, cerebral palsy, or multiple sclerosis. In such cases, muscle spasms may be localized or spread throughout the entire body. **Dystonia** is a symptom characterized by abnormal muscle tension starting in one area of the body and progressing to other areas. Dystonic contractions often appear in places such as the eyes, face, neck, torso, spine, hips, and limbs. Cervical dystonia is a genetic disorder where neck muscles stiffen causing extreme discomfort and an abnormal posture.

dys = abnormal
tonia = tension

Fast Facts Muscle Spasms

- Over 12 million people worldwide have muscle spasms.
- Muscle spasms severe enough for drug therapy are generally found in clients who have had other debilitating disorders such as stroke, injury, neurodegenerative diseases, and cerebral palsy.

ANTISPASMODIC DRUGS

Antispasmodic drugs relieve symptoms of muscular stiffness and rigidity. They improve mobility in cases where clients have restricted movements.

30.2 The purpose of antispasmodic drugs is to improve mobility.

The occurrence of muscle spasms represents a disruption of the normal way that motor neural pathways and spinal reflexes function. The uncoordinated actions of muscle groups are medically referred to as **spasticity**. With spasticity, some muscles are overactive; others are underactive.

The goal of drug therapy in this case is to improve the client's ability to move around. In many cases, treatment is needed so clients can perform normal daily activities, referred to as ADLs or *activities of daily living*. Medications often allow clients to regain flexibility or to engage in simple activities like grooming, eating, turning, moving their heads, or sitting up.

Occasionally, antispasmodic medications worsen the client's ability to move. In these cases, medications are often withheld or used on a more limited basis. For example, important muscles necessary for standing upright might require a measure of rigidity, even if they are not reacting normally. In this instance, it would be the role of the physical or occupational therapist to offer other forms of therapy that might help the client to position, stretch, or strengthen selected muscle groups.

Concept review 30.1

- Give several reasons why muscle spasms develop. What is the main goal of antispasmodic therapy?

30.3 Many antispasmodic drugs treat spasticity at the level of the central nervous system.

Drugs work to relieve muscle spasms by several mechanisms. Many drugs treat spasticity by acting at the level of the central nervous system. This means that their antispasmodic effects are generated within the brain and/or spinal cord. These effects usually stem from inhibition of upper motor neuron activity, sedation, or alteration of simple reflexes. Centrally acting medications used for spasticity are summarized in Table 30.1.

NATURAL ALTERNATIVES

Black Cohosh for Muscle Spasms

Black cohosh (*Cimicifuga racemosa*) is an herb found in the rich upland woods of North America from Ontario to Georgia. Its name, *racemosa,* the means "to drive away." Folklore has it that black cohosh was once used as an insect repellent to drive away insects. Today it is used to treat muscle spasms, among other ailments. It is commonly used to relief muscle cramps in dysmenorrhea. Black cohosh is purported to affect the female reproductive system the same way as estrogen but without unpleasant side effects or cancer risks.

For full effectiveness in general muscle relaxation, it is often combined with other tranquilizing herbs such skullcap, passionflower, or valerian. The user has to be careful, however, because larger doses of these herbs can produce nausea, vomiting, and other signs of toxicity. Only someone trained to understand the limitations of these natural products should use black cohosh. Additionally, this herb should not be taken during pregnancy. ■

Antispasmodic drugs may be used alone or in combination with other medications. Commonly used centrally acting medications are baclofen (Lioresal), tizanidine (Zanaflex), and benzodiazepines such as diazepam (Valium), clonazepam (Klonopin), and lorazepam (Ativan).

Baclofen produces its effect by a mechanism that is not fully known. This drug is structurally similar to the inhibitory neurotransmitter gamma amino butyric acid (GABA). Thus, it inhibits neuronal activity within the brain and possibly the spinal cord, although there is some question as to whether the spinal effects of baclofen are associated with GABA. Common side effects of baclofen are drowsiness, dizziness, weakness, and fatigue.

DRUG PROFILE:
Cyclobenzaprine (Cycloflex, Flexeril)

Actions:

Cyclobenzaprine relieves muscle spasms of local origin without interfering with general muscle function. This medication depresses motor activity by actions primarily in the brain stem but with limited effects occurring also in the spinal cord. It increases circulating levels of norepinephrine, blocking presynaptic uptake. Its mechanism of action is similar to tricyclic antidepressants (Chapter 9 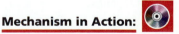). Therapeutically, it causes muscle relaxation in cases of acute muscle spasticity, but it is not effective in cases of cerebral palsy or diseases of the brain and spinal cord. This medication is meant to provide therapy only for two to three weeks.

Adverse Effects:

Adverse reactions to cyclobenzaprine include drowsiness, dizziness, dry mouth, rash, and tachycardia. One reaction, although rare, is swelling of the tongue. Alcohol, phenothiazines, and MAO inhibitors increase the risk of these unfavorable reactions.

Mechanism in Action:

Cyclobenzaprine relaxes skeletal muscle and prevents local muscle spasms, alleviating pain. These effects are produced by depression of motor activity originating at the level of the brain stem and spinal motor neurons. Cyclobenzaprine also increases circulating levels of norepinephrine in the bloodstream, and causes potent anticholinergic activity throughout the nervous system.

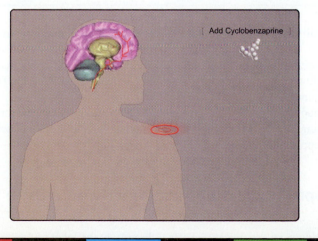

TABLE 30.1	Centrally Acting Antispasmodic Drugs	
DRUG	**ROUTE AND ADULT DOSE**	**REMARKS**
(Pr) cyclobenzaprine hydrochloride (Cycloflex, Flexeril)	PO; 10–20 mg bid-qid (max 60 mg/day).	Short-term relief of muscle spasms associated with acute muscloskeletal conditions; not for cerebral palsy or central nervous system diseases.
baclofen (Lioresal)	PO; 5 mg tid (max 80 mg/day).	May be administered orally or by an implantable pump, which infuses medication directly into the subarachnoid space.
carisoprodol (Soma)	PO; 350 mg tid.	CNS depressant; does not inhibit motor activity like other conventional muscle relaxers; muscle relaxation seems to be related to sedation.
chlorphenesin (Maolate)	PO; 800 mg tid until effective; reduce to 400 mg qid or less.	Often used in conjunction with physical therapy in cases of musculoskeletal injury and pain.
chlorzoxazone (Paraflex, Parafon Forte)	PO; 250–500 mg tid-qid (max 3 grams/day).	Depresses nerve transmission in the brain and spinal cord, possibly by sedation; not effective for cerebral palsy.
clonazepam (Klonopin)	PO; 0.5 mg tid (max 20 mg/day).	Benzodiazepine usually taken in combination with other drugs; used for the relief of skeletal muscle spasms; primarily for seizure disorders.
diazepam (Valium)	PO; 4–10 mg bid-qid IM/IV; 2–10 mg, repeat if needed in 3–4 hrs; IV pump; administer emulsion at 5 mg/min.	Benzodiazepine used for the relief of skeletal muscle spasms associated with cerebral palsy, partial paralysis.
lorazepam (Ativan)	PO; 1–2 mg bid-tid (max 10 mg/day).	Benzodiazepine used for extreme muscle tension.
metaxalone (Skelaxin)	PO; 800 mg tid-qid × max of 10 days.	For acute musculoskeletal conditions; causes it effect through sedation.
methocarbamol (Robaxain)	PO; 1.5 grams qid × 2–3 days, then reduce to 1 gram qid.	Adjunct to physical therapy for acute musculoskeletal disorders and tetanus.
orphenadrine citrate (Banflex, Flexon, Myolin, Norflex)	PO; 100 mg bid.	IM/IV forms available.
tizanidine (Zanaflex)	PO; 4–8 mg tid-qid (max 36 mg/day).	To relax muscle tone associated with spasticity.

Tizanidine is a centrally acting $alpha_2$ adrenergic-agonist inhibiting motor neurons mainly at the level of the spinal cord. Clients receiving high doses report being drowsy. Thus, it also affects some neural activity in the brain. One undesirable effect of tizanidine is hallucinations, which have been reported by a few clients. The most frequent side effects are dry mouth, fatigue, tiredness, dizziness, and sleepiness.

As mentioned in Chapters 7 and 8 ⊂⊃ , benzodiazepines inhibit both sensory and motor neuron activity by enhancing the effects of GABA. Common adverse side effects include drowsiness and ataxia (loss of coordination).

30.4 Some antispasmodic drugs act directly on muscle tissue.

Four important drugs produce an antispasmodic effect directly at the level of the neuromuscular junction as shown in Figure 30.1. These are Botulinum toxin type A (Botox, Dysport), Botulinum

FIGURE 30.1

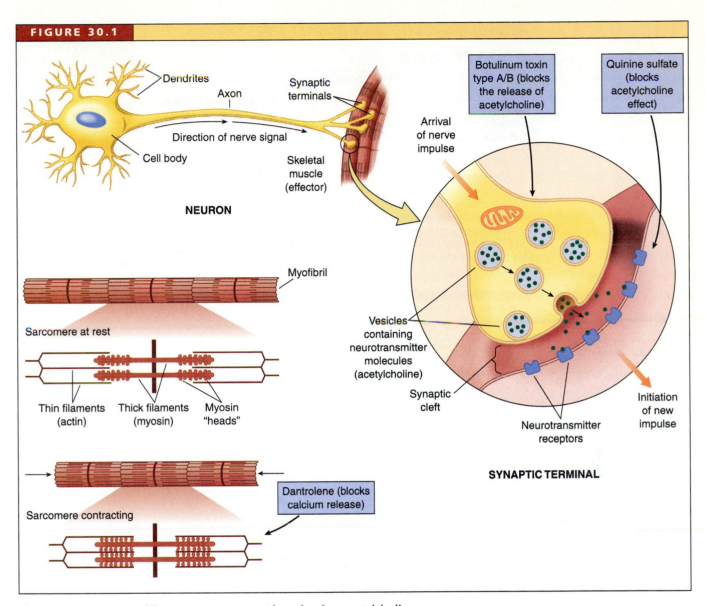

The motor neuron enables motor movement by releasing acetylcholine

toxin type B (Myobloc), dantrolene sodium (Dantrium), and quinine sulfate (Quinamm, Quiphile). These drugs are summarized in Table 30.2.

Botulinum toxin is an unusual drug because, in higher quantities, it acts a poison. *Clostridium botulinum* is the bacteria responsible for food poisoning or botulism. However, at lower doses this drug is safe and effective as a muscle relaxant. It produces its effect by blocking the release of acetylcholine from cholinergic nerve terminals (Chapter 6 ⊂⊃).

Because of the extreme weakness associated with this medication, physical therapists often focus on therapies that improve muscle strength. To circumvent major problems with mobility or posture, Botulinum toxin is often applied to small muscle groups. Sometimes, Botulinum is administered along with centrally acting oral medications to increase functional use of a range of muscle groups.

One drawback to Botulinum is its delayed and limited effects. The treatment is mostly effective within six weeks and lasts only for three to six months. Another drawback is pain; Botulinum is injected directly into the muscle. Pain associated with injections is usually blocked by a local anesthetic (Chapter 12 ⊂⊃).

Concept review 30.2

■ Identify two general ways that antispasmodic drugs relieve muscle spasms and symptoms of spasticity.

DRUG PROFILE:
Dantrolene Sodium (Dantrium)

Actions:

Many clients have muscle spasms of the head and neck area. Dantrolene (Dantrium) is often used for this kind of disorder. It directly relaxes muscle spasms by interfering with the release of calcium ions from storage areas inside the muscle cells. It does not affect cardiac or smooth muscle. Dantrolene is especially useful for muscle spasms when they occur after spinal cord injury or stroke and in cases of cerebral palsy and multiple sclerosis. It is sometimes used for the treatment of muscle pain after heavy exercise.

Adverse Effects:

Adverse effects include muscle weakness, dizziness, blurred vision, diarrhea, tachycardia, and erratic blood pressure. Dantrolene should not be taken with alcohol or other CNS depressants. Verapamil (Calan) and other calcium channel blockers taken with dantrolene increase the risk of ventricular fibrillation and cardiovascular collapse. Clients with impaired cardiac or pulmonary function or hepatic disease should not take this drug.

TABLE 30.2	Antispasmodic Drugs Acting Directly on Skeletal Muscles	
DRUG	**ROUTE AND ADULT DOSE**	**REMARKS**
Botulinum toxin Type A (Botox, Dysport)	25 units injected directly into target muscle (max 30 day dose should not exceed 200 units).	May be used in cases of cerebral palsy, multiple sclerosis, and traumatic brain or spinal cord injury; may also used for strabismus (crossed eyes); sometimes used for excessive sweating and wrinkles.
Botulinum toxin Type B (Myobloc)	2500–5000 units per dose injected directly into target muscle; doses should be divided among muscle groups.	May be used in cases of cervical dystonia.
Pr dantrolene sodium (Dantrium)	PO; 25 mg qd; increase to 25 mg bid-qid; may increase every 4–7 days up to 100 mg bid-tid.	Hydantoin-like medication; also for the treatment of malignant hyperthermia; IV form available.
quinine sulfate (Quinamm, Quiphile)	PO; 260–300 mg at hs.	Antimalarial drug; for nocturnal leg cramps or congenital tonic spasms.

HYPOCALCEMIA

Hypocalcemia, or lowered levels of calcium in the blood, is associated with a range of problems including poor nutrition, muscle spasms, convulsions, and endocrine and bone disorders.

30.5 Proper functioning of nerves, muscles, and bones depends on calcium and vitamin D.

One of the most important minerals in the body, responsible for proper nerve and muscle function, is calcium. Calcium disorders are often associated with vitamin D disorders. Certain skeletal, nutritional, and endocrine conditions are caused by calcium and vitamin D disorders.

FIGURE 30.2

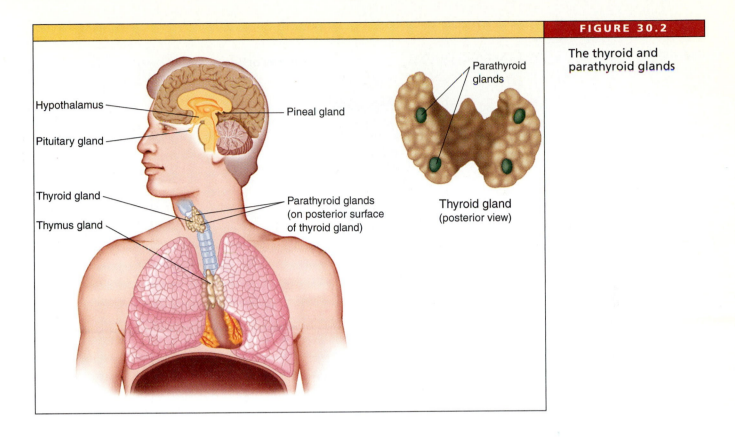

The thyroid and parathyroid glands

Hypothalamus

Pituitary gland

Thyroid gland

Thymus gland

Pineal gland

Parathyroid glands (on posterior surface of thyroid gland)

Parathyroid glands

Thyroid gland (posterior view)

Levels of calcium in the bloodstream are controlled by two endocrine glands: the parathyroid glands and the thyroid gland. Parathyroid hormone (PTH) comes from the parathyroid glands; calcitonin, sometimes called *thyrocalcitonin,* comes from the thyroid gland as shown in Figure 30.2.

One of the functions of PTH is to stimulate a population of bone cells called *osteoclasts,* which accelerate the process of bone resorption. **Bone resorption** is the act of bone demineralization, or breaking down of bone into smaller mineral components. After bone resorption, calcium is released into the blood and the levels of calcium subsequently rise. The opposite of this process is **bone deposition**, which is bone building. This process is stimulated by the hormone calcitonin.

Both PTH and calcitonin control calcium metabolism in the body by influencing three major targets: the bones, kidneys, and gastrointestinal (GI) tract. The GI tract is mainly influenced by parathyroid hormone and involves vitamin D.

Vitamin D is a fat soluble vitamin. It is unique among vitamins in that the body is able to synthesize it from precursor molecules. In the skin, the inactive form of vitamin D, called **cholecalciferol**, is synthesized from an important precursor, cholesterol. Exposure of the skin to sunlight or ultraviolet light stimulates an increase of cholecalciferol in the bloodstream. Cholecalciferol can also be ingested from dietary products such as milk or other foods fortified with vitamin D. Figure 30.3 shows the metabolism of vitamin D.

After being absorbed into the blood stream, cholecalciferol is converted into an intermediate vitamin form called **calcifediol**. Calcifediol is transported to the kidneys where enzymes further transform this substance into **calcitriol**, which is the active form of vitamin D.

Parathyroid hormone stimulates the formation of calcitriol at the level of the kidneys. After being released from the kidneys, calcitriol increases calcium absorption from the GI tract. Dietary calcium is absorbed much better in the presence of active vitamin D and parathyroid hormone. The more calcium absorbed across the intestinal wall, the higher levels of calcium found in the bloodstream.

The importance of proper calcium balance in the body cannot be understated. Calcium ion influences the excitability of all neurons. Whenever calcium concentrations are too high (hypercalcemia), sodium permeability decreases across cell membranes. This is a dangerous state because nerve conduction depends upon the proper influx of sodium into cells.

hyper = *elevated*
hypo = *lowered*
calc = *calcium*
emia = *blood level*

FIGURE 30.3

Pathway for vitamin D
activation and action

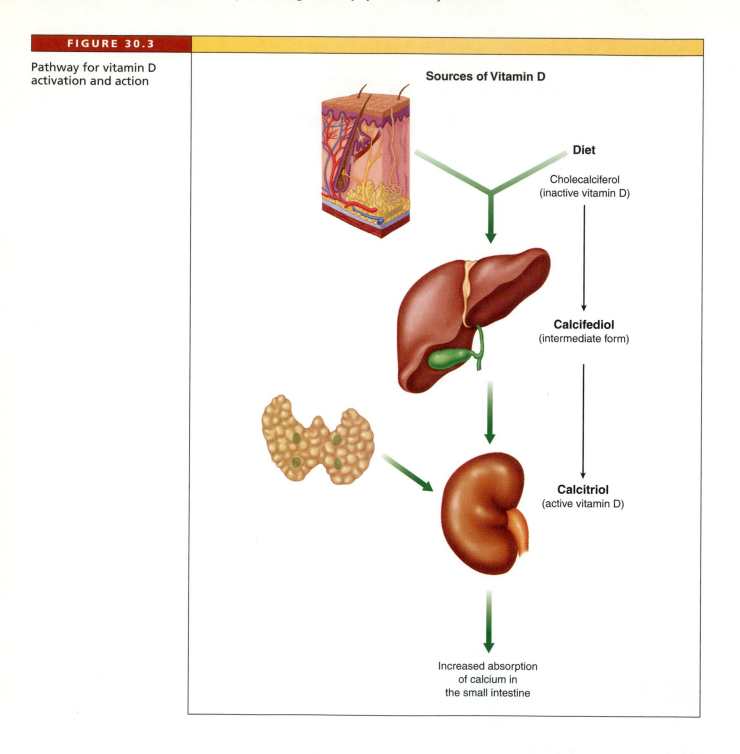

Sources of Vitamin D

Diet

Cholecalciferol
(inactive vitamin D)

Calcifediol
(intermediate form)

Calcitriol
(active vitamin D)

Increased absorption
of calcium in
the small intestine

   Whenever calcium levels in the blood stream are too low (hypocalcemia), cell membranes become extremely excitable. If this situation becomes severe, the client may have convulsions or muscle spasms. Prolonged muscle spasms are referred to as **tetany**.
   Calcium is also important for the normal functioning of other body processes such as blood coagulation and myocardial activity. Refer to Unit III to review how some drugs affect calcium activity related to hypertension, heart failure, and dysrhythmias. Figure 30.4 summarizes the effects of parathyroid hormone and calcitonin in the body.

Concept review 30.3

▪ Give examples where unusually low or high levels of blood calcium affect normal body functioning.

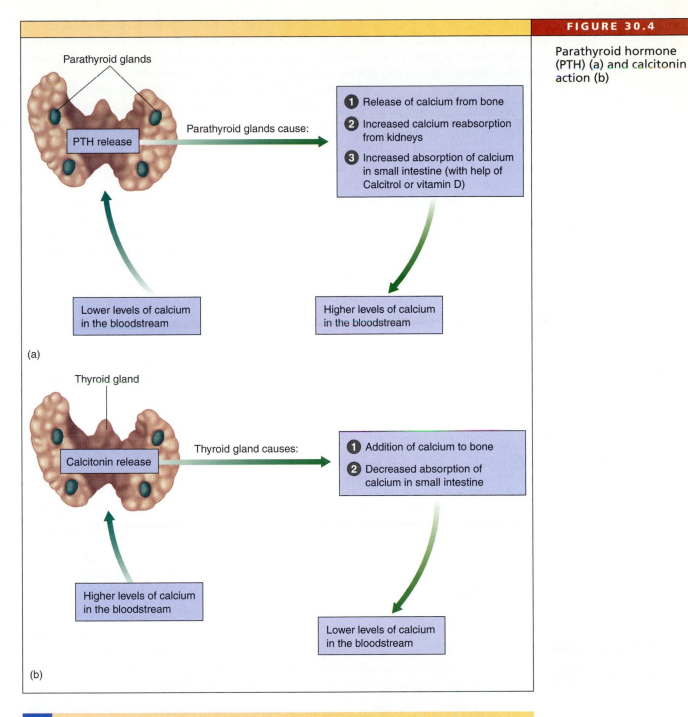

FIGURE 30.4

Parathyroid hormone (PTH) (a) and calcitonin action (b)

CALCIUM SUPPLEMENTS AND VITAMIN D THERAPY

Calcium supplements and vitamin D therapy are used to restore the critical balance of calcium in certain nutritional, hormonal, or bone disorders.

30.6 Calcium supplements and vitamin D therapy are useful in treating osteomalacia, rickets, and hypocalcemia.

Osteomalacia, referred to as rickets in children, is a disorder characterized by softening of bones without alteration of basic bone structure. The cause of osteomalacia and rickets is usually a lack of vitamin D and calcium in the diet. These disorders may also be caused by kidney failure or malabsorption of calcium from the GI tract. Symptoms include hypocalcemia, muscle weakness, muscle spasms, and diffuse bone pain, especially in the hip area. Clients may also experience pain in the arms, legs, and spinal column. Classic signs of rickets in children include bowlegs and a pigeon breast. Children may also develop a slight fever and become restless at night.

Tests performed to verify osteomalacia include bone biopsy, bone x-ray, computerized tomography (CT) scan of the vertebral column, and determination of serum calcium, phosphate, and vitamin D levels. Many of these tests are routine for bone disorders and are performed as needed to determine the extent of bone health.

In extreme cases, surgical correction of disfigured limbs may be required. Drug therapy for children and adults consists of calcium supplements and vitamin D. A summary of drugs used for these conditions is provided in Table 30.3.

There are two major forms of calcium: complexed and elemental. Most calcium supplements come in the form of complexed calcium. They are often compared on the basis of their ability to release elemental calcium into the bloodstream. The greater the ability of complexed calcium to release elemental calcium, the more potent is the supplement. Elemental calcium may be obtained from dietary sources such as dark green vegetables, canned salmon, and fortified products including tofu, orange juice, and milk.

Inactive, intermediate, and active forms of vitamin D are also available as medications. The amount of vitamin D a client needs will often vary depending upon how much he or she is exposed to sunlight.

Concept review 30.4

■ Identify the major drug therapies used for osteomalacia, rickets, and hypolcalcemia.

WEAK AND FRAGILE BONES

Two important disorders characterized by weak and fragile bones are osteoporosis and Paget's disease. Although these disorders are not the same, they share many of the same symptoms.

30.7 Osteoporosis is a disorder characterized by weak and fragile bones.

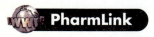

OSTEOPOROSIS AND RELATED BONE DISEASES NATIONAL RESOURCE CENTER

Osteoporosis is a condition where bones become brittle and are susceptible to fracture. Osteoporosis occurs for two major reasons. The first is menopause, which occurs in women after the age of 50. The second is disruption of the normal bone rebuilding process. The elderly are especially at risk for osteoporosis. The risk factors for this disorder follow.

- high alcohol consumption
- anorexia nervosa
- smoking
- lack of exercise
- onset of menopause in women (low levels of estrogen in the bloodstream)
- testosterone deficiency in men, particularly in the elderly
- poor nutrition (lack of appropriate vitamin D and calcium in the diet)
- age, obesity, low muscle strength

PharmLink

NATIONAL OSTEOPOROSIS FOUNDATION

When women reach menopause, estrogen levels decline in the bloodstream (Chapter 29 ⊂⊃). When estrogen blood levels are low, bones become weak and fragile. One theory is that normal levels of estrogen may naturally limit the life span of *osteoclasts,* bones cells that resorb bone. When estrogen levels become low, osteoclast activity is not controlled as before, and bone demineralization

DRUG PROFILE:
Calcium Gluconate (Kalcinate)

Actions:

Calcium gluconate is a supplement designed to increase calcium blood levels. It is effective in cases of hypocalcemic tetany. It may also be used in cases of pregnancy, growth during childhood, and in cases of osteoporosis.

Adverse Effects:

The most common adverse effect of calcium gluconate is hypercalcemia, brought on by taking too much of this supplement. Symptoms include nausea, vomiting, thirst, constipation, lethargy, and psychosis. IV administration of calcium may cause hypotension, bradycardia, dysrhythmia, and cardiac arrest.

TABLE 30.3	Calcium Supplements and Vitamin D Therapy	
DRUG	**ROUTE AND ADULT DOSE (ALL DOSES ARE IN TERMS OF ELEMENTAL CALCIUM.)**	**REMARKS**
Calcium Supplements		
Pr calcium gluconate (Kalcinate)	PO; 1–2 g bid-qid.	1 gram calcium gluconate equals 90 mg (4.5 mEq) elemental calcium; IV form available.
calcium acetate (Phos-Ex, PhosLo)	PO; 1–2 g bid-tid.	1 gram calcium acetate equals 250 mg (12.6 mEq) elemental calcium.
calcium carbonate (BioCal, Calcite-500, others)	PO; 1–2 g bid-tid.	1 gram calcium carbonate equals 400 mg (20 mEq) elemental calcium.
calcium chloride	IV; 0.5–1 g qd q 3 days.	1 gram calcium chloride equals 272 mg (13.6 mEq) elemental calcium; may be irritating to body tissues.
calcium citrate (Citracal)	PO; 1–2 g bid-tid.	1 gram calcium citrate equals 210 mg (12 mEq) elemental calcium.
calcium gluceptate	IV; 1.1–4.4 gram qd IM; 0.5–1.1 gram qd.	1 gram calcium gluceptate equals 82 mg (4.1 mEq) elemental calcium.
calcium lactate	PO; 325 mg-1.3 g tid with meals.	1 gram calcium lactate equals 130 mg (6.5 mEq) elemental calcium.
calcium phosphate tribasic (Posture)	PO; 1–2 g bid-tid.	1 gram calcium phosphate equals 390 mg 1(19.3 mEq) elemental calcium.
Vitamin D Supplements		
Pr calcitriol (Calcijex, Rocaltrol)	PO; 0.25 μg qd.	For hypocalcemia in chronic renal failure and with hypoparathyroidism.
ergocalciferol (Deltalin, Calciferol)	PO/IM; 25–125 μg qd × 6–12 weeks.	For osteomalacia; also used for vitamin D-dependent rickets and hypoparathyroidism.
calcifediol (Calderol)	PO; 50–100 μg qd or qod.	For metabolic bone disease and hypocalcemia associated with chronic kidney failure.

DRUG PROFILE:

Calcitriol (Calcijex, Rocaltrol), Active Vitamin D

Actions:

Calcitriol is the active form of vitamin D. It promotes the intestinal absorption of calcium and elevates serum levels of calcium. This medication is used in cases where clients have poorly functioning kidneys or have an imbalance of PTH. Calcitriol reduces bone resorption and is useful in treating rickets.

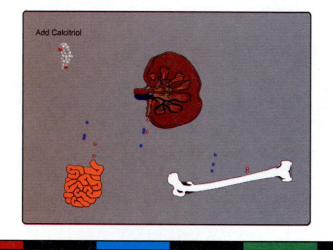

Add Calcitriol

Adverse Effects:

Common side effects include hypercalcemia, headache, weakness, dry mouth, thirst, increased urination, and muscle or bone pain. Thiazide diuretics may enhance effects of vitamin D, causing hypercalcemia. Too much vitamin D may cause dysrhythmia in clients receiving cardiac glycosides.

Mechanism in Action:

Calcitriol is an active form of vitamin D, responsible for increasing calcium absorption. Calcium is important for the proper functioning of the muscular, skeletal, and nervous systems. All three systems, as well as organs of the endocrine and renal system, play a critical role in maintaining a proper balance of calcium in the bloodstream.

is accelerated, resulting in bone weakness. In women with osteoporosis, fractures usually occur in the hips, wrists, forearms, or spine.

Among other clients, osteoporosis is mainly due to a disrupted pattern of bone rebuilding. Simply stated, bone resorption outpaces bone deposition. As a result, many clients develop weak bones. In some cases, the lack of dietary calcium, vitamin D, or physical inactivity contribute to osteoporosis. Medications such as corticosteroids, some anti-seizure medications, and immunosuppressive drugs may lower calcium levels in the bloodstream, making the disorder worse.

Fast Facts Osteoporosis

- Osteoporosis is the most prevalent bone disorder in America.
- On a yearly basis, 28 million clients are either diagnosed with osteoporosis or are considered to be at extreme risk for this disorder.
- Women are four times more likely to develop osteoporosis than men. Many women with osteoporosis are of postmenopausal age.
- After the age of 50, one out of every two women and one out of every eight men are likely to develop a fracture related to osteoporosis.

Concept review 30.5

- Identify two important disorders characterized by weak and fragile bones.

INHIBITORS OF BONE RESORPTION

Drugs that inhibit bone resorption strengthen bones by increasing their mass and density. Some inhibitors of bone resorption have other therapeutic uses, for example, estrogens and cholesterol-lowering drugs.

30.8 Weak and fragile bones are improved by drugs that inhibit bone resorption.

Many drug treatments are available for weak and fragile bones. These include calcium and vitamin D therapy, estrogen replacement therapy, estrogen receptor modulators, statins, slow-release sodium fluoride, biphosphonates, and calcitonin. Many of these treatments are also used for other bone disorders or conditions unrelated to the skeletal system. In cases of osteoporosis, calcium supplements and vitamin D therapy help to maintain bone density and reduce the risk of fractures. These treatments have already been discussed.

Estrogen replacement therapy (ERT) is one of the most common treatments for osteoporosis in postmenopausal women. One drawback to ERT, however, is the increased risk of uterine cancer. Practitioners reduce this risk by prescribing estrogen with progesterone. As discussed in Chapter 29 ⬭, progesterone produces a thick cervical mucous and protects the uterine lining. Women who take long-term ERT have a higher incidence of thromboembolic disease and breast cancer.

An alternative to ERT is use of selective estrogen receptor modulators (SERMs). These drugs provide the same protection against uterine or breast cancer as progesterone, and reduce the risk of cardiovascular disease. However, SERMs do not reduce the incidence of blood clots (Table 30.4).

Tamoxifen (Nolvadex) is another alternative to ERT. It provides the benefit of increasing bone density without the risk of uterine cancer. Tamoxifen blocks the effects of estrogen on breast tissue, but it has the opposite effect on bone tissue. It mimics the effect of estrogen, reducing the risk of bone fracture. While vaginal bleeding may occur with this medication, the incidence of blood clots is less compared to other drugs.

Statins are drugs used to treat hyperlipidemia (Chapter 19 ⬭). Although they are not routinely used for the treatment of osteoporosis, these medications may be effective in reducing the incidence of bone fractures in some women who have osteoporosis.

Slow-release sodium fluoride seems to be helpful in reducing symptoms of osteoporosis. When given to postmenopausal women, this drug increases bone mass with continued therapy.

The most common treatment for osteoporosis, other than ERT, is a family of drugs called biphosphonates. These medications are structurally similar to endogenous biphosphates: organic salts found within the body. Biphosphonates block bone resorption by inhibiting osteoclast activity. Common drugs are etidronate (Didronel), alendronate (Fosamax) and tiludronate (Skelid). Pamidronate (Aredia) is provided as an injectable drug. These drugs strengthen bones with continued use. Adverse effects are gastrointestinal problems such as nausea, vomiting, abdominal pain, and esophageal irritation. Biphosphonate drugs are summarized in Table 30.5.

Calcitonin therapy is most often given to clients who are not able to take estrogen or biphosphonate therapy. Calcitonin inhibits bone resorption and prevents fractures resulting from low bone density. Calcitonin is available as a nasal spray, or it may be injected. It comes from two sources: human and salmon (synthetic polypeptide). The pharmacological actions of both drugs are similar, but calcitonin-salmon is more potent and lasts longer (Table 30.5).

Concept review 30.6

■ What are the major drug therapies used for osteoporosis?

TABLE 30.4	Risks of ERT, ERT with Progesterone, and SERMS Compared		
	RISKS		
	UTERINE CANCER	BLOOD CLOTS	BREAST CANCER
ERT	✔		✔
ERT with progesterone		✔	
SERMs		✔	

DRUG PROFILE:
Raloxifene (Evista)

Actions:

Raloxifene is a selective estrogen receptor modulator (SERM). It decreases bone resorption and increases bone mass and density by acting through the estrogen receptor. Raloxifene is primarily used for the prevention of osteoporosis in postmenopausal women. This drug also reduces serum total cholesterol and LDL (low-density lipoproteins) without lowering HDL (high-density lipoproteins) or triglycerides.

Adverse Effects:

Common side effects are hot flashes, migraine headache, flu-like symptoms, endometrial disorder, breast pain, and vaginal bleeding. Clients should not take cholesterol-lowering drugs or estrogen replacement therapy at the same time with this medication.

TABLE 30.5	Common Bone Resorption Inhibitor Drugs of Importance for Bone Disorders	
DRUG	**ROUTE AND ADULT DOSE**	**REMARKS**
Hormonal Agents		
Pr raloxifene hydrochloride (Evista)	PO; 60 mg qd.	Selective estrogen receptor modulator; mimics the effects of estrogen on bone.
tamoxifen citrate (Nolvadex)	PO; 10–20 mg qd-bid.	Traditionally used for breast carcinoma, but mimics the effects of estrogen on the bone; competes with estrogen in reproductive areas.
calcitonin- human (Cibacalcin); Calcitonin-salmon (Calcimar; Miacalcin)	Paget's disease: SC; human, 0.5 mg qd SC/IM; salmon, 100 IU qd; hypercalcemia: SC/IM: salmon, 4 IU/kg bid IU = international units.	Used commonly for hypercalcemia and Paget's disease.
Biphosphonates		
Pr etidronate disodium (Didronel)	PO; 5–10 mg/kg qd × 6 months or 11–20 mg/kg qd × 3 months.	For Paget's disease.
alendronate sodium (Fosamax)	osteoporosis treatment: PO; 10 mg qd; osteoporosis prevention: PO; 5 mg qd; Paget's disease: PO; 40 mg qd × 6 months.	For osteoporosis and Paget's disease.
pamidronate disodium (Aredia)	IV; 15–90 mg in 1000 ml NS or D5W over 4–24 hours.	For Paget's disease and moderate hypercalcemia of malignancy.
risedronate sodium (Actonel)	PO; 30 mg qd at least 30 minutes before the first drink or meal of the day × 2 months.	For Paget's disease.
tiludronate disodium (Skelid)	PO; 400 mg qd taken with 6–8 ounces of water 2 hours before or after food × 3 months.	For Paget's disease.

PAGET'S DISEASE

Paget's disease is a chronic debilitating disorder characterized by enlarged and abnormal bones. With this disorder, the process of abnormal bone resorption and bone formation occurs continually. Because of the excessive bone turnover, the new bone is very weak and brittle. Deformity and fractures may also develop. Clients often experience pain and inflammation of the joints. Symptoms include aching of the hips and femurs, headaches, facial pain, and hearing loss if bones around the ear cavity are affected. Nerves along the spinal column may be pinched due to compression between the vertebrae.

Paget's disease is sometimes confused with osteoporosis because many of the symptoms are similar. In fact, many of the medical treatments for osteoporosis are also similar to Paget's disease. However, the cause of Paget's disease is quite different. With Paget's disease, the enzyme *alkaline phosphatase* is elevated in the bloodstream because of the extensive bone turnover. Alkaline phosphatase is responsible for liberating minerals—mainly phosphate—from the chemical complexes making up the bone. Other minerals such as calcium are also liberated because of their close association with phosphate. Therefore, Paget's disease is usually confirmed by early detection of this enzyme in the blood. If diagnosis is made early enough, symptoms can be treated successfully. If diagnosis is made late in the progress of the disease, permanent skeletal abnormalities may develop, and other disorders may appear including arthritis, kidney stones, and heart disease.

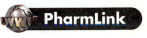

THE PAGET FOUNDATION

30.9 Paget's disease is treated by drug therapies similar to those used for weak and fragile bones.

Treatment for Paget's disease includes biphosphonates and calcitonin. The pharmacologic goals are to slow the rate of bone resorption and encourage the deposition of strong bone. Surgery may be indicated in cases of severe bone deformity, degenerative arthritis, or fracture. Clients with Paget's disease should maintain adequate dietary sources of calcium and vitamin D on a daily basis. Adequate exposure to sunlight is also important.

Concept review 30.7

▪ What major defect other than weak and fragile bones does Paget's disease have? Identify the two main drug therapies used for this disorder.

DRUG PROFILE:

Etidronate (Didronel)

Actions:

Etidronate slows down bone resorption and new bone growth in clients with Paget's disease. Effects may begin one to three months after therapy starts and continue for months after therapy is stopped. This drug lowers serum alkaline phosphatase, the enzyme associated with bone turnover, without any major adverse effects. Etidronate may also be used to prevent osteoporosis and PTH-induced bone resorption.

Adverse Effects:

Common side effects of etidronate are diarrhea, nausea, and a metallic or altered taste perception. Calcium supplements may decrease absorption of etidronate; therefore, concomitant use of these drugs should be avoided. Food-drug interactions are common, especially with milk and other dairy products.

NATURAL ALTERNATIVES

Glucosamine and Chondroitin for Osteoarthritis

Glucosamine sulfate is natural substance that is an important building block of cartilage. With aging, glucosamine is lost with the natural thinning of cartilage. As cartilage wears down, joints lose their normal cushioning ability, resulting in the pain and inflammation of osteoarthritis.

Glucosamine sulfate is sold as a non-prescription dietary supplement. Some studies have shown it to be more effective than a placebo in reducing mild arthritis and joint pain. It is purported to promote cartilage repair in the joints. Although reliable long-term studies are not available, glucosamine is marketed as a safe and inexpensive alternative to prescription anti-inflammatory drugs.

Chondroitin sulfate is another dietary supplement purported to promote cartilage repair. It is a natural substance that forms part of the matrix between cartilage cells. Chondroitin is usually combined with glucosamine in specific arthritis formulas. ■

ARTHRITIC DISORDERS AND GOUT

arthr = joint
itis = associated disease, often linked with inflammation

osteo = bone
arthritis = joint disease

Osteoarthritis is painful disorder caused by erosion of cartilage at articular joint surfaces. **Rheumatoid arthritis** is an equally painful inflammatory joint disorder caused by an attack of the body's own immune system. **Gout** is a second major inflammatory disorder caused by the buildup of uric acid within the blood or joint cavities.

30.10 Arthritis is one of the major problems affecting mobility.

Osteoarthritis is a degenerative disease characterized by wearing away of cartilaginous joints. Joints within the fingers, spine, hips, and knees are especially susceptible. Symptoms of osteoarthritis include muscle spasms, localized pain and stiffness, joint and bone enlargement, and limited movement. Osteoarthritis is sometimes called *non-inflammatory-type arthritis* because it is not accompanied by the inflammation normally associated with other rheumatic disorders.

The causes of osteoarthritis are not understood, although symptoms seem to be associated with genetic and immune-related factors occurring mainly after the age of 40. Because of its predominant occurrence among elderly clients, many consider this to be a normal part of the aging process. Middle-age clients who are extremely active and obese clients are at high risk for this disorder.

rheuma = watery discharge
toid = associated

Unlike osteoarthritis which is considered an age-onset, degenerative condition, rheumatoid arthritis is a systemic autoimmune disorder. It is characterized by inflammation of multiple joints. In some cases, inflammation may be minor, or in others, many joints may be inflamed, causing the client extreme discomfort. Rheumatoid arthritis is disfiguring and occurs at an earlier age than osteoarthritis. Symptoms include tenderness, swelling, dull aching pain, and stiffness. At times, symptoms may undergo remission or worsen depending on the levels of circulating autoantibodies in the bloodstream.

auto = self-directed
anti = against
bodies = things

Autoantibodies are proteins called *rheumatoid factors* released by B lymphocytes connected with the humoral immune response (Chapter 20 ⬤▭). Autoantibodies activate, complement, and draw other leukocytes into the area, where they attack normal cells. This results in persistent injury and the formation of inflammatory fluid within the joints, one cause of discomfort. Joint capsules, tendons, ligaments, and skeletal muscles may also be affected. Another cause of discomfort is major damage to other structural body components. Rheumatoid nodules or lesions may appear on the skin's surface or internal body organs. Clients may develop systemic manifestations including infections, pulmonary disease, pericarditis, abnormal numbers of blood cells, and symptoms of metabolic dysfunction such as fatigue, anorexia, and weakness.

Fast Facts Arthritic Disorders and Gout

- Between 20 and 40 million clients in the U.S. are affected by osteoarthritis.
- After age 40, more than 90% of the population has symptoms of osteoarthritis in major weight-bearing joints. After 70 years of age, almost all clients have symptoms of osteoarthritis.
- One percent of the world's population has rheumatoid arthritis. Rheumatoid arthritis most often affects clients between 30 and 50 years of age. Women are three to five times more likely to develop rheumatoid arthritis than men.
- Between 1% and 3% of the U.S. population is affected by gout. Most of the clients are men between the ages of 30 and 60. Most of the women are affected after menopause.

Concept review 30.8

- Identify the two major types of arthritis. What are the general differences between these two disorders?

ANTIARTHRITIC DRUGS

Antiarthritic disease-modifying drugs mainly suppress autoimmunity. Examples include antimalarial agents, gold compounds, sulfasalazine, minocycline, and penicillamine.

30.11 Drug therapy for arthritis depends upon the nature of the disorder.

Pharmacotherapy for osteoarthritis includes a wide variety of medications including aspirin, acetaminophen, nonsteroidal anti-inflammatory drugs (NSAIDs), and analgesics. Because these medications have already been covered (Chapters 11 and 20 ⊂⊃⊂⊃), they are not discussed again. Pain management is the most specific from of therapy for this disorder. Examples of pain medications used for osteoarthritis are listed below.

- topical pain relievers (capsaicin cream and balms)
- NSAIDS, including aspirin
- acetaminophen; acetaminophen and tramadol (Ultram)
- COX-2 inhibitors

Mild pain relief is provided through the use of aspirin, NSAIDs, COX-2 inhibitors, and acetaminophen. Stronger pain relief may be provided by analgesics such as tramadol mixed with acetaminophen or antidepressants. Nonpharmacological treatments for pain include manipulation, mild heat, meditation, visualization, and distraction techniques. Knowledge of proper body

ON THE JOB

Physical Therapist Assistants (PTAs) and Drug Therapies

Physical therapist assistants work under the supervision of licensed physical therapists. These healthcare professionals must utilize skills from a number of areas including knowledge of muscle movement, neurological approaches, and principles of therapeutic exercise. Principles of joint motion and gait are studied as a means of preparing to help clients with minor or major mobility problems. A knowledge of drug therapies is also important because rarely are joint, bone, or muscle therapies applied exclusive of drug therapy. Physical therapist assistants may perform duties in a variety of clinical settings. Thus, a familiarity with basic, important drug actions and their side effects helps to ensure a higher level of proficiency and better outcome for the client. The physical therapist assistant is are a critical component of the entire medical treatment team. ■

mechanics and posturing may offer some benefit. Physical or occupational therapists are usually very active in helping clients minimize pain through these approaches. Surgical techniques such as joint replacement and reconstructive surgery sometimes offer the most significant benefit in cases where other methods are not effective.

Treatment for rheumatoid arthritis is provided by several classes of medications.

- NSAIDS
- COX-2 inhibitors
- corticosteroids
- disease-modifying drugs: hydroxychloroquine (Plaquenil), gold salts, sulfasalazine (Azulfidine), D-penicillamine (Cuprimine)

DRUG PROFILE:
Hydroxychloroquine Sulfate (Plaquenil)

Actions:

Hydroxychloroquine is commonly prescribed for rheumatoid arthritis and lupus erythematosus. Symptoms of these disorders include severe inflammation, bone erosion, tissue wasting, and destruction of muscles and joints. This drug suppresses unfavorable symptoms mainly caused by tissue damage. For full effectiveness, hydroxychloroquine is most often prescribed with salicylates and glucocorticoids; it is also used for prophylaxis and treatment of malaria (Chapter 22).

Adverse Effects:

Adverse symptoms include blurred vision, GI disturbances, loss of hair, headache, and mood and mental changes. Hydroxychloroquine should be avoided during pregnancy. Antacids with aluminum and magnesium may prevent absorption. This drug interferes with the client's response to rabies vaccine.

TABLE 30.6	Disease-Modifying Drugs of Importance for Rheumatoid Arthritis	
DRUG	**ROUTE AND ADULT DOSE**	**REMARKS**
Pr aurothioglucose (Gold thioglucose, Solganal)	IM; 10 mg wk 1, 25 mg wk 2; then 50 mg/wk to a cumulative dose of 1 g.	Gold salt.
auranofin (Ridaura)	PO; 3–6 mg qd-bid; may increase up to 3 mg tid after 6 mo if tolerated and needed.	Gold salt.
gold sodium thiomalate (Myochrysine)	IM; 10 mg wk 1, 25 mg wk 2; then 25–50 mg/wk to a cumulative dose of 1 g.	Gold salt; expected side effects with administration: flushing, dizziness, fainting.
Pr hydroxychloroquine sulfate (Plaquenil Sulfate)	PO; 400–600 mg qd.	Also for acute malaria and malaria suppression.
penicillamine (Cuprimine, Depen)	PO; 125–250 mg qd; (max 1–1.5 g/day).	Also used to promote increased excretion of excess copper; used to limit urinary excretion of cystine.
sulfasalazine (Azulfidine)	PO; 250–500 mg qd (max 8 g/day).	Also for ulcerative colitis.

- immunosuppressants: methotrexate (Rheumatrex), leflunomide (Arava), azathioprine (Imuran), cyclosporine (Neoral), cyclophosphamide (cytoxan)

- tumor necrosis factor blockers: etanercept (Enbrel), infliximab (Remicade)

Anti-inflammatory drugs, glucocorticoids, immunosuppressants, and tumor necrosis factor agents were discussed in Chapter 20 ⬤▭⬤. A number of disease-modifying drugs for autoimmunity are important antiarthritic agents and are shown in Table 30.6.

Disease-modifying drugs alter the course of autoimmune progression. They are taken as a third course of treatment after pain and anti-inflammatory medications. Glucocorticoids are taken as a second approach to control inflammation. Disease-modifying drugs are often taken along with immunosuppressant drugs to suppress the autoimmune response. Several months may be required before maximum therapeutic effects are achieved. Because these drugs can be particularly toxic, clients should be closely monitored. Adverse effects vary depending on the type of drug.

Concept review 30.9

- Identify the major drug therapies for osteoarthritis and rheumatoid arthritis.

URIC ACID-INHIBITORS

Uric acid-inhibiting drugs inhibit the accumulation of uric acid within the blood or uric acid crystals within the joints.

30.12 Gout is treated by medications that prevent a buildup of uric acid.

Gout is a metabolic disorder characterized by the accumulation of uric acid in the bloodstream or joint cavities. This can occur due to increased metabolism of the nucleic acids, deoxyribonucleic acid (DNA), and ribonucleic acid (RNA) or reduced natural excretion of uric acid by the kidneys. Gout may be classified as primary, secondary, or gouty arthritis.

Primary gout is caused by elevated blood levels of uric acid or hyperuricemia. This particular kind of gout may be caused by inborn or genetic malfunction. Uric acid is the final breakdown product of DNA and RNA metabolism. One well-known step, the conversion of hypoxanthine to uric acid, is helped by the enzyme xanthine oxidase, the target for some uric acid-inhibitors. Allopurinol, for example, blocks the formation of uric acid by inhibiting xanthine oxidase.

hyper = elevated
uric = uric acid
emia = blood level

Secondary gout may be caused by drugs that interfere with uric acid excretion, for example, thiazide diuretics, aspirin, cyclosporine, and ethanol when ingested on a chronic basis. Diabetic ketoacidosis, kidney failure, and diseases connected with a rapid cell turnover (leukemia, hemolytic anemia, and polycythemia) may also cause secondary gout.

Acute gouty arthritis occurs when needle-shaped uric acid crystals quickly accumulate in the joints resulting in red, swollen, and inflamed tissue. Attacks often occur in the nighttime and may be triggered by diet, injury, or other stresses. Gouty arthritis most often occurs in the big toes, heels, ankles, wrists, fingers, knees, and elbows.

Medications for gout and gouty arthritis include uric acid-inhibitors such as colchicine, probenecid (Benemid), sulfinpyrazone (Anturan), and allopurinol (Lopurin). Probenecid and

DRUG PROFILE:
Colchicine

Actions:

Colchicine inhibits inflammation and reduces pain associated with gouty arthritis. It may be taken prophylactically for acute gout or taken in combination with other uric acid-inhibiting agents. Colchicine works by inhibiting the synthesis of microtubules, subcellular structures responsible for helping white blood cells infiltrate an area.

Adverse Effects:

Side effects such as nausea, vomiting, diarrhea, and gastrointestinal upset are more likely to occur at the beginning of therapy. These side effects are related to disruption of microtubules responsible for cell proliferation. Colchicine may also directly interfere with the absorption of vitamin B_{12}.

TABLE 30.7	Uric Acid-Inhibiting Drugs of Importance for Gout and Gouty Arthritis	
DRUG	**ROUTE AND ADULT DOSE**	**REMARKS**
Pr colchicine	PO; 0.5–1.2 mg followed by 0.5–0.6 mg q1–2 h until pain relief (max 4 mg/ attack).	For acute gouty attack; may cause gastric upset at higher doses; IV form available.
allopurinol (Lopurin, Zyloprim)	primary: oral; 100 mg qd; may increase by 100 mg/wk; (max 800 mg/day) secondary: oral; 200–800 mg qd for 2–3 d or longer.	For primary hyperuricemia, secondary hyperuricemia, and prevention of gout flare-up.
probenecid (Benemid, Probalan)	PO; 250 mg bid × 1 wk; then 500 mg bid (max 3g/d).	For gout; also used as an adjunct for penicillin or cephalosporin therapy.
sulfinpyrazone (Anturan)	PO; 100–200 mg bid for 1 wk; then increase to 200–400 mg bid.	For gout; also used for inhibition of platelet aggregation.

sulfinpyrazone increase the excretion of uric acid and are thus called uricosuric drugs. These are summarized in Table 30.7. When uric acid accumulation is blocked, the symptoms associated with gout diminish. Pain medications and antiinflammatory agents may also be taken for this disorder. These include NSAIDS, glucocorticoids (prednisone, cortisone,) and adrenocorticotropic hormone (ACTH).

Concept review 30.10

■ What are the differences between gouty arthritis and other arthritic disorders? How do these differences influence drug therapy?

CLIENT TEACHING

Clients taking antispasmodic drugs or drugs for bone or joint disorders need to know the following:

1. Most antispasmodic drugs produce side effects such as drowsiness and dizziness. Therefore, CNS depressants and alcohol should be avoided.

2. When receiving treatment for problems with mobility, it often takes several weeks for effectiveness to begin. Be willing to follow the advice of your healthcare practitioner to achieve full therapeutic effect.

3. When taking calcium or vitamin D supplements, be aware of the signs and symptoms of hypercalcemia. You should check with your healthcare practitioner or pharmacist before taking supplements of any kind. In some cases, only proper diet and sunshine are needed for successful therapy.

4. Zinc-rich food products (nuts, seeds, tofu, and legumes) may interfere with calcium absorption. Calcium may react with some foods or interfere with the absorption of iron and biphosphonates.

5. When taking medication, you should be familiar with the risks and long-term effects of vitamin D therapy, corticosteroids, estrogen replacement therapy, and estrogen receptor modulators. Report any unfavorable symptoms such as bone pain, restricted mobility, inflammation, or fracture to your healthcare practitioner. Communicate about muscle pain, as muscles that have not been moved for a while may feel stiff and tender.

6. Know how to use a nasal pump if taking calcitonin by this method. Be aware that some vitamins may interfere with the pharmacological effects of calcitonin.

7. Some medications cause GI discomfort. Drugs like this can be administered after meals or with milk to minimize discomfort.

8. When taking some antigout medications, drink plenty of fluids to avoid kidney stones. To ensure proper fluid balance, monitor intake and output of fluids.

9. When taking probenecid, avoid taking aspirin for pain because it interferes with probenecid's action. Take acetaminophen instead.

10. Be careful when taking sulfa drugs because they may produce unfavorable reactions. ■

CHAPTER REVIEW

Core Concepts Summary

30.1 Muscle spasms occur for a variety of reasons.

Muscle spasms occur for many reasons, including cerebral palsy, multiple sclerosis, traumatic brain or spinal cord injury, stroke, and dementia. Spasms may also accompany acute musculoskeletal injury, dystonia, or congenital myotonic disorders. When muscle spasms occur, many areas of the body may be affected, including the head, neck, trunk, and limbs.

30.2 The purpose of antispasmodic drugs is to improve mobility.

In many cases, antispasmodic drugs provide enough mobility for clients to engage in daily ac-

tivities such as grooming, sitting up, or turning the head. Careful consideration must be given to determine whether general mobility will be enhanced or hindered by drug therapy, such as when treating major standing or postural muscles.

30.3 Many antispasmodic drugs treat spasticity at the level of the central nervous system.

Many drugs improve mobility by inhibiting neurons in the brain and spinal cord. Some of these drugs work directly through inhibition of motor pathways; others work by causing sedation. One of the major side effects of centrally acting medications is drowsiness.

30.4 Some antispasmodic drugs act directly on muscle tissue.

A few drugs act directly at the neuromuscular level by inhibiting the effect of the natural neurotransmitter acetylcholine. Weakness and fatigue are major symptoms of these drugs.

30.5 Proper functioning of nerves, muscles, and bones depends on calcium and vitamin D.

Adequate levels of calcium in the body are necessary to properly transmit nerve impulses, to prevent muscle spasms, and to provide stability and movement. Adequate levels of vitamin D, parathyroid hormone, and calcitonin are also necessary for these functions.

30.6 Calcium supplements and vitamin D therapy are useful in treating osteomalacia, rickets, and hypocalcemia.

Symptoms or disorders resulting from improper levels of calcium or vitamin D are hypocalcemia, osteomalacia, and rickets. All of these conditions may be treated by drugs that restore calcium and vitamin D.

30.7 Osteoporosis is a disorder characterized by weak and fragile bones.

Osteoporosis is the most common type of disorder associated with weak and fragile bones. There are several causes of this disorder, including menopause and overactivity of the bone resorption process. Risks for osteoporosis are well known.

30.8 Weak and fragile bones are improved by drugs that inhibit bone resorption.

Most drugs treat weak and fragile bones by inhibiting the process of bone resorption. Two main categories of drugs are hormonal agents and biphosphonates. Hormonal agents include estrogen replacement therapy, estrogen modulator drugs, and calcitonin. Additional drug approaches are vitamin D therapy, statins, and slow-release fluoride.

30.9 Paget's disease is treated by drug therapies similar to those used for weak and fragile bones.

The bones of Paget's disease clients, in addition to being weak and fragile, are abnormal because of the continuous turnover of irregular bone. Biphosphonates and calcitonin are two major drug therapies used for Paget's disease.

30.10 Arthritis is one of the major problems affecting mobility.

Two major forms of arthritis are osteoarthritis and rheumatoid arthritis. Osteoarthritis is a non-inflammatory type disorder in which joint surfaces degenerate. Rheumatoid arthritis is an inflammatory autoimmune disorder.

30.11 Drug therapy for arthritis depends upon the nature of the disorder.

For osteoarthritis, the main drug therapy is pain medication that includes aspirin, acetaminophen, NSAIDs, COX-2 inhibitors, and stronger analgesics. Drug therapy for rheumatoid arthritis includes NSAIDs, COX-2 inhibitors, glucocorticoids, immunosuppressants, and disease-modifying drugs.

30.12 Gout is treated by medications that prevent a buildup of uric acid.

Gout and gouty arthritis are disorders characterized by a buildup of uric acid either in the blood or in the joint cavities. Drug therapy for these conditions centers around agents that inhibit uric acid buildup or enhance its excretion.

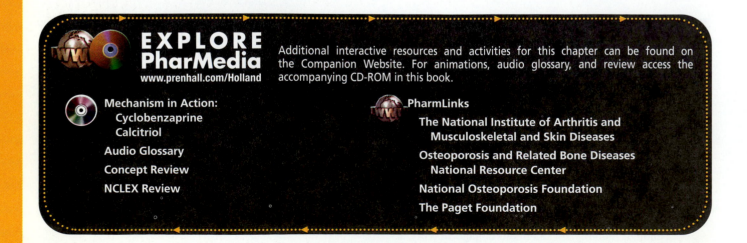

31 Drugs for Skin Disorders

CORE CONCEPTS

31.1 Three layers of skin provide protection to the body.

31.2 The major causes of skin disorders are injury, aging, inherited factors, and other medical conditions.

SKIN PARASITES

Scabicides and Pediculicides

31.3 Scabicides and peducilicides treat parasitic mite and lice infestation.

SUNBURN AND MINOR IRRITATION

Drugs for Sunburn and Minor Irritation

31.4 The goal of drug therapy for sunburn is to eliminate discomfort until healing occurs.

ACNE AND ACNE-RELATED DISORDERS

Drugs for Acne and Acne-related Disorders

31.5 Problems of acne and rosacea are treated by a combination of OTC and prescription drugs.

DERMATITIS AND ECZEMA

Topical Glucocorticoids

31.6 Topical glucocorticoids are used mainly to treat dermatitis and related symptoms.

PSORIASIS

Drugs for Psoriasis

31.7 Several topical and systemic medications are used to treat psoriatic symptoms.

OBJECTIVES

After reading this chapter, the student should be able to:

1. Identify important skin layers and explain how superficial skin cells must be replaced after they become damaged or lost.

2. Describe major symptoms associated with stress and injury to the skin versus those associated with a client's changing age or health.

3. Identify important drug therapies for the following disorders, distinguishing between topical and systemic medications.

   a. scabies (mites) and *Pediculus* (lice) infestation
   b. sunburn, minor irritations, and insect bites
   c. acne and acne-related disorders (blackheads, whiteheads, rosacea)
   d. dermatitis (eczema, contact dermatitis, seborrheic dermatitis, stasis dermatitis)
   e. psoriasis

4. Identify the major actions of the following types of drugs as they pertain to treatment of skin disorders: scabicides, pediculicides, topical anesthetics, antibiotics, retinoids, keratolytic agents, glucocorticoids, emollients, and psoralens.

5. Describe popular treatments used in conjunction with available drug therapies for skin disorders.

PharMedia
www.prenhall.com/holland

Additional interactive resources and activities for this chapter can be found on the Companion Website. For animations, audio glossary, and review access the accompanying CD-ROM in this book.

closed comedomes (KOME-eh-domes): commonly called whiteheads, this type of acne develops just beneath the surface of the skin / *page 514*

dermatitis (dur-mah-TIE-tiss): inflammatory condition of the skin characterized by itching and scaling / *page 517*

eczema (ECK-zih-mah): also called *atopic* dermatitis, a skin disorder with unexplained symptoms of inflammation, itching, and scaling / *page 515*

emollients (ee-MOLE-ee-ents): agents used to soothe and soften the skin / *page 518*

erythema (ear-ih-THEE-mah): redness associated with skin irritation / *page 509*

keratinization (keh-RAT-en-eye-zay-shun): development of the stratum corneum or horny layer of epithelial tissue / *page 514*

keratolytic agents (keh-RAT-oh-lih-tik): drugs used to promote shedding of old skin / *page 515*

open comedomes: type of acne where sebum has plugged the oil gland; commonly called blackheads / *page 514*

papules (PAP-yools): inflammatory bumps without pus that swell, thicken, and become painful / *page 514*

pediculicides (puh-DIK-you-lih-sides): medications that kill lice / *page 511*

pruritus (proo-RYE-tus): itching symptom associated with dry, scaly skin / *page 509*

psoralen (SORE-uh-len): drug used along with phototherapy for the treatment of psoriasis and other severe skin disorders / *page 518*

pustules (PUSS-chools): inflammatory bumps with pus / *page 514*

retinoids (RETT-ih-noydz): vitamin A-like compounds used in the treatment of severe acne and psoriasis / *page 515*

retinol (RETT-ih-nall): chemical name for vitamin A / *page 516*

rosacea (roh-ZAY-shee-uh): skin disorder characterized by clusters of papules / *page 514*

scabicides (SKAY-bih-sides): drugs that kill scabies mites / *page 511*

scabies (SKAY-beez): skin disorder caused by the female mite burrowing into the skin and laying eggs / *page 511*

seborrhea (seb-oh-REE-ah): condition characterized by overactivity of oil glands / *page 514*

The integumentary system consists of the skin, hair, nails, sweat glands, and oil glands. The largest of all organs is the skin. Because of its large surface area, it normally provides an effective barrier between extreme conditions in the outside environment and the body's internal organs. At times, however, external conditions become too extreme or conditions within the body change, resulting in unhealthy skin. When this happens, either the body's natural defense system must try to correct the problem or therapy may be provided to improve the skin's condition. The relationship between the integumentary system and other body systems is depicted in Figure 31.1.

The purpose of this chapter is to examine the broad scope of skin disorders and the medications used for skin therapy. Particular attention is given to drugs that are of direct benefit to lice and mite infestation, sunburn, acne, inflammation, and dry, scaly skin. Pharmarotherapy of these conditions provides the basis for a more complete understanding of the many drugs applied to the skin's surface.

31.1 Three layers of skin provide protection to the body.

The skin has three major layers: the epidermis, dermis, and a subcutaneous layer called the hypodermis. Each layer is distinct in form and function and provides the basis for how drugs are injected or applied to the surface of the skin (Chapter 3 ⬤▬⬤). The most superficial skin layer is the epidermis. Depending on its thickness, the epidermis has either four or five sublayers. The strongest and outermost sublayer is the stratum corneum, or horny layer. It is called this because of the abundance of the protein keratin, also found in the hair, hooves, and horns of many vertebrate mammals. Not every part of the skin has a large amount of keratin—only those areas that are subject to mechanical stress, for example, the soles of the feet and the palms of the hands.

The deepest sublayer of the epidermis is the stratum germanitivum. It supplies the epidermis with new cells after older, superficial cells have been damaged or lost by normal wear. Cells must migrate over their lifetime to the outermost layers of the skin, where they eventually fall off. As these cells are pushed to the surface, they are flattened and covered with a

FIGURE 31.1

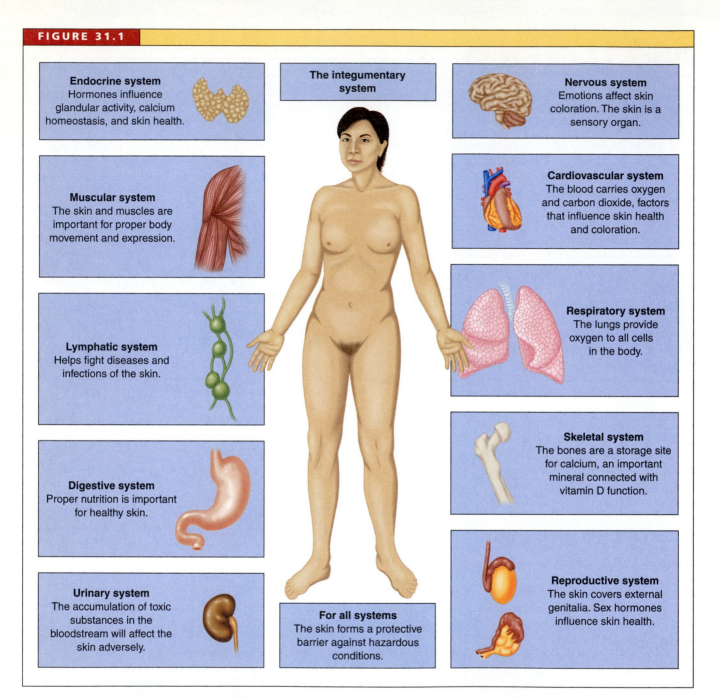

Endocrine system
Hormones influence glandular activity, calcium homeostasis, and skin health.

Muscular system
The skin and muscles are important for proper body movement and expression.

Lymphatic system
Helps fight diseases and infections of the skin.

Digestive system
Proper nutrition is important for healthy skin.

Urinary system
The accumulation of toxic substances in the bloodstream will affect the skin adversely.

The integumentary system

For all systems
The skin forms a protective barrier against hazardous conditions.

Nervous system
Emotions affect skin coloration. The skin is a sensory organ.

Cardiovascular system
The blood carries oxygen and carbon dioxide, factors that influence skin health and coloration.

Respiratory system
The lungs provide oxygen to all cells in the body.

Skeletal system
The bones are a storage site for calcium, an important mineral connected with vitamin D function.

Reproductive system
The skin covers external genitalia. Sex hormones influence skin health.

The integumentary system (skin) and how the other body systems affect it

water-insoluble material, forming a protective seal. The average time it takes for a cell to move from the germanitivum layer to the outer body surface is about three weeks. Specialized cells within the deeper layers of the epidermis called *melanocytes* secrete the dark pigment melanin, which offers a degree of protection from the sun's ultraviolet rays.

The next major layer of skin, the dermis, is made up of dense, irregular connective tissue, named this way because of its irregular arrangement of thick protein fibers. The dermis provides a foundation for the epidermis and appendages such as hair and nails. Most receptor nerve endings, sweat glands, oil glands, and blood vessels are found within the dermis.

The deepest of the skin layers is the subcutaneous layer, or hypodermis. This layer is composed mainly of adipose tissue or fat that cushions, insulates, and provides a source of energy for the body. The hypodermis is involved with the maintenance of body homeostasis, temperature regulation, and metabolism.

31.2 The major causes of skin disorders are injury, aging, inherited factors, and other medical conditions.

Common disorders of the skin may affect one or more of the skin layers. Skin, that is dry, cracked, scaly, or worn represents a disturbance in the outermost skin layer. Pruritus, or itching, is a symptom often associated with dry, scaly skin, or it may be a symptom of infestation as with mites and lice. The thick, horny layer is designed to protect the skin and keep it from drying out.

prur = itching
itus = condition

Some forceful or noxious stresses may damage deeper layers of the epidermis. When this happens, the role of the germanitivum layer is to replace any skin that might be lost or damaged due to special stresses.

Burns are a unique type of stress that may affect all layers of the skin. They are classified according to the degree of skin damage. First degree burns affect only the outer layers of the epidermis, are characterized by redness, and are analogous to sunburn. Second degree burns affect most of the epidermis and part of the dermis, resulting in inflammation and blisters. Third degree burns are full-thickness burns; all layers of the skin are damaged. With full-thickness burns, the skin cannot regenerate, and skin grafting is required.

Inflammation, a characteristic of burns and other traumatic disorders, occurs when damage to the skin is extensive. Signs accompanying inflammation include erythema or redness, irritation, and pain. A larger group of symptoms including bleeding, bruises, and infections may accompany trauma to deeper tissues. Common symptoms of stress or skin injury are shown in Table 31.1.

eryth = red
ema = appears

TABLE 31.1	Symptoms Associated with Stress or Injury to the Skin
SYMPTOM	**DESCRIPTION**
sunburn	The sun's hazardous rays may damage the skin; also, prolonged sun exposure may cause some types of skin cancer.
rash	Exposure to wet conditions for long periods may cause rash; examples are an infant's wet diaper or someone staying in a wet bathing suit for too long.
crusty and cracked areas	These may be caused by lack of moisture, extremely dry conditions, or hot temperatures; areas affected by lack of moisture include the lips, corners of the mouth, nose, between the fingers and toes, and joint areas.
inflammation and redness	Tissue damage almost always results in inflammation; other signs may also accompany inflammation as with some allergies, drugs, insect bites, stings, and plant toxins.
blisters and calluses	Improperly fitting shoes or clothing may cause mechanical stress and abrasion leading to these symptoms.
bruises, scrapes, and small-impact injuries	Increased physical activity sometimes wears away at the skin and results in minor skin damage.
cuts, abrasions, and larger wounds	These signs may accompany more dramatic stress, such as sudden trauma or serious accidental injury.
irritated areas	Burning and itching are common symptoms of irritated skin; many chemical agents (for example, household or industrial detergents, greases, and volatile organic agents) may cause skin irritation.
sores and lesions	Lack of attention to an area of the body for a long time may cause unhealthy skin, as with elderly, bed-ridden clients or clients who are wheel-chair-bound.
infections and infestations	There are many types of bacterial, fungal, parasitic, and viral infections that occur throughout the body; ticks, lice, and mites are common problems associated with hairy skin.

TABLE 31.2	Signs and Symptoms Associated with a Client's Changing Health, Age, or Weakened Immune System
SYMPTOM	**DESCRIPTION**
discoloration of the skin	Discoloration is often a useful sign of another medical disorder (for example, anemia, cyanosis, fever, jaundice, and Addison's disease); some medications have photosensitive properties, making a client's skin sensitive to the sun and causing erythema.
delicate skin, wrinkles, and hair loss	Many degenerative changes occur in the skin; some are found in elderly clients; others are genetically related (fragile epidermis, wrinkles, reduced activity of oil and sweat glands, male pattern baldness, poor blood circulation); hair loss may also be linked to some medical procedures, for example radiation and chemotherapy.
seborrhea/oily skin and bumps	This condition is usually associated with a younger age group; examples include cradle cap in infants and an oily face, chest, arms, and back in teenagers and young adults; pustules, cysts, papules, and nodules represent lesions connected with oily skin.
scales, patches, and itchy areas	Some symptoms may be related to a combination of genetics, stress, and immunity; others symptoms may be related to a fast turnover of skin cells; some symptoms develop for unknown reasons.
warts, skin marks, and moles	Some skin marks are congenital; others are acquired or may be linked to environmental factors.
tumors	Tumors may be genetic or may occur because of exposure to harmful agents or conditions.

Not all skin disorders are associated with a stressful environment. Many common skin disorders are related to inherited factors or the normal aging process. Sometimes the skin may appear unhealthy because of another medical condition, or in some cases, the reason for skin irritation may be unclear and indirect. Common symptoms associated with a range of conditions are shown in Table 31.2.

As shown in Table 31.3, the reasons for skin conditions are many. They can be grouped based on whether they are infectious disorders, inflammatory disorders, or cancer-related disorders.

TABLE 31.3	Classification of Skin Disorders
DISORDER	**EXAMPLE**
infectious disorders	Bacterial infections such as boils, impetigo, infected hair follicles; fungal infections such as ring worm, athlete's foot, jock itch, nail infection; parasitic infections such as mosquito bites, ticks, mites, lice; viral infections such as cold sores, fever blisters (herpes simplex), chicken pox, warts, shingles (herpes zoster), measles (rubeola), and German measles (rubella).
inflammatory disorders	Injury and exposure to the sun such as sunburn and other environmental stresses; disorders marked by a combination of overactive glands, increased hormone production, and/or infection such as acne, blackheads, whiteheads, rosacea; disorders marked by itching, cracking, and discomfort such as eczema (atopic dermatitis), other forms of dermatitis (contact dermatitis, seborrheic dermatitis, stasis dermatitis), and psoriasis.
skin cancers	There are several types of malignant skin cancers: squamous cell carcinoma, basal cell carcinoma, and malignant melanoma. Malignant melanoma is the most dangerous. Other types of cancer (benign type) include keratosis and keratoacanthoma.

Although there are many skin disorders, a limited number are less debilitating and warrant only intermittent drug therapy. A few irritating disorders are of particular importance to clients who require healthcare on a walk-in basis. Examples include lice infestation, sunburn with minor irritation, and acne. Eczema, dermatitis, and psoriasis are more serious disorders requiring therapy for a longer time. Figure 31.2 shows examples of regions in the body where irritating symptoms are most likely to occur.

Fast Facts Skin Disorders

- An estimated 3 million people with new cases of lice infestation are treated each year in the U.S.
- Nearly 17 million people in the U.S. have acne, making it the most common skin disease.
- More than 15 million people in the U.S. have symptoms of dermatitis.
- Ten percent of infants and young children experience symptoms of dermatitis. Roughly 60% of these infants continue to have symptoms into adulthood.
- Psoriasis affects between one and two percent of the U.S. population. This disorder occurs in all age groups—adults mainly—affecting about the same number of men as women.

Concept review 31.1

- Identify the three skin layers protecting the body. Give examples of layers specifically affected by minor or major external stresses. What skin disorders are not related to the external environment? How would you categorize most skin disorders?

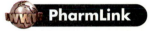

NATIONAL INSTITUTE OF ALLERGIES AND INFECTIOUS DISEASES

SKIN PARASITES

Common skin parasites include mites and lice. Mites cause a skin disorder called scabies, based on their scientific name, *Sarcoptes scabiei.* Scabies is an eruption of the skin caused by the female mite burrowing into the skin and laying eggs. This causes intense itching most commonly between the fingers, extremities, and around the trunk and pubic area. Scabies is readily spread among family members and sexual partners.

Lice, scientific name *Pediculus,* are another type of skin parasite readily passed on by infected clothing or close personal contact. Lice often infest the pubic area or the scalp and lay eggs that attach to body hairs.

SCABICIDES AND PEDICULICIDES

Scabicides are pharmacological agents that kill mites; pediculicides kill lice. Either treatment may be effective for both types of parasites. The choice of drug often depends on where the infestation has occurred.

31.3 Scabicides and pediculicides treat parasitic mite and lice infestation.

Three important drugs kill lice and mites. These are lindane (Kwell, Scabene), sometimes referred to by its chemical name, gamma benzene hexachloride, crotamiton (Eurax), and permethrin (Nix). Unlike lindane or crotamiton, permethrin is an insecticide and should be rinsed from the body within ten minutes after being applied. Permethrin is most often applied to the pubic or scalp area. Clients should be cautioned against applying any lice or mite medication to the mouth, open skin lesions, or eyes.

FIGURE 31.2

Anatomic distribution of common skin disorders: (a) contact dermatitis due to footwear; (b) or cosmetics; (c) seborrheic dermatitis; (d) acne; (e) scabies; (f) sunburn

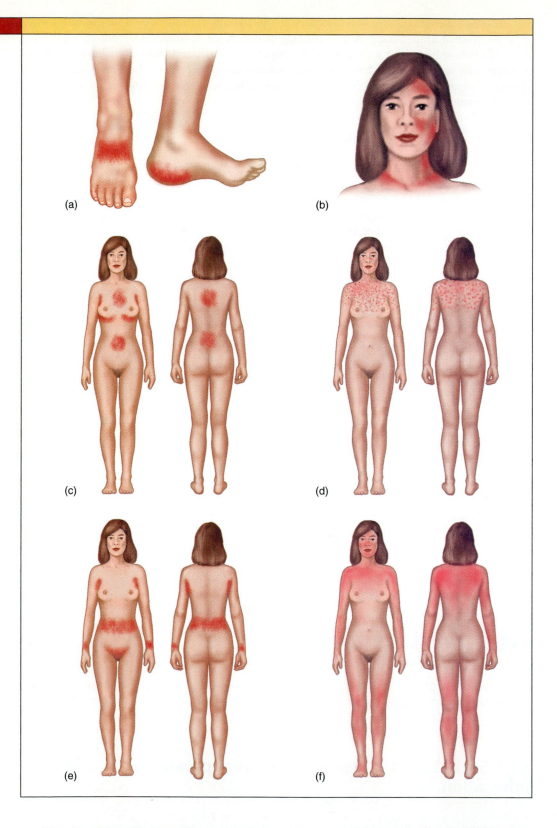

Lice lay eggs called *nits*. Fine-toothed nit combs are useful in removing nits after the lice have been killed. Clients should comb the infested area after the hair has been dried. In order to ensure that drug therapy using lindane, crotamiton, or permethrin is effective, clients should inspect hair shafts daily for at least one week after treatment. Because nits may be present in bedding and other upholstery material, all material coming in close contact with the client is either washed or treated with medication.

DRUG PROFILE:
Lindane (Kwell)

Actions:

Lindane for mites is marketed as a cream or lotion. Lindane for head lice is available as a shampoo. Lindane cream or lotion takes longer to produce its effect; therefore, it is usually left on the body for about 8 to 12 hours before rinsing. Lindane shampoo is usually applied and left on for at least five minutes before rinsing. Clients should be aware that penetration of the skin with mites causes itching, which lasts for up to two or three weeks even after the parasites have been killed. Thus, a persistent itch is not unusual. Lindane kills mites and lice by over-stimulating their nervous system.

Adverse Effects:

If lindane is accidentally ingested in high enough doses, symptoms may include restless-ness, dizziness, tremors, or convulsions. If inhaled, lindane may cause headaches, nausea, vomiting, or irritation of the ears, nose, or throat. A substantial number of lice and mite strains have become resistant to lindane; therefore, one should check carefully over the course of several weeks to make sure the medication is working.

Concept review 31.2

- Name examples of medications used to treat mite and lice infestations. What precautions should be taken when using these medications?

SUNBURN AND MINOR IRRITATION

Sunburn is a common problem among the general public that is associated with factors such as light skin complexion and lack of proper sun protection. Nonpharmacological approaches to sun protection include the appropriate use of sunscreens, sunglasses, and sufficient clothing. Limiting the amount of time spents directly in the sun is essential to avoiding sunburn. Many dangers result from sun exposure, including eye injury and skin cancer. Some of these disorders may not appear until years after the exposure.

DRUGS FOR SUNBURN AND MINOR IRRITATION

Drugs for sunburn and minor irritation include mild lotions and topical anesthetic medications. These are meant to provide temporary relief of painful symptoms.

31.4 The goal of drug therapy for sunburn is to eliminate discomfort until healing occurs.

Pharmacological treatments for sunburn may not be necessary; alternative methods can be employed to control pain, and inflammation. In cases where pharmacological intervention is necessary, topical anesthetics such as benzocaine (Solarcaine, others), dibucaine (Nupercainal), and tetracaine (Pontocaine) may be applied. Some of these medications may also provide minor relief from insect bites and pruritis. In cases of more prolonged sun exposure, more potent pain medications may be administered (Chapters 11 and 20 ⊂⊃), and tetanus toxoid may be administered to prevent infection (Chapter 21 ⊂⊃).

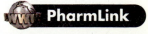

THE AMERICAN ACADEMY OF DERMATOLOGY

DRUG PROFILE:
Benzocaine (Solarcaine and Others)

Actions:

Benzocaine provides temporary relief for pain and discomfort in cases of sunburn, pruritis, minor wounds, and insect bites. Its pharmacological action is caused by local anesthesia of skin receptor nerve endings. Preparations are also available to treat the skin and other areas such as the ear, mouth, throat, rectal, and genital areas.

Adverse Reactions:

Benzocaine should not be used for treatment of clients with open lesions, traumatized mucosal areas, or a history of drug sensitivity. Benzocaine may interfere with the activity of some antibacterial sulfonamides. Clients should use preparations only in areas of the body for which the medication is intended.

Concept review 31.3

■ What is the major purpose of drugs used to treat sunburn, insect bites, and related injuries? What major class of drugs would be used for this purpose?

ACNE AND ACNE-RELATED DISORDERS

sebor = oil
rhea = flow

Acne is a common condition found most often in adolescents and young adults. The disorder usually begins one or two years before puberty and is caused by overproductive oil glands or seborrhea. Acne is also caused by abnormal keratinization or development of the horny layer of the epithelial tissue. This activity results in blocked oil glands. Administration of androgens or testosterone-like hormones may cause extensive acne by increasing keratinization and the production of sebum (oil). Following this, the bacterium *Propionibacterium acnes* grows within gland openings and modifies the sebum into an acidic and irritating substance. As a result, small inflamed bumps appear on the surface of the skin.

Blackheads, or open comedomes, are a type of acne in which sebum has plugged the oil gland, causing it to become black because of the presence of melanin granules. Whiteheads, or closed comedomes, are a type of acne that develop just beneath the surface of the skin and appear white rather than black. In more severe cases of acne, deeper bumps called *nodules* may appear and become very painful because of the intense inflammation and pus found within pore pockets.

Another related skin disorder characterized by inflammation without pus is rosacea. Unlike pimples or pustules, the technical name given to pus-filled bumps, rosacea is characterized by small papules or inflammatory bumps without pus that swell, thicken, and become very painful. Associated with rosacea is swelling that occurs just beneath the surface of the skin. Sometimes the face of a client with rosacea takes on a flushed appearance, particularly around the nose and cheek area. Rosacea is exacerbated by many factors including sunlight, stress, increased temperature, and agents that dilate facial blood vessels including alcohol, spicy foods, and warm beverages.

DRUGS FOR ACNE AND ACNE-RELATED DISORDERS

Most acne drugs slow down the turnover of skin cells, especially those surrounding pore openings. Some inhibit bacterial growth because they are combined with antibiotics such as doxycycline and tetracycline. Some drugs must be used carefully because of their ability to dramatically reduce oil gland activity and skin cell turnover.

31.5 Problems of acne and rosacea are treated by a combination of OTC and prescription drugs.

Benzoyl peroxide (Benzaclin, Benzamycin, and others) is the main OTC medication used to treat acne-related disorders. This medication may be dispensed as a lotion, cream, or gel and is available in various concentrations. Benzoyl peroxide decreases symptoms of acne by inhibiting bacterial growth and suppressing the turnover of skin cells at the pore's opening. Sometimes benzoyl peroxide is combined with antibiotics in order to directly fight bacterial infections. Important medications for acne-related disorders are summarized in Table 31.4.

Retinoids are vitamin A-like compounds. Vitamin A seems to provide improved resistance to bacterial infection by reducing oil production and the occurrence of clogged pores; however, retinoids are not recommended during pregnancy because of possible harmful effects to the fetus. A common reaction to retinoids is sensitivity to sunlight.

Prescription medications for acne include adapalene (Differin), a retinoid-like compound, and related compounds such as azelaic acid (Alzelex), sulfacetamide (Klaren), and tretinoin (Retin-A). Tretinoin is sometimes used for wrinkle removal. When acne is particularly severe, resorcinol, salicylic acid, or sulfur may be used as additional treatments to promote shedding of old skin. These are called keratolytic agents.

kerato = horny layer
lytic = loosening

Some drugs may be taken in combination with or in lieu of other acne medications, including doxycycline (Vibramycin and others), tetracycline (Achromycin), and ethinyl estradiol (Estinyl, Feminone). Doxycycline and tetracycline are antibiotics. Ethinyl estradiol is an estrogen commonly found in birth control medications.

Concept review 31.4

■ What is the major purpose of drugs used to treat acne and related skin conditions? Give examples of both topical and systemic medications. Which medications are OTC, and which are prescription medications?

DERMATITIS AND ECZEMA

Eczema, also called *atopic dermatitis,* is a skin disorder with symptoms resembling an allergic reaction, including inflammation, itching, and rash. Long-term itching and scaling may cause the skin to appear thickened and leathery. Exposure to environmental irritants may make these symptoms worse. Other conditions, including stress, too little or too much moisture, and extreme temperature fluctuations, may worsen symptoms. Blisters and other lesions may also develop. In infants and small children, lesions usually begin on the face and progress to other parts of the body. The skin may become raw and infected from scratching.

atopic = out of place

NATURAL ALTERNATIVES

Burdock Root for Acne and Eczema

Burdock root, *Arcticum lappa,* comes from a thick, flowering plant sometimes found on the roadsides of Britain and North America. It contains several active substances such as bitter glycosides and flavenoids, and it has a range of properties in the body: anti-infective, diuretic, mild laxative, and skin detoxifier. It is sometimes described as an attacker of skin disorders from within because it fights bacterial infections, reduces inflammation, and treats some stages of eczema, particularly the dry and scaling phases. Some claim that it is also effective against boils and sores.

In many cases, burdock root is combined with other natural products for a better range of effectiveness. Such products include sarsaparilla (*Smilax officinalis*), yellow dock (*Rumex crispus*), licorice root (*Glycyrrhiza glabra*), echinacea (*Echinacea purpurea*), and dandelion (*Taraxacum officinale*). ■

DRUG PROFILE:
Isotretinoin/13-Cis-Retinoic Acid (Accutane)

Actions:

The principal action of isotretinoin is regulation of skin growth and turnover. As cells from the germanitivum grow toward the skin's surface, skin cells are lost from the pore openings, and their replacement is slowed down. Isotretinoin also decreases oil production by reducing the size and number of oil glands. This drug is most often used in cases of cystic acne or severe keratinization disorders.

Adverse Effects:

Isotretinoin is a highly toxic metabolite of **retinol** or vitamin A. Therefore it must be used carefully. Common effects are conjunctivitis (visual disturbance), dry mouth, inflammation of the lip, dry nose, increased serum concentrations of triglycerides (by 50 to 70%), bone and joint pain, and photosensitivity. Liver function, serum glucose, and serum triglyceride tests should be performed when taking isotretinoin. Vitamin A supplements should be avoided. Clients should not take this drug while pregnant.

TABLE 31.4	Drugs for Acne and Acne-related Disorders
DRUG	**REMARKS**
Acne-related drugs	
OTC Medication—Topical Preparation	
benzoyl peroxide (Benzaclin, Benzamycin, others)	Often combined with erythromycin or clindamycin to fight bacterial infection; refer to Chapter 21 🔗 .
Prescription Medication—Topical Preparations	
adapalene (Differin)	Retinoid-like compound used to treat acne formation.
azelaic acid (Alzelex)	For mild to moderate inflammatory acne.
sulfacetamide sodium (AK-Sulf, Cetamide)	For sensitive skin; sometimes combined with sulfur to promote peeling, as in the condition rosacea; also used for conjunctivitis.
tretinoin (Retin-A, others)	Used to prevent clogging of pore follicles; also used for the treatment of acute promyelocytic leukemia and wrinkles.
Prescription Medication—Oral Preparations	
🅟🆁 isotretinoin/13-cis-retinoic acid (Accutane)	For acne with cysts or acne formed in small, rounded masses; category X drug.
doxycycline (Doryx, Vibramycin)	Antibiotic; refer to Chapter 21 🔗 .
tetracycline hydrochloride (Achromycin, Panmycin, Sumycin)	Antibiotic; refer to Chapter 21 🔗 .
ethinyl estradiol (Estinyl)	Oral contraceptives are sometimes used for acne treatment; combination drugs may be helpful, for example, ethinyl estradiol plus norgestimate (Ortho Tri-Cyclen -28).

Contact dermatitis is a delayed type of allergic reaction resulting from exposure to specific allergens, for example, perfume, cosmetics, detergents, latex, or jewelry. Accompanying the allergic reaction may be various degrees of cracking, bleeding, or small blisters.

Seborrheic dermatitis is a disorder caused by overactive oil glands. This condition is sometimes seen in newborns and in teenagers after puberty. Oily and scaly patches of skin appear in areas of the face, scalp, chest, back, or pubic area. Bacterial infection or dandruff may accompany these symptoms.

Stasis dermatitis is seen more commonly in older women. It is found primarily in the lower extremities. Redness and scaling may be observed in areas where venous circulation is impaired or where deep venous blood clots have formed.

TOPICAL GLUCOCORTICOIDS

Topical glucocorticoids or corticosteroids are used in cases of dermatitis and eczema to treat symptoms of inflammation, burning, and pruritis. In conjunction with other medical therapies, topical corticosteroids are also used for the treatment of psoriasis.

dermat = skin
itis = inflammation

31.6 Topical glucocorticoids are used mainly to treat dermatitis and related symptoms.

Topical glucocorticoids are the most effective treatment for dermatitis. As shown in Table 31.5, there are many varieties of glucocorticoids supplied at different levels of potency. Creams, lotions, solutions, gels, and pads are specially formulated to cross skin membranes. These medications are especially intended for the relief of local inflammation and itching. In cases of long-term use, however, adverse affects such as irritation, redness, and thinning of the skin membranes may occur. If absorption occurs, topical glucocorticoids may produce undesirable systemic effects including adrenal insufficiency, mood changes, serum imbalances, and bone defects as discussed in Chapter 20 ⟲ .

TABLE 31.5	Topical Glucocorticoids Used to Treat Dermatitis and Related Symptoms
GENERIC NAME	**TRADE NAMES**
Highest level of potency	
betamethasone	Benisone, Diprosone, Valisone
clobetasol	
diflorasone	Florone, Maxiflor, Psorcon
Middle level of potency	
amcinonide	Cyclocort
desoximetasone	Topicort, Topicort LP
fluocinonide	Lidex, Lidex-E
halcinonide	Halog
mometasone	Elocon
triamcinolone	Aristocort, Kenelog, others
Lower level of potency	
clocortilone	Cloderm
fluocinolone	Symalar
flurandrenolide	Cordran
fluticasone	Flonase
hydrocortisone	Hytone, Locoid, Westcort
Lowest level of potency	
aclometasone	Aclovate
desonide	DesOwen, Tridesilon
dexamethasone	Decaderm, Decadron

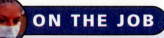

ON THE JOB

Massage Therapists

Licensed massage therapists are a vital part of the hospital team working to restore the health of a client's skin, muscles, and other superficial body structures. Most therapists in this field declare that, without a doubt, the total mental and physical well-being of the client is dependent upon that part of the body that separates external stresses from the body's internal health—the skin. When there is an imbalance produced by unhealthy stressors, the therapist must identify them and offer some means of assistance. In related situations, knowledge of drugs used directly for skin therapy may not be as important as drugs used by the client for other disorders. A broad knowledge of pharmacology is essential for responsible client care. ▪

PSORIASIS

Psoriasis is a chronic disorder characterized by red patches of skin covered with flaky, silver-colored scales. The silver-colored scales are called *plaques*. The reason for the appearance of plaques is an extremely fast skin turnover rate. The skin reacts as if it has been injured, but skin cells reach the surface much more quickly than usual, in about four days, which is six to seven times faster than usual. The reason for this kind of reaction is not known, although scientists believe that it may be a genetic immune reaction. Plaques are ultimately shed from the skin's surface, while the underlying skin becomes inflamed and irritated.

DRUGS FOR PSORIASIS

emolli = to soften
ent = causing

Because psoriatic symptoms may be extreme, numerous drugs are employed to soothe the client's symptoms including **emollients**, topical glucocorticoids, and immunosuppressant medications.

31.7 Several topical and systemic medications are used to treat psoriatic symptoms.

Drugs used for the treatment of psoriasis include many topical and systemic medications. Examples are provided in Table 31.6. One of the main treatments for psoriasis is topical glucocorticoids, which reduce the inflammation associated with fast skin turnover. Other agents applied topically are retinoid-like compounds such as calcipotriene (Dovonex) and tarzarotene (Tazorac). These drugs provide the same benefits as topical glucocorticoids, but they are much less toxic. Calcipotriene produces elevated levels of calcium in the blood stream, so this medication is not used on an extended basis.

Systemic medications for psoriasis include acitreten (Soriatane) and etretinate (Tegison). These drugs are taken orally to inhibit skin cell growth. Methotrexate (Amethopterin and others) produces similar effects in the body (Chapter 23 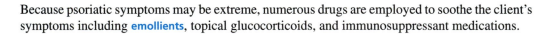). Other medications used for different disorders, but which provide relief of severe psoriatic symptoms, are hydroxyurea (Hydrea) and cyclosporine (Sandimmune, Neoral). Hydroxyurea is a sickle cell anemia medication. Cyclosporine is an immunosuppressive agent that was discussed in Chapter 20 .

Skin therapy techniques may be used with or without other psoriasis medications. These include various forms of tar treatment (coal tar) and a material called *anthralin*. Both substances are applied to the skin's surface. Tar and anthralin inhibit DNA synthesis and arrest abnormal cell growth.

UVB (ultraviolet B) and UVA (ultraviolet A) phototherapy are techniques used in cases of severe psoriasis. UVB therapy is less hazardous than UVA therapy. UVB light has a wavelength similar to sunlight; it reduces widespread lesions that normally resist topical treatments. With close supervision, this type of phototherapy can be administered at home. Keratolytic pastes are often applied between treatments. The second type of phototherapy is often referred to as PUVA therapy because **psoralens** are often administered in conjunction with phototherapy. Psoralens are

TABLE 31.6	Drugs for Psoriasis and Related Disorders	
DRUG	**ROUTE AND ADULT DOSE**	**REMARKS**
Topical Medications		
calcipotriene (Dovonex)	Topically to lesions qd-bid.	Synthetic form of vitamin D$_3$; may raise the level of calcium in the body to unhealthy levels.
tazarotene (Tazorac)	Acne: Apply thin film to clean dry area qd; plaque psoriasis: apply thin film qd in the evening.	Topical retinoid; less toxic than corticosteroids.
Systemic Medications		
acitretin (Soriatane)	PO; 10–50 mg qd with the main meal.	Retinoid; category X drug.
etretinate (Tegison)	PO; 0.75–1 mg/kg qd (max 1.5 mg/kg/day).	Second-generation retinoid; category X drug.
methotrexate (Amethopterin, Folex, Rheumatrx)	PO: 2.5–5 mg bid × 3 doses each week (max 25–30 mg/week).	Also for rheumatoid arthritis and neoplasia; see Chapter 23.
hydroxyurea (Hydrea)	PO; 80 mg/kg q 3 days or 20–30 mg/kg qd.	Unlabeled use for psoriasis; also used for sickle cell anemia.
cyclosporine (Sandimmune, Neoral)	PO; 1.25 mg/kg bid (max 4 mg/kg/day).	Immunosuppressant drug; see Chapter 20.

oral or topical agents that, when exposed to UV light, produce a photosensitive reaction. This reaction seems to provide benefit to the client by reducing the number of lesions, but unpleasant side effects such as headache, nausea, and skin sensitivity still occur, limiting the effectiveness of this therapy. Immunosuppressant drugs such as cyclosporine are not used in conjunction with PUVA therapy because they increase the risk of skin cancer.

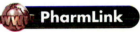

PharmLink

THE NATIONAL PSORIASIS FOUNDATION

Concept review 31.5

- In most cases, which drug category is used to treat symptoms of dermatitis and psoriasis? What other drug therapies and techniques are used to provide a measure of relief for these symptoms?

CLIENT TEACHING

Clients taking medications for skin disorders need to know the following:

1. Inform family members, sexual partners, and any other persons with whom you have close contact about skin infestations. Treat clothes, bed linens, and personal items properly to avoid reinfestation.
2. Be informed and understand the proper way to apply medication or to remove nits if necessary. Scabicides and pediculicides should not be applied to the face, mouth, open skin lesions, or the eyes.
3. For acne and related disorders, apply medication only to areas where it is supposed to be applied. Follow instructions in package inserts and do not deviate from the precautions communicated by medical staff.
4. Do not share your skin medication with family or friends. Be familiar with medication side effects, especially if you have a more severe skin disorder or are taking retinoids or retinoid-like compounds.
5. Use your medication only during the time for which it is intended. With extended use, some medications (for example, corticosteroids) may cause adverse side effects. Take a medication suitable for your disorder: avoid those that are too potent or not potent enough.
6. Give medications a chance to work. Some systemic medications must be taken exactly as prescribed without skipping or stopping early.
7. Avoid contact with agents that are known to cause allergy or dermatitis. Try to avoid scratching, if possible. For severe skin disorders, see a dermatologist. ■

CHAPTER REVIEW

 Core Concepts Summary

31.1 Three layers of skin provide protection to the body.

Three layers of skin protect the body: the epidermis, dermis, and hypodermis. The most superficial layer is the epidermis, where skin cells are replenished every three weeks. New cells arise from the bottom layer, called the germanitivum, and are pushed to the outermost layer.

31.2 The major causes of skin disorders are injury, aging, inherited factors, and other medical conditions.

Many symptoms are associated with skin stress and injury. Others are associated with a client's changing age or health. Skin disorders fit into three main categories: infectious, inflammatory, and cancerous disorders.

31.3 Scabicides and peducilicides treat parasitic mite and lice infestation.

Mites affect the skin and hair, while lice remain localized in hairy regions of the body. Both conditions are treatable with medications. Scabicides kill mites; pediculicides kill lice.

31.4 The goal of drug therapy for sunburn is to eliminate discomfort until healing occurs.

Local anesthetics are the primary medication used to treat mild sunburn and irritation. Often drugs are used for temporary relief of minor discomfort, and in some cases, drugs may not be needed at all.

31.5 Problems of acne and rosacea are treated by a combination of OTC and prescription drugs.

Blackheads, whiteheads, and rosacea are disorders in which pores become blocked, inflamed, or infected because of accelerated skin processes. Topical drugs for acne are those that inhibit bacterial growth (antibiotics) or promote shedding of old skin (keratolytic agents). Vitamin A-like compounds (retinoids) provide an improved resistance to bacterial infections by reducing oil production and the occurrence of clogged pores.

31.6 Topical glucocorticoids are used mainly to treat dermatitis and related symptoms.

Dermatitis is treated by agents that reduce symptoms of inflammation, itchiness, flaking, cracking, bleeding, and lesions. Topical corticosteroids are the primary drug treatment for dermatitis. Potency depends on the type of drug formulation and whether it is packaged as a cream, lotion, solution, gel, or pad.

31.7 Several topical and systemic medications are used to treat psoriatic symptoms.

Psoriasis is a chronic disorder characterized by extreme discomfort and flaky areas called plaques. The treatments for psoriasis include topical glucocorticoids, retinoid-like compounds, drugs that arrest skin cell growth, and immunosuppressants. Skin therapy techniques are also used, including keratolytic agents, coal tar, anthralin, psoralens, and phototherapy.

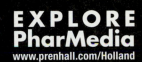 **EXPLORE PharMedia**
www.prenhall.com/Holland

Additional interactive resources and activities for this chapter can be found on the Companion Website. For animations, audio glossary, and review access the accompanying CD-ROM in this book.

Audio Glossary
NCLEX Review
Concept Review

 PharmLinks

National Institute of Allergies and Infectious Diseases
The American Academy of Dermatology
The National Psoriasis Foundation

32 Drugs for Eye and Ear Disorders

CORE CONCEPTS

32.1 Knowledge of basic eye anatomy is fundamental for an understanding of eye disorders and drug therapy.

GLAUCOMA

32.2 Glaucoma is one of the leading causes of blindness.

32.3 Glaucoma therapy centers on adjusting the circulation of aqueous humor.

Drugs that Increase the Outflow of Aqueous Humor

32.4 Some anti-glaucoma medications increase the outflow of aqueous humor.

Drugs that Decrease the Formation of Aqueous Humor

32.5 Other anti-glaucoma medications decrease the formation of aqueous humor.

Cycloplegic and Mydriatic Drugs

32.6 Drugs provide relief for minor eye conditions and are used for eye exams.

EAR CONDITIONS

Otic Preparations

32.7 Otic preparations treat infections, inflammation, and ear wax buildup.

OBJECTIVES

After reading this chapter, the student should be able to:

1. Describe important eye anatomy underlying glaucoma development.

2. Identify the major risk factors associated with glaucoma.

3. Explain how intraocular pressure is associated with nerve damage in the eye.

4. Compare and contrast the two principle types of glaucoma and explain their reasons for development.

5. Explain two major mechanisms by which drugs reduce intraocular pressure.

6. Identify examples of important drugs responsible for treating glaucoma and explain their basic actions and adverse effects.

7. Identify examples of drugs that dilate or constrict pupils, relax ciliary muscles, constrict ocular blood vessels, or moisten eye membranes.

8. Identify examples of drugs that treat ear infections, earaches, or a build-up of ear wax.

PharMedia
www.prenhall.com/holland

Additional interactive resources and activities for this chapter can be found on the Companion Website. For animations, audio glossary, and review access the accompanying CD-ROM in this book.

The eye is one of the most precious sensory organs. A simple scratch can cause the client almost unbearable discomfort. Other eye disorders may be more bearable, but are extremely dangerous— including glaucoma, one of the leading causes of blindness. The first part of this chapter covers various drugs used for the treatment of glaucoma. Drugs used routinely by ophthalmic practitioners are also discussed. The remaining part of the chapter covers examples of drugs used for treatment of ear disorders, including infections, inflammation, and the build-up of ear wax.

32.1 Knowledge of basic eye anatomy is fundamental for an understanding of eye disorders and drug therapy.

To understand eye disorders and drug action, one must be familiar with basic eye anatomy. As shown in Figure 32.1, a watery fluid called *aqueous humor* is found in the anterior cavity of the eye. The anterior cavity has two major subcavities: the anterior chamber and the posterior chamber. In the posterior chamber, aqueous humor originates from an important muscle structure called the *ciliary body*. From there, aqueous humor flows through the pupil and into the anterior chamber. Within the anterior chamber and around the periphery is a network of spongy connective tissue called the *trabecular meshwork*. Connected with trabecular meshwork is an opening called the canal of Schlemm, the location where aqueous humor drains from the anterior cavity.

trabecular = strut-like

GLAUCOMA

Glaucoma is one of the most dreaded eye disorders. In some cases, glaucoma is genetic; in other cases, glaucoma may be caused by non-genetic factors including eye injury and disease. Some medications may contribute to the development of glaucoma, including long-term use of topical glucocorticoids, some antihypertensives, antihistamines, and antidepressants. The major risk factors associated with glaucoma include high blood pressure, migraine headaches, refractive disorders such as nearsightedness or farsightedness, and older age.

32.2 Glaucoma is one of the leading causes of blindness.

Tests such as tonometry may confirm the presence of glaucoma. Tonometry is an ophthalmic technique for measuring increased pressure inside the eye. Other routine refractory and visual field

FIGURE 32.1

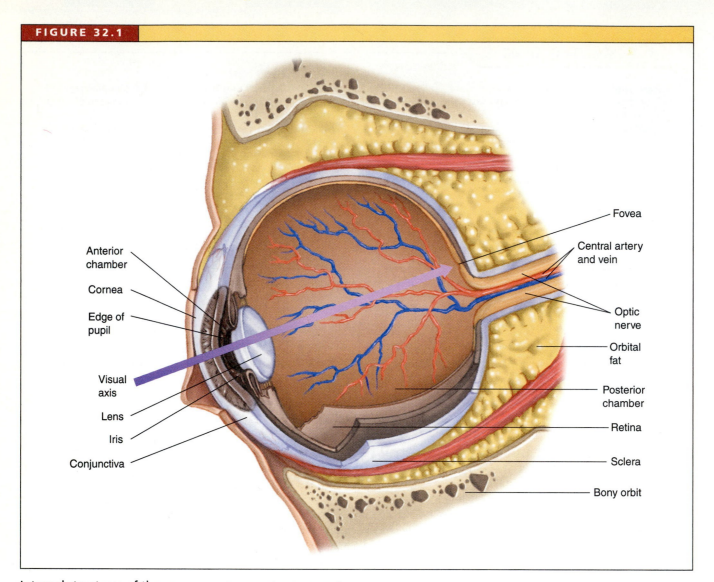

Anterior chamber

Cornea

Edge of pupil

Visual axis

Lens

Iris

Conjunctiva

Fovea

Central artery and vein

Optic nerve

Orbital fat

Posterior chamber

Retina

Sclera

Bony orbit

Internal structures of the eye   *SOURCE: Pearson Education/PH College*

tono = pressure
metry = measurement

tests may uncover glaucoma signs. One problem with testing is that clients with glaucoma typically do not experience symptoms and therefore do not schedule regular eye exams. In some cases, glaucoma occurs so gradually that clients do not notice a problem until later in the disease process.

Fast Facts Glaucoma

- Worldwide, over 5 million people have lost their vision as a result of glaucoma. More than 50,000 are in the U.S.
- Clients of African heritage are affected more by glaucoma than any other group.
- Glaucoma is most common in clients over 60 years of age.
- Acute glaucoma is often caused by head trauma, cataracts, tumors, or hemorrhage.
- Chronic simple glaucoma accounts for 90% of all glaucoma cases.

intra = inside
ocular = eye

Glaucoma is characterized by increased pressure inside the eyeball, termed *intraocular pressure* (IOP). The reason why IOP develops is because the flow of aqueous humor becomes blocked. Over time, pressure around the optic nerve can build, leading to blindness. In some cases, eye injury may be sudden, but in most cases it is gradual.

FIGURE 32.2

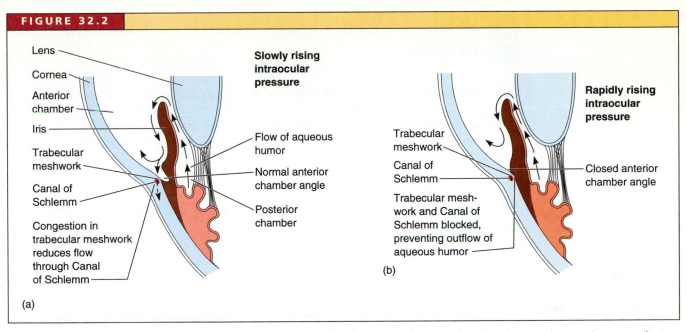

(a)

(b)

Forms of primary adult glaucoma: (a) in chronic open-angle glaucoma, the anterior chamber angle remains open, but drainage of aqueous humor through the canal of Schlemm is impaired; (b) in acute angle-closure glaucoma, the angle of the iris and anterior chamber narrows, obstructing the outflow of aqueous humor   *SOURCE: Pearson Education/PH College.*

As shown in Figure 32.2, the two principal types of glaucoma are closed-angle glaucoma and open-angle glaucoma. Both disorders result from the same problem: a build-up of aqueous humor. Pressure inside the anterior cavity, places pressure on posterior cavity, leading to progressive damage of the optic nerve. The difference between these two disorders lies with how quickly the IOP develops.

Closed-angle glaucoma, sometimes referred to as *acute glaucoma,* is usually caused by stress, impact injury, or medications. Pressure inside the anterior chamber increases suddenly because the iris is pushed over the area where the aqueous fluid normally drains. Symptoms include intense headaches, difficultly concentrating, bloodshot eyes, and blurred vision.

Open-angle, or *chronic simple glaucoma,* is the most common type of glaucoma. With this disorder, intraocular pressure develops more slowly. It is called "open-angle" because the iris does not cover the trabecular meshwork.

32.3 Glaucoma therapy centers on adjusting the circulation of aqueous humor.

There are several approaches to glaucoma therapy. In cases of acute glaucoma, conventional or laser surgery might be performed to return the iris back to its original position. Most therapies are designed to reduce the amount of aqueous humor formation as quickly as possible or to unblock its drainage. Drug therapy for glaucoma works by two mechanisms: either by increasing the outflow of aqueous humor at the canal of Schlemm or by decreasing the formation of aqueous humor at the ciliary body.

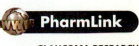

GLAUCOMA RESEARCH FOUNDATION

Concept review 32.1

▪ Which components of the eye are specifically affected by glaucoma? Why is glaucoma such a dreaded eye disease? Drug therapy for glaucoma centers around which major approach?

DRUGS THAT INCREASE THE OUTFLOW OF AQUEOUS HUMOR

Drug increasing the outflow of aqueous humor include miotics, sympathomimetics, prostaglandins, and prostamides. **Miotics** are drugs that cause the pupils to constrict. Sympathomimetics are drugs that mimic activation of the sympathetic nervous system (Chapter 6 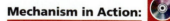). Prostaglandins and prostamides are chemical agents that change vascular permeability in selected body tissues.

32.4 Some anti-glaucoma medications increase the outflow of aqueous humor.

miosis = shortening

Drugs that increase the outflow of aqueous humor are sometimes used to treat glaucoma. Miotic drugs produce an effect like acetylcholine; sympathomimetic drugs produce an effect like norepinephrine. Acetylcholine normally causes constriction of pupils or **miosis**. Norepinephrine causes dilation of pupils or **mydriasis**. Although no anti-glaucoma agents are intended to directly alter pupil diameter, they often produce this effect because of their physiological properties. Prostaglandins do not affect pupil diameter at all, but rather directly dilate the trabecular meshwork within the anterior chamber. One of the drawbacks of prostaglandins, however, is that they change the pigmentation of the eyes. A related class of drugs called *prostamides* also directly affects the trabecular meshwork but with less dramatic effects on iris pigmentation. Although their long-term effectiveness remains to be established, prostamides represent a promising class of drug for the treatment of open angle glaucoma. Drugs that increase the outflow of aqueous humor are summarized in Table 32.1.

DRUG PROFILE:
Pilocarpine (Adsorbocarpine, Ocusert, and Others)

Actions:

Pilocarpine is supplied as eye drops or by slow-release delivery system (Ocusert). It directly acts at cholinergic receptor sites, similar to the neurotransmitter acetylcholine. Pilocarpine reduces IOP by stimulating ciliary muscles and pulling them away from the anterior filtration site. With eye drops, miosis occurs within 10–30 minutes; IOP is reduced within 60 minutes. Miosis remains from four to eight hours, and IOP remains low for several hours longer. With the Ocusert delivery system, effects can last up to seven days.

Adverse Effects:

Vision may be temporarily reduced in poorly illuminated areas. Ophthalmic solutions cause local irritation. Systemic effects are rare. However, if high doses of pilocarpine enter the general circulation, cholinergic effects such as nausea, salivation, sweating, hypotension bradycardia, and bronchoconstriction may occur.

Mechanism in Action:

Pilocarpine is used for the treatment of glaucoma. It relieves pressure in the eye caused by poor drainage of aqueous humor. Pilocarpine causes the pupils to constrict and the ciliary muscles to contract, which facilitates the outflow of fluid. These effects are mediated by activation of muscarinic-type acetylcholine receptors.

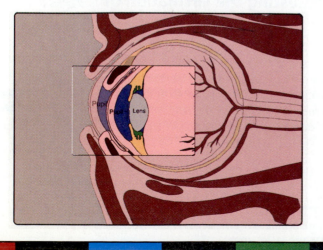

TABLE 32.1	Anti-glaucoma Drugs that Increase the Outflow of Aqueous Humor	
DRUG	**ROUTE AND ADULT DOSE**	**REMARKS**
Miotics, Direct-Acting Cholinergic Agonists		
Pr pilocarpine hydrochloride (Adsorbocarpine, Isopto Carptine, and others)	acute glaucoma: 1 drop 1–2% solution every 5–10 minutes for 3–6 doses; chronic glaucoma: 1 drop 0.5–4% solution every 4–12 hours.	Ophthalmic solution; cholinergic-agonist; may be prescribed as an ocular therapeutic system, a slow release delivery method (Ocusert, other names); Ocusert effects can last up to 7 days.
acetylcholine chloride (Miochol)	0.5–2 ml 1% intraocular solution instilled into eye.	Intraocular treatment before surgery; cholinergic-agonist.
carbachol (Isopto Carbachol, Miostat)	1–2 drops 0.75–3% solution in lower conjunctival sac q 4h – tid.	Ophthalmic solution; cholinergic-agonist; less useful in glaucoma than other drugs; causes stinging of the eyes.
Miotics, Cholinesterase Inhibitors		
demecarium bromide (Humorsol)	1–2 drops 0.125–0.25% solution 2 × per week.	Ophthalmic solution; longer acting medication (2–3 days).
echothiophate iodide (Phosphaline Iodide)	1 drop 0.03–0.25% solution qd-bid.	Ophthalmic solution; must be prepared immediately before use because of instability.
physostigmine sulfate (Eserine sulfate)	1 drop 0.25–0.5% solution qd-qid.	Ophthalmic solution; also constricts ciliary muscle, decreasing intraocular pressure.
Sympathomimetics		
dipivefrin HCl (Propine)	1 drop 0.1% solution bid.	Ophthalmic solution; converted to epinephrine in the eye.
epinephrine borate (Ipinal, Eppy/N)	1–2 drops 0.25–2% solution qd-bid.	Ophthalmic solution; causes mydriasis.
Prostaglandins and Prostamides		
bimatoprost (Lumigan)	1 drop 0.03% solution qd in the evening.	Ophthalmic solution; prostamide; approved by the FDA, March 2001.
latanoprost (Xalatan)	1 drop (1.5 mg) solution qd in the evening.	Ophthalmic solution; prostaglandin.
travoprost (Travatan)	1 drop 0.004% solution qd in the evening.	Ophthalmic solution; prostamide; approved by the FDA, March 2001, maximum effect after about 12 h.
unoprostone isopropyl (Rescula)	1 drop 0.15% solution bid.	Ophthalmic solution; prostaglandin.

Acetylcholine chloride (Miochol), carbachol (Isopto Carbachol, Miostat), and pilocarpine (Adsorbocarpine, Isopto Carptine, and others) are cholinergic agonists. These directly activate the cholinergic receptor, producing various responses in the eye including miosis and decreased IOP. Demecarium bromide (Humorsol), echothiophate iodide (Phosphaline iodide), and physostigmine sulfate (Eserine sulfate) are indirect-acting cholinergic agonists. These produce essentially the same effects as direct-acting drugs, except that they block cholinesterase, the enzyme responsible for breaking down the natural neurotransmitter acetylcholine. When acetylcholine activity is prolonged, this dilates the trabecular meshwork so the canal of Schlemm can absorb more aqueous humor. When more aqueous humor is absorbed, IOP is reduced. Side effects, however, include temporary cycloplegia or blurred vision and accommodation defects.

Dipivefrin (Propine) and epinephrine borate (Ipinal and others) are sympathomimetic drugs. Dipiverdin is converted to epinephrine; epinephrine produces mydriasis, increased outflow of

cyclop = round eye
plegia = paralysis

aqueous humor, and the subsequent fall of IOP. As discussed in Chapter 18 , when epinephrine is released into the general circulation, it increases blood pressure and heart rate.

Bimatoprost (Lumigan), latanoprost (Xalatan), travoprost (Travatan), and unoprostone isopropyl (Rescula) also increase aqueous humor outflow. Their main side effect is heightened pigmentation, usually brown color of the iris in clients with lighter colored eyes. These medications cause cycloplegia, local irritation, and stinging of the eyes. Because of these effects, prostaglandins are normally administered just before the client goes to bed. Although prostaglandins can be irritating to the eyes, they usually do not prevent the client from falling asleep.

DRUGS THAT DECREASE THE FORMATION OF AQUEOUS HUMOR

Beta-adrenergic blockers, alpha$_2$ adrenergic agonists, carbonic anhydride inhibitors, and osmotic diuretics are drug classes that decrease the formation of aqueous humor. Beta-blockers do not alter pupil diameter or produce cycloplegic effects. Similarly, alpha$_2$ agonists produce fewer ocular symptoms. For clients who cannot use beta-blocking agents, carbonic anhydrase inhibitors and osmotic diuretics are other alternatives.

32.5 Other anti-glaucoma medications decrease the formation of aqueous humor.

Drugs from a variety of classes decrease the formation of aqueous humor. These are summarized in Table 32.2. Beta-blocking agents are used more often than the other anti-glaucoma medications. These include betaxolol (Beta Optic), carteolol (Ocupress), levobunolol (Betagan), metipranolol (OptiPranolol), and timolol (Timoptic, Timoptoc XE). The exact mechanism by which these drugs produce their effects is not fully understood. However, they all reduce IOP effectively without the ocular side effects associated with miotoic and sympathomimetic drugs. Systemic beta-blocker effects can be problematic; however, the doses of beta-blockers used for glaucoma treatment are generally not high enough to enter the general circulation. Systemic side effects may include bronchoconstriction, bradycardia, and hypotension.

Alpha$_2$-adrenergic-agonists are less frequently prescribed than the other anti-glaucoma medications. These medications include apraclonidine (Iopidine) and brimonidine (Alphagan). They produce minimal cardiovascular and pulmonary side effects. The most significant side effects of these drugs are headache, drowsiness, dry mucosal membranes, blurred vision, and irritated eyelids.

Carbonic anhydrase inhibitors may be administered topically or systemically to reduce IOP. Usually these medications are used as a second choice if beta-blockers are not effective. Examples include acetazolamide (Diamox), brinzolamide (Azopt), dichlorphenamide (Duranide, Oratrol), dorzolamide (Trosopt), and methazolamide (Neptazane). These medications are more effective in cases of open angle glaucoma. Clients must be cautioned when taking these medications because they are sulfonamides—agents that may cause an allergic reaction. All of these drugs are diuretics, which means they can reduce IOP rather quickly and dramatically alter serum electrolytes with continuous treatment.

Osmotic diuretics are most often used in cases of eye surgery or acute closed-angle glaucoma. Examples include glycerin anhydrous (Ophthalagen), isosorbide (Ismotic), mannitol (Osmitrol), and urea (Ureaphil and others). Because they have an ability to reduce plasma volume very quickly (Chapter 27), they are very effective in reducing the formation of aqueous humor. Unpleasant side effects include headache, tremors, dizziness, dry mouth, fluid and electrolyte imbalance, and thrombophlebitis or venous clot formation near the site of IV administration.

thrombo = *clot*
phleb = *vein*
itis = *inflammation*

Concept review 32.2

▪ Describe two major approaches for controlling intraocular pressure in glaucoma clients. What major drug classes are used in each case?

DRUG PROFILE:
Acetazolamide (Diamox)

Actions:

Acetazolamide produces its diuretic effect by inhibiting carbonic anhydrase activity in the proximal renal tubule. In the eye, inhibition of carbonic anhydrase reduces the rate of aqueous humor formation and consequently lowers IOP. Acetazolamide is particularly effective in treating open-angle glaucoma and for preoperative treatment of acute closed-angle glaucoma. Acetazolamide is also used to treat seizures, edema, high altitude sickness, hydrocephalus, and renal impairment.

Adverse Effects:

Side effects include fatigue and muscle weakness. Clients often feel numbness or tingling in the extremities, lips, facial muscles, or anus. Hypocalcemia and metabolic acidosis are common side effects. Acetazolamide is contraindicated in cases where clients are hypersensitive to sulfonamides. Potassium loss in the urine tends to be greatest during the earliest part of acetazolamide therapy and is accelerated by drugs such as amphotericin B and corticosteroids. Renal excretion of many drugs may be decreased. Renal excretion of lithium and phenobarbital may be increased.

CYCLOPLEGIC AND MYDRIATIC DRUGS

Cycloplegic and mydriatic drugs are commonly used to examine the eyes, treat discomfort, and for surgical procedures.

32.6 Drugs provide relief for minor eye conditions and are used for eye exams.

Drugs for minor irritation and injury come from a broad range of classes including antimicrobials, local anesthetics, glucocorticoids, and nonsteroidal anti-inflammatory drugs (NSAIDs). In each case, a range of drug preparations may be employed including drops, salves, optical inserts, and injectable formulations. Some agents only provide moisture to the eye's surface. Others are designed to penetrate and affect a specific area of the eye.

Some drugs are specifically designed to examine the eyes of clients. These include cycloplegic drugs to relax ciliary muscles and mydriatic drugs to dilate the pupils. One has to be

NATURAL ALTERNATIVES

Aloe Vera for Improving Eye and Ear Health

For centuries, *Aloe vera* has been hailed as the "medicine plant" because of its ability to treat burns, cuts, scrapes, rashes, and abrasions. It has a reputation for treating inflammation, acid indigestion, and even lowering blood cholesterol. *Aloe* may be able to treat eye irritation and conjunctivitis in addition to many other disorders.

One does not have to put *Aloe* directly into the eyes to obtain its therapeutic effect. The benefit comes from treating areas around the eyes, including the bridge of the nose and the outside of the eyelids and cheeks. The skin around the ears may also be treated. The antiseptic properties of *Aloe* probably come from a plethora of agents found within its sap and leaves. Many agents have a reputation for killing microorganisms, including salicylic acid, urea nitrogen, cinnamonic acid, phenols, sulphur, and lupeol. Other groups of agents that qualify as substances with healing properties include plant sterols, immune modulating peptides, anti-inflammatory fatty acids, and viscous-like polysaccharides. ▪

TABLE 32.2	Anti-glaucoma Drugs that Decrease the Formation of Aqueous Humor	
DRUG	**ROUTE AND ADULT DOSE**	**REMARKS**
Beta-Adrenergic Blockers		
betaxolol (Beta optic)	1 drop 0.5% solution bid.	Ophthalmic solution; available as ophthalmic suspension; beta$_1$-blocker; reduces blood pressure, heart rate.
carteolol (Ocupress)	1 drop 1% solution every bid.	Ophthalmic solution; nonspecific beta-blocker; causes bronchoconstriction.
levobunolol (Betagan)	1–2 drops 0.25–0.5% solution qd-bid.	Ophthalmic solution; nonspecific beta-blocker.
metipranolol (OptiPranolol)	1 drop 0.3% solution bid.	Ophthalmic solution; nonspecific beta-blocker.
timolol (Timoptic, Timoptoc XE)	drops: 1–2 drops of 0.25–0.5% solution qd-bid gel (salve): apply qd.	Ophthalmic solution; nonspecific beta-blocker.
Alpha$_2$-Adrenergic Agonists		
apraclonidine (Iopidine)	1 drop 0.5% solution bid.	Ophthalmic solution.
brimonidine tartrate (Alphagan)	1 drop 0.2% solution tid.	Ophthalmic solution.
Carbonic Anhydrase Inhibitors		
(Pr) acetazolamide (Diamox)	PO; 250 mg qd-qid.	Oral diuretic; sulfonamide; Also for seizures, high altitude sickness, and renal impairment.
brinzolamide (Azopt)	1 drop 1% solution tid.	Ophthalmic solution; sulfonamide.
dichlorphenamide (Duranide, Oratrol)	PO; 100–200 mg followed by 100 mg bid.	Oral sulfonamide.
dorzolamide hydrochloride (Trusopt)	1 drop 2% solution tid.	Ophthalmic solution; sulfonamide.
methazolamide (Neptazane)	PO; 50–100 mg bid or tid.	Oral sulfonamide; less diuretic activity than acetazolamide.
Osmotic Diuretics		
glycerin anhydrous (Ophthalagen)	PO; 1–1.8 g/kg 1–1.5 h before ocular surgery; may repeat q5h.	Often used for eye surgery in cases of injury.
isosorbide (Ismotic)	PO; 1–3 g/kg bid – qid.	Used before and after eye surgery.
mannitol (Osmitrol)	IV; 1.5–2 mg/kg as a 15–25% solution over 30–60 minutes.	Raises osmotic pressure causing diuresis; IV medication.
urea (Ureaphil)	IV; 1–1.5 g/kg of 30% solution infused slowly over 1–2.5 h at a rate not to exceed 4 ml/min (max 120 g/24h).	For cases of prolonged surgery to reduce intracranial and intraocular pressure associated with head injury.

especially careful with anticholinergic mydriatics because these drugs can worsen the condition of clients with glaucoma by impairing aqueous humor outflow and thereby increasing IOP. In addition, cholinergic-agonists have the potential for producing unfavorable central side effects in adults such as confusion, unsteadiness, or drowsiness. Children generally become restless and spastic. Examples of cycloplegic, mydriatic, and lubricant drugs are listed in Table 32.3.

TABLE 32.3	Drugs of Importance for Eye Examinations and Moistening Eye Membranes	
DRUG	**ROUTE AND ADULT DOSE**	**REMARKS**
Mydriatics: Sympathomimetics		
hydroxyamphetamine (Paredrine)	1 drop 1% solution before eye exam.	Used to dilate pupils in closed-angle glaucoma.
phenylephrine hydrochloride (Mydfrin, Neo-Synephrine)	1 drop 2.5 or 10% solution before eye exam.	Decongestant and vasoconstriction properties; smaller doses provide temporary relief of eye redness; Also for pupil dilation in closed-angle glaucoma.
Cycloplegics: Anticholinergics		
atropine sulfate (Isopto Atropine, others)	1 drop 0.5% solution qd.	Also provided as ointment; should not be administered to clients with glaucoma; effects may be prolonged.
cyclopentolate (Cyclogyl, Pentalair)	1 drop 0.5–2% solution 40–50 minutes before procedure.	Not for glaucoma clients; causes burning and irritation; possible central side effects with higher doses.
homatropine (Isopto Homatropine, others)	1–2 drops 2 or 5% solution before eye exam.	Not for glaucoma clients; effects may be prolonged after treatment.
scopolamine hydrobromide (Isopto Hyoscine)	1–2 drops 0.25% solution 1 hour before eye exam.	Not for glaucoma clients; effects may be prolonged after treatment; possible central side effects with higher doses.
tropicamide (Mydriacyl, Tropicacyl)	1–2 drops 0.5–1% solution before eye exam.	Not for glaucoma clients; central side effects with higher doses.
Lubricants Causing Ocular Vasoconstriction		
naphazoline hydrochloride (Albalon Allerest, ClearEyes, others)	1–3 drops 0.1% solution every 3–4 hours prn.	OTC and prescription medications available.
oxymetazoline hydrochloride (OcuClear, Visine LR)	1–2 drops 0.025% solution qid.	OTC and prescription medications available.
tetrahydrozoline hydrochloride (Collyrium, Murine Plus, Visine, others)	1–2 drops 0.05% solution bid-tid.	Primarily OTC medication.
General Purpose Lubricants		
lanolin alcohol (Lacri-lube)	Apply a thin film to the inside of the eyelid.	Mixed with mineral oil and petroleum jelly as a salve.
methylcellulose (Methulose, Visculose, others)	1–2 drops prn.	Artificial tear solution.
polyvinyl alcohol (Liquifilm. others)	1–2 drops prn.	Artificial tear solution.

Concept review 32.3

■ List examples of commonly used drugs for minor eye irritation and injury. What are the major actions of cycloplegic and mydriatic drugs?

FIGURE 32.3

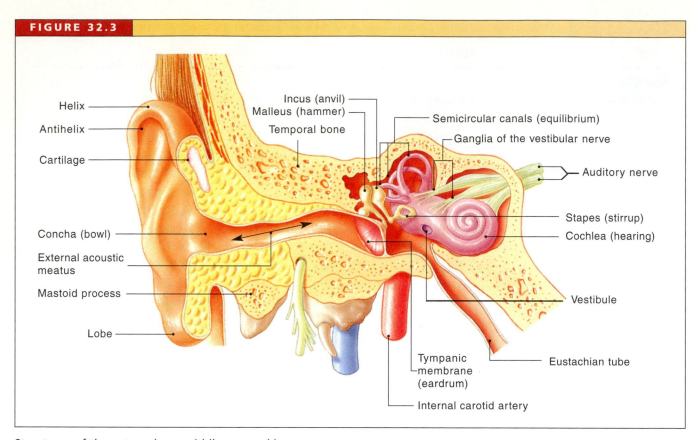

Structures of the external ear, middle ear, and inner ear   *SOURCE: Pearson Education/PH College.*

EAR CONDITIONS

The ear has two major sensory functions: hearing and maintenance of equilibrium and balance. Three important structural areas—the outer ear, middle ear, and inner ear—carry out these functions.

ot = ear
itis = inflammation

Otitis, inflammation of the ear, most often occurs in the outer and middle ear compartments. **External otitis,** commonly called *swimmer's ear,* is inflammation of the outer ear; **otitis media** is inflammation of the middle ear. Outer ear infections are most often associated with water exposure. Middle ear infections are most often associated with upper respiratory infections, allergies, or auditory tube irritation. Of all ear infections, the most difficult ones to treat are inner ear infections. **Mastoiditis,** or inflammation of the mastoid sinus, can be a serious problem because if left untreated, it can result in hearing loss.

OTIC PREPARATIONS

Combination drugs effectively treat many different types of ear conditions including infections, earaches, edema, and ear wax.

32.7 Otic preparations treat infections, inflammation, and ear wax buildup.

The basic treatment for ear infection is essentially the same as in all places of the body: antibiotics. Topical antibiotics in the form of ear drops may be administered for external ear infections. Systemic antibiotics (Chapter 12) may be needed in cases where outer ear infections are

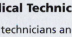

ON THE JOB

Ophthalmic Medical Technicians

Ophthalmic medical technicians and technologists are trained to perform diagnostic tests and to administer many medications under the direct supervision of an ophthamologist. They must be familiar with ocular anatomy, eye diseases, and ophthalmic pharmacology. They often work closely with clients and are responsible for helping communicate risk factors associated with various eye diseases including glaucoma. They also help clients to understand the side effects of medications given by the ophthamologist during an eye exam. They gather important information that will become a part of the client's medical record, and may assist in ophthalmic surgery in a hospital or clinic setting. This profession requires a higher level of expertise involving drugs that particularly affect general eye health. ■

extensive or in cases of middle or inner ear infections. Medications for pain, edema, and itching may also be necessary. Glucocorticoids are often combined with antibiotics or with other drugs when inflammation is present. Examples of these drugs are listed in Table 32.4.

Mineral oil, ear wax softeners, and commercial products are also used for proper ear health. When ear wax accumulates, it narrows the ear canal, and may interfere with hearing. This is especially true for older clients who are not able to properly take care of themselves. Healthcare providers working with the elderly are trained to take appropriate measures when removing impacted ear wax.

PharmLink

U.S. NATIONAL LIBRARY OF MEDICINE

Concept review 32.4

■ Identify areas of the ear where microbial infections are most likely. What kind of otic preparations treat infections, inflammation, and ear wax buildup?

TABLE 32.4	Otic Preparations for General Ear Health or Removal of Ear Wax	
DRUG	**ROUTE AND ADULT DOSE**	**REMARKS**
aluminum sulfate and calcium acetate (Domeboro)	2 drops 2% solution tid-qid.	For general ear infections and the prevention of swimmer's ear; may be administered using an ear wick; OTC medication.
acetic Acid and hydrocortisone (Vosol HC)	3 to 5 drops in the affected ear q 4h-qid × 24 hours, then 5 drops tid-qid.	Combination of acetic acid and glucocorticoid; for general ear infections and inflammation; prescription medication.
benzocaine and antipyrine (Auralgan)	Fill ear canal with solution tid × 2 or 3 days.	For acute otitis media and the removal of ear wax; reduces earache associated with the infection; prescription medication.
carbamide peroxide (Debrox)	1–5 drops 6.5% solution bid × 4 days.	To soften, loosen, and remove excessive ear wax; OTC medication.
ciprofloxacin hydrochloride and hydrocortisone (Cipro)	3 drops of the suspension instilled into the affected ear bid × 7 days.	Combination of fluoroquinolone antibiotic and glucocorticoid; for ear infections and inflammation; prescription medication.
polymixin B, neomycin and hydrocortisone (Cortisporin)	4 drops in ear tid-qid.	Combination of antibiotics and glucocorticoid; for general ear or mastoid infections and inflammation; some clients may develop dermatitis as a result of sensitivity to neomycin; prescription medication.
triethanolamine polypeptide oleate 10% condensate (Cerumenex)	Fill ear canal with solution; wait 10–20 minutes.	Drug dissolved in propylene glycerol; breaks apart ear wax; small risk of sensitivity; OTC medication.

CLIENT TEACHING

Clients taking medications for eye and ear disorders need to know the following:

1. Have regular eye exams after the age of 40.
2. If you are at risk for glaucoma, do not exert yourself by straining or lifting heavy objects. Any effort that might produce eyestrain should be avoided.
3. Tell your practitioner about any allergies or sensitivities, including sulfa drugs.
4. Do not take OTC medications that "get the red out" for periods of time greater than 24 hours. Use eye lubricants instead. Persistent irritation should be reported immediately to your practitioner.
5. Take precautions to keep the ear canal dry when you have to remain in or around water for an extensive time. Use appropriate earplugs or a bathing cap.
6. Apply 2% acetic acid to the ear canal after swimming. Acetic acid acts as a drying agent and restores the ear canal to its normal acidic condition.
7. Avoid using glucocorticoids for long periods of time. They could cause eye or ear damage.
8. Use a bulb syringe approved for removing debris and warm water rather than by placing objects like cotton swabs in the ear canal. Use cerumen dissolving agent responsibly. ▪

CHAPTER REVIEW

 Core Concepts Summary

32.1 Knowledge of basic eye anatomy is fundamental for an understanding of eye disorders and drug therapy.

The anterior cavity of the eye is the focal point where aqueous humor is circulated. Aqueous humor originates from the ciliary body located in the posterior chamber and drains into the canal of Schlemm found in the anterior chamber.

32.2 Glaucoma is one of the leading causes of blindness.

Glaucoma develops because the flow of aqueous humor in the anterior eye cavity becomes disrupted, leading to increasing intraocular pressure (IOP). Two principle types of glaucoma are closed-angle glaucoma and open-angle glaucoma.

32.3 Glaucoma therapy centers on adjusting the circulation of aqueous humor.

Glaucoma therapy generally works by increasing the outflow of aqueous humor or decreasing aqueous humor formation.

32.4 Some anti-glaucoma medications increase the outflow of aqueous humor.

Drugs that increase the outflow of aqueous humor include miotics, sympathomimetics, prostaglandins, and prostamides.

32.5 Other anti-glaucoma medications decrease the formation of aqueous humor.

Medications that decrease the formation of aqueous humor include beta-blockers alpha$_2$-adrenergic agonists, carbonic anhydrase inhibitors, and osmotic diuretics. The beta-adrenergic blockers are the most commonly prescribed drug class.

32.6 Drugs provide relief for minor eye conditions and are used for eye exams.

Mydriatic or pupil-dilating drugs and cyclopegic or ciliary muscle relaxing drugs are routinely used for eye examinations. Some drugs constrict local blood vessels. Others lubricate the eyes.

32.7 Otic preparations treat infections, inflammation, and ear wax buildup.

Combination drugs provide relief of ear conditions associated with the outer, middle, and inner ear. Drugs include antibiotics, corticosteroids, and ear wax dissolving agents.

EXPLORE PharMedia
www.prenhall.com/holland

Additional interactive resources and activities for this chapter can be found on the Companion Website. For animations, audio glossary, and review access the accompanying CD-ROM in this book.

Mechanism in Action:
   Pilocarpine
Audio Glossary
NCLEX Review
Concept Review

PharmLinks
   Glaucoma Research Foundation
   U.S. National Library of Medicine

APPENDIX A: References

General References

Audesirk, T., Audesirk, G., & Beyers, B. E. (2000). *Biology: Life on earth* (6th ed.). New Jersey: Prentice-Hall.

Beers, M. H. & Berkow, R., (Eds.). (2001). *Merck manual: Diagnosis and therapy* (17th ed.). Whitehouse Station, NJ: Merck & Co., Inc.

Krogh, D. (2000). *Biology: A guide to the natural world.* New Jersey: Prentice-Hall.

LeMone, P., & Burke, K. M. (2000). *Medical-surgical nursing: Critical thinking in client care* (2nd ed.). New Jersey: Prentice-Hall.

Martini, F. H. (2001). *Fundamentals of human anatomy and physiology* (5th ed.). New Jersey: Prentice-Hall.

Mulvihill, M. L., Zelman, P., Holdaway, P., Tompary, E., & Turchany, J. (2001). *Human diseases: A systemic approach* (5th ed.). New Jersey: Prentice Hall.

Medical Economics Staff (Ed.). (2002). *Physician's desk reference.* (56th ed.). Montvale: Medical Economics.

Medical Economics Staff (Ed.). (2001). *Physician's desk reference for non-prescription drugs and dietary supplements.* Montvale: Medical Economics.

Rice, J. (1999). *Medical terminology with human anatomy.* New Jersey: Prentice-Hall.

Silverthorn, D. U. (1998). *Human physiology: An integrated approach.* New Jersey: Prentice-Hall.

Wilson, B. A., Shannon, M. T., & Strang, C. L. (2002). *Nurse's drug guide 2002.* New Jersey: Prentice-Hall.

CHAPTER 1
Introduction to Pharmacology: Drug Regulation and Approval

Bond, C. A., Raehl, C. L., & Franke, T. (2001). Medication errors in United States hospitals. *Pharmacotherapy, 21*(9), 1023–1036.

Brown, S. D., & Landry, F. J. (2001). Recognizing, reporting, and reducing adverse drug reactions, *South Med J, 94*(4), 370–373.

Carrico, J. M. (2000). Human Genome Project and pharmacogenomics: Implications for pharmacy. *J Am Pharm Assoc 40*(1), 115–116.

Gaither, C. A., Kirking, D. M., Ascione, F. J., & Welage, L.S. (2001). Consumers' views on generic medications. *J Am Pharm Assoc 41*(5), 729–736.

Kacew, S. (1999). Effects of over-the-counter drugs on the unborn child: What is known and how should this influence prescribing? *Paedriatr Drugs 1*(2), 75–80.

Kohn, L. T., Corrigan, J. M., & Donaldson, M. S. (Eds.) (1999). *To err is human: Building a safer system.* Washington, DC: The National Academy of Sciences, National Academy Press.

Lazarou, J., Pomeranz, B. H., & Corey, P. N. (1998). Incidence of adverse drug reactions in hospitalized patients. *JAMA 279*(15), 1200–1205.

Newton, G. D., Pray, W. S., & Popovich, N. G. (2001). New OTC drugs and devices 2000: A selective review. *J Am Pharm Assoc 41*(2), 273–282.

Nies, A. S. (2001). Principles of therapeutics. In Hardman, J. G., Limbird, L. E. & Goodman, A. G. (Eds.), *The pharmacological basis of therapeutics* (pp. 45–66). New York: McGraw-Hill.

Olsen, D. P. (2000). The patient's responsibility for optimum healthcare. *Dis Manage Health Outcomes 7*(2), 57–65.

Phillips, K. A., Veenstra, D. L., Oren, E., Lee, J.K., & Sardee, W. (2001). Potential role of pharmacogenomics in reducing adverse drug reactions: A systematic Review. *JAMA 286*, 2270–2279.

CHAPTER 2
Drug Classes, Schedules, and Categories

Brass, E. P. (2001). Drug therapy: Changing the status of drugs from prescription to over-the counter availability. *N Engl J Med 345*, 810–816.

Smith, S. F., Duell, D. J., & Martin, B. C. (2000). *Clinical nursing skills* (5th ed.). New Jersey: Prentice-Hall.

CHAPTER 3
Methods of Drug Delivery

Berman, A., Snyder, S., Kozier, B., & Erb, G. (2002). *Kozier and Erb's techniques in clinical nursing* (5th ed.). New Jersey: Prentice-Hall.

Smith, S. F., Duell, D. J., & Martin, B. C. (2002). *Photo atlas of nursing skills.* New Jersey: Prentice-Hall.

CHAPTER 4
What Happens After a Drug Has Been Administered

Bateman, D. N. (2001). Introduction to pharmacokinetics and pharmacodynamics. *J of Toxicol: Clin Toxicol 39*(3), 207.

Consider racial, ethnic, and cultural differences in cardiovascular drug effectiveness. (2001). *Prog Cardiovasc Nurs 16*(4), 152–160+.

Levy, R. H., Thummel, K. E., Trager, W. F., Hansten, P. D., & Eichelbaum, M. (Eds.). (2000). *Metabolic drug interactions.* Philadelphia: Lippinott Williams & Wilkins.

Ross, E. M., & Kenakin, T. P. (2001). Pharmacodynamics: Mechanisms of drug action and the relationship between drug concentration and effect. In Hardman, J. G., Limbird, L. E., & Goodman, A. G. (Eds.), *The pharmacological basis of therapeutics* (p. 31–44). New York: McGraw-Hill.

Wilkinson, G. R. (2001). The dynamics of drug absorption, distribution, and elimination. In Hardman, J. G., Limbird, L. E., & Goodman, A. G. (Eds.), The pharmacological basis of therapeutics (pp. 3–30). New York: McGraw-Hill.

CHAPTER 5
Substance Abuse

Haseltine, E. (2001). The unsatisfied mind: Are reward centers in your brain wired for substance abuse? *Discover 22*(11), 88.

Jason, L. A., Davis, M. I., Ferrari, J. R., & Bishop, P. D. (2001). A review of research and implications for substance abuse recovery and community research. *J of Drug Educ 31*(1), 1–28.

Manoguerra, A. S. (2001). Methamphetamine abuse. *J of Toxicol: Clinic Toxicol 38*(2), 187.

Naegle, M. A., & D'Avanzo, C. E. (2001). *Addictions and substance abuse: Strategies for advanced practice nursing.* New Jersey: Prentice-Hall.

O'Brien, C. P. (2001). Drug addiction and drug abuse. In Hardman, J. G., Limbird, L. E., & Goodman, A. G. (Eds.), *The pharmacological basis of therapeutics* (p. 621–642). New York: McGraw-Hill.

Sindelar, J. L., & Fiellin, D. A. (2001). Innovations in treatment for drug abuse: Solutions to a public health problem. *Ann Rev of Pub Health 22*, 249.

Wasilow-Mueller, S., & Erickson, C. K. (2001). Drug abuse and dependency: Understanding gender differences in etiology and management. *J Am Pharm Assoc 41*(1), 78–90.

CHAPTER 6
Drugs for Disorders Associated with the Autonomic Nervous System

Hoffman, B. B., and Taylor, P. (2001). Neurotransmission: The autonomic and somatic motor nervous systems. In Hardman, J. G., Limbird, L. E., & Goodman, A. G. (Eds.), *The pharmacological basis of therapeutics* (pp. 115–154). New York: McGraw-Hill.

CHAPTER 7
Drugs for Anxiety, Daytime Sedation, and Insomnia

Baldessarini, R. J. (2001). Drugs and the treatment of psychiatric disorders: Depression and anxiety disorders. In Hardman, J. G., Limbird, L. E., & Goodman, A. G. (Eds.), *The pharmacological basis of therapeutics* (pp. 447–484). New York: McGraw-Hill.

Charney, D. S., Mihic, J., & Harris, A. (2001). Hypnotics and sedatives. In Hardman, J. G., Limbird, L. E., & Goodman, A. G. (Eds.), *The pharmacological basis of therapeutics* (pp. 399–428). New York: McGraw-Hill.

Fontaine, K. L., & Fletcher, J. S. (1999). *Mental health nursing* (4th ed.). New Jersey: Prentice-Hall.

Gorman, J. N. (2001). Generalized anxiety disorder. *Clin Corner 3*(3), 37–46.

Lippmann, S., Mazour, I., & Shahab, H. (2001). Insomnia: Therapeutic approach. *South Med J 94*(9), 866–873.

Smock, T. K. (2001). *Physiological psychology: A neuroscience approach.* New Jersey: Prentice-Hall.

Vitiello, M. V. (2000). Effective treatment of sleep disturbances in older adults. *Clin Corner 2*(5), 16–27.

CHAPTER 8
Drugs for Seizures

Bourdet, S. V., Gidal, B. E., & Alldredge, B. K. (2001). Pharmacologic management of Epilepsy in the elderly. *J Am Pharm Assoc 41*(3), 421–436.

Landover, M. D. (1999). *Epilepsy: A report to the nation* [On-line]. Available: http://www.efa.org/epusa/nation/nation/html

McNamera, J. O. (2001). Drugs effective in the therapy of the epilepsies. In Hardman, J. G., Limbird, L. E., & Goodman, A. G. (Eds.), *The pharmacological basis of therapeutics* (pp. 521–548). New York: McGraw-Hill.

Schachter, S. C. (2000). The next wave of anticonvulsants: Focus on levetiracetam, oxcarbazepine, and zonisamide. *CNS Drugs 14*(3), 229–249.

Tatum, W. O., Galvez, R., Benbadis, S., & Carrazana, E. (2000). New antiepileptic drugs: Into the new millennium. *Arch Fam Med 9*, 1135–1141.

Winkelman, C. (1999). Pharmacology update: A review of pharmacodynamics and pharmacokinetics in seizure management. *J of Neurosci Nur 31*(1), 50–53.

CHAPTER 9
Drugs for Behavioral/Emotional Disorders, Mood Disorders, and Psychoses

American Academy of Pediatrics. (2000). Diagnosis and evaluation of the child with attention deficit-hyperactivity disorder. *Pediatrics 105*(5), 1158–1170.

Baldessarini, R. J. (2001). Drugs and the treatment of psychiatric disorders: Depression and anxiety disorders. In Hardman, J. G., Limbird, L. E., & Goodman, A. G. (Eds.), *The pharmacological basis of therapeutics* (pp. 447–484). New York: McGraw-Hill.

Baldessarini, R. J., & Tarazi, F. I. (2001). Drugs and the treatment of psychiatric disorders: Psychosis and mania. In Hardman, J. G., Limbird, L. E. & Goodman, A. G. (Eds.), *The pharmacological basis of therapeutics* (pp. 485–520). New York: McGraw-Hill.

Brown, C. S., Markowitz, J. S., Moore, T. R., & Parker, N. G. (1999). Atypical antipsychotics: Part II. Adverse effects, drug interactions, and costs. *Ann Pharmacother 33*, 210–217.

Burns, M. J. (2001). The pharmacology and toxicology of atypical antipsychotic agents. *J of Toxicol: Clin Toxicol 39*(1), 1.

Canales, P. L., Olsen, J., Miller, A. L., & Crismon, M. L. (1999). Role of antipsychotic polypharmacotherapy in the treatment of schizophrenia. *CNS Drugs 12*, 179–188.

Desai, H. D., & Jann, M. W. (2000). Major depression in woman: A review of the literature. *J Am Pharm Assoc 40*(4), 525–537.

Emslie, G. J., & Mayes, T. L. (1999). Depression in children and adolescents: a guide to diagnosis and treatment. *CNS Drugs 11*(3), 181–189.

Markowitz, J. S., Brown, C. S., & Moore, T. R. (1999). Atypical antipsychotics: Part I. Pharmacology, pharmacokinetics, and efficacy. *Ann Pharmacother 33*, 73–85.

Nelson, J. C. (2000). Augmentation strategies in depression. *J Clin Psych 61*, 13–19.

Owen, W., & Castle, D. J. (1999). Late-onset schizophrenia: Epidemiology, diagnosis, management, and outcomes. *Drugs and Aging 15*(2), 81–89.

Tandon, R., Milner, K., & Jibson, M. D. (1999). Antipsychotics from theory to practice: Integrating clinical and basic data. *J Clin Psychiatry 8*, 21–28.

Vitiello, B. (2001). Psychopharmacology for young children: Clinical needs and research opportunities. *Pediatrics 108*(4), 983.

CHAPTER 10
Drugs for Parkinson's Disease and Dementia

Cummings, J. L. (2000). Treatment of Alzheimer's disease. *Clinic Corner 3*(4), 27–39.

Dooley, M., & Lamb, H. M. (2000). Donepezil: A review of its use in Alzheimer's disease. *Drugs and Aging 16*(3), 199–226.

Hristove, A. H., & Koller, W. C. (2000). Early Parkinson's disease: What is the best approach in treatment? *Drugs Aging 17*(3), 165–181.

Lambert, D., & Waters, C. H. (2000). Comparative tolerability of the new generation antiparkinson agents. *Drugs and Aging 16*(1), 55–65.

Olanow, C. W., & Tatton, W. G. (1999). Etiology and pathogenesis of Parkinson's Disease. *Ann Rev Neurosci 2*, 123–144.

Standaert, D. G., & Young, A. B. (2001). Treatment of central nervous system degenerative disorders. In Hardman, J. G., Limbird, L. E. & Goodman, A. G. (Eds.), *The pharmacological basis of therapeutics* (pp. 549–568). New York: McGraw-Hill.

CHAPTER 11
Drugs for the Control of Pain and Fever

Bannwarth, B. (1999). Risk-benefit assessment of opioids in chronic noncancer pain. *Drug Safety 21*(4), 283–296.

Barkin, R. L., & Barkin, D. (2001). Pharmacologic management of acute and chronic pain: Focus on drug interactions and patient-specific pharmacotherapeutic selection. *South Med J 94*(8) 756–812.

Broadbent, C. (2000). The pharmacology of acute pain—Part 3. *Nursing Times 96*(26), 39.

elt-Hansen, P., DeVries, P., & Sexena, P. R. (2000). Triptans in migraine: A comparative review of pharmacology, pharmacokinetics, and efficacy. *Drugs 60*(6), 1259–1287.

Glajchen, M. (2001). Chronic pain: Treatment barriers and strategies for clinical practice. *J Am Board Fam Pract 14*(3), 178–183.

Guay, D. R. P. (2001). Adjunctive agents in the management of chronic pain. *Pharmacotherapy 21*(9), 1070–1081.

Gunsteuin, H., & Akil, H. (2001). Opioid analgesics. In Hardman, J. G., Limbird, L. E., & Goodman, A. G. (Eds.), *The pharmacological basis of therapeutics* (pp. 569–620). New York: McGraw-Hill.

Khouzam, H. R. (2000). Chronic pain and its management in primary care. *South Med J 93*(10), 946–952.

Tepper, S. J., & Rapoport, A. M. (1999). The triptans: A summary. *CNS Drugs 12*(5), 403–417.

CHAPTER 12
Drugs for Local and General Anesthesia

Catterall, W. A., & Mackie, K. Local anesthetics. In Hardman, J. G., Limbird, L. E., & Goodman, A. G. (Eds.), *The pharmacological basis of therapeutics* (pp. 367–384). New York: McGraw-Hill.

Colbert, B. J., & Mason, B. J. (2001). *Integrated cardiopulmonary pharmacology.* New Jersey: Prentice-Hall.

Evers, A., & Crowder, C. M. (2001). General anesthetics. In Hardman, J. G., Limbird, L. E., & Goodman, A. G. (Eds.), *The pharmacological basis of therapeutics* (pp. 337–366). New York: McGraw-Hill.

Nagelhout, J. J., Nagelhout, K., & Zaglaniczny, V. H. (2001). *Handbook of nurse anesthesia* (2nd ed.). Philadelphia: W. B. Saunders.

Omoigui, S. (1999). Sota Omogui's Anesthesia drugs handbook (3rd ed.). Hawthorne, CA: State of the Art Technologies.

Stoelting, R. K. (1999). Pharmacology and physiology in anesthetic practice (3rd ed.). Philadelphia: Lippincott, Williams, and Wilkins.

Waugaman, W. R., Foster, S. D., & Rigor, B. M. (1999). *Principles and practice of nurse anesthesia* (3rd ed.). New Jersey: Prentice-Hall.

CHAPTER 13
Drugs for Coagulation Disorders

Alligood, K. A., & Iltz, J. L. (2001). Update on antithrombotic use and mechanism of action. *Prog in Card Nurs 16*(2), 81–85.

Blackwell, S., & Hendrix, P. C. (2001). Common anemias: What lies beneath. *Clinic Rev 11*(3), 530–62.

Hiatt, W. R. (2001). Drug therapy: Medical treatment of peripheral arterial disease and claudication. *N Engl J Med 344*, 1608–1621.

Majerus, P. W., & Tollefson, D. M. (2001). Anticoagulant, thrombolytic, and antiplatelet drugs. In Hardman, J. G., Limbard, L. E. & Goodman, A. G. (Eds.), *The pharmacological basis of therapeutics* (p. 1519–1538). New York: McGraw-Hill.

Vasant, B. P., & Moliterno, D. J. (2000). Glycoprotein IIb/IIIa antagonist and fibrinolytic agents: New therapeutic regimen for acute myocardial infarction. *J Invasive Cardiol 12*(B), 8B–15B.

CHAPTER 14
Drugs for Hypertension

Braunwald, E., Zipes, D. P., & Libby, P. (Eds.). (2001). *Heart disease: A textbook of cardiovascular medicine* (6th ed.). Philadelphia: W. B. Saunders.

Colbert, B. J., & Mason, B. J. (2001). *Integrated cardiopulmonary pharmacology*. New Jersey: Prentice-Hall.

Dabrow, A. (1999). Managing hypertension. *Nursing 99*. Mar: 41.

Mazzolai, L., & Burnier M. (1999). Comparative safety and tolerability of angiotensin II receptor antagonists. *Drug Safety 21*(1), 22–23.

Oates, J. A., & Brown, N. J. (2001). Antihypertensive agents and the drug therapy of hypertension. In Hardman, J. G., Limbard, L. E., & Goodman, A. G. (Eds.), *The pharmacological basis of therapeutics* (pp. 871–900). New York: McGraw-Hill.

Oparil, S. (2000). Essential Hypertension. Part II; treatment, Circulation 101(4), 1524–1539.

Weir, M. R. (2000). When antihypertensive monotherapy fails: Fixed-dose combination therapy. *South Med J 93*(6), 548–556.

CHAPTER 15
Drugs for Heart Failure

Albrant, D. H. (2001). Drug treatment protocol: Management of chronic systolic heart failure. *J Am Pharm Assoc 41*(5), 672–681.

Gomberg-Maitland, M., Baran, D. A., & Fuster, V. (2001). Treatment of congestive heart failure: Guidelines for the primary care physician and the heart failure specialist. *Arch Intern Med 161*, 342–352.

Jamali, A. H., Tang, A. H. W., Khot, U. N., & Fowler, M. B. (2001). The role of angiotensin receptor blockers in the management of chronic heart failure. *Arch Intern Med 161*, 667–672.

Ooi, H., & Colucci, W. (2001). Pharmacological treatment of heart failure. In Hardman, J. G., Limbard, L. E., & Goodman, A. G. (Eds.), *The pharmacological basis of therapeutics* (pp. 901–932). New York: McGraw-Hill.

Opie, L. H., & Gersh, B. J. (Eds.). (2001). *Drugs for the heart* (5th ed.). Philadelphia: W. B. Saunders.

Sperelakis, N., Kurachi, Y., Terzic, A., & Cohen, M. (Eds.). (2001). *Heart physiology and pathophysiology* (4th ed.). San Diego: Academic Press.

Steering Committee and Membership of the Advisory Council to Improve Outcomes Nationwide in Heart Failure. (1999). Consensus recommendations for the management of chronic heart failure. *Am J Cardiol 83*(2A), 1A–38A.

Van Bakel, A. B., & Chidsey, G. (2000). Management of advanced heart failure. *Clinic Corner 3*(2), 25–35.

CHAPTER 16
Drugs for Dysrhythmias

Falk, R. H. (2001). Medical progress: Atrial fibrillation. *N Eng J Med 344*, 1067–1078.

Huikuri, H. V., Castellanos, A., & Myerburg, R. J. (2001). Medical progress: Sudden death due to cardiac arrhythmias. *N Eng J Med 345*, 1473–1482.

Morrill, P. (2000). Pharmacotherapeutics of positive inotropes. *AORN-Journal 71*(1), 173–178, 181–185.

Podrid, P. J., & Kowey, P. R. (Eds.). (2001). Cardiac arrhythmia: Mechanisms, diagnosis, and management (2nd ed.). Philadelphia: Lippincott, Williams, and Wilkins.

Roden, D. M. (2001). Antidysrhythmic drugs. In Hardman, J. G., Limbard, L. E., & Goodman, A. G. (Eds.), *The pharmacological basis of therapeutics* (pp. 933–970). New York: McGraw-Hill.

CHAPTER 17
Drugs for Chest Pain, Myocardial Infarction, and Stroke

Ambrose, J., & Dangas, G. (2000). Unstable angina: Current concepts of pathogenesis and treatment. *Arch Int Med 160*, 25–237.

Deedwania, P. C. (2000). Silent myocardial ischemia in the elderly. *Drugs and Aging 16*(5), 381–389.

Kerins, D. M., Robertson, R. M., & Robertson, D. (2001). Drugs used for the treatment of myocardial ischemia. In Hardman, J. G., Limbard, L. E., & Goodman, A. G. (Eds.), *The pharmacological basis of therapeutics* (pp. 843–870). New York: McGraw-Hill.

Kreisberg, R. A. (2000). Overview of coronary heart disease and selected risk factors. *Clin Rev,* Spring, 4–9.

Larsen, J. A., Kadish, A. H., & Schwartz, J. B. (2000). Proper use of antiarrhythmic therapy for reduction of mortality after myocardial infarction. *Drugs and Aging 16*(5), 341–350.

Levine, G. N., Ali, M. N., & Schafer, A. I. (2001). Antithrombotic therapy in patients with acute coronary symptoms. *Arch Intern Med 161*, 937–948.

Priglinger, U., & Huber, K. (2000). Thrombolytic therapy in acute myocardial infarction. *Drugs and Aging 16*(4), 301–312.

Sarti, C., Kaarisalo, M., & Tuomilehto, J. (2000). The relationship between cholesterol and stroke: Implications for hyperlipidemic therapy in older patients. *Drugs and Aging 17*(1), 33–51.

CHAPTER 18
Drugs for Acute Shock and Anaphylaxis

Baumgartner, J. D., & Calandra, T. (1999). Treatment of sepsis: Past and future avenues. *Drugs 57*(2), 127–132.

Jurewicz, M. A. (2000). Anaphylaxis: When the body overreacts. *Nursing 2000 30*(7), 58–61.

Mower-Wade, D., Bartley, M. K., & Chiari-Allwein, J. L. (2000). Shock: Do you know how to respond? *Nursing 2000 30*(10), 34–39.

Neugut, A. I., Ghatak, A. T., & Miller, R. L. (2001). Anaphylaxis in the United States: An investigation into its epidemiology. *Arch Intern Med 161*, 15–21.

von Rosensteil, N., von Rosensteil, I., & Adam, D. (2001). Management of sepsis and septic shock in infants and children. *Paediatr Drugs 3*(1), 9–27.

CHAPTER 19
Drugs for Lipid Disorders

Beaird, S. L. (2000). HMG-CoA reductase inhibitors: Assessing differences in drug Interactions and safety profiles. L Am Pharm Assoc 40(5), 637–644.

Expert Panel on Detection, Evaluation, and Treatment of High Blood Cholesterol in Adults. (2001). Executive summary of the third report of the national cholesterol education panel (NCEP). *JAMA* 285, 2486–2497.

Harper, C. R., & Jacobsen, T. A. (2001). The fats of life: The role of omega-3 fatty acids in the prevention of coronary heart disease. *Arch Intern Med* 161, 2185–2192.

Illingworth, D. R. (2000). Management of hypercholesterolemia. *Med Clin North Am 84*(1), 23–42.

Kreisberg, R. A. (2000). Art and science of statin use. *Clin Rev,* Spring, 47–51.

Mahley, R. W., & Bersot, T. P. (2001). Drug therapy for hypercholesterolemia and dyslipidemia. In Hardman, J. G., Limbard, L. E., & Goodman, A. G. (Eds.), *The pharmacological basis of therapeutics* (pp. 971–1002). New York: McGraw-Hill.

Oberman, A. (2000). Role of lipids in the prevention of cardiovascular disease. *Clin Rev,* Spring, 10–15.

Robinson, A. W., Sloan, H. L., & Arnold, G. (2001). Use if niacin in the prevention and management of hyperlipidemia. *Prog Cardiovasc Nurs 16*(1), 14–20.

Young, K. L., Allen, J. K., & Kelly, K. M. (2001). HDL Cholesterol: Striving for healthier levels. *Clin Rev 11*(5), 50–61.

CHAPTER 20
Drugs for Inflammation, Allergies, and Immune Disorders

Capriotti, T. (2001). Monoclonal antibodies: Drugs that combine pharmacology and biotechnology. *MedSurg Nursing 10*(2), 89.

Fitzgerald, G. A., & Patrono, C. (2001). Drug therapy: The coxibs, selective inhibitors of cyclooxygenase-2. *N Engl J Med 345,* 433–442.

Hawkey, L. M., & Hawkey, C. J. (1999). COX-2 inhibitors. *Lancet* 353, 307–314.

Jackson, L. M., & Hawkey, C. J. (2000). COX-2 selective nonsteroidal anti-inflammatory drugs: Do they really offer any advantages? *Drugs 59*(6), 1207–1216.

Krensky, A. M., Strom, T. B., & Bluestone, J. A. (2001). Immunomodulators: immunosuppressive agents, toleragens, and immunostimulants. In Hardman, J. G., Limbard, L. E., & Goodman, A. G. (Eds.), *The pharmacological basis of therapeutics* (pp. 1463–1484). New York: McGraw-Hill.

Phelan, D., Jacobsen, R. M., & Poland, G. A. (2001). Current adult and pediatric vaccine recommendations. *Infect Med 18*(8), FV6–FV14.

Roberts, L. J., & Morrow, J. D. (2001). Analgesic-antipyretic and anti-inflammatory agents employed in the treatment of gout. In Hardman, J. G., Limbard, L. E. & Goodman, A. G. (Eds.), *The pharmacological basis of therapeutics* (pp. 687–732). New York: McGraw-Hill.

Slater, J. W., Zechnich, A. D., & Haxby, D. G. (1999). Second-generation antihistamines: A comparative review. *Drugs 57*(1), 31–47.

CHAPTER 21
Drugs for Bacterial Infections

Centers for Disease Control and Prevention. (1998). *Guidelines for treatment of sexually transmitted diseases.* MMWR 47, RR 1.

Chambers, H. F. (2001). Antimicrobial agents: The aminoglycosides. In Hardman, J. G., Limbard, L. E., & Goodman, A. G. (Eds.), *The pharmacological basis of therapeutics* (pp. 1219–1239). New York: McGraw-Hill.

Diekema, D., & Jones, R. (2001). Oxazolidinones: A review. *Drugs 59*(1), 7–16.

Gilbert, D. N., Moellering, R. C., & Sande, M. A. (2001). *The Sanford guide to antimicrobial therapy 2001* (31st ed.). Hyde Park, VT: Antimicrobial Therapy, Inc.

Hellinger, W. C. (2000). Confronting the problem of increasing antibiotic resistance. *South Med J 93*(9), 842–848.

Petri, W. A. (2001). Antimicrobial agents: Penicillins, cephalosporins, and other beta-lactam antibiotics. In Hardman, J. G., Limbard, L. E., & Goodman, A. G. (Eds.), *The pharmacological basis of therapeutics* (pp. 1189–1218). New York: McGraw-Hill.

Petri, W. A. (2001). Antimicrobial agents: Sulfonamides, Trimethoprim-Sulfamethasoxazole, Quinolones, and agents for urinary tract infections. In Hardman, J. G., Limbard, L. E. & Goodman, A. G. (Eds.), *The pharmacological basis of therapeutics* (pp. 1171–1188). New York: McGraw-Hill.

Petri, W. A. (2001). Drugs used in the chemotherapy of tuberculosis, *Mycobacterium avium* complex disease, and leprosy. In Hardman, J. G., Limbard, L. E., & Goodman, A. G. (Eds.), *The pharmacological basis of therapeutics* (pp. 1273–1294). New York: McGraw-Hill.

Sheff, B. (2001). Taking aim at antibiotic-resistant bacteria. *Nursing 2001 31*(11), 62–68.

Small, P. M., & Fujiwara, P. I. (2001). Medical progress: Management of tuberculosis in the United States. *N Engl J Med* 345, 189–200.

Tortora, G. J., Funke, B. R., & Case, C. L. (2001). *Microbiology: An introduction* (7th ed.). Menlo Park, CA: Benjamin Cummings.

Virk, A., & Steckelberg, J. M. (2000). Clinical aspects of antimicrobial resistance. *Mayo Clin Proc* 75, 200–214.

CHAPTER 22
Drugs for Fungal, Viral, and Parasitic Infections

Bennet, J. E. (2001). Antimicrobial agents: Antifungal agents. In Hardman, J. G., Limbard, L. E., & Goodman, A. G. (Eds.), *The pharmacological basis of therapeutics* (pp. 1295–1312). New York: McGraw-Hill.

Goldschmidt, R. H., & Dong, B. J. (2001). Treatment of AIDS and HIV-related conditions. *J Am Board Fam Pract* 14(4) 283–309.

Hayden, F. G. (2001). Antimicrobial agents: Antiviral agents (nonretroviral). In Hardman, J. G., Limbard, L. E., & Goodman, A. G. (Eds.), *The pharmacological basis of therapeutics* (pp. 1313–1348). New York: McGraw-Hill.

HIV Panel on Clinical Practices for Treatment of HIV Infection. (2000).Guidelines for the use of antiretroviral agents in HIV-infected adults and adolescents. Washington DC: U. S. Department of Health and Human Services. Available: http://www.hivatis.org/guidelines/adult/Feb0501/

Lewis, R. E., & Kontoyiannis, D. P. (2001). Rationale for combination antifungal therapy. *Pharmacotherapy 21*(8s), 149s–164s.

Pray, W. S. (2001). Treatment of vaginal fungal infections. *U. S. Pharmacist 26*(9).

Raffanti, S. P., & Haas, D. W. (2001). Antimicrobial agents: Antiretroviral agents. In Hardman, J. G., Limbard, L. E., & Goodman, A. G. (Eds.), The pharmacological basis of therapeutics (pp. 1349–1380). New York: McGraw-Hill.

Tracy, J. W., & Webster, L. T. (2001). Drugs used in the chemotherapy of protozoal Infections: Malaria. In Hardman, J. G., Limbard, L. E., & Goodman, A. G. (Eds.), *The pharmacological basis of therapeutics* (pp. 1069–1096). New York: McGraw-Hill.

Zappa, A. J. (1999). The role of the pharmacist in the management of HIV/AIDS. *Dis Manage Health Outcomes* 6(1) 19–28.

CHAPTER 23
Drugs for Neoplasia

Buzdar, A. U. (2000). Tamoxifen's clinical applications: Old and new. *Arch Fam Med* 9 906–912.

Chabner, B. A., Ryan, D. P., Paz-Ares, L., Garcia-Carbonero, R., & Calabresi, P. (2001). Antineoplastic agents. In Hardman, J. G., Limbard, L. E., & Goodman, A. G. (Eds.), *The pharmacological basis of therapeutics* (pp. 1389–1460). New York: McGraw-Hill.

Dalton, R. R., & Kallab, A. M. (2001). Chemoprevention of breast cancer. *South Med J 94*(1), 7–15.

Moran, P. (2000). Cellular effects of cancer chemotherapy administration. *J of Infusion Nur 23*(1), 44.

Wood, L. (2001). Antineoplastic agents. *J of Infusion Nur 24*(1), 48.

CHAPTER 24
Drugs for Pulmonary Disorders

Barnes, P. J. (1998). Efficacy of inhaled corticosteroids in asthma. *J Allergy Clin Immunol 102*, 531–538.

Drazen, J. M., Israel, E., & O'Byrne, P. M. (1999). Treatment of asthma with drugs modifying the leukotriene pathway. *N Engl J Med 340*, 197–206.

Fink, J. (2000). Metered dose inhalers, dry powder inhalers, and transitions. *Respir Care 45*, 623–635.

Kelly, H. W. (1998). Comparison of inhaled corticosteroids. *Ann Pharmacother 32*, 220–232.

Staniforth, A. D. (2001). Contemporary management of chronic stable angina. *Drugs and Aging 18*(2), 109–121.

Undem, B. J., & Lichtenstein, L. M. (2001). Drugs used in the treatment of asthma. In Hardman, J. G., Limbard, L. E., & Goodman, A. G. (Eds.), *The pharmacological basis of therapeutics* (pp. 733–754). New York: McGraw-Hill.

CHAPTER 25
Drugs for Gastrointestinal Disorders

Brown, G. J. E., & Yeomans, N. D. (1999). Prevention of the gastrointestinal adverse effects of nonsteroidal anti-inflammatory drugs: The role of proton pump inhibitors. *Drug Safety 21*(6), 503–512.

Glazer, G. (2001). Long-term pharmacotherapy of obesity 2000: A review of efficacy and safety. *Arch Intern Med 161*, 1814–1824.

Gordon, C. R., & Shupak, A. (1999). Prevention and treatment of motion sickness in children. *CNS Drugs 12*(5), 369–381.

Heber, D. (1999). Pharmacotherapy in the treatment of obesity. *Clin Corner 2*(3), 33–42.

Hoogerwerf, W. A., & Pasricha, P. J. (2001). Agents used for the control of gastric acidity and treatment of peptic ulcers and gastroesophageal reflux disease. In Hardman, J. G., Limbard, L. E., & Goodman, A. G. (Eds.), *The pharmacological basis of therapeutics* (pp. 1005–1020). New York: McGraw-Hill.

Jafri, S., & Pasricha, P. J. (2001). Agents used for diarrhea, constipation, and inflammatory bowel disease; agents used for biliary and pancreatic disease. In Hardman, J. G., Limbard, L. E., & Goodman, A. G. (Eds.), *The pharmacological basis of therapeutics* (pp. 1037–1058). New York: McGraw-Hill.

Pasricha, P. J. (2001). Prokinetic agents, antiemetics, and agents used in irritable bowel syndrome. In Hardman, J. G., Limbard, L. E., & Goodman, A. G. (Eds.), *The pharmacological basis of therapeutics* (pp. 1021–1036). New York: McGraw-Hill.

Pray, W. S. (2000). Diarrhea: Causes and self-care treatments. *U. S. Pharmacist 25*(11).

CHAPTER 26
Vitamins, Minerals, and Herbs

Astin, J. A. (1998). Why patients use alternative medicine: Results of a national study. *JAMA 279*, 1548–1553.

Eisenberg, D. M., Davis, R. B., Ettner, S. L., Appel, S., Wilkey, S., Van Rompay, M., & Kessler, R. C. (1998). Trends in alternative medicine use in the United States, 1990–1997. *JAMA 280*, 1569–1575.

Fontaine, K. L. (2000). *Healing practices: Alternative therapies for nursing.* New Jersey: Prentice-Hall.

Goldman, P. (2001). Herbal medicines today and the roots of modern pharmacology. *Ann of Int Med 135*(8), 594–597.

Hardy, M. L. (2000). Herbs of special interest to women. *Am Pharm Assoc 40*(2), 234–242.

Hatcher, T., Dokken, D., & Sydnor-Greenberg, N. (2000). Exploring complementary and alternative medicine in pediatrics: Parents and professionals working together for new understanding. *Pediatric Nursing 26*(4), 383.

Hatcher, T. (2001). The proverbial herb. *AJN 101*(2), 36.

Levine, M., Rumsey, S. C., Daruwala, R., Park, J. B., & Wang, Y. (1999). Criteria and recommendations for vitamin C intake. *JAMA 281*, 1415–1423.

Marcus, R., & Coulston, A. M. (2001). Fat-soluble vitamins: Vitamin A, K, and E. In Hardman, J. G., Limbard, L. E., & Goodman, A. G. (Eds.), *The pharmacological basis of therapeutics* (pp. 1773–1792). New York: McGraw-Hill.

Marcus, R., & Coulston, A. M. (2001). Water-soluble vitamins: The vitamin B complex and ascorbic acid. In Hardman, J. G., Limbard, L. E., & Goodman, A. G. (Eds.), *The pharmacological basis of therapeutics* (pp. 1753–1772). New York: McGraw-Hill.

McDermott, J. H. (2000). Antioxidant nutrients: Current dietary recommendations and research update. *J Am Pharm Assoc 40*(6), 785–799.

Murch, S. J., KrishnaRaj, S., & Saxena, P. K. (2000). Phytopharmaceuticals: Problems, limitations, and solutions. *Sci Rev of Alt Med 4*(2), 33–37.

Medical Economics Staff (Ed.). (2000). *Physician's desk reference for herbal medicines* (2nd ed.). Montvale: Medical Economics.

Tyler, V. E. (2000). Product definition deficiencies in clinical studies of herbal medicines. *Sci Rev of Alt Med 4*(2), 17–21.

White, L. B., & Foster, S. (2000). *The herbal drugstore.* Emmaus, PA: Rodale.

CHAPTER 27
Drugs for Kidney, Acid-Base, and Electrolyte Disorders

Chio, P. T. L., Yip, G., Quinonez, L. G., & Cook, D. J. (1999). Crystalloids vs colloids in fluid resuscitation: A systemic review. *Crit Care Med 27*(1), 200–203.

Jackson, E. K. (2001). Diuretics. In Hardman, J. G., Limbard, L. E., & Goodman, A. G. (Eds.), *The pharmacological basis of therapeutics* (pp. 757–788). New York: McGraw-Hill.

Josephson, D. L. (1999). *Intravenous fluid therapy for nurses: Principles and practice.* Albany: Delmar.

Rose, B. D. (2000). *Clinical physiology of acid-base and electrolyte disorders* (5th ed.). New York: McGraw-Hill.

Wilmore, D. (2000). Nutrition and metabolic support in the 21st century. *J of Parenteral & Enteral Nutr 4*(1), 1–4.

CHAPTER 28
Drugs for Endocrine Disorders

American Diabetes Association. (2000). Clinical practice recommendations. *Diabetes Care 23*, Suppl. 1, S1–S16.

American Diabetes Association. (2001). Standards of care. Diabetes Care 24, Suppl. 1, S33–S43.

Bell, D. S. H., & Ovalle, F. (2000). Management of type 2 diabetes. *Clin Rev*, Spring, 93–96.

Chehade, J. M., & Mooradian, A. D. (2000). A rational approach to drug therapy of type 2 diabetes mellitus. *Drugs 60*(1), 95–113.

Davis, S. N. & Granner, D. K. (2001). Insulin, oral hypoglycemic agents, and the pharmacology of the endocrine pancreas. In Hardman, J. G., Limbard, L. E., & Goodman, A. G. (Eds.), *The pharmacological basis of therapeutics* (pp. 1679–1714). New York: McGraw-Hill.

Demester, N. (2001). Diseases of the thyroid: A broad spectrum. *Clin Rev 11*(7), 58–64.

Farwell, A. P., & Braverman, L. E. (2001). Thyroid and antithyroid drugs. In Hardman, J. G., Limbard, L. E., & Goodman, A. G. (Eds.), *The pharmacological basis of therapeutics* (pp. 1563–1596). New York: McGraw-Hill.

Harrigan, R. A., Nathan, M. S., & Beattie, P. (2001). Oral agents for the treatment of type 2 diabetes mellitus: Pharmacology, toxicity, and treatment. *Ann of Emer Med 38*(1), 68.

Margioris, A, N., & Chrousos, G. P. (Eds.). (2001). *Adrenal disorders.* New Jersey: Humana Press.

Mokdad, A. H., Bowman, B. A., Ford, E. S., Vinicor, F., Marks, J. S. & Koplan, J. P. (2001). The continuing epidemics of obesity and diabetes in the United States. *JAMA* 286, 1195–1200.

Parker, K. L., & Schimmer, B. P. (2001). Pituitary hormones and their hypothalamic releasing factors. In Hardman, J. G., Limbard, L. E., & Goodman, A. G. (Eds.), *The pharmacological basis of therapeutics* (pp. 1541–1562). New York: McGraw-Hill.

Winqvist, O., Rorsman, F., & Kampe, O. (2000). Autoimmune adrenal insufficiency: Recognition and management. *BioDrugs 13*(2), 107–114.

CHAPTER 29
Drugs for Disorders and Conditions of the Reproductive System

Basaria, S., & Dobs, A. S. (1999). Risk versus benefits of testosterone therapy in elderly men. *Drugs and Aging 15*(2), 131–142.

Frackiewicz, E. J., & Shiovitz, T. M. (2001). Evaluation and management of premenstrual syndrome and premenstrual dysphoric disorder. *J Am Pharm Assoc 41*(3), 437–447.

Loose-Mitchell, D. S., & Stancel, G. M. (2001). Estrogens and progestins. In Hardman, J. G., Limbard, L. E., & Goodman, A. G. (Eds.), *The pharmacological basis of therapeutics* (pp. 1597–1634). New York: McGraw-Hill.

Nelson, A. (2000). Contraceptive update Y2K: Need for contraception and new contraceptive options. *Clinic Corner 3*(1), 48–62.

Rozenberg, S., Vasquez, J. B., Vandromme, J., & Kroll, M. (1998). Educating patients about the benefits and drawbacks of hormone replacement therapy. *Drugs and Aging 13*(1), 33–41.

Shepherd, J. E. (2001). Effects of estrogen on cognition, mood, and degenerative brain diseases. *J Am Pharm Assoc 41*(2), 221–228.

Snyder, P. J. (2001). Androgens. In Hardman, J. G., Limbard, L. E., & Goodman, A. G. (Eds.), *The pharmacological basis of therapeutics* (pp. 1635–1648). New York: McGraw-Hill.

Vermeulen, A. (2001). Androgen replacement therapy in the aging male: a critical Evaluation. & Clin Endocrinol metab 86, 2380–2390.

CHAPTER 30
Drugs for Muscle Spasms and Bone Disorders

Cashman, J. N. (2000). Current pharmacotherapeutic strategies in rheumatic diseases and other pain states. *Clin Drug Invest* 19 Suppl. 2, 9–20.

Clemett, D. & Goa, K. L. (2000). Celecoxib: A review of its use in osteoarthritis, rheumatoid arthritis, and acute pain. *Drugs 59*(4), 957–980.

Jelley, M. J., & Wortmann, R. (2000). Practical steps in the diagnosis and management of gout. *BioDrugs 14*(2), 99–107.

Lacki, J. K. (2000). Management of the patient with severe refractory rheumatoid arthritis: Are the newer treatment options worth considering? *BioDrugs 13*(6), 425–435.

Marcus, R. (2001). Agents affecting calcification and bone turnover: Calcium, phosphate, parathyroid hormone, vitamin D, calcitonin, and other compounds. In Hardman, J. G., Limbard, L. E., & Goodman, A. G. (Eds.), *The pharmacological basis of therapeutics* (pp. 1715–1744). New York: McGraw-Hill.

Orwoll, E. S. (1999). Osteoporosis in men. *New Dimen in Osteopor 1*(5), 2–8, 12.

Prestwood, K. M. (2000). Prevention and treatment of osteoporosis. *Clinic Corner 2*(6), 34–44.

Roberts, L. J. & Morrow, J. D. (2001). Analgesic-antipyretic and anti-inflammatory agents employed in the treatment of gout. In Hardman, J. G., Limbard, L. E., & Goodman, A. G. (Eds.), *The pharmacological basis of therapeutics* (pp. 687–732). New York: McGraw-Hill.

Watts, N. B. (1999). Treatment of postmenopausal osteoporosis. *New Dimen in Osteopor 1*(4), 2–6.

CHAPTER 31
Drugs for Skin Disorders

Roos, T. C., & Merk, H. F. (2000). Important drug interactions in dermatology. *Drugs 59*(2), 181–192.

Feldman, S. (2000). Advances in psoriasis treatment. *Dermat Online 6*(1), 4.

Wyatt, E. L., Sutter, S. H., & Drake, L. A. (2001). Dermatological pharmacology. In Hardman, J. G., Limbard, L. E., & Goodman, A. G. (Eds.), *The pharmacological basis of therapeutics* (pp. 1795–1818). New York: McGraw-Hill.

CHAPTER 32
Drugs for Eye and Ear Disorders

APhA drug treatment protocols: Management of pediatric acute otitis media. *J Am Pharm Assoc 40*(5), 599–608.

Brook, I. (1999). Treatment of otitis externa in children. *Paediatr Drugs 1*(4), 283–289.

Camras, C. B., & Tamesis, R. R. (1999). Efficacy and adverse effects of medications used in the treatment of glaucoma. *Drugs and Aging 15*(5), 377–388.

Hoyng, P. F. J., & van Beek, L. M. (2000). Pharmacological therapy for glaucoma: A review. *Drugs 59*(3), 411–434.

Leibovitz, E., & Dagan, R. (2001). Otitis media therapy and drug resistance: Management principles. *Infect Med 18*(4), 212–216.

Leibovitz, E., & Dagan, R. (2001).). Otitis media therapy and drug resistance: Current concepts and new directions. *Infec Med 18*(5), 263–270.

Moroi, S. E., & Lichter, P. R. (2001). Ocular pharmacology. In Hardman, J. G., Limbard, L. E., & Goodman, A. G. (Eds.), *The pharmacological basis of therapeutics* (pp. 1821–1848). New York: McGraw-Hill.

Pray, S. (2001). Swimmer's ear: An ear canal infection. *U. S. Pharmacist 26*(8).

U.S. Drug Name	Canadian Drug Name
acebutolol hydrochloride (Sectral)	Monitan
acetaminophen (Tylenol)	Albenal, Atasol, Campain, and others
acetazolamide (Diamox) **Pr**	Acetazolam, Apo-Asetazolamide
acetohexamide (Dymelor)	Dimelor
albuterol (Proventil, Salbutamol) **Pr**	Gen-Salbutamol, Novosalmol
allopurinol (Lopurin, Zyloprim)	Alloprin, Apo-allopurinol
altretamine, hexamethylmelamine (Hexalen)	Hexastat
aminophylline (Truphylline)	Paladron, Corophyllin
amitriptyline hydrochloride (Elavil)	Apo-amitripyline, Levate, Novotriptyn
amoxicillin (Amoxil, Trimox, Wymox)	Apo-Amoxi
amphojel, basaljel	Alugel
ampicillin (Polycillin, Omnipen) **Pr**	Novoampicillin, Penbritin
asparaginase (Elspar)	Kidrolase
aspirin (ASA and others) **Pr**	Novasen, Astrin, Entrophen, and many others
atenolol (Tenormin)	Apo-Atenolol
atropine sulfate (Isopto Atropine, others)	Atropair
bacampicillin hydrochloride (Spectrobid)	Penglobe
benztropine mesylate (Cogentin)	Apo-Benzotropine, Bensylate, PMS Benzotropine
betamethasone (Celestone, Betacort, and many others)	Betnelan, Betaderm, and many others
bretylium tosylate (Bretylol)	Bretylate
brompheniramine maleate (Codimal A, Dimetapp)	Dimetane
carbamazepine (Tegretol)	Apo-carbamazine, Mazepine
carbenicillin indanylna (Geocillin, Geopen)	Geopen Oral
calcium carbonate (BioCal, Calcite-500, others)	Apo-Cal, Calsan, Caltrate
cephalexin (Keflex)	Ceporex , Novo-Lexin
cetirizine (Zyrtec)	Reactine
chloramphenicol (Chlorofair, Chloromycetin, Chloroptic, Fenicol)	Novochlorocap, Pentamycetin
chlordiazepoxide hydrochloride (Librium)	Libritab Medilium, Novopoxide
chlorthalidone (Hygroton)	Novothalidone, Uridon
chlorpropamide (Chloronase, Diabinese, Glucamide)	Apo-Chlorpropamide, Novopropamide
chloral hydrate (Noctec)	Novochlorhydrate
chlordiazepoxide hydrochloride (Librium)	Medilium, Novopoxide
chlorpheniramine maleate (Chlor-Trimeton and others)	Chlor-Tripolon, Novopheniram
chlorprothixene (Taractan)	Tarasan
chlorpromazine hydrochloride (Thorazine) **Pr**	Largactil, Novochlorpromazine
chlorthalidone (Hygroton)	Novothalidone
cimetidine (Tagamet) **Pr**	ApoCimetidine, Novocimetinel, Peptol
cisplatin (Platinol)	Abiplatin
clindamycin hydrochloride (Cleocin)	Dalacin T
clonazepam (Klonopin)	Rivotril
clonidine hydrochloride (Catapres)	Dixaril
clorazepate dipotassium (Tranxene)	Novoclopate
clotrimazole (Gyne-Lotrimin, Mycelex, Femizole)	Canesten, Clotrimaderm, Myclo-Gyne
cloxacillin (Tegopen)	Apo-Cloxi, Novocloxin

U.S. Drug Name	Canadian Drug Name
codeine	Paveral
colchicine **Pr**	Novocolchicine
colestipol (Colestid)	Cholestabyl
cyclizine hydrochloride (Marezine)	Marzine
cyclophosphamide (Cytoxan, Neosar) **Pr**	Procytox
cyproheptadine hydrochloride (Periactin)	Vimicon
danazol (Danocrine)	Cyclome
dexamethasone (Decadron, Dexasone, Hexadrol, Maxidex)	Deronil, Oradexon
dextroamphetamine sulfate (Dexedrine)	Oxydess II
diazepam (Valium) **Pr**	Apo-Diazepam, Diazemuls, E-Pam
diethylstilbestrol (DES, Stilbestrol)	Honval
diltiazem (Cardizem, Dilacor, Tiamate, Tiazac)	Apo- Dilitaz
dimenhydrinate (Dramamine)	Apo-Dimenhydrinate, Gravol
diphenhydramine hydrochloride (Benadryl and others) **Pr**	Allerdryl
dipyridamole (Persantine)	Apo-Dipyridamole
disopyramide phosphate (Norpace, Nopamide)	Rythmodan
docusate (Surfak, Dialose, Colace)	Regulax
dopamine hydrochloride (Dopastat, Intropin)	Revimine
doxepin hydrochloride (Sinequan)	Tridapin
doxycycline hyclate (Doryx, Doxy, Monodox, Vibramycin)	Apo-Doxy, Doxycin
econazole nitrate (Spectazole)	Esostatin
epinephrine (Adrenalin, Bronkaid, Primatene)	SusPhrine
ergocalciferol (Deltalin, Calciferol)	Ostoforte, Radiostol
ergotamine tartrate (Ergostat)	Gynergen
erythromycin (E-mycin, Erythrocin) **Pr**	Novorythro, Eryhtromid, Apo-Erythro-S
estradiol valerate (Delestrogen, Duragen-10, Valergen)	Femogex
flucytosine (Ancobon)	Ancotil
fluoxymesterone (Halotestin)	Ora-Testryl
flurazepam (Dalmane)	Apo-Flurazepam, Novoflupam
furosemide (Lasix) **Pr**	Furomide
gentamicin sulfate (Garamycin, G-mycin, Jenamicin) **Pr**	Cydomycin
glyburide (DiaBeta, Micronase, Glynase)	Euglucon
griseofulvin (Fulvicin)	Grisovin-FP
haloperidol (Haldol)	Peridol
heparin sodium (Heplock) **Pr**	Calcilean, Hepalean
hydralazine hydrochloride (Apresoline)	Novo-Hylazin
hydrocodone bitartrate (Hycodan)	Robidone
hydrocortisone (Cetacort, Cortaid, Solu-cortef) **Pr**	Rectocort, Cortiment
hydrochlorothiazide (Hydrodiuril, HCTZ) **Pr**	Apo-Hydro, Urozide
hydroxyzine (Atarax, Vistaril)	Apo-Hydroxyzine
ibuprofen (Advil, Motrin, and many others) **Pr**	Amersol
imipramine hydrochloride (Tofranil)	Impril, Novopramine
indapamide (Lozol)	Lozide
isoniazid (INH, Laniazid, Nydrazid, Teebaconin) **Pr**	Isotamine, PMS Isoniazid

U.S. Drug Name	Canadian Drug Name
isosorbide dinitrate (Isordil, Sorbitrate, Dilatrate SR)	Coronex, Novosorbide
ketoprofen (Actron, Orudis, Oruvail)	Rhodis
lidocaine hydrochloride (Xylocaine)	Xylocard
lithium carbonate (Eskalith) **Pr**	Carbolith, Duralith, Lithizine
lorazepam (Ativan)	Apo-Lorazepam
loxapine succinate (Loxitane)	Loxapac
meclizine (Antivert, Bonine)	Bonamine
methyldopa (Aldomet)	Apo-methyldopa
methyltestosterone (Android, Testred)	Metandren
metoclopramide (Reglan)	Emex, Maxeran
metoprolol tartrate (Toprol, Lopressor)	Betaloc, Norometoprol, Apo-metoprolol
morphine sulfate (Astramorph PF, Duramorph, and others)	Epimorph, Statex
mylanta, Maalox Plus, Gelusil, Rulox	Diovol
naproxen (Naprosyn; Anaprox)	Apo-Naproxen, Naxen, Novonaprox
nifedipine (Procardia, Aldalat) **Pr**	Apo-Nifed, Novo-Nifedin
nitrofurantoin (Furadantin, Furalan, Furantoin, Marobid, Macrodantin)	Apo-Nitrofurantoin, Nephronex, Novofuran
norethindrone acetate	Aygestin, Norlutate
nystatin (Mycostatin, Nilstat, Nystex)	Nadostine, Nyaderm
omeprazole (Prilosec) **Pr**	Losec
oxazepam (Serax)	Ox-pam, Zapex
oxymetazoline hydrochloride (Afrin/12 hr, Neo-Synephrine/12 hr and others)	Nafrine
penicillin G sodium/potassium (Pentids) **Pr**	Megacillin
penicillin V (PenVee K, Veetids, Betapen VK)	Apo-Pen VK, Nadopen-V
pentamidine isothionate (Pentam 300, Nebupent)	Pentacarinat
pentobarbital sodium (Nembutal)	Novopentobarb
phenylephrine hydrochloride (Mydfrin, Neo-Synephrine)	AK-Dilate Dionephrine
pilocarpine hydrochloride (Adsorbocarpine, Isopto Carptine, others) **Pr**	Pilocarpine, Miocarpine
prednisolone (Delta-Cortef, Keypred, Prelone, and others)	Diopred, Inflamase, Pediapred
prednisone (Deltasone, Meticoten)	Apo-Prednison, Winpred
primidone (Mysoline)	Apo-Primidone
probenecid (Benemid, Probalan)	Benuryl
procarbazine hydrochloride (Matulane)	Natulan
prochlorperazine (Compazine)	Prorazin, Stemetil
procyclidine hydrochloride (Kemadrin)	Procyclid
promethazine (Pentazine, Phenazine, Phenergan, others)	Histantil
propranolol hydrochloride (Inderal) **Pr**	Apo-Propranolol, Detensol, Novopranol
propoxyphene hydrochloride (Darvon)	Novopropoxyn
propoxyphene napsylate (Darvon-N)	
propylthiouracil (PTU) **Pr**	Propyl-Thyracil
protriptyline hydrochloride (Vivactil)	Triptil
psyllium muciloid (Metamucil, Naturcil)	Karasil
pyrazinamide	Tebrazid
quinidine gluconate (Duraquin, Quinaglute)	Apo-Quinidine, Novoquinidin
quinidine sulfate (Quinidex) **Pr**	Quinidine polygalacturonate (Cardioquin)
quinine sulfate (Quinamm)	Novoquinine
ranitidine (Zantac)	APO-ranitidine
rifampin (Rifidin, Rimactane)	Rofact
Riopan, Lowsium	Losopan
scopolamine (Hyoscine, Transderm Scop)	Transderm V
secobarbital (Seconal) **Pr**	Novosecobarb
spironolactone (Aldactone) **Pr**	Novospiroton
sulfasalazine (Azulfidine)	PMS sulfasalazine, others
sulfinpyrazone (Anturan)	Antazone, Anturane, others
tamoxifen citrate (Nolvadex)	Nolvadex-D, Tamofen
testosterone (Andro 100, Histerone, Testoderm) **Pr**	Malogen
testosterone enanthate (Andro LA, Delatest, Delatestryl)	Malogex
tetracycline hydrochloride (Achromycin, Panmycin, Sumycin) **Pr**	Novotetra
theophylline (Theo-dur)	Pulmophylline and Somophyllin-12
thioguanine (TG)	Lanvis
thioridazine hydrochloride (Mellaril)	Novoridazine
tolbutamide (Orinase)	Mobenol, Novo-Butamide
trifluoperazine hydrochloride (Stelazine)	Novoflurazine, Solazine, Terfluzine
trihexyphenidyl hydrochloride (Artane)	Aparkane, Apo-Trihex, Novohexidyl
tripelennamine hydrochloride (PBZ-SR, Pelamine)	Pyribenzamine
Tums	Apo-Cal
valproic acid (Depakene)	Epival
verapamil hydrochloride (Calan, Isoptin, Verelan)	Novo-Veramil, Nu-Verap
vinblastine sulfate (Velban)	Velbe
warfarin sodium (Coumadin) **Pr**	Warfilone

Note: Drugs indicated by **Pr** *are profiled within the text.*

Indexing style is as follows: **Profile drugs appear in boldface, GENERIC IN BOLDFACE, SMALL CAPS.** NON-PROFILE DRUGS APPEAR IN SMALL CAPS, REGULAR TYPE. <u>Drug classifications appear underlined.</u> Diseases and disorders appear in blue. *(Phonetic pronunciations for generic drugs appear in italics within parentheses.)* Information in tables is denoted with a "t" after the page number. Information in figures is denoted with a "f" after the page number.

READ THIS LICENSE CAREFULLY BEFORE OPENING THIS PACKAGE. BY OPENING THIS PACKAGE, YOU ARE AGREEING TO THE TERMS AND CONDITIONS OF THIS LICENSE. IF YOU DO NOT AGREE, DO NOT OPEN THE PACKAGE. PROMPTLY RETURN THE UNOPENED PACKAGE AND ALL ACCOMPANYING ITEMS TO THE PLACE YOU OBTAINED THEM. *THESE TERMS APPLY TO ALL LICENSED SOFTWARE ON THE DISK EXCEPT THAT THE TERMS FOR USE OF ANY SHAREWARE OR FREEWARE ON THE DISKETTES ARE AS SET FORTH IN THE ELECTRONIC LICENSE LOCATED ON THE DISK:*

1. GRANT OF LICENSE and OWNERSHIP: The enclosed computer programs and data ("Software") are licensed, not sold, to you by Pearson Education, Inc. ("We" or the "Company") and in consideration of your purchase or adoption of the accompanying Company textbooks and/or other materials, and your agreement to these terms. We reserve any rights not granted to you. You own only the disk(s) but we and/or our licensors own the Software itself. This license allows you to use and display your copy of the Software on a single computer (i.e., with a single CPU) at a single location for academic use only, so long as you comply with the terms of this Agreement. You may make one copy for back up, or transfer your copy to another CPU, provided that the Software is usable on only one computer.

2. RESTRICTIONS: You may not transfer or distribute the Software or documentation to anyone else. Except for backup, you may not copy the documentation or the Software. You may not network the Software or otherwise use it on more than one computer or computer terminal at the same time. You may not reverse engineer, disassemble, decompile, modify, adapt, translate, or create derivative works based on the Software or the Documentation. You may be held legally responsible for any copying or copyright infringement which is caused by your failure to abide by the terms of these restrictions.

3. TERMINATION: This license is effective until terminated. This license will terminate automatically without notice from the Company if you fail to comply with any provisions or limitations of this license. Upon termination, you shall destroy the Documentation and all copies of the Software. All provisions of this Agreement as to limitation and disclaimer of warranties, limitation of liability, remedies or damages, and our ownership rights shall survive termination.

4. LIMITED WARRANTY AND DISCLAIMER OF WARRANTY: Company warrants that for a period of 60 days from the date you purchase this SOFTWARE (or purchase or adopt the accompanying textbook), the Software, when properly installed and used in accordance with the Documentation, will operate in substantial conformity with the description of the Software set forth in the Documentation, and that for a period of 30 days the disk(s) on which the Software is delivered shall be free from defects in materials and workmanship under normal use. The Company does not warrant that the Software will meet your requirements or that the operation of the Software will be uninterrupted or error-free. Your only remedy and the

Company's only obligation under these limited warranties is, at the Company's option, return of the disk for a refund of any amounts paid for it by you or replacement of the disk. THIS LIMITED WARRANTY IS THE ONLY WARRANTY PROVIDED BY THE COMPANY AND ITS LICENSORS, AND THE COMPANY AND ITS LICENSORS DISCLAIM ALL OTHER WARRANTIES, EXPRESS OR IMPLIED, INCLUDING WITHOUT LIMITATION, THE IMPLIED WARRANTIES OF MERCHANTABILITY AND FITNESS FOR A PARTICULAR PURPOSE. THE COMPANY DOES NOT WARRANT, GUARANTEE OR MAKE ANY REPRESENTATION REGARDING THE ACCURACY, RELIABILITY, CURRENTNESS, USE, OR RESULTS OF USE, OF THE SOFTWARE.

5. LIMITATION OF REMEDIES AND DAMAGES: IN NO EVENT, SHALL THE COMPANY OR ITS EMPLOYEES, AGENTS, LICENSORS, OR CONTRACTORS BE LIABLE FOR ANY INCIDENTAL, INDIRECT, SPECIAL, OR CONSEQUENTIAL DAMAGES ARISING OUT OF OR IN CONNECTION WITH THIS LICENSE OR THE SOFTWARE, INCLUDING FOR LOSS OF USE, LOSS OF DATA, LOSS OF INCOME OR PROFIT, OR OTHER LOSSES, SUSTAINED AS A RESULT OF INJURY TO ANY PERSON, OR LOSS OF OR DAMAGE TO PROPERTY, OR CLAIMS OF THIRD PARTIES, EVEN IF THE COMPANY OR AN AUTHORIZED REPRESENTATIVE OF THE COMPANY HAS BEEN ADVISED OF THE POSSIBILITY OF SUCH DAMAGES. IN NO EVENT SHALL THE LIABILITY OF THE COMPANY FOR DAMAGES WITH RESPECT TO THE SOFTWARE EXCEED THE AMOUNTS ACTUALLY PAID BY YOU, IF ANY, FOR THE SOFTWARE OR THE ACCOMPANYING TEXTBOOK. BECAUSE SOME JURISDICTIONS DO NOT ALLOW THE LIMITATION OF LIABILITY IN CERTAIN CIRCUMSTANCES, THE ABOVE LIMITATIONS MAY NOT ALWAYS APPLY TO YOU.

6. GENERAL: THIS AGREEMENT SHALL BE CONSTRUED IN ACCORDANCE WITH THE LAWS OF THE UNITED STATES OF AMERICA AND THE STATE OF NEW YORK, APPLICABLE TO CONTRACTS MADE IN NEW YORK, AND SHALL BENEFIT THE COMPANY, ITS AFFILIATES AND ASSIGNEES. HIS AGREEMENT IS THE COMPLETE AND EXCLUSIVE STATEMENT OF THE AGREEMENT BETWEEN YOU AND THE COMPANY AND SUPERSEDES ALL PROPOSALS OR PRIOR AGREEMENTS, ORAL, OR WRITTEN, AND ANY OTHER COMMUNICATIONS BETWEEN YOU AND THE COMPANY OR ANY REPRESENTATIVE OF THE COMPANY RELATING TO THE SUBJECT MATTER OF THIS AGREEMENT. If you are a U.S. Government user, this Software is licensed with "restricted rights" as set forth in subparagraphs (a)-(d) of the Commercial Computer-Restricted Rights clause at FAR 52.227-19 or in subparagraphs (c)(1)(ii) of the Rights in Technical Data and Computer Software clause at DFARS 252.227-7013, and similar clauses, as applicable.

Should you have any questions concerning this agreement or if you wish to contact the Company for any reason, please contact in writing: Prentice-Hall, New Media Department, One Lake Street, Upper Saddle River, NJ 07458.

QUICK GUIDE TO SPECIAL FEATURES

continued on next page

QUICK GUIDE TO SPECIAL FEATURES (continued)